Metabolic Polymorphisms and Susceptibility to Cancer

International Agency for Research on Cancer

The International Agency for Research on Cancer (IARC) was established in 1965 by the World Health Assembly, as an independently financed organization within the framework of the World Health Organization. The headquarters of the Agency are at Lyon, France.

The Agency conducts a programme of research concentrating particularly on the epidemiology of cancer and the study of potential carcinogens in the human environment. Its field studies are supplemented by biological and chemical research carried out in the Agency's laboratories in Lyon, and, through collaborative research agreements, in national research institutions in many countries. The Agency also conducts a programme for the education and training of personnel for cancer research.

The publications of the Agency are intended to contribute to the dissemination of authoritative information on different aspects of cancer research. Information about IARC publications and how to order them is available via the Internet at: http://www.iarc.fr/

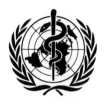

INTERNATIONAL AGENCY FOR RESEARCH ON CANCER
WORLD HEALTH ORGANIZATION

Metabolic Polymorphisms and Susceptibility to Cancer

Edited by
Paolo Vineis, Núria Malats, Matti Lang, Angelo d'Errico,
Neil Caporaso, Jack Cuzick and Paolo Boffetta

IARC Scientific Publications No. 148

International Agency for Research on Cancer
Lyon, France
1999

Published by the International Agency for Research on Cancer,
150 cours Albert-Thomas, 69372 Lyon cedex 08, France

Distributed by Oxford University Press, Walton Street, Oxford OX2 6DP, UK
(fax: +44 1865 267782) and in the USA by Oxford University Press, 2001 Evans Road, Carey,
NC 27513 (fax: +1 919 677 1303). All IARC publications can also be ordered directly from IARC*Press*
(fax: +33 04 72 73 83 02; e-mail: press@iarc.fr).

IARC Library Cataloguing in Publication Data

Metabolic polymorphisms and susceptibility to cancer / editors, P. Vineis ... [et al.]

(IARC scientific publications; 148)

1. Disease susceptibility – genetics
2. Neoplasms - genetics
3. Polymorphism (genetics)
I. Vineis, Paolo II. Series

ISBN 92 832 2148 6   (NLM Classification: W1)
ISSN 0300-5085

Printed in France

Contents

Contributors

Dr Simone Benhamou
INSERM U351
Unit of Cancer Epidemiology
Institut Gustave-Roussy
39, rue Camille Desmoulins
94805 Villejuif cedex
France

Dr Brunhilde Blömeke
Molecular Epidemiology Section
Laboratory of Human Carcinogenesis
NCI Bldg 37, Room 2C16
37 Convent Drive, MSC 4255
Bethesda, MD 20892-4255
USA

Dr Paolo Boffetta
Unit of Environmental Cancer Epidemiology
International Agency for Research on Cancer
150 cours Albert-Thomas
F-69372 Lyon cedex 08
France

Dr Christine Bouchardy
Geneva Cancer Registry
55 boulevard de la Cluse
CH-1205 Geneva
Switzerland

Dr Paul Brennan
Unit of Environmental Cancer Epidemiology
International Agency for Research on Cancer
150 cours Albert-Thomas
F-69372 Lyon cedex 08
France

Dr Neil Caporaso
Genetic Epidemiology Branch
National Cancer Institute
6130 Executive Boulevard
Rockville, MD 20892
USA

Dr Francesca Crosti
Ospedale Policlinico- IRCCS
Scientific Directorate
Via F. Sforza 28
I-20122 Milan
Italy

Dr Jack Cuzick
Department of Mathematics
Imperial Cancer Research Fund
PO Box No. 123
Lincoln's Inn Fields
GB - London WC2A 3PX
United Kingdom

Dr Angelo d'Errico
Environmental Protection Agency for
Piedmont Region
Epidemiology Unit
V. Sabaudia 164,
I-10095 Grugliasco (Turin)
Italy

Dr Andrew N. Freedman
Genetic Epidemiology Branch
National Cancer Institute
NIH/NCI/EPN 400
6130 Executive Boulevard
Bethesda, MD 20892-7360
USA

Dr Anthony A. Fryer
Clinical Biochemistry Research Group
Centre for Cell and Molecular Medicine
Keele University School of
Postgraduate Medicine
North Staffordshire Hospital
Stoke-on-Trent ST4 7QB
United Kingdom

Dr Montserrat Garcia-Closas
Division of Cancer Epidemiology and Genetics
National Cancer Institute
NIH/NCI/EPN 418
6130 Executive Boulevard
Bethesda, MD 20892-7364
USA

Dr Seymour Garte
Department of Environmental Medicine
NYU Medical Center
550 First Avenue
New York, NY 10016
USA
and Scientific Director
Genetics Research Institute
Milan-Italy

Dr Pierre Hainaut
Unit of Molecular Carcinogenesis
International Agency for Research on Cancer
150, cours Albert-Thomas
F-69372 Lyon cedex 08
France

Dr Ari Hirvonen
Molecular Epidemiology Group
Department of Industrial Hygiene
and Toxicology
Finnish Institute of Occupational Health
Topeliuksenkatu 41 a A
FIN-00250 Helsinki
Finland

Dr Evelyne Jacqz-Aigrain
INSERM U120
and Department of Clinical Pharmacology
Hôpital Robert Debré
F-75019 Paris
France

Dr Peter W. Jones
Department of Mathematics
Keele University
North Staffordshire Hospital
GB - Stoke-on-Trent
United Kingdom

Dr F.F. Kadlubar
Division of Molecular Epidemiology
National Center for Toxicological Research
Jefferson, AR 72097
USA

Dr Kaname Kawajiri
Department of Biochemistry
Saitama Cancer Center Research Institute
818 Komuro, Ina
Saitama 362
Japan

Dr Maria Teresa Landi
Genetic Epidemiology Branch
EPN 400-6130 Executive Boulevard
Bethesda, MD 20892
USA

Dr Matti Lang
Dept of Pharmaceutical Biosciences
Faculty of Pharmacy
Uppsala University
Box 578
S-751 23 Uppsala
Suede

Dr N.P. Lang
Arkansas Cancer Research Center
University of Arkansas for Medical Sciences
Little Rock, AR 72205
USA

Dr Jay Lubin
Division of Cancer Epidemiology and Genetics
National Cancer Institute
NIH/NCI/EPN 418
6130 Executive Boulevard
Bethesda, MD 20892-7364
USA

Dr Núria Malats
Institut Municipal d'Investigació Mèdica
Carrer del Dr. Aiguader, 80
E-08003 Barcelona
Espagne

Dr Neil Pearce
Wellington Asthma Research Group
Wellington School of Medicine
PO Box 7343 Wellington
New Zealand

Dr Olavi Pelkonen
Department of Pharmacology and Toxicology
University of Oulu
Kajaanintie 52 D
FIN-90220 Oulu
Finland

Dr Hannu Raunio
Department of Pharmacology and Toxicology
University of Oulu
Kajaanintie 52 D
FIN-90220 Oulu
Finland

Dr Arja Rautio
Department of Pharmacology and Toxicology
University of Oulu
Kajaanintie 52 D
FIN-90220 Oulu
Finland

Dr Nathaniel Rothman
Division of Cancer Epidemiology and Genetics
National Cancer Institute
NIH/NCI/EPN 418
6130 Executive Boulevard
Bethesda, MD 20892-7364
USA

Dr Peter G. Shields
Molecular Epidemiology Section
Laboratory of Human Carcinogenesis
NCI Bldg 37, Room 2C16
37 Convent Drive, MSC 4255
Bethesda, MD 20892-4255
USA

Dr Rashmi Sinha
Genetic Epidemiology Branch
National Cancer Institute
NIH/NCI/EPN 400!
6130 Executive Boulevard
Bethesda, MD 20892
USA

Dr Gillian Smith
ICRF Molecular Pharmacology Unit
Biomedical Research Centre
University of Dundee
Ninewells Hospital & Medical School
GB - Dundee DD1 9SY
United Kingdom

Dr Kazuhiro Sogawa
Department of Chemistry
Graduate School of Science
Tohoku University
Aoba-ku
Sendai 980-77
Japan

Dr Walter T. Stewart
Department of Epidemiology
School of Hygiene and Public Health
Johns Hopkins University
Baltimore, MD 21205
USA

Dr Richard C. Strange
Centre for Cell and Molecular Medicine
Keele University School of
Postgraduate Medicine
North Staffordshire Hospital
Thornburrow Drive, Hartshill
GB - Stoke-on-Trent ST4 7QB
United Kingdom

Dr Michael J. Stubbins
GLP Clinical Genotyping Laboratory
Glaxo Wellcome Research and Development
Building 2, GC25, Park Road, Ware
Hertfordshire SG12 0DP
United Kingdom

Dr Kirsi Vähäkangas
Department of Pharmacology and Toxicology
University of Oulu
52-D Kajaninitie
SF-90220 Oulu
Finland

Dr Paolo Vineis
Cancer Epidemiology Unit
University of Turin
Via Santena, 7
I-10126 Turin
Italy

Dr C. Roland Wolf
ICRF Molecular Pharmacology Unit
Biomedical Research Centre
University of Dundee
Ninewells Hospital & Medical School
GB - Dundee DD1 9SY
United Kingdom

Foreword

The study of interactions between genes and environmental exposures has expanded considerably in recent years. Highly penetrant genes that are involved in familial cancer have been identified but they are likely to account for only a relatively small proportion of total cancers. Other predisposing genes have low penetrance, resulting in a moderate increase in the risk of specific cancers, but they are widespread in the general population. This is true of the so-called metabolic polymorphisms, i.e. polymorphisms of genes encoding for enzymes involved in the metabolism of carcinogens or anti-carcinogens. Although the individual increase in cancer risk in carriers of a specific polymorphism is in most cases small, the importance of such genes can be considerable both at the population level and in individuals with a particular environmental exposure. Scientific interest in metabolic poly-morphisms is based on the possibility of identifying population subgroups that are at elevated risk of developing environmentally-induced cancer. However, such studies raise both methodological prob-lems, related to study design and analysis, and ethical problems related to the practical use that can be made of genetic information. The present volume, which deals thoroughly with these problems, represents the first attempt to collect a comprehensive set of contributions from scientists in different disciplines on metabolic polymorphisms and their role in the evolution of human cancers.

Paul Kleihues
Director, IARC

Acknowledgements

The editors thank Drs D. Bell, G.G. Chabot, U. Meyer, R. Montesano, G. Romeo, R. Saracci and E. Taioli for help in reviewing the contributions to this volume, and Mrs M. Geesink, Mme M Garroni-Pichelingat and Mrs S. Rosi for secretarial help.

Metabolic Polymorphisms and Susceptibility to Cancer
W. Ryder
IARC Scientific Publications No. 148
International Agency for Research on Cancer, Lyon, 1999

Chapter 1. Why study metabolic susceptibility to cancer?

Paolo Vineis, Núria Malats and Paolo Boffetta

Therapies have only modest effectiveness in reducing the death burden due to cancer. Among adult males in Europe, only four relatively uncommon cancers (testis, larynx, penis and Hodgkin's disease) have a five-year survival rate exceeding 50%; in women the situation is better, eight cancers (breast, cervix, corpus uteri, Hodgkin's disease, larynx, oral cavity, vagina and chronic lymphatic leukaemia) having five-year survival rates above this level (Berrino *et al.*, 1995). From 1991 to 1994, mortality rates from cancer declined by 1% in the USA, but between 1970 and 1994, when the "war on cancer" was heavily funded, the rates increased by 6% (Bailar & Gornick, 1997). In Europe, age-adjusted incidence rates increased by 8.7% in men between 1970 and 1990, although in women they decreased by 1.4% in this period; excluding lung cancer, the increase among men was 5.7% and the decrease among women was 5.4% (Tomatis *et al.*, 1997).

In the developed countries the overall picture seems to be slowly improving, since we are beginning to see a decline in cancer mortality in the younger generations. However, this phenomenon appears to be related more to preventive efforts (anti-smoking campaigns, improved working conditions and dietary habits) than to the success of therapies. In the developing countries it is very likely that there will be increasing incidence and mortality rates due to the diffusion of Western lifestyles, particularly tobacco-smoking (Pisani *et al.*, 1993).

Prevention is clearly the best way to reduce cancer mortality in developed countries and to avoid a large-scale cancer epidemic in developing countries (Bailar & Gornick, 1997; Tomatis *et al.*, 1997). Several attempts have been made to estimate how many cancers could be prevented on the basis of current knowledge. In industrialized countries the overall estimate is at least 50% (Tomatis *et al.*, 1997). It is important to realize that the sum of the proportions attributable to the different risk factors may well exceed 100% because of multiple pathways in the carcinogenic process. In other words, the fact that 90% or more of lung cancers are due to tobacco does not mean that only 10% are attributable to all other causes. In addition, the concept of interaction is exemplified by the carcinogenic potency of complex mixtures and by the importance of host-environment interactions. Even in the case of a disease with a clear "necessary cause" like tuberculosis the genetic background is highly significant in modifying the risk (Table 1).

Table 1. Effect of genetic relatedness on host response to *M. tuberculosis* in families with an index case (Evans, 1993)	
Relation of family member to index case	**% of exposed and susceptible individuals showing clinical manifestations of tuberculosis**
Spouse	7.1
Half-sibling	11.9
Dizygotic twin	25.5
Monozygotic twin	83.3

Interactions may occur in many different ways. They can involve different carcinogenic exposures (as in mixtures), simultaneous exposure to causal and protective factors (for example, smoking and high intake of fruit and vegetables), and both external and "host" factors. A special class of interaction between external exposures and "host" factors is represented by gene-environment interactions, including metabolic polymorphism. By metabolic polymorphism we mean a variable ability, shown by subgroups in populations or by single individuals, to metabolize chemical carcinogens (a more formal definition is given in subsequent Chapters).

The incorporation of the study of metabolic polymorphisms into cancer epidemiology is particularly important for at least three reasons : (a) the identification of a subpopulation of subjects who are more susceptible to chemically-induced cancer would increase the power of epidemiological studies; (b) the suspicion of the role of an etiological agent is strengthened by the knowledge of the enzyme involved in its metabolism; (c) polymorphisms may be particularly significant in relation to low-level exposures, influencing the process of risk assessment and of setting "tolerable" limits of exposure, which should take individual susceptibility into account.

We can think of genetic susceptibility as a spectrum encompassing a range of intermediate situations between two extremes. On one side we have monogenic, high-penetrance conditions such as inherited mutations of the BRCA1 or the APC gene. In this case the lifetime cumulative risk of cancer among the carriers of the mutations is very high, of the order of 50-90%. However, such mutations are rare in the general population, so that only a small fraction of the cancers in question (breast or colon cancers in the example above) can be attributed to inherited traits. The other extreme is represented by metabolic polymorphisms: in this case we deal with very frequent mutations (of the order of 40-50% of the population, as with N-acetyltransferase 2 slow acetylator alleles and GSTM1 null in Caucasians), but the increase in risk is modest. In the latter example, the individual risk is increased by a small amount but the proportion of cancers attributable to the genetic trait may be high. However, a further difference must be

kept in mind: the type of genetic susceptibility represented by metabolic polymorphisms is such that it requires chemical exposure to be effective, i.e. it is an example of modification (or modulation) of the effect of an external exposure. This is not necessarily true for genes such as BRCA1, p53 or APC, which seem to act at a more basic level of the cell cycle. In fact we do not know how most high-penetrance genes work, but they may well modulate other factors. However, the difference is important on practical grounds, because to prevent chemically induced cancer the only realistic solution is to eliminate carcinogens from the environment, whereas genetic susceptibility related to familial cancer requires a different approach. A confusion between the two approaches may create considerable practical and ethical problems (see Chapter 24).

This book is structured to cover different points of view on the application of metabolic polymorphisms in cancer epidemiology. However, most of the concepts discussed can be applied to other fields, either in chronic pathologies (as in cardiovascular, neurodegenerative and inflammatory diseases) or acute conditions (as with occupational and environmental toxicity).

Firstly, the book gives an overview of the main aspects of metabolic polymorphisms at the genotype and phenotype levels. The nomenclature introduced by the authors is usually based on the terms used in the original papers. However, Chapter 2 extends the suggestion of a standardized nomenclature by Vatsis et al. (1995) and Daly et al. (1996) to all the gene polymorphisms discussed in the book. If agreement were reached, this could be adopted for future studies. Chapter 4 deals with the selection strategy for the genes in the studies.

The second part of the book covers the main issues in designing, analysing, and interpreting epidemiological studies involving metabolic polymorphisms: correspondence between genotype and phenotype, misclassification problems, new study designs, and conceptual and practical aspects of interaction, effect modification, subgroup analyses, and sample size. Chapter 13 describes and gives the sources of the main laboratory methods for determining genetic polymorphisms.

The third part is more technical, being devoted to the main polymorphisms so far identified as being associated with cancer: Ah receptor, P450 1A1, P450 1A2, P450 2A subfamily, P450 2D6, glutathione-S-transferases, N-acetyltransferases and a miscellaneous group of enzymes of interest in connection with cancer susceptibility. Chapter 22 provides some examples of gene-gene interaction between enzymes and discusses its interpretation from a biological point of view. Chapter 23 presents a detailed review of the epidemiological evidence and a meta-analysis of the risk of selected cancers associated with polymorphisms in selected enzymes, and of methodological issues related to these studies. The Annex contains tables relating to this review. Although the field is evolving rapidly we believe that enough evidence is available for some general conclusions to be drawn.

The fourth part deals with some general matters, including ethical and social concerns.

The present book refers only to genetic polymorphisms that are related to metabolic enzymes involved in the metabolism of carcinogens. Other types of genetic susceptibility to cancer are not included, for example germ-line mutations of the p53 gene, BRCA1 and BRCA2, or variability in DNA repair capacity. Finally, some polymorphisms considered in the literature to be associated with cancer but not with exogenous or endogenous carcinogen metabolism are not covered in the book, among them multiple drug resistance complex (Md complex), blood group ABO polymorphism, tumour necrosis factor beta gene (TNF-beta), HLA polymorphisms, and vitamin D receptor.

References

Bailar, J.C. & Gornick, H.L. (1997) Cancer undefeated. *N. Engl. J. Med..*, 336, 1569-1574

Berrino, F., Sant, M., Verdecchia, A., Capocaccia, R., Hakulinen, T. & Esteve, J., eds, (1995) *Survival of cancer patients in Europe.* Lyon, IARC (IARC Scientific Publication No. 132)

Daly, A.K., Brockmöller, J., Broly, F., Eichelbaum, M., Evans, W.E., Gonzalez, F.J., Huang, J.D., Idle, J.R., Ingelman-Sundberg, M., Ishizaki, T., Jacqz-Aigrain, E., Meyer, U.A., Nebert, D.W., Steen, V.M., Wolf, C.R. & Zanger, U.M. (1996) Nomenclature for human CYP2D6 alleles. *Pharmacogenetics,* 6, 193-201

Evans, A.S. (1993) *Causation and disease.* New York, Plenum Medical Books

Pisani, P., Parkin, D.M. & Ferlay, J. (1993) Estimates of the worldwide incidence of eighteen major cancers in 1985: implications for prevention and projections of future burden. *Int. J. Cancer,* 55, 891-903

Tomatis, L., Huff, J., Hertz-Picciotto, I., Sandler, D.P., Bucher, J., Boffetta, P., Axelson, O., Blair, A., Taylor, J., Stayner, L. & Barrett, J.C. (1997) Avoided and avoidable risks of cancer. *Carcinogenesis,* 18, 97-105

Vatsis, K.P., Weber, W.W., Bell, D.A., Dupret, J.M., Evans, D.A., Grant, D.M., Hein, D.W., Lin, H.J., Meyer, U.A. & Relling, M.V. (1995) Nomenclature for N-acetyltransferases. *Pharmacogenetics,* 5, 1-17

Corresponding author
Paolo Vineis
Unit of Cancer Epidemiology,
S. Giovanni Battista Hospital and University of Torino,
Italy

Metabolic polymorphisms and Susceptibility to Cancer
W. Ryder
IARC Scientific Publications No. 148
International Agency for Research on Cancer, Lyon, 1999

Chapter 2. A nomenclature system for metabolic gene polymorphisms

Seymour Garte and Francesca Crosti

A nomenclature system for all human metabolic gene polymorphisms is suggested. This system should replace the various nomenclatures used in the literature to describe polymorphisms in many of the cytochrome P450 (CYP) genes, as well as the glutathione S-transferase (GST) and N-acetyltransferase (NAT) genes. The system is based on two published papers proposing nomenclatures for the various alleles of CYP2D6 and NAT. The gene name is followed by an asterisk, followed by an arabic number designating the specific polymorphism in chronological order of first publication. The final number may be followed by letters A,B, etc. when allelic subtypes exist. A table is presented showing nomenclature for 72 polymorphisms in 12 genes, including detailed descriptions and commonly used previous designations.

As research into the structure and function of genetic polymorphisms in human metabolic genes continues to accelerate, the problem of consistent and logical nomenclature also grows. For certain genes such as CYP1A1 and CYP2E1 there is already a considerable potential for confusion due to the widely differing nomenclature systems used by various authors. In extreme cases it is even possible that the same symbol can refer to different polymorphisms in different publications. Of course, the problem is not unique to this field, and many attempts to produce useful and universal nomenclature systems have been made for certain gene families and genetic variant alleles. For example, the cytochrome P450 genes were successfully incorporated into a system of nomenclature which includes information on substrate specificity in a logical and highly systematic way. At the present time the CYP[number][letter][number] system (e.g. CYP1A1) is almost universally used in the literature.

The purpose of this Chapter is to suggest a logical and consistent system of metabolic gene polymorphism nomenclature that can be used with any gene. The system proposed here is based on the two publications, each dealing with a specific metabolic gene, proposing a nomenclature for metabolic gene polymorphisms (Vatsis *et al.*, 1995; Daly *et al.*, 1996). Table 1 illustrates the proposed nomenclature for the polymorphisms in the *CYP1A1, GSTM1, GSTT1, CYP2E1* and *AHR*

genes. For completeness we have also included the nomenclature for *NAT2, CYP2D6, CYP2A6, CYP2C9, CYP2C18* and *CYP2C19*, although these have been previously published, and for complete details on these gene polymorphisms we recommend the reader to consult the above-mentioned publications. Table 1 lists examples of previously used nomenclature for each allele along with selected references; the lists of such alternative names and references for some of these alleles are neither complete nor comprehensive but are included simply for illustrative purposes. It should be noted that some of the restriction fragment length polymorphisms (RFLP) described may be markers of functional mutations, generated at the same time, but not identical with the diagnostic mutation. Because of recombination, such markers may not always completely define a particular allele.

For each allele the new name includes the gene name in capital italic letters, followed by an asterisk and an Arabic number representing the polymorphism without spaces. In some cases a letter is used after the final number to distinguish subtypes of a single allele. A recent paper describing a system for naming the various complex polymorphisms of the N-acetyltransferase (*NAT*) genes suggested a numbering system based on chronological discovery of each allele (Vatsis *et al.*, 1995). This is a logical approach for polymorphism nomenclature, because systems based on function or location would probably be insufficiently flexible to deal with the variety of potential gene polymorphisms already known and yet to be discovered. A system based on chronology has the advantage of being highly flexible, especially with regard to the very likely event that many more polymorphisms will be described in the future in these genes. Whenever possible, therefore, the sequence of the allele numbers should follow the publication date. Consequently, for all the genes discussed here it is expected that authors will name new polymorphisms with the next available number upon first publication of the discovery and/or application of a new polymorphism. It is also hoped that errors or corrections related to Table 1 will be brought to the attention of the editors, and that further updates of the entire metabolic gene nomenclature will be published regularly.

Specific metabolic gene polymorphisms
CYP1A1

The *CYP1A1* gene, discussed by Kawajiri in Chapter 15 of this volume, contains four significant polymorphisms, all resulting from point mutations. The polymorphisms and the resulting alleles have been designated by various systems. In an attempt to clarify the situation, and to enable a simplified method of naming alleles with multiple mutations, we previously suggested a nomenclature system (Garte et al., 1996) that used C for the wild type allele, M for the original Msp1 RFLP, E for the exon 7 polymorphism, and A for the African specific Msp1 RFLP in intron 7. This system had the advantage of allowing for simple genotype designations, and also provided some information regarding the position of the mutation(s). However, it lacked the flexibility required to deal with new polymorphisms, such as another Msp 1 RFLP in exon 7 which was recently discovered (Cascorbi et al., 1996). According to the new proposed system, as shown in Table 1, the C allele = *CYP1A1*1*, M = *CYP1A1*2*, E = *CYP1A1*3*, A = *CYP1A1*4*, and the new Msp1 RFLP = *CYP1A1*5*. A similar nomenclature has been described by Cascorbi et al., (1996), except that these authors use *2A and *2B for the alleles *2 and *3. The rationale given for their choice of CYP1A1 nomenclature is that these two alleles are tightly linked. Actually, while

there is a close association between these two point mutations in Asians, the linkage is less common in Caucasians, and does not exist at all in Africans (Garte et al., 1996).

GSTs

The polymorphisms in the *GST* genes are thoroughly discussed in Chapter 19 by Strange and Fryer. The nomenclature used by these authors for *GSTM1* alleles is similar to that proposed here, except for the use of letters rather than numbers to distinguish the two *GSTM1* non-deleted alleles. In order to retain maximum consistency with these previous designations, and still follow the rules of the proposed system, the *A and *B alleles will be called *1A and *1B respectively. The null or deleted allele, termed *GSTM1*0* by Strange and Fryer, is now *GSTM1*2*. In those cases where authors do not distinguish between the A and B variants of the *GSTM1* present (or wild type) allele, it is appropriate to use *GSTM1*1*, which is then distinguished from the null allele *GSTM1*2*. The same rules are applied to the other *GST* genes, as shown in Table 1.

CYP2E1

This gene represents one of the most confusing cases of polymorphism nomenclature in the current literature. For example there are two Rsa 1 RFLPs, one of which results in the loss of a restriction site and is always accompanied by a Pst 1 RFLP. This allele is designated *CYP2E1*3*, following the wild type (*CYP2E1*1*), and a Taq 1 RFLP in intron 7 (*CYP2E1*2*). The other three RFLPs are listed in Table 1.

AHR

As discussed in Chapter 14 by Garte and Sogawa the polymorphism picture for the Ah receptor gene in humans is currently quite fluid and subject to rapid change. As a consequence the polymorphisms listed in Table 1 for this gene will probably be incomplete by the time of publication of the present volume, and should be considered as only a starting point for *AHR* gene nomenclature.

Table 1. Nomenclature for metabolic gene polymorphisms

GENE	NAME	DESCRIPTION TYPE	POSITION	RFLP OTHER	PREVIOUS NAMES	AUTHORS
AHR	AHR*1	wt				
	AHR*2	fs ins T#2498				Itoh & Kamataki (1993); Ema et al. (1994)
	AHR*3	?	?			Jones et al. (1994)
	AHR*4	pm G->A	exon 10 Arg->Lys cod. 554	MspI RFLP	A2	Kawajiri et al. (1995)
CYP1A1	CYP1A1*1	wt			w, A	Nebert & Gonzalez (1987)
	CYP1A1*2	pm T->C,	#6235 3' non-coding	Msp1 RFLP, cut,	m1, B, M	Kawajiri et al. (1990); Petersen et al. (1991)
	CYP1A1*3	pm A->G,	#4889 Ile->Val exon 7	BsrDI RFLP, non cut	m2, G, E	Hayashi et al. (1991); Hirvonen et al. (1992)
	CYP1A1*4	pm T->C	cod. 462 #5639 intron 7	Msp1 RFLP, cut. African Specific	AA, m3, A	Crofts et al. (1993)
	CYP1A1*5	pm C->A	#4887 exon 7 cod. 461 Thr->Asn	Bsal RFLP, non-cut,	m4	Cascorbi et al. (1996)
CYP2A6	CYP2A6*1	wt				
	CYP2A6*2	pm T->A	cod. 160, exon 3 Leu->His	Xcm1 RFLP	v1	Fernandez-Salguero et al. (1995)
	CYP2A6*3	Gene conversion with CYP2A7		Dde1 RFLP	v2	Daly et al. (1996); Fernandez-Salguero et al. (1995)
CYP2C9	CYP2C9*1	wt				
	CYP2C9*2	pm C->T	cod. 144 Arg->Cys		R144C	Daly et al. (1996); Stubbins & Wolf (1999)
	CYP2C9*3	pm A->C	cod. 359 Ile->Leu		Leu359	Daly et al. (1996); Stubbins & Wolf (1999)
CYP2C18	CYP2C18*1	wt	5' flank	Dde RFLP non-cut		Tsuneoka et al. (1996)
	CYP2C18*2	?				
CYP2C19	CYP2C19*1	wt				
	CYP2C19*2	pm G->A	#681, exon 5	BamH1 RFLP, non-cut	m1	De Morais et al. (1994a)
	CYP2C19*3	pm G->A	#636, exon 4		m2	De Morais et al. (1994b)

Table 1 (Contd). Nomenclature for metabolic gene polymorphisms

GENE	NAME	DESCRIPTION TYPE	POSITION	RFLP OTHER	PREVIOUS NAMES	AUTHORS
CYP2D6	CYP2D6*1A	wt				See Daly et al. (1996) for details
	CYP2D6*1B	pm G->A	#3916			
	CYP2D6*2	pm G->C	#1749			
		pm C->T	#2938			
		pm G->C	#4268			
	CYP2D6*3	del A	#2637			
	CYP2D6*4A	pm C->T	#188			
		pm C->A	#1062			
		pm A->G	#1072			
		pm C->G	#1085			
		pm G->C	#1749			
		pm G->A	#1934			
		pm G->C	#4268			
	CYP2D6*4B	pm C->T	#188			
		pm C->A	#1062			
		pm A->G	#1072			
		pm C->G	#1085			
		pm G->A	#1934			
		pm G->C	#4268			
	CYP2D6*4C	pm C->T	#188			
		pm G->C	#1749			
		pm G->A	#1934			
		pm T->C	#3975			
		pm G->C	#4268			
	CYP2D6*4D	pm C->T	#188			
		pm C->T	#1127			
		pm G->C	#1749			
		pm G->A	#1934			
		pm G->C	#4268			
	CYP2D6*5	gene del.				
	CYP2D6*6A	del T	#1795			
	CYP2D6*6B	del T	#1795			
	CYP2D6*7	pm G->A	#2064			
		pm A->C	#3023			
	CYP2D6*8	pm G->C	#1749			
		pm G->T	#1846			
		pm C->T	#2938			
		pm G->C	#4268			
	CYP2D6*9	del	#2701-2703			
		or del	#2702-2704			

Table 1 (Contd). Nomenclature for metabolic gene polymorphisms

GENE	NAME	DESCRIPTION TYPE	POSITION	RFLP OTHER	PREVIOUS NAMES	AUTHORS
	CYP2D6*10A	pm C->T	#188			
		pm G->C	#1749			
		pm G->C	#4268			
	CYP2D6*10B	pm C->T	#188			
		pm G->C	#1749			
		pm G->C	#4268			
	CYP2D6*10C	pm C->T	#188			
		pm C->T	#1127			
		pm G->C	#1749			
		pm G->C	#4268			
		coversion to CYP2D7 in exon 9				
	CYP2D6*11	pm G->C	#971			
		pm C->T	#1749			
		pm C->T	#2938			
		pm G->C	#4268			
	CYP2D6*12	pm G->A	#212			
		pm G->C	#1749			
		pm C->T	#2938			
		pm G->C	#4268			
	CYP2D6*13	fs	exon 1 = CYP2D7			
	CYP2D6*14	pm C->T	#188			
		pm G->A	#1846			
		pm C->T	#2938			
		pm G->C	#4268			
		ins T	#226			
	CYP2D6*15	fs	exon 1-7 = CYP2D7			
	CYP2D6*16	pm C->T	#1111			
	CYP2D6*17	pm G->C	#17266			
		pm C->T	#2938			
		pm G->C	#4268			
CYP2E1	CYP2E1*1	wt			c1, w, H, C, A2	
	CYP2E1*2	pm C->G	#9930 intron 7	Taq1 RFLP, cut	A1	McBride et al. (1987)
	CYP2E1*3	pm C->T	#1019	Pst1 cut, RFLPs, Rsa1 non-cut	c2, m	Watanbe et al. (1990)
		pm G->C	#1259, 5' flanking			
	CYP2E1*4	pm T->A	#7668 intron 6	Dra1 RFLP, non-cut	D	Uematsu et al. (1991a); Uematsu et al. (1991b)
	CYP2E1*5	pm	intron 5	Rsa1 RFLP cut	I	Uematsu et al. (1991b)
	CYP2E1*6	pm		Msp1 RFLP cut		Uematsu et al. (1991c)

9

Table 1 (Contd). Nomenclature for metabolic gene polymorphisms

GENE	NAME	DESCRIPTION TYPE	POSITION	RFLP OTHER	PREVIOUS NAMES	AUTHORS
GSTM1	GSTM1*1A	wt.			A, GSTM1*A	DeJong et al. (1988); Brockmöller et al. (1994)
	GSTM1*1B	pm	exon 7		B, GSTM1*B	DeJong et al. (1988); Brockmöller et al. (1994)
	GSTM1*2	gene del.			0, null, GSTM1*0	Seidegard et al. (1988)
GSTM3	GSTM3*1	wt.			A	Inskip et al. (1995)
	GSTM3*2	3bp del.	intron 6	MnlI RFLP, non-cut	B	Inskip et al. (1995)
GSTT1	GSTT1*1	wt				
	GSTT1*2	gene del.			null	Pemble et al. (1994)
NAT2	NAT2*4	wt				See Vatsis et al. (1995) for details
	NAT2*5A	pm T->C	#341			
		pm C->T	#481			
	NAT2*5B	pm T->C	#341			
		pm C->T	#481			
		pm A->G	#803			
	NAT2*5C	pm T->C	#341			
		pm A->G	#803			
	NAT2*6A	pm C->T	#282			
		pm G->A	#590			
	NAT2*6B	pm G->A	#590			
	NAT2*7A	pm G->A	#857			
	NAT2*7B	pm C->T	#282			
		pm G->A	#857			
	NAT2*12A	pm A->G	#803			
	NAT2*12B	pm C->T	#282			
		pm A->G	#803			
	NAT2*13	pm C->T	#282			
	NAT2*14A	pm G->A	#191			
	NAT2*14B	pm C->T	#282			
		pm G->A	#191			
	NAT2*17	pm A->C	#434			
	NAT2*18	pm A->C	#845			

Abbreviations and explanations:

wt: wild type
pm: point mutation
del.: deletion
fs: frame shift
#: nucleotide no.

ins.: insertion
cod.: codon
cut: the polymorphic form is spliced by the enzyme
non-cut: the polymorphic form is not spliced by the enzyme

References

Brockmöller, J., Kerb, R., Drakoulis, N., Staffeldt, B. & Roots, I. (1994) Glutathione S transferase M1 and its variants A and B as host factors of bladder cancer susceptibility: a case control study. *Cancer Res.*, 54, 4103-4111

Cascorbi, I., Brockmöller J. & Roots, I.A. (1996) C4887A polymorphism in exon 7 of human CYP1A1, population frequency, mutation linkages, and impact on lung cancer susceptibility. *Cancer Res.*, 56, 4965-4969

Crofts, F., Cosma, G.N., Taioli, E., Currie, D.C., Toniolo, P.T. & Garte, S.J. (1993) A novel CYP1A1 gene polymorphism in African-Americans. *Carcinogenesis*, 14, 1729-1731

Daly, A.K., Brockmöller, J., Broly, F., Eichelbaum, M., Evans, W.E., Gonzalez, F.J., Huang, J.D., Idle, J.R., Ingelman-Sundberg, M., Ishizaki, T., Jacqz-Aigrain, E., Meyer, U.A., Nebert, D.W., Steen, V.M., Wolf, C.R. & Zanger, U.M. (1996) Nomenclature for human CYP2D6 alleles. *Pharmacogenetics,* 6, 193-201

De Morais, S.M.F., Wilkinson, G.R., Blaisdell, J., Nakamura, K., Meyer, U.A. & Goldstein, J.A. (1994a) The major genetic defect responsible for the polymorphism of S-mephenytoin metabolism in humans. *J. Biol. Chem.*, 269, 15419-15422

De Morais, S.M.F., Wilkinson, G.R., Blaisdell, J., Meyer, U.A., Nakamura, K. & Goldstein, J.A. (1994b) Identification of a new genetic defect responsible for the polymorphism of (S)-mephenytoin metabolism in Japanese. *Mol. Pharmacol.*, 46, 594-598

DeJong, J.L., Chang, C., WongPeng, J., Knutsen, T. & Tu, C.D. (1988) The human liver glutathione S-transferase gene superfamily: expression and chromosome mapping of H_b subunit cDNA. *Nucleic Acids Res.*, 16, 8541-8554

Ema, M., Ohe, N., Suzuki, M., Mimura, J., Sogawa, K., Ikawa, S. & Fujii-Kuriyama,Y. (1994) Dioxin binding activities of polymorphic forms of mouse and human arylhydrocarbon receptors. *J. Biol. Chem.*, 269 (44), 27337-27343

Fernandez-Salguero, P., Hoffman, S.M.G., Cholerton, S., Mohrenweiser, H., Raunio, H., Rautio, A., Pelkonen, O., Huang, J.D., Evans, W.E., Idle, J.R. & Gonzalez, F.J. (1995) A genetic polymorphism in coumarin 7-hydroxylation: sequence of the human CYP2A genes and identification of variant CYP2A6alleles. *Am. J. Hum. Genet.*, 57, 651-660

Garte, S.J., Trachman, J., Crofts, F., Toniolo, P., Buxbaum, J., Bayo, S. & Taioli, E. (1996) Distribution of composite CYP1A1 genotypes in Africans, African-Americans and Caucasians. *Hum. Hered.*, 46, 121-127

Hayashi, S., Watanabe, J., Nakachi, K. & Kawajiri, K. (1991) Genetic linkage of lung cancer-associated Msp1 polymorphism with amino acid replacement in the haeme-binding region of the human cytochrome P450IA1 gene. *J. Biochem. (Tokyo)*, 110, 407-411

Hirvonen, A., Pursianen, K.H., Karjalainen, A., Anttila, S. & Vainio, H. (1992) Point mutational Msp1 and Ile-Val polymorphism closely linked in the CYP1A1 gene: lack of association with susceptibility to lung cancer in a Finnish study population. *Cancer Epidemiol. Biomarkers Prev.*, 1, 485-489

Inskip, A., Elexperu-Carimuaga, J., Buxton, N., Dias, P.S., MacIntosh, J., Campbell, D., Jones, P.W., Yengi, L., Talbot, J.A. & Strange, R.C. (1995) Identification of polymorphism at the glutathione S-transferase GSTM3 locus: evidence for linkage with GSTM1A. *Biochem. J.*, 312, 713-716

Itoh, S. & Kamataki, T. (1993) Ah receptor cDNA: analysis for highly conserved sequences. *Nucleic Acids Res.*, 21, 3578

Jones, J.E., Huckaby, C.S., Stafford, M.D. & Linnoila, R.I. (1994) An MspI RFLP of the human AHR gene. *Hum. Mol. Genet.*, 3(11), 2083

Kawajiri, K., Nakachi, K., Imai, K.,Yoshii, A., Shinoda, N. & Watanabe, J. (1990) Identification of genetically high-risk individuals to lung cancer by DNA polymorphisms of the cytochrome P4501A1 gene. *FEBS*, 263, 131-133

Kawajiri, K., Watanabe, J., Eguchi, H., Nakachi, K., Kiyohara, C. & Hayashi, S. (1995) Polymorphisms of human Ah receptor gene are not involved in lung cancer. *Pharmacogenetics*, 5(3), 151-158

McBride, O.W., Umeno, M., Belboin, H.V. & Gonzalez, F.J. (1987) A taq I polymorphism in the human P450IIEI gene on chromosome 10 (CYPZE). *Nucleic Acids Res.*, 15, 10071

Nebert, D.W. & Gonzalez, F.J. (1987) P450 genes: structure, evolution, and regulation. *Annu. Rev. Biochem.*, 56, 945-993

Pemble, S., Schroeder, K.R., Spencer, S.R., Meyer, D.J., Hallier, E., Bolt, H.M., Ketterer, B. & Taylor J.B. (1994) Human glutathione S-transferase theta (GSTT1) cDNA cloning and the characterization of a genetic polymorphism. *Biochem. J.*, 300, 271-276

Petersen, D.D., McKinney, C.D., Ikeya, K., Smith, H.H., Bale, A.E., McBride, O.W. & Nebert, D.W. (1991) Human CYP1A1 gene: cosegregation of the enzyme inducibility phenotype and an RFLP. *Am. J. Hum. Genet.*, 48, 720-725

Seidegard, J., Voracheck, W.R., Pero, R.W. & Pearson, W.R. (1988) Hereditary differences in the expression of the human glutathione transferase activity on trans-stilbene oxide are due to a gene deletion. *Proc. Natl. Acad. Sci. USA*, 85, 7293-7297

Stubbins, M.J. & Wolf, C.R. (1999) Additional polymorphisms and cancer. In: Vineis, P., Malats, N., Lang, M., d'Errico, A., Caparaso, N., Cuzick, J. & Boffetta, P., eds, *Metabolic Polymorphisms and Susceptibility to Cancer*. (IARC Scientific Publications No. 148). Lyon, International Agency for Research on Cancer, pp. 271-302

Tsuneoka, Y., Matsuo, Y., Okuyama, E., Watanbe, Y. & Ichikawa, Y. (1996) Genetic analysis of the cytochrome P-450IIC18 (CYP2C18) gene and a novel member of the CYP2C family. *FEBS Lett.*, 384, 281-284

Uematsu, F., Kikuchi, H., Motomiya, M., Abe, T., Sagami, I., Ohmachi, T., Wakui, R. & Watanabe, M. (1991a) Association between restriction fragment length polymprophism of the human cytochrome P450IIE1 gene and susceptibility to lung cancer. *Jpn J. Cancer Res.*, 82, 254-256

Uematsu, F., Kikuchi, H., Ohmachi, T., Sagami, I., Motomiya, M., Kamataki, T., Komori, M. & Watanabe, M. (1991b) *Nucleic Acids Res.*, 19, 2803

Uematsu, F., Kikuchi, H., Abe, T., Motomiya, M., Ohmachi, T., Sagami, I. & Watanabe, M. (1991c) Msp I polymorphism of the human CYP2E gene. *Nucleic Acids Res.*, 19, 5797

Vatsis, K.P., Weber, W.W., Bell, D.A., Dupret, J.M., Evans, D.A.P., Grant, D.M., Hein, D.W., Lin, H.J., Meyer, U.A., Relling, M.V., Sim, E., Suzuki, T. & Yamazoe, Y. (1995) Nomenclature for N-acetyltransferases. *Pharmacogenetics*, 5, 1-17

Watanabe, J., Hayashi, S.I., Nakachi, K., Imai, K., Suda, Y., Sekine, T. and Kawajiri, K. (1990) Pst L and RSA i RFLP in complete linkage dysequilibrium at the CYP2E gene. *Nucleic Acids Res.*, 18, 7194

Corresponding author
Seymour Garte
Environmental and Occupational Health Sciences Institute, UMDNJ,
170 Frelinghuysen Road,
Piscataway, NJ, USA

and

Sci. Dir.
Genetics Research Institute
Milan, Italy

Metabolic Polymorphisms and Susceptibility to Cancer
W. Ryder
IARC Scientific Publications No. 148
International Agency for Research on Cancer, Lyon, 1999

Chapter 3. Metabolism of xenobiotics and chemical carcinogenesis

Matti Lang and Olavi Pelkonen

In order to avoid the accumulation of harmful xenobiotics in cells, living organisms have developed ways for their elimination. Multiple xenobiotic metabolizing enzymes with variable but partially overlapping catalytic properties play a key role in the elimination process. These enzymes are encoded by superfamilies of genes which, during the course of evolution, have evolved in a way that has made it possible for the different species to survive and take advantage of different habitats and diet containing a variable composition of harmful xenobiotics. As a result of this evolutionary process, species have achieved capacities to metabolize xenobiotics which are appropriate for their survival but which may differ considerably from those of other species. This evolutionary process may also explain the interethnic and interindividual variability of drug metabolism in humans.

Because many carcinogens are substrates of drug-metabolizing enzymes it is reasonable to assume that humans have a variable capacity to activate or inactivate carcinogens. This has been shown to be the case. It appears that most of the carcinogen-metabolizing enzymes are inducible by xenobiotics: they respond to environmental stimuli and therefore vary in their activity. Furthermore, many of the encoding genes are polymorphic and multiple allelic variants relevant for the phenotype may exist in human populations.

Analysis of the genetic variability that affects the capacity to metabolize carcinogens in humans has shown that a few members of the cytochrome P450, glutathione S-transferase and N-acetyltransferae gene families may play an important role in chemical carcinogenesis. Yet for several enzymes such a role has not been established until now, although their catalytic properties and expression in human tissues suggest that such a role should exist. More studies on the role of individual enzymes in chemical carcinogenesis are therefore warranted.

Living organisms are exposed to a vast number of foreign chemicals from various environmental sources. Many of these compounds are relatively small and lipophilic and therefore could easily accumulate in cells and quickly reach toxic or lethal concentrations unless excluded. To avoid such accumulation and toxicity under chemical stress it has been necessary for the living organisms to develop ways of eliminating xenobiotics and preventing their accumulation. This is achieved mainly by means of enzymes that can recognize xenobiotics and convert them to water-soluble forms which are easily excreted.

The enzymatic reactions of xenobiotic metabolism can be divided into two distinct phases. On entering cells, drugs are first metabolized by the phase I enzymes, often in an oxidation reaction, which introduce a functional, typically electrophilic, centre into the molecule. The creation of a reactive centre allows phase II enzymes to introduce a hydrophilic moiety (such as a glutathione or acetyl group) into the molecule, and this usually results in a sufficiently water-soluble and easily excretable product. Depending on the structure of the parent compound, adequate solubility in water may be obtained already after phase I reactions. In some cases, phase II reactions may be possible without phase I metabolism.

In most cases the toxicity of the molecule is reduced during the course of metabolism. In some cases, however, it may be increased. This occurs especially after the phase I reaction where, as a result of oxidation, reactive electrophilic intermediates are formed. The toxic effects of the reactive intermediates depend on their structure.

Typically, however, their targets are nucleophilic macromolecules of the cell, and many of them are genotoxic and potentially carcinogenic. Indeed, it is well known that most chemical carcinogens need metabolic activation in order to exert their carcinogenic properties.

It may seem surprising that enzymes that have evolved to protect organisms from foreign chemicals may increase the toxicity of some of them. However, it should be borne in mind that the activation reactions represent only a small portion of foreign chemicals encountered by animals. Furthermore, the role of the enzymes is to solve an acute problem: that of lethal accumulation of xenobiotics, whereas carcinogenic processes are long-lasting and usually affect animals only after their reproductive stage. Therefore, it is possible that chemical carcinogenesis does not play a strong role in the evolutionary selection of populations. (For reviews on drug and carcinogen metabolism see Nebert *et al.*, 1981 and Gonzalez & Gelboin, 1994).

Because the number of foreign chemicals that living organisms are exposed to is practically unlimited, it is reasonable to assume that a large number of enzymes is needed to recognize and metabolize all the different structures. This is indeed the case. Investigations conducted during the last several years have shown that some of the key enzyme systems such as the cytochrome P450s (CYPs) and the glutathione S-transferases (GSTs) consist of large superfamilies of enzymes with different but overlapping substrate specificities. Importantly, it has also been shown that the CYPs are one of the fastest evolving gene systems of living organisms. This has probably been necessary for various species to adapt to different habitats and diet. Such flexibility has undoubtedly increased the chances of evolving species to take advantage of and cope with diets consisting of varying combinations of noxious chemicals.

As a result of the adaptation and relatively fast evolution of the encoding genes, different species have essential differences in the composition and catalytic properties of their drug-metabolizing enzymes. This is also why the profile of human drug metabolism is different from those of other species and why, even among human beings, considerable interethnic and interindividual differences occur in the structures of encoding genes. It is worth noting that genetic polymorphism of human drug-metabolizing enzymes is almost the rule rather than the exception, and it may not be obvious what advantages this confers. As the decisive factor in adaptation is the survival of the species, rather than all individuals, one possibility is that a high number of allelic variants, as with the CYP2D6 gene, somehow improves the chances of survival of at least certain individuals when dramatic environmental changes take place.

The very reason for interindividual variability in the capacity to activate or inactivate carcinogens and thus for individuals to be more or less protected against chemical carcinogenesis therefore lies in the fast-evolving nature by many and frequent modifications of the various genes encoding for drug-metabolizing enzymes (Nebert *et al.*, 1982). It should be noted that although the driving force behind the evolution of drug-metabolizing enzymes is probably exposure to compounds of natural origin, such as plant alkaloids, the enzymes just as easily recognize and metabolize man-made compounds, for example newly synthesized drugs that did not exist when the genes encoding for the human enzymes attained their final structure and composition.

An overview is presented below of the catalytic properties and regulation of the most important enzymes of human carcinogen metabolism. Many of these enzymes or their corresponding genes will be dealt with in more detail in later Chapters summarizing investigations on their potential role in carcinogenesis.

The cytochrome P450 (CYP) superfamily

The cytochrome P450s (CYPs) comprise the principal enzyme system catalysing various phase I oxidation reactions of xenobiotics including the metabolic activation of carcinogens. CYPs exist in most living organisms and have evolved into a superfamily of genes which, according to a recent review, has almost 500 members. For classification and communication purposes a nomenclature system has been developed where the individual genes and gene products have been arranged in families and subfamilies based on their sequence homology. For example, *CYP1A2* denotes member 2 in family 1, subfamily A (and CYP1A2 denotes the corresponding gene product). For more details concerning the CYP superfamily, see Nelson *et al.* (1996).

Based on investigations into the evolution of the CYP superfamily it seems that the early forms already appeared about 3.5 billion years ago, probably before the prokaryote/eukaryote divergence. The functions of the early forms were possibly to metabolize endogenous compounds such as steroids and fatty acids, rather than xenobiotics. The first xenobiotic metabolizing forms may have appeared about 400-500 million years ago, to metabolize noxious chemicals found in plants. Nebert, Gonzalez and their coworkers have proposed that "plant-animal warfare" has been the driving force in the evolution of the CYP superfamily. Plants produce toxins for their protection and animals evolve enzymes to eliminate them. As a result of this warfare, which has been going on for hundreds of millions of years, various forms of CYP enzymes have appeared in the different species seeking new habitats and diet as part of their strategies of survival. For a review of this subject, see Gonzalez & Gelboin (1994).

Human CYPs involved in carcinogen metabolism

Of the various CYP enzymes expressed in humans, only those belonging to families 1-3 seem to play a significant role in carcinogen metabolism (Guengerich et al., 1991).

The CYP1 gene family

CYP1A1 is the principal enzyme metabolizing polycyclic aromatic hydrocarbons (PAHs), such as benzo(a)pyrene and dimethylbenzanthracene. Several of these compounds are considered to be important carcinogens and they are present in, e.g. tobacco smoke and urban air. Some PAHs may require more than one metabolic step for their activation and in many of the reactions CYP1A1 plays a role, although some other CYPs may also participate. The enzyme is found in several extrahepatic tissues but seems to be absent from the liver.

The expression of the enzyme is regulated transcriptionally by the aromatic hydrocarbon (Ah) receptor, a cytosolic transcription factor which, upon ligand-binding, is activated and translocates to the nucleus where it binds to the Ah-responsive element of the CYP1A1 gene. Genetic polymorphisms of the CYP1A1 gene have been described

and some studies suggest their association with cancer (see Chapter 15 by Kawajiri).

CYP1A2, despite its rather high homology with CYP1A1, has an essentially different and broad substrate specificity including such structurally diverse compounds as nitrosamines, heterocyclic arylamines (some of which are important food mutagens) and aflatoxin B1. Unlike CYP1A1, this enzyme is liver specific and cannot be detected in extrahepatic tissues. The expression of CYP1A2 is regulated by the Ah receptor but the regulation does not seem to be identical to that of CYP1A1. It has also been proposed that posttranscriptional events may play a role in its regulation.

So far no genetic polymorphism has been found for the CYP1A2 gene but using the specific substrate, caffeine, great interindividual variability has been found in its in vivo activity. The reasons for this variability are not known but they could include genetic as well as environmental factors such as inducers in the diet or tobacco smoke. A genetic polymorphism of the gene itself or of a transacting regulatory factor explaining the interindividual variability should not be ruled out (for reviews on CYP1A1 and CYP1A2, see Gonzalez & Gelboin (1994) and Guengerich & Shimada (1991)).

CYP1B1: A novel CYP enzyme was recently cloned and characterized which appears to belong to subfamily 1B. It exhibits arylhydrocarbon hydroxylase (AHH) activity, is expressed in many human tissues, and the expression seems to be regulated by TCDD, possibly via the Ah receptor. Its properties are similar to those of CYP1A1 (Shen et al , 1994; Sutter et al., 1994). No detailed studies have been conducted on the regulation of this enzyme, nor on its possible role in carcinogen metabolism.

The CYP2 gene family

The CYP2 gene family is the largest family of CYPs, consisting of several subfamilies. A vast number of structurally diverse compounds are recognized and metabolized by the various CYP2 enzymes, and the modes of regulation of the enzymes are complex. Essential differences may exist both in the catalytic properties and regulation of the members in different subfamilies and also between members within one subfamily (Nelson et al , 1996).

CYP2A6 metabolizes several carcinogens, including some nitrosamines and aflatoxin B1. In this respect it shares catalytic properties with CYP1A2, CYP2E1 and CYP3A4. CYP2A6 also seems to be the major catalyst of nicotine metabolism (Raunio *et al.*, Chapter 17).

In vivo studies using coumarin as a specific diagnostic substrate have shown large interindividual variablility in the expression of CYP2A6 (Camus *et al.*, 1993; Rautio *et al.*, 1992). This has been confirmed by determining the levels of the CYP2A6 protein in human liver specimens and by determining the microsomal coumarin 7-hydroxylase activity of human liver (Camus *et al.*, 1993). Based on some animal studies and our unpublished observations in humans it seems that the enzyme is also expressed in some extrahepatic tissues (Béréziat *et al.*, 1995).

A genetic polymorphism of the human CYP2A6 gene has been reported (Fernandez-Salguero *et al.*, 1995). It seems likely that the alterations in the CYP2A6 gene structure affect the catalytic properties of the enzyme but the relationship between the phenotype and the genotype have not been well established, particularly with respect to carcinogen metabolism. Little information is as yet available on the possible association of the CYP2A6 polymorphism and cancer.

CYP2B6 is able to activate at least aflatoxin B1 and some other carcinogens (Gonzalez & Gelboin, 1994, and reference 2 therein). As in the case of CYP2A6, the interindividual variability in the expression of CYP2B6 is large. The counterparts of this enzyme, CYP2B1 and CYP2B2, are known to be induced by phenobarbital and related compounds. It is uncertain whether or not the human enzyme is subject to similar regulation. Genetic polymorphism of *CYP2B6* has not been reported and its role in human carcinogenesis has remained unclear.

The **CYP2C** subfamily has at least four members expressed in human liver, namely CYP2C8, CYP2C9, CYP2C18 and CYP2C19 (reviewed by Smith *et al.*, 1995). Many compounds, including several clinically used drugs, are substrates of these enzymes. The *CYP2C19* gene polymorphism was discovered on the basis of the polymorphic distribution of mephenytoin metabolism in human populations. Approximately 5% of Caucasians and 20-25% of Orientals have the *CYP2C19* gene defect, leading to poor metabolism (Wilkinson *et al.*, 1989).

Despite their wide range of substrate specificity

and abundance in the liver, the CYP2C enzymes do not seem to have a significant role in carcinogen metabolism. This possibility should, however, not be ruled out.

CYP2D6 metabolizes several important clinically used drugs (Smith *et al.*, 1995) but there is little evidence for it having a role in carcinogen activation. Crespi *et al.* (1991) reported some evidence that CYP2D6 activates NNK [4-(methylnitrosamino)-1-(3-pyridyl)-1-butanone], a nitrosamine derived from tobacco smoke which is a potent carcinogen. This result is often referred to as evidence for the contribution of the CYP2D6 to carcinogen activation and lung cancer. This should be interpreted with caution, however, because only indirect evidence based on a mutagenisis assay is available, and because other CYPs such as CYP1A2 and CYP2A3 (CYP2A6) seem to be more prominent than CYP2D6 in NNK activation. Furthermore, it is not clear whether CYP2D6 is expressed in human lung.

With debrisoquine as a substrate, a high interindividual variability in CYP2D6 activity has been observed *in vivo*. In addition, there is a distinct group of slow metabolizers: about 5-7% of the Caucasian population and a few individuals with an extremely high metabolic rate. All these variations are due to genetic alterations in the encoding gene. In the case of the ultrarapid metabolizers a gene multiplication has been demonstrated (Johansson *et al.*, 1993).

There have been several attempts to link the *CYP2D6* polymorphism to increased cancer risk, in particular with respect to lung cancer and leukaemia (Wolf *et al.*, 1992). Some evidence exists but the role of CYP2D6 in carcinogenesis has remained controversial (see Chapter 18 by Smith & Wolf).

CYP2E1 metabolizes many low-molecular-weight toxins and carcinogens, such as nitrosamines, ethanol, benzene, carbon tetrachloride, vinyl chloride and acrylonitriles (Guengerich *et al.*, 1991). A few of the substrates are also inducers of CYP2E1. Furthermore, the enzyme is induced, e.g. during fasting or diabetes, possibly by some endogeneously formed compounds.

The fact that CYP2E1 is able to metabolize a large number of compounds with different structures indicates that its active site does not fit well any particular structure; the substrates, therefore, may not have a high affinity for the enzyme. This seems to be the case since typically high concentrations of substrates are needed in enzymatic assay to reach the Vmax conditions (Guengerich *et al.*, 1991). The loose substrate binding is also consistent with the fact that in the oxidation reactions catalysed by CYP2E1 relatively large amounts of activated oxygen "leak" out of the active site and do not reach the substrate to be oxidized. It is possible that this oxygen activation is one of the mechanisms by which CYP2E1 plays a role in hepatotoxicity (Dai *et al.*, 1993).

CYP2E1 is expressed at high levels in the liver and at lower levels in several extrahepatic tissues. Its mode of regulation is complex, involving transcriptional as well as postranscriptional events (Eliasson *et al.*, 1992). As compared to other CYP2 subfamilies, CYP2E is simple, only one gene having been identified so far (Song *et al.*, 1986). Several polymorphisms have been identified at the CYP2E1 locus by RFLP analysis.

In a study by Uematsu *et al.* (1991), CYP2E1 polymorphism was associated with lung cancer in a Japanese population. However, it has not been possible to show this association in other populations or for other cancers. This is somewhat surprising, given the central role played by CYP2E1 in the metabolism of various carcinogens and toxins. An explanation for this could lie in the complex regulation of the expression of CYP2E1, where postranscriptional events such as protein stabilization seem essential, making it difficult to relate the genotype to the phenotype.

CYP2F1 has been identified in human lung and low-level expression has been found in liver. Little information is available about its role in carcinogen metabolism (Nhamburo *et al.*, 1990; Ritter *et al.*, 1991).

The CYP3 gene family
CYP3A: At least three members of this subfamily, CYP3A4, CYP3A5 and CYP3A7 are expressed in humans, CYP3A4 perhaps being the most abundant single CYP enzyme expressed in the liver. CYP3A4 and CYP3A5 share catalytic properties and play an important role in the metabolism of both clinically used drugs and carcinogens such as aflatoxin B1, 6-aminochrysene and benzo(a)pyrene.

High interindividual variation has been found in the expression of the CYP3As. Part of this variability is due to the polymorphism of CYP3A5 which has been shown *in vivo* by the bimodal distribution of nifedipine metabolism in human populations. This polymorphism is also indicated by the fact that only about 20% of humans seem to express the CYP3A5 in the liver. The genetic basis for this polymorphism is not yet clear (Gonzalez & Gelboin, 1994; Smith *et al.*, 1995).

The glutathione S-transferase (GST) superfamily
As a result of various oxidation reactions catalysed by the phase I enzymes, many xenobiotics are transformed into reactive electrophilic intermediates which readily attack nucleophilic targets in cells such as proteins and nucleic acids. Reactive electrophiles may also arise from endogenous processes initiated by, e.g., respiration, inflammation or ionizing radiation which produce reactive oxygen species (ROS), including superoxide radicals and hydroxy radicals.

In order to survive it is necessary for living organisms to protect themselves from these electrophilic compounds. Of the several detoxification systems used for protection, one of the most efficient in the elimination of electrophiles is that of reduced glutathione (GSH) and glutathione S-transferases (GSTs). Glutathione is a nucleophilic tripeptide which serves as a target for the electrophiles instead of the cellular macromolecules. The role of the catalysing enzymes (GSTs) is to facilitate the reaction (which also may occur non-enzymatically in cells) by binding the GSH, lowering its pKa at the active site, and bringing the electrophilic substrate close to the enzyme-bound GSH. In this connection it has been found that the various GSTs have a highly specific binding site for GSH, whereas binding sites for the electrophilic substrates display broad but overlapping substrate specificities (Adang *et al.*,1989).

Evolution
GSTs can be found in most living organisms, including primitive forms of life such as bacteria, yeast, fungi and plants. In the most developed species, for example in humans, a multitude of enzymes are expressed (Buetler & Eaton, 1992; Mannervik *et al.*, 1985). On the basis of their structural homology the genes have been arranged in families or classes analogous to those of the cytochrome P450 system. According to this system, five classes of GSTs are expressed in mammals: cytosolic GSTalpha, GSTmu, GSTpi,

GSTtheta and the microsomal GSTmic. Sequence comparisons suggest that the ancestral form belonged to class theta GSTs and that GSTsigma was the class that diverged from the ancestral gene (theta and sigma are abundant in non-vertabrate species). Of the four cytosolic GSTs expressed in mammals, it appears that GSTmu diverged from the ancestral gene before the alpha and pi GSTs (Hayes & Pulford, 1995).

Human GSTs: their expression and catalytic properties
It has recently been estimated that there are at least 20 human GST enzymes. For GSTalpha, five different genes encoding for A1, A2, A3, A4 and A5 have been identified. A1 and A2 are expressed mainly in the liver and the active enzymes consist of homodimeric and heterodimeric forms of these two subunits. An enzyme consisting of subunits A3 and A5 is expressed in several tissues including skin, as well as a homodimeric enzyme consisting of subunit A4 (Del Boccio *et al.*, 1987; Singhal *et al.*, 1994; Stockman *et al.*, 1985).

Class mu (GSTM) is also expressed in the liver but, because of a gene deletion resulting in a polymorphism, only in some individuals. In addition to the deletion, two allelic forms of the GSTM gene exist. The variants, GSTM1A and GSTM1B differ only by one amino acid and can form homodimers and heterodimers which seem to have similar catalytic properties (Wildersten *et al.*, 1991). In addition to hepatic forms of GSTM, sub-units M2, M3, M4 and M5 have been identified which are expressed in several extrahepatic tissues; it is possible that other forms of mu class GSTs exist which have not yet been characterized (Hussey & Hayes,1993; Ross *et al.*, 1993).

Class pi (GSTP) is expressed in several extra-hepatic tissues. On the basis of structural analyses of the purified enzyme from several organs it seems that only one gene product belongs to this family which results in a homodimeric enzyme: GSTP1-1 (Marcus *et al.*, 1978). Recently, allelic variants of the GSTP1 gene have been reported. Their significance for the expression and catalytic properties of the enzyme is discussed in Chapter 19 by Strange and Fryer.

Class theta (GSTT) consists of two gene products expressed in the liver as homodimeric enzymes, GSTT1-1 and GSTT2-2. GSTT1 seems to be polymorphic, resulting in different catalytic properties between the wild type and the mutated genotype (Pemble *et al.*, 1994).

In addition to the cytosolic enzymes, two forms of microsomal GSTs exist. Comparison of the structures reveals major differences between the cytosolic and microsomal forms, suggesting separate origins of the encoding genes (DeJong *et al.*, 1988; Welsh *et al.*, 1994). It is not entirely clear what role the microsomal forms play in the detoxification of electrophilic xenobiotics.

Catalytic properties of human GSTs
Among several detoxification systems the GSTs comprise one of the most efficient in the protection of organisms against electrophilic substances causing oxidative stress. Most GST enzymes have a remarkably broad substrate specificity and their catalytic properties therefore largely overlap (Mannervik & Danielson, 1988). In general terms the numerous substrates can be described as compounds with variable structures where electrophilic centres have been created by carbon, nitrogen, sulphur, oxygen or halogen atoms. Typically, such compounds include unsaturated carbonyls, organic thiocyanates, arene oxides and various halogen compounds (Chasseaud, 1979; Jakoby, 1978; Mannervik, 1985). The substrates can also originate from endogenous processes, e.g. the oxidation of fatty acids. A large number of these compounds have been identified as genotoxic or carcinogenic. (For more details on the catalytic properties of human GSTs, see Hayes & Pulford, 1995.)

Regulation of expression of GST genes
Several of the substrates of GSTs may also act as their inducers, analogously to the CYP system. The modes of regulation of the various GST genes seem to be extremely complex where both transcriptional and posttranscriptional events are involved.

Several regulatory elements, such as the glucocorticoid-responsive element, the xenobiotic-responsive element, the antioxidant-responsive element and the barbie-box-like sequences have been identified in the 5'-regulatory sequences of the genes. Not much is known about the factors contributing to the postranscriptional regulation of the genes or to their tissue specific expression (see Hayes & Pulford, 1995).

Because of their central role in the detoxification of various reactive electrophiles, many of which are carcinogens, it can be assumed that the GSTs play an important part in the protection of humans against chemical carcinogenesis. Several studies have been conducted in order to demonstrate this; they are reviewed in Chapter 19 by Strange and Fryer.

N-acetyltransferases (NATs)

These enzymes catalyse the metabolism of xenobiotics and carcinogens by transferring an acetyl group to the compounds in question. As compared to the CYPs and GSTs the variety of molecules the NATs metabolize is limited, consisting mainly of aromatic and heterocyclic amines and hydrazines. However, several of these are strong carcinogens, and since some of them are used in industrial processes, e.g. in the rubber and dye industries, while some may be formed during cooking or cigarette smoking, they may be highly relevant to human cancer. The NATs comprise one of the major enzyme systems catalysing their metabolism, and it is therefore reasonable to assume that the NATs play a role in human carcinogenesis. For more details, see Smith *et al.* (1995).

Metabolism of carcinogens by human NATs and their role in carcinogenesis

Much of the evidence on the role of human NATs in carcinogenesis has been obtained in studies on bladder cancer. Epidemiological studies in which bladder cancer patients and controls with high exposure to aromatic amines were analysed for their NAT phenotype have shown that the slow acetylator phenotype is associated with an increased risk of bladder cancer (Cartwright *et al.*, 1982). This suggests that acetylation has a protective role in bladder carcinogenesis. This is also consistent with the facts that (i) for smokers the level of 4-aminophenyl haemoglobin adducts is higher among slow acetylators than among fast acetylators (Vineis *et al.*, 1990) and (ii) for smokers or workers exposed to aromatic amines the urine of slow acetylators is more mutagenic than that of fast acetylators (Sinues *et al.*, 1992). This indirect evidence suggests that acetylation reactions inactivate carcinogens, at least in the case of bladder cancer.

In spite of this evidence the role of NATs in human carcinogenesis is not straightforward. First, the fast acetylation phenotype does not appear to protect against colon cancer; indeed, the contrary appears true (Smith *et al.*, 1995). Second, at least in some *in vitro* systems, NAT seems to activate carcinogens (Grant *et al.*, 1992). In this connection it has been found that, with regard to some carcinogens, NAT may actually catalyse O-acetylation, which appears to be an activating step, instead of the normal N-acetylation (Hein, 1988). Furthermore, the enzymatic steps in the acetylation reactions are often not well understood in detail, leaving the possibility open that activation, in addition to inactivation reactions, may sometimes take place. It could therefore be that, while NATs contribute to chemical carcinogenesis, their role depends on the type of exposure (type of reaction catalysed), the type of tissue or cancer in question, and other metabolic pathways that compete for the substrates with the NATs, such as the CYP1A2-catalysed hydroxylation reactions (activation) of heterocyclic amines (Kadlubar *et al.*, 1992).

Polymorphism of human NATs

Various phenotyping studies have established that NAT activity is polymorphically expressed in human populations. Three genes have recently been identified which belong to the human NAT family: a pseudogene and two functional genes, NAT1 and NAT2. Both functional genes appear to be polymorphic (Smith *et al.*, 1995). It is likely that both genes contribute to the polymorphic phenotype but it is not yet clear what is the contribution of the two gene products to the metabolism of various carcinogens or to carcinogen metabolism in different tissues. However, the recently developed methodologies for analysing the genotypes of both NAT1 and NAT2 should make it possible to correlate the genotypes to the phenotyes in the case of different exposures as well as to study the association of genotypes to different cancers. (For more details see Chapter 20 by Hirvonen.)

Conclusions

- During the course of evolution, living organisms have developed superfamilies of genes which are responsible for the metabolism of xenobiotics.

- Due to the rapid evolution of these gene super-families there is great interspecies and interindividual variability in their structure and function.

- Consequently, humans have significant interindividual differences in their capacity to activate and inactivate carcinogens.

- Several population studies have shown that variability in carcinogen metabolism is a risk factor in chemical carcinogenesis.

- As many enzymes contribute to the this metabolism, further studies are desirable on the link between individual enzymes and the risk of cancer.

References

Adang, A.E., Meyer, D.J., Brussee, J., Van der Gen, A., Ketterer, B. & Mulder, G.J. (1989) Interaction of rat glutathione S-transferases 7-7 and 8-8 with gamma-glutamyl- or glycyl-modified glutathione analogues. *Biochem. J.*, 264, 759-764

Béréziat, J.-C., Raffalli, F., Schmezer, P., Frei, E., Geneste, O. & Lang, M.A. (1995) Cytochrome P450 2A of nasal epithelium: regulation and role in carcinogen metabolism. *Mol. Carcinogenesis*, 14, 130-139

Buetler, T.M. & Eaton, D.L. (1992) Glutathione S-transferase: amino acid sequence comparison, classification and phylogenetic relationship. *Environ. Carcinogen. Ecotoxicol. Rev.*, C10, 181-203

Camus, A.-M., Geneste, O., Honkakoski, P., Béréziat, J.-C., Henderson, C.J., Wolf, C.R., Bartsch, H. & Lang, M.A. (1993) High variability of nitrosamine metabolism among individuals: role of cytochromes P450 2A6 and 2E1 in the dealkylation of *N*-nitroso dimethylamine and *N*-nitroso diethylamine in mice and humans. *Mol. Carcinogen.*, 14, 130-139

Cartwright, R.A., Glashan, R.W., Rogers, H.J., Ahmad, R.A., Barham-Hall, D., Higgins, E. & Kahn, M.A. (1982) Role of N-acetyltransferase phenotypes in bladder carcinogenesis; a pharmacogenetic epidemiological approach to bladder cancer. *Lancet*, ii, 842-845

Chasseaud, L.F. (1979) The role of glutathione and glutathione S-transferases in the metabolism of chemical carcinogens and other electrophilic agents. *Adv. Cancer Res.*, 29, 175-274

Crespi, C.L., Penman, B.W., Steimel, D.T., Gelboin, H.V. & Gonzalez, F.J. (1991) The development of a human cell line stably expressing human CYP3A4: role in the metabolic activation of aflatoxin B1 and comparison to CYP1A2 and CYP2A3. *Carcinogenesis*, 12, 355-359

Dai, Y., Rashba, Step, J. & Cederbaum, A.I. (1993) Stable expression of human cytochrome P4502E1 in HepG2 cells: characterization of catalytic activities and production of reactive oxygen intermediates. *Biochemistry*, 32, 6928-6937

DeJong, J.L., Morgenstern, R., Jornvall, H., DePierre, J.W. & Tu, C.P. (1988) Gene expression of rat and human microsomal glutathione S-transferases. *J. Biol. Chem.*, 263, 8430-8436

Del Boccio, G., Di Ilio, C., Alin, P., Jörnvall, H. & Mannervik, B. (1987) Identification of a novel glutathione transferase in human skin homologous with class alpha glutathione transferase 2-2 in the rat. *Biochem. J.*, 244, 21-25

Eliasson, E., Mkrtchian, S. & Ingelman-Sundberg, M. (1992) Hormone- and substrate-regulated intracellular degradation of cytochrome P450 (2E1) involving MgATP-activated rapid proteolysis in the endoplasmic reticulum membranes. *J. Biol. Chem.*, 267, 15765-15769

Fernandez-Salguero, P., Hoffmann, S.M.G., Cholerton, S., Mohrenweiser, H., Rautio, H., Rautio, A., Pelkonen, O., Huang, J., Evans, W.E., Idel, J.R. & Gonzalez, F.J. (1995) A genetic polymorphism in coumarin 7-hydroxylation: sequence of the human *CYP2A* gene and identification of variant *CYP2A6* alleles. *Am. J. Genet.*, 57, 651-660

Gonzalez, F.J. & Gelboin, H.V. (1994) Role of human cytochrome P450 in the metabolic activation of chemical carcinogens and toxins. *Drug Metab. Rev.*, 26, 165-183

Grant, D.M., Josephy, P.D., Lord, H.L. & Morrison, L.D. (1992) *Salmonella typhimurium* strains expressing human arylamine N-acetyltransferases: metabolism and mutagenic activation of aromatic amines. *Cancer Res.*, 52, 3961-3964

Guengerich, F.P., Kim, D.H. & Iwasaki, M. (1991) Role of human cytochrome P-450 IIE1 in the oxidation of many low-molecular-weight cancer suspects. *Chem. Res. Toxicol.*, 4, 168-179

Guengerich, F.P. & Shimada, T. (1991) Oxidation of toxic and carcinogenic chemicals by human cytochrome P450 enzymes. *Chem.Res.Toxicol.*, 4, 391-407

Hayes, J.D. & Pulford, D.J. (1995) The glutathione S-transferase supergene family: regulation of GST and the contribution of the isoenzymes to cancer chemoprotection and drug resistance. *Crit. Rev. Biochem. Mol. Biol.*, 30, 445-600

Hein, D.W. (1988) Acetylator genotype and arylamine-induced carcinogenesis. *Biochim. Biophys. Acta*, 948, 37-66

Hussey, A.J. & Hayes, J.D. (1993) Human Mu-class glutathione S-transferases present in liver, skeletal muscle and testicular tissue. *Biochim. Biophys. Acta*, 1203, 131-141

Jakoby, W.B. (1978) The glutathione S-transferases: a group of multifunctional detoxification proteins. *Adv. Enzymol.*, 46, 383-414

Johansson, I., Lundqvist, E., Bertilsson, L., Dahl, M.L., Sjoqvist, F. & Ingelman-Sundberg, M. (1993) Inherited amplification of an active gene in the cytochrome P450 CYP2D locus as a cause of ultrarapid metabolism of debrisoquine. *Proc. Natl. Acad. Sci. USA*, 90, 11825-11829

Kadlubar, F.F., Buetler, M.A., Kaderlik, K.R., Chou, H.C. & Lang, N.P. (1992) Polymorphisms for aromatic amine metabolism in humans: relevance for human carcinogenesis. *Environ. Health Perspect.*, 98, 69-74

Mannervik, B. (1985) The isoenzymes of glutathione transferase. *Adv. Enzymol.*, 57, 357-417

Mannervik, B., Alin, P., Guthenberg, C., Jensson, H., Tahir, M.K., Warholm, M. & Jornvall, H.(1985) Identification of three classes of cytosolic glutathione transferase common to several mammalian species: correlation between structural data and enzymatic properties. *Proc. Natl. Acad. Sci. USA*, 82, 7202-7206

Mannervik, B. & Danielson, U.H. (1988) Glutathione transferases - structure and catalytic activity. *CRC Crit. Rev. Biochem.*, 23, 283-337

Marcus, C.J., Habig, W.H. & Jakoby, W.B. (1978) Glutathione transferase from human erythrocytes. Nonidentity with the enzymes from liver. *Arch. Biochem. Biophys.*, 188, 287-293

Nebert, D.W., Eisen, H.J., Negishi, M., Lang, M., Hjelmeland, L.M. & Oakey, A.B. (1981) Genetic mechanism controlling the induction of polysubstrate monooxygenase (P-450) activities. *Ann. Rev. Pharmacol. Toxicol.*, 21, 431-462

Nebert, D.W., Negishi, Lang, M., Hjelmeland, L.M. & Eisen, H.J. (1982) The Ah locus, a multigene family necessary for survival in a chemically adverse environment: comparison with the immune system. *Adv. Genet.*, 21, 1-52

Nelson, D.R., Koymans, L., Kamataki, T., Stegeman, J.J., Feyereisen, R., Waxman, D.J., Waterman, M.R., Gotoh, O., Coon, M.J., Estabrook, R.W., Gunsalus, I.C. & Nebert, D.W. (1996) P450 superfamily: update on new sequences, gene mapping, accession numbers and nomenclature. *Pharmacogenetics*, 6, 1-42

Nhamburo, P.T., Kimura, S., McBride, O.W., Kozak, C.A., Gelboin, H.V. & Gonzalez, F.J. (1990) The human CYP2F gene subfamily: identification of a cDNA encoding a new cytochrome P450, cDNA-directed expression, and chromosome mapping. *Biochemistry*, 29, 5491-5499

Pemble, S., Schroeder, K.R., Spencer, S.R., Meyer, D.J., Hallier, E., Bolt, H.M., Ketterer, B. & Taylor, J.B. (1994) Human glutathione S-transferase theta (GSTT1): cDNA cloning and the characterization of a genetic polymorphism. *Biochem. J.*, 300, 271-276

Rautio, A., Kraul, H., Kojo, A., Salmela, E. & Pelkonen, O. (1992) Interindividual variability of coumarin 7-hydroxylatoin in health volunteers. *Pharmacogenetics*, 2, 227-233

Ritter, J.K., Owens, I.S., Negishi, M., Nagata, K, Sheen, Y.Y., Gillette, J.R. & Sansame, H. (1991) Mouse pulmonary cytochrome P450 naphthalene hydroxylase: cDNA cloning, sequence and expression in *Saccharaomyces cerevisiae*. *Biochemistry*, 30, 11430-11437

Ross, V.L. & Board, P.G. (1993) Molecular cloning and heterologous expression of an alternatively spliced human Mu class glutathione S-transferase transcript. *Biochem. J.*, 294, 373-380

Shen, Z., Wells, R.L. & Elkind, M.M. (1994) Enhanced cytochrome P450 (*Cyp1b1*) expression, aryl hydrocarbon hydroxylase activity, cytotoxicity and transformation of C3H 10T1/2 cells by dimethylbenz(a)anthracene in conditioned medium. *Cancer Res.*, 54, 4052-4056

Singhal, S.S., Zimniak, P., Sharma, R., Srivastava, S.K., Awasthi, S. & Awasthi, Y.C. (1994) A novel glutathione S-transferase isozyme similar to GST 8-8 of rat and mGSTA4-4 (GST 5.7) of mouse is selectively expressed in human tissues. *Biochim. Biophys. Acta*, 1204, 279-286

Sinues, B., Perez, J., Bernal, M.L., Saenz, M.A., Lanuza, J. & Bartolome, M. (1992) Urinary mutagenicity and N-acetylation phenotype in textile industry workers exposed to arylamines. *Cancer Res.*, 52, 4885-4889

Smith, G., Stanley, L.A., Sim, E., Strange, R.C. & Wolf, C.R. (1995) Metabolic polymorphisms and cancer susceptibility. *Cancer Surv.*, 25, 27-65

Song, B.J., Gelboin, H.V., Park, S.S., Yang, C.S. & Gonzalez, F.J. (1986) Glutathione S-transferase delta is composed of two distinct subunits (B1 and B2). *Biochem. J.*, 227, 457-465

Stockman, P.K., Beckett, G.J. & Hayes, J.D. (1985) Identification of a basic hybrid glutathione S-transferase from human liver. Complementary DNA and protein sequences of ethanol-inducible rat and human cytochrome P-450s. Transcriptional and post-transcriptional regulation of the rat enzyme. *J. Biol. Chem.*, 261, 16689-16697

Sutter, T.R., Tang, Y.M., Hayes, Yu-Yuan, P.W., Jabs, E.W., Li, X., Hong, Y., Cody, C.W. & Greenblatt, W.F. (1994) Complete cDNA sequence of a human dioxin-inducible mRNA identifies a new gene subfamily of cytochrome P450 that maps to chromosome 2. *J. Biol. Chem.*, 269, 13092-13099

Uematsu, F., Kikuchi, H., Motomiya, M., Abe, T., Sagami, I., Ohmachi, T., Wakui, A., Kanamaru, R. & Watanabe, M. (1991) Association between restriction fragment length polymorphism of the human cytochrome P450IIE1 gene and susceptibility to lung cancer. *Jpn. J. Cancer Res.*, 82, 254-256

Vineis, P., Caporaso, N., Tannenbaum, S.R., Skipper, P.L., Glogowski, J., Bartsch, H., Coda, M., Talaska, G. & Kadlubar, F. (1990) Acetylation phenotype, carcinogen-haemoglobin adducts, and cigarette smoking. *Cancer Res.*, 50, 3002-3004

Welsh, D.J., Creely, D.P., Hauser, S.D., Mathis, K.J., Krivi, G.G. & Isakson, P.C. (1994) Molecular cloning and expression of leukotriene-C_4 synthase. *Proc. Natl. Acad. Sci. USA*, 91, 9745-9749

Widersten, M., Pearson, W.R., Engström, A. & Mannervik, B. (1991) Heterologous expression of the allelic variant Mu-class gluthathione transferase μ and *Biochem. J.*, 276, 519-524

Wilkinson, G.R., Guengerich, F.P. & Branch, R.A. (1989) Genetic polymorphism of S-mephenytoin hydroxylation. *Pharmacol. Ther.*, 43, 53-76

Wolf, C.R., Smith, C.A., Gough, A.C., Moss, J.E., Vallis, K.A., Howard, G., Carey, F.J., Mills, K., McNee, W, Carmichael, J. & Spurr, N.K. (1992) Relationship between the debrisoquine hydroxylase polymorphism and cancer susceptibility. *Carcinogenesis*, 13, 1035-1038

Corresponding author

Matti A. Lang
Department of Biochemistry,
Faculty of Pharmacy,
University of Uppsala,
Biomedical Centre,
Uppsala, Sweden

Metabolic Polymorphisms and Susceptibility to Cancer
W. Ryder
IARC Scientific Publications No. 148
International Agency for Research on Cancer, Lyon, 1999

Chapter 4. Selection of candidate genes for population studies

Neil Caporaso

A broad view of genetic susceptibility in humans suggests that high-penetrance hereditary genes cause a number of relatively uncommon tumours in the familial setting, while common cancers are influenced by multiple susceptibility loci. Early investigations of the latter category focused on the role of genes in the metabolism of carcinogens (activation, detoxification) while current and planned studies extend to genes with diverse mechanisms involving DNA repair, cell cycle control, nutrient metabolism and other processes. The present report considers some methodological issues pertinent to the study of the common genes, focusing in particular on the selection of appropriate candidates for study.

A central issue in population studies that consider putative genetic risk factors is the selection of appropriate candidate genes for study. The 'susceptibility genes' of interest in this connection overlap but differ in many respects from the 'human disease genes' or high penetrance genes that have been identified for a variety of rare cancers and a subset of common cancers. Typically, the high penetrance disease genes are uncommon (i.e. have a low gene frequency, typically less or much less than 1%), when present confer a high relative and absolute risk, and have been identified and studied in the family setting (Caporaso & Goldstein, 1995) (Table 1).

Two general approaches have been used to identify candidate genes potentially involved in familial cancers: the functional approach and the positional approach. In the *functional approach*, used in many early studies, a known biochemical basis for pathogenesis is exploited to generate a

gene product or to perform functional complementation cloning. For example, the addition of certain fragments of human chromosomes to cell lines from individuals who have various DNA repair defects can produce a repair competent phenotype (Auerbach *et al.*, 1998). This method led to the identification of Fanconi's anaemia. Pharmacogenetic approaches are related in that heritable differences in enzymes thought to have a function relevant to the condition of interest are selected as candidates. A gene product that is known to control a metabolic transformation crucial to carcinogenesis, such as activation of benzo(a)pyrene by CYP1A1 or the Ah receptor, would draw attention to the gene for study in relation to susceptibility to cancer where that agent is a known risk factor.

More commonly the 'forward genetics' approach is not applicable since a responsible metabolic pathway is not known. Particularly for

Table 1. Genes: single and susceptibility		
Factor	Single	Susceptibility
Gene frequency	Rare	Common (>1%)
Study setting	Family	Population
Study type	Linkage	Association
Penetrance	High	Low
Absolute/relative risk	High	Low
Population-attributable risk	Low	High
Role of environment	Modest	Critical

the rare cancers that exhibit Mendelian patterns of inheritance, 'reverse genetics' *positional approaches* have achieved notable successes. The term 'positional' refers to their dependence on the chromosomal location of the gene.

Positional strategies fall loosely into three categories. Linkage studies are an increasingly common method of identifying disease loci. This approach relies on locating genes through recognizing their cosegregation with marker alleles. This method requires a sufficient number of well-characterized families with the disease of interest, biological specimens (i.e. germline DNA from affected and unaffected individuals in the kindreds, a postulated genetic mechanism (i.e. autosomal dominant/recessive), a set of polymorphic markers, and a statistical approach to detect evidence for linkage (i.e. elevated LOD scores (LOD = log of odds; a value over 3 is generally accepted as evidence). A second method used to identify tumour-suppressor genes involves the detection of loss of heterozygosity. In this approach, paired normal and tumour tissues are examined for polymorphic markers. The loss of signal in target (usually, but not always tumour) tissue compared to normal tissue, if consistently observed in a particular chromosome region, is taken as evidence that a 'second hit' has occurred at a critical region representing an important gene (Wistuba *et al.*, 1997). Finally, the identification of chromosome abnormalities in tumour tissue may implicate a particular area (Nowell & Hungerford, 1960).

Once a subchromosomal region is identified by one of these approaches, further work is required to identify particular candidate genes within the area. Both the increasing repertoire of molecular approaches and the number of human genes that are mapped have rendered this stage of the process more tractable. Once identified, evidence to implicate a gene in pathogenesis can involve a variety of approaches: mutation screening (identifying mutations of the genes in individuals with the condition in question), demonstration of restoration of a normal phenotype when transfection of the cloned normal allele is introduced into a cell line with the mutant phenotype, or production of a mouse model of the disease using gene targeting to introduce the defective mutation.

The present paper considers aspects of the study of the more common, low penetrance genes postulated to play a role in many or even most common diseases. These genes are characterized by high allele frequency (1% to 90% or more), low relative and absolute risk, but potentially high population-attributable risk (Caporaso & Goldstein, 1995). Can the methods used to identify the family cancer genes be applied to the study of the susceptibility genes? The answer is mixed. Linkage analysis approaches face power constraints when the genotypic relative risk (GRR) is small. Risch & Merikangas (1996) observed that even under ideal conditions, i.e. a closely linked marker locus that is highly informative, the number of families required to detect a GRR of 2 would be around 2500, which would be prohibitive. Thus approaches based on association are likely to be required to examine candidate gene hypotheses involving low to modest relative risks. Hybrid approaches such as 'association mapping', exploiting linkage disequilibrium to identify candidate areas, require detailed genetic maps (thousands of evenly spaced genetic markers) and automated techniques to characterize polymorphic markers in pooled specimens. This approach, which should become feasible in the next few years, is likely to have improved power over linkage approaches (Lander & Kruglyak, 1995; Barcellos *et al.*, 1997).

The steadily increasing list of known genes, the improved technical means of extracting genetic information, and the diminishing quantities of biological material required to read the genetic record permit expanding opportunities to perform DNA studies. Automated or chip-based genotype recognition systems can be expected to further facilitate the acquisition of genetic information.

It is worth reflecting on the historical context of studies on susceptibility genes to better understand both the general direction of the field and the implications for newer studies. Only a decade ago, early studies of this type required laborious phenotype determinations in order to establish the innate activity of one gene. Examples include the work of Lower *et al.* (1979) on the acetylation phenotype and bladder cancer in workers occupationally exposed to aryl amines, the study of

Kellerman *et al.* (1973) on aryl hydrocarbon hydroxylase inducibility in lung cancer, and the work of Ayesh *et al.* (1984) on debrisoquine metabolism in lung cancer. In each of these studies, the effort required for phenotype determination imposed methodological limitations. For example, it was difficult and expensive to carry out phenotyping on substantial numbers of subjects, and bias was possible through exclusion of the sickest subjects who did not meet clinical criteria. A distinct advantage of the phenotyping approach is that the functional nature of the gene is established by the phenotyping operation. In theory this approach avoids the problem of absent underlying functional genetic variation

or of mutations being too numerous or diverse to identify by genotyping. Some of the contrasts between the phenotyping era, the early genotyping phase, and the anticipated future course of studies are presented in Table 2.

In view of the new opportunities offered by current technologies, some discussions of criteria for gene selection are worth considering. This is particularly relevant, as current technologies offer enhanced ability to test multiple genes. There are pitfalls, however, notably a predictable increase in false positives due to multiple comparisons. This implies that function and biological plausibility are increasingly critical in guiding the interpretation of findings.

Table 2. Historical evolution of the study of common genes and cancer			
	Phenotyping	**Early genotyping**	**Future genotyping**
Period	1974-1987	1987-present	Future
Number of genes	One	One to a few	Many per study
Type of genes	Metabolic polymorphisms (phenotype)	Metabolic polymorphisms (genotype)	Wide variety of gene categories (genotype with enhanced functional information)
Study design	Case and control series	Case-control	Cohort
Analysis	Main effect of gene	Main effect of gene	Gene-environment interaction
Investigator	Laboratory scientist	Epidemiologist	Interdisciplinary genetic epidemiologist
Mechanism	Metabolic activation	Metabolic activation, as well as: - metabolic deactivation - oncogene polymorphisms	All previous categories, plus: - DNA repair, - hormone and vitamin disposition, - cell cycle control, - neurotransmitter polymorphisms, - infection susceptibility, - disposition of lipids, - receptor polymorphisms
Limiting factors	Difficulty and inherent bias of phenotyping in field setting	Early genotyping often inadequate functional information	- multiple comparisons - ethical constraints
Advantages	Implicit is some information on function of measured trait	Avoids phenotyping and attendant sources of bias	- increasingly facile genotyping - non-invasive biospecimen collection - interdisciplinary approach - larger study size advantages of cohort design - studies exploit the human genome map, i.e. linkage disequilibrium mapping

The following are proposed as criteria for evaluating candidate genes for population studies.

1. Interindividual variation in the trait exists in the population

The historic rationale for considering hereditary differences in metabolic polymorphisms as being important in cancer etiology are the existence of substantial phenotypic differences between individuals (Lower et al., 1979). These differences may be manifest as wide variation in urine or serum measurements of a metabolite (e.g. isoniazid, procainamide or sulfamethazine and the acetylation phenotype) (Drayer & Reidenberg, 1977), a 'metabolic ratio' (debrisoquine to 4-hydroxydebrisoquine in urine) (Gonzalez & Idle, 1994), or protein or mRNA directly detectable in liver or other relevant organ. The original meaning of a phenotype was a clinically recognizable state, but in the present context the focus is on 'biochemical' or 'molecular' phenotypes. Without important variation in a phenotype in the population, the rationale for examining a genotype would be weak. There are a great number of pharmacological factors (i.e. differences in absorption, distribution and excretion) and environmental factors (e.g. influence of age, gender, other drugs, physiological state, presence of disease) that can contribute to such variability. This variation must be eliminated to the greatest possible degree or by study design or controlled in the analysis.

Important interindividual variation is often manifest as clinical consequences following administration of the medications that are dependent on the particular pathway. For example, hereditary variation in hydralazine (NAT2) metabolism may explain susceptibility to systemic lupus erythematosus (Grant, 1993). Severe neurotoxicity following 5-fluorouracil administration is related to dihydropyrimidine dehydrogenase variation (Tuckman et al., 1985). The pharmacogenetic literature contains many further examples (Kalow, 1962). Precise definition of the phenotype is vital because misclassification degrades the power to detect important differences. Selection of the proper measure to characterize it is also critical; for example, head size differs between phenylketonurics and normal individuals but this trait does not distinguish individuals with and without phenylketonuria as well as plasma phenylalanine measurements. Using the more precise laboratory study to define the phenotype permits a much clearer distinction of affected and non-affected individuals (Bogardus & Lillioja, 1992).

2. The gene is involved in a process related to carcinogenesis

While a complete inventory of all the processes that contribute to carcinogenesis remains to be elucidated, certain pathways unquestionably participate in neoplastic transformation. Early studies established that carcinogens require metabolic activation, and it was proposed that genetic control of activation (Ayesh et al., 1984; Kellerman et al., 1973) or elimination (Seidegard et al., 1986; Lower et al., 1979) might account for variation in tobacco-related cancer susceptibility. A broader appreciation of human carcinogenesis suggests other categories of genes that may control processes of equal relevance (Table 3). These include genes involved with DNA repair, chromosome stability, the activity of oncogene or tumour suppressor genes, cell cycle control or signal transduction, influence on hormonal or vitamin metabolism pathways, immune function, and neurotransmitter action.

The experience of the last few years provides ample evidence that our understanding of all the processes that influence carcinogenesis is incomplete. Thus apoptosis, telomerases, obesity, and addiction (behaviour) are all influenced by genetic variation and are likely to yield basic insights relevant to cancer during the next few years through investigations into the genetic determinants.

In addition, unusual genetic mechanisms have begun to be studied in the context of malignancy, including imprinting (Feinberg et al., 1995), non-chromosomal inheritance, epigenetic mechanisms (e.g. methylation), and transgenerational effects (Tomatis, 1994).

The implications of genes that act at more than one biological hierarchical level need to be anticipated. For instance, if one gene acts to alter the disposition of carcinogens in tobacco smoke, and another (or the same one) acts to alter the likelihood that an individual will smoke, the analysis needs to take this into account. CYP2A6 and CYP2D6 are plausible candidates that have possible roles in both nicotine metabolism and nitrosamine activation.

3. The trait exhibits an inheritance pattern consistent with Mendelian transmission

Variability in a trait may be observed in the general population and there may be a plausible reason to consider a relation to cancer. The next step is a demonstration that variation has a genetic basis. Family studies that demonstrate a pattern of inheritance consistent with Mendelian transmission are required to establish that a phenotype is genetic in origin, e.g. as demonstrated in kindreds with debrisoquine-deficient metabolizers (Evans et al., 1980). It has become routine in many studies to confirm that transmission of purported variants exhibits a pattern consistent with Mendelian transmission by demonstrating it in commercially available DNA from multigeneration kindreds. In animals, controlled matings can be used to study the genetic transmission of traits. In human populations the proportion of offspring with the observed trait (or genotype) can be compared with that expected under a particular genetic hypothesis, an approach formally known as segregation analysis.

Supportive evidence for a genetic basis for variation can also be provided by twin studies, demonstrating that concordance of a particular trait is significantly greater between monozygotic than dizygotic twins. A demonstration that a particular trait exhibits a distribution in the population consistent with the predictions of Hardy-Weinberg equilibrium is another piece of supporting evidence.

Certain phenotypes such as "mutagen sensitivity" have exhibited strong associations with smoking-related cancers (Spitz & Hsu, 1994; Spitz et al., 1995) but the precise nature of this 'host susceptibility' factor remains incompletely understood. Demonstrating that population variability is consistent with a genetic origin is no substitute for the demonstration of a clear pattern of inheritance in families. Lacking a genetic basis, phenotypes remain vulnerable to the classic criticisms when associations with diseases are reported, i.e. covariates linked with disease are responsible for phenotypic variation, or treatment or secondary metabolic consequences of the condition present in the host biases the phenotype measurement,

resulting in misclassification. The latter problem is typical of case-control studies but is avoided in cohort studies if phenotyping is performed prior to the onset of disease.

4. Gene action exists in the relevant organ

Genes exhibit differential expression. The demonstration of gene expression in the organ or tissue of interest can lend plausibility to the hypothesis of a putative role in tumorigenesis. Alternatively, expression in the liver allows one to postulate that a carcinogen is activated in that organ, and that a carcinogenic product is eventually transported to the relevant organ. Thus, CYP1A1 is largely absent from the liver but present in the lung, lending some plausibility to disease associations focused on pulmonary pathology. CYP2D6 is expressed in the brain, giving rise to hypotheses suggesting an influence on behaviour. At least one recent report finds no evidence of expression in the lung (Kivisto et al., 1997), arguing against a role in lung cancer. GSTM1 null genotype has been epidemiologically associated with lung cancer and exhibits at least some expression in the lung (Nakajima et al., 1995; Anttila et al.,1993), although the highest pulmonary expression by a member of the GST family may be GSTP1. Various explanations have been offered for the weak but consistent finding of an association of GSTM1 null genotype with lung cancer, e.g. close linkage to a gene with similar function which is expressed in the lung (i.e. GSTM3), expression in the nasal mucosa (Gervasi et al., 1991), or a more systematic role of the gene in preventing lipid peroxidation and secondary promotion, pulmonary localization not being critical. The epidemiological and mechanistic findings must ultimately be reconciled in order to provide a coherent explanation.

5. Gene location and characterization

The location and characterization of the gene contributes to our understanding in a number of ways. The structure of the gene may reveal similarities with other genes which suggest function or parallels with other organisms. The existence of pseudogenes may create difficulties in designing assays that are specific for the sequence of interest. For example, the nuclear enzyme poly (ADP-ribose) polymerase functions in DNA repair and recombination. Bhatia *et al.* (1990) reported an association of a polymorphism of a related gene, probably a pseudogene, with various tumours. The finding may implicate the locus as a site of a nearby tumour suppressor gene rather than involvement of the specific gene itself in tumour susceptibility. The location of the mutation itself in relation to the gene locus also has significance. Most mutations of pathological significance occur in the coding sequence, with tandem repeats and CpG dinucleotides being favoured as particular hot spots. Mutations in intragenic noncoding and regulatory sequences may also result in altered function. The extent to which a mutation alters function may also depend on the precise effect on expression (reduced, abolished, augmented or ectopic), the degree to which the phenotype is expressed in the heterozygote, the proportion of cells in which the mutant gene is present (hereditary mutations are present in all cells, somatic changes usually only in a few), and occasionally the parental origin of the mutation (i.e. imprinting). (Miyagawa, 1998).

6. Polymorphisms and mutation

Detectable variation in a particular gene ranges from deletion of the entire gene, through missense and nonsense mutations that are highly likely to ablate function, to single base-pair changes that result in amino acid changes. Changes in base pairs at degenerate codons are the least likely to impact on function, along with minor intronic changes. Variable repeat polymorphisms in intronic (presumably regulatory) areas have been widely studied (examples are H ras vtr, the androgen receptor, and dopamine transporter protein).

The absence of a functional role for a genetic variant that has an otherwise convincing association with disease implies that an observed association is due to a) the observed variant being in linkage disequilibrium with some other truly functional gene, b) the variant having a non-obvious regulatory role, or c) chance.

7. Gene-gene interaction

In general, genes act in concert to exert effects. Genes often act in pathways, and therefore effects on one gene may induce compensatory changes in others. Critical pathways may have redundan-

cies. This is the case, for example, for the p450 genes that exhibit overlapping substrate specificities. As mentioned earlier, genes may act at different hierarchical levels in the organism, i.e. gene (regulation of transcription), biochemical (activation of carcinogen), organ (specific toxicity) or organism (alteration of behaviour). Only a limited number of studies have examined the combined effects of two or more genes. The best example is the combined effect of CYP1A1 and GSTM1 in relation to lung cancer risk in Asians (Nakachi, 1993). The underlying complexity suggests that it is not surprising that studies of single genes and common cancers have not always yielded consistent findings. Considering multiple genes is more realistic biologically and should provide a more complete view of susceptibility in future studies in which there are both adequate numbers of subjects and technologies for multiple genotyping.

Certain biological effects are reasonably well established as dependent on one particular gene. For instance, CYP2D6 seems to exert complete control of the metabolic fate of a variety of medications. Consistent with this, metabolic consequences in deficient metabolizers are observed when these drugs are administered, i.e. side-effects at relatively low doses. However, even for model substrates of CYP2D6 such as dextromethorphan, some influence of other genes is likely (Ducharme *et al.*, 1996). Given that multiple genes with overlapping substrate specificities influence the fate of single distinct moieties, it seems highly likely that the complex mixture of carcinogens in tobacco smoke depends on an array of polymorphic genes for its ultimate effects. A good example is NNK, a nitrosamine carcinogen that may be activated by one of many p450s, including CYP2A6 and CYP2D6. The overlapping specificities of p450 enzymes are consistent with the observation that these enzymes vary commonly without obvious ill effects in the population. Since inactivating mutations are at least occasionally present for a number of p450s the particular gene cannot be essential for life; inactivating mutations would otherwise be under strong negative selection and redundant pathways would be even more common.

With regard to chronic diseases and, particularly, malignancy, it seems that we must invoke a complex of genes and exogenous exposure combinations to alter risk. Thus for the metabolic polymorphisms, combinations of Phase 1 genes, combinations of Phase 2 genes, and Phase 1 and Phase 2 genes together may influence cancer risk in unexpected ways. To date, the best-studied genes with possible joint effects are CYP1A1 and GSTM1. There is at least some suggestion of both effect modification (Kihara *et al.*, 1995; Nakachi, 1993) in the population data as well as biological interaction (Vaury *et al.*, 1995).

8. Animal models

Animal work is increasingly providing important information relevant to genetic factors in humans and has probably been underutilized as a source of candidate genes. Animal models provide distinct advantages, among them the ability to control for numerous sources of variability, directly administer carcinogens, perform detailed genetic studies including controlled matings, obtain available tissue from all organs, and precisely fit numbers to power requirements. On the other hand, most animal work has focused on the 'familial' cancer genes because of their clear mechanistic relationship with cancer, rather than the subtler but more common effects of polymorphisms that influence metabolism. Closer working relationships and interdisciplinary training can clearly benefit the field, and epidemiological studies on highly plausible genes of interest which have inadequate functional information (e.g. CYP1A1 and CYP2E1) would be greatly facilitated by further animal work. Knockout mice will provide invaluable adjunct information to answer some of these questions (Nebert & Duffy,1997). In addition, new 'susceptibility' loci being reported from animal studies can be expected to serve as a fertile source of new ideas for human evaluation. Animal work can often provide important confirmation that a hypothesized susceptibility gene is a plausible candidate for human study. For example, the demonstration that gastrointestinal adenomas in mice with fully penetrant mutations of the APC gene were blocked by sulindac administration provides important support for the potential chemopreventive role of this medication, suggests that the mechanism involves decreased apoptosis in enterocytes, and encourages further investigation of this class of drugs in humans (Boolbol *et al.*,1996).

Animal work suggests that modifier loci can alter the effects of major cancer genes. An example is provided by the modifier locus for the APC gene, demonstrated in the multiple intestinal neoplasia (Min) mouse (Dietrich *et al.*, 1993). This work hints that susceptibility gene studies might profitably focus on the question of whether any of the susceptibility genes modify penetrance in individuals in kindreds with 'rare' mutations of cancer genes (e.g. Brca1 and breast cancer).

Murine cancer models parallel the human situation to a greater or lesser degree. For example, the NZB mouse exhibits a genetically regulated clonal proliferation of aneuploid cells resembling human chronic lymphocytic leukaemia. The CLL-like mice do not, however, exhibit involvement of the lymph nodes or liver as in the human disease (Philips *et al.*, 1992). Nevertheless, studying this model is likely to provide insights into the pathogenesis of the disorder as well as new candidate genes for human study, once the mouse locus is mapped.

It is also interesting to note that the genetics of certain tumours are quite well established in murine models. For example, genetic susceptibility to lung tumours has been well documented in mice for over a half century (Dragani *et al.*, 1995). A possible candidate based on homology with an implicated mouse locus is K-ras. K-ras mutations are frequently observed in human adenocarcinoma, although to date no specific heritable susceptibility locus has been demonstrated.

Finally, it appears that for tumours that have been well studied in the murine model, multiple susceptibility loci exist. This is certainly the case for lung (Dragani *et al.*, 1995) and has also been demonstrated for hepatocarcinogeneis in mice (Manenti *et al.*, 1994). In humans, where exposures are more varied, the genetics are more complex, and familial clustering is not apparent or rare (as is the case for most human tumours), it would seem plausible to suppose that susceptibility loci are also multiple.

9. Human studies: gene frequency

Investigators should know or determine the gene frequencies of the relevant alleles prior to formal association testing, because power calculations depend on this variable. There is a trade-off between the prevalence of the gene and the magnitude of risk that may be detected by a particular study size. The more common a variant, the less likely it is to exhibit a strong association, but generally the more power there is to establish an association of a given magnitude. An example of this is the CYP2D6 gene that has a deficient genotype frequency of around 7% in European Caucasians, 4% in American Blacks, and 1% or less in Asians. Other factors being equal, there is moderate power to detect a given effect in Caucasians, weak power in an African-American population, and poor power in an Asian population.

10. Human studies: genotype-phenotype

The function of the genetic variants selected for study is of central importance. Unfortunately, functional information is often not available or is incomplete. Kellerman first studied the relationship of aryl hydrocarbon hydroxylase inducibility to lung cancer in 1974. This trait is dependent on CYP1A1, and polymorphisms in this gene have been described. Nevertheless, the precise relationship of the various polymorphisms to the phenotype remains incompletely understood. In the case of CYP1A1 there is some evidence that other genes in the same pathway such as the arnt receptor or Ah receptor play a role in influencing inducibility (Micka *et al.*, 1997). It is possible for measurement of the phenotype to be imprecise (measurement error) or non-specific (i.e. influenced by more than one gene), or for environmental factors to interfere (e.g. CYP1A2). For certain genes the proposed phenotype (i.e. CYP2E1 and chlorzoxazone) and genotype exhibit an irregular correspondence.

Methodological problems arise if the phenotype-genotype relationship is unknown. Particularly, in the absence of a facile measure of function the dominance relationship of the gene and directionality of the hypothesized association are unknown. Without this information, statistical power is weakened. For example, assuming a simple two-allele system, the risk group may be a genotype (AA, AB, or BB), presence/absence of the polymorphism (e.g. AA and AB vs. BB; implicit in this choice is some knowledge of the dominance relationship), or gene frequency (frequency of A) to examine in relation to disease. When multiple alleles are present these choices grow more complex and the danger of post-hoc assignment influencing findings becomes acute. It has been suggested that, in

certain cases, heterozygotes may be the at-risk group, compared to both homozygotes. Such a possibility may be suggested by marked deviation from Hardy-Weinberg equilibrium conditions.

11. Human studies: relationship to disease

Ultimately, *in vitro* and animal findings must be confirmed in humans to establish their significance for human health and disease. It can be anticipated that interpretation of the vast genetic information derived from the Human Genome Project will require large well-designed studies in human populations. It is often poorly understood that genes that have been studied in families also require specific study in the general population (frequency permitting) to establish whether and to what degree they are associated with risk in that setting.

The point with regard to candidate gene selection is that findings from epidemiological studies comprise another category of evidence to focus both laboratory and population studies in the future on particular genes.

12. Ethnic variation

The polymorphic genes that involve metabolic polymorphisms almost universally exhibit important ethnic and racial variation. Ethnic variability is important for a number of reasons. First, gene frequency in the ethnic group targeted for study must be known in order to perform power calculations and estimate the size of the study needed. For example, a study of the relationship of CYP2D6-deficient metabolizers to a condition of interest would have reasonable power in a Caucasian population where 7% of subjects are poor metabolizers, but would be impossible in an Asian population where 1% or less are deficient metabolizers. Second, qualitatively different gene variants imply that different functional variants exist and possibly predominate in different ethnic groups. Studying a 'new' ethnic group with variants important in a different group may therefore miss the critical sources of variation. Third, population stratification (also known as ethnic admixture) is a potential source of bias. The classic example is the apparent association of the Gm 3,5,13,14 haplotype with non-insulin dependent diabetes in an admixed population of Pima Indians. When the analysis was stratified according to the degree of Indian ancestry the association disappeared (Knowler et al., 1988). Population stratification can be thought of as a confounding issue, and the problem should be greatly minimized by the usual measures for the control of confounding, including proper control selection and adjustment for ethnicity. Methods that use relatives of cases as controls can theoretically eliminate this problem (e.g. the transmission disequilibrium test (Spielman et al., 1993)). However, the choice of relative controls poses difficulties in population-based studies. For example, enrolling parents of subjects with solid tumours, which typically have a median age of onset in the 60s, is typically not feasible. Fourth, the geographical variation that underlies ethnic variation probably holds important clues to the factors that drive this type of variation and may suggest determinants of disease susceptibility. The relationship of sickle cell disease/trait and malaria is the classic example.

Table 3. Categories of genes studied in relation to cancer susceptibility		
Gene type	**Examples**	**Cancer**
Phase 1	CYP1A1 (Kellerman et al., 1973)	Lung, others
	CYP1A2 (Lang et al., 1994)	Colon, lung
	CYP2A6 (Gullsten et al., 1997)	Liver
	CYP2C9 (London et al., 1997)	Lung
	CYP2D6 (Ayesh et al., 1984)	Lung, bladder
	CYP2E1 (Uematsu et al., 1991, Hildesheim et al.,1997)	Lung, NPC
Phase 2	GSTM1 (Seidegard et al., 1986)	Lung, bladder, others
	GSTT1 (Chen, H. et al., 1996)	Myelodysplasia
	Epoxide hydrolase (Heckbert et al., 1992)	Lung
	NAD(P)H quinone oxidoreductase (Schulz et al., 1997)	Lung, kidney
	NAT1 (Bell et al., 1995)	Colon, bladder
	NAT2 (Lower et al., 1979; Cascorbi et al., 1996)	Bladder, lung, others
Oncogene polymorphism	H-ras vtr (Krontiris et al., 1985)	Lung, breast, others
Tumour suppressor gene	p53 (Murata et al., 1996)	Various
	APC	Various
Nutrition	Vitamin D polymorphism (Taylor et al., 1996)	Prostate
	Methylene-tetrahydrofolate reductase (Chen et al., 1996)	Colon
	Ethanol (Harty et al., 1997)	Oral cavity
DNA repair	Bleomycin sensitivity phenotype (Spitz & Hsu, 1994; Spitz et al., 1995)	Lung, head and neck
Behaviour	DRD2 (Comings et al., 1994)	No cancer studies to date
	Serotonin receptor (Lerman et al., 1998)	No cancer studies to date
Inflammation	COX-2 (prostaglandin synthesis) (Boolbol et al., 1996)	No cancer studies to date
Hormone	Testosterone (Maenpaa et al., 1993)	Prostate, breast
	5 alpha reductase (Reichardt et al., 1995)	Prostate
	Aromatase	Breast
	Androgen receptor (Irvine et al., 1995)	Prostate
Immune	HLA	Lymphoproliferative (?)
Medications and xenobiotics	Chemotherapeutic agents	Various
	Dioxin	Various
Miscellaneous	Blood groups	Stomach
	Apolipoprotein	Stomach

Conclusions

A number of criteria for the selection of candidate genes have been offered and placed loosely in the historical context. None of them are absolute but none should be ignored. A promising epidemiological finding should stimulate laboratory efforts, while a new gene implicated in an animal model should be considered for study in the appropriate human condition. Findings that lack either the population or the laboratory component require cautious interpretation. It is likely that the complete picture of most malignancies will involve multiple genes and complex biological interactions.

A few predictions can be offered in the light of trends observed over the past years. Larger studies that include exposure information and incorporate numbers of genetic markers (increasingly available from work related to the Human Genome Project) are anticipated in the next few years. For the first time there should be opportunities to examine gene-gene and gene-environment interaction in an appropriate setting, i.e. of adequate power and with relevant exposure information.

The problem of multiple comparisons should be dealt with by sequentially performing studies in multiple populations. Even large settings can be expected to have a 'hypothesis generating' component. In spite of the proliferating genetic approaches, traditional epidemiological designs will remain the mainstay (i.e. association studies rather than family-based linkage/sib-pair designs) because power and exposure information are needed to detect the relatively modest effects of these genes.

References

Anttila, S., Hirvonen, A., Vainio, H., Husgafvel-Pursiainen, K., Hayes, J.D. & Ketterer, B. (1993) Immunohistochemical localization of glutathione S-transferases in human lung. *Cancer Res.*, 53, 5643-5648

Auerbach, A.D., Buchwald, M. & Joenje, H. Fanconi anemia. (1998) In: Vogelstein, B. & Kinzler, K.W., eds. *The genetic basis of human cancer*. New York, McGraw Hill, pp. 317-332

Ayesh, R., Idle, J.R., Richie, J.C., Crothers, M.J. & Hetzel, M.R. (1984) Metabolic oxidation phenotypes as markers for susceptibility to lung cancer. *Nature*, 312, 169-170

Barcellos, L.F., Klitz, W., Field, L.L., Tobias, R., Bowcock, A.M., Wilson, R., Nelson, M.P., Nagatomi, J. & Thomson, G. (1997) Association mapping of disease loci by use of a pooled DNA genomic screen. *Am. J. Hum. Genet.*, 61, 734-747

Bhatia, K.G., Cherney, B.W., Hupppi, K., Magrath, I.T., Cossman, J., Sausville, E., Barriga, F., Johnson, B., Gause, B. & Bonney, G. (1990) A deletion linked to a poly(ADP-ribose) polymerase gene on chromosome 13q33-qter occurs frequently in a normal black population as well as in multiple tumour DNA. *Cancer Res.*, 50, 5406-5413

Bell, D.A., Stephans, E.A., Castranio, T., Umbach, D.M., Watson, M., Deakin, M., Elder, J., Hendrickse C., Duncan, H. & Strange, R.C. (1995) Polyadenylation polymorphism in the acetyltransferase 1 gene (NAT1) increases risk of colorectal cancer. *Cancer Res.*, 55, 3537

Bogardus, C. & Lillioja, S. (1992) Pima Indians as a model to study the genetics of NIDDM *J. Cell.Biochem.*, 48, 337-343

Boolbol, S.K., Dannenberg, A.J., Chadburn, A., Martucci, C., Guo, X.J., Ramonetti, J.T., Abreu-Goris, M., Newmark, H.L., Lipkin, M.L., DeCrosse, J.J. & Bertagnolli, M.M. (1996) Cyclooxygenase-2 overexpression and tumour formation are blocked by sulindac in a murine model of familial adenomatosis polyposis. *Cancer Res.*, 56, 2556-2560

Caporaso, N. & Goldstein, A. (1995) Cancer genes: single and susceptibility: exposing the difference. *Pharmacogenetics*, 5, 59-63

Cascorbi, I., Brockmöller, J., Mrozikiewicz, P.M., Bauer, S., Loddenkemper, R. & Roots, I. (1996) Homozygous rapid arylamine N-acetyltransferase (NAT2) genotype as susceptibility factor for lung cancer. *Cancer Res.*, 56, 3961-3966

Chen, H., Sandler D.P., Taylor, J.A., Shore, D.L., Liu, E., Bloomfield, C.D. & Bell D.A. (1996) Increased risk of myelodysplastic syndromes in individuals with glutathione theta 1 (GSTT1) gene defect. *Lancet*, 347, 295-297

Chen, J., Giovannucci, E., Kelsey, K., Rimm, E.B., Stampfer, M.J., Colditz, G.A., Spiegelman, D., Willett, W.C. & Hunter, D.J. (1996) A methylenetetrahydrofolate reductase polymorphism and the risk of colorectal cancer. *Cancer Res.*, 56, 4862-4864

Comings, D.E., Muhleman, D., Ahn, C., Gysin, R. & Flanagan, S.D. (1994) The dopamine D2 receptor gene: a risk factor for substance abuse. *Drug Alcohol Depend.*, 34, 175-180

d'Errico, A., Taioli, E., Xiang, C. & Vineis, P. (1996) Genetic metabolic polymorphisms and the risk of cancer: a review of the literature. *Biomarkers*, 1, 174-177

Dietrich, W.F., Lander, E.S., Smith, J.S., Moser, A.R., Gould, K.A., Luongo, C., Borenstein, N. & Dove, W. (1993) Genetic Identification of Mom-1, a major modifier locus affecting min-induced intestinal neoplasia in the mouse. *Cell*, 75, 631-639

Dragani, T.A., Manenti, G. & Pierotti, M.A. (1995) Genetics of murine lung tumors. *Advances Cancer Res.*, 67, 83-112

Drayer, D.E. & Reidenberg, M.M. (1977) Clinical consequences of polymorphic acetylation of basic drugs. *Clin.Pharmacol. Ther.*, 22(3), 251-258

Ducharme, J., Abdullah, S. & Wainer, I.W. (1966) Dextromethorphan as an *in vivo* probe for the simultaneous determination of CYP2D6 and CYP3A activity. *J. Chromatogr.*, 678, 113-128

Evans, D.A.P., Mahgoub, A., Sloan, T.P., Idle, J.R. & Smith, R.L. (1980) A family and population study of the genetic polymorphism of debrisoquine oxidation in a white British population. *J. Med. Genet.*,17, 102-105

Feinberg, A.P., Rainier, S. & DeBaun, M.R. (1995) Genomic imprinting, DNA methylation, and cancer. *J. Natl. Cancer Inst.*, 17, 21-26

Gervassi, P.G., Longo, V., Naldi, F., Panattoni, G. & Ursino, F. (1991) Xenobiotic-metabolizing enzymes in human respiratory nasal mucosa. *Biochem. Pharmacol.*, 41, 177-184

Gonzalez, F.J. & Idle, J.R. (1994) Pharmacogenetic phenotyping and genotyping. *Clin. Pharmacokinet.*, 26, 59-70

Grant, D.M. (1993) Molecular genetics of the N-acetyltransferases. *Pharmacogenetics*, 3, 45-50

Gullsten, H., Agundez, J.A.G., Benitez, J., Laara, E., Ladero, J.M., Diaz-Rubio, M., Fernandez-Salguero, P., Gonzalez, F., Rautio, A., Pelkonen, O. & Raunio, H. (1997) CYP2A6 gene polymorphism and risk of liver cancer and cirrhosis. *Pharmacogenetics*, 7, 247-250

Harty, L.C., Caporaso, N.E., Hayes, R.B., Winn, D.M., Bravo-Otero, E., Blot, W.J., Brown, L.M., Armenian, H.K., Fraumeni, J.F.F. & Shields, P.G. (1997) Alcohol dehydrogenase 3 genotype and risk of oral and pharyngeal cancers. *J. Natl. Cancer Inst.*, 89, 1698-1705

Heckbert, S.R., Weiss, N.S., Hornung, S.K., Eaton, D.L. & Motulsky, A.G. (1992) Glutathione S transferase and epoxide hydrolase activity in human leukocytes in relation to risk of lung cancer and other smoking-related cancers. *J. Natl. Cancer Inst.*, 84, 414-421

Hildesheim, A., Anderson, L.M., Chen, C.-J., Brinton, L.A., Daly, A.K., Reed, C.D., Chen, I.-H., Caporaso. N.E., Hsu, M.-M., Chen, J.-Y., Idle, J.R., Hoover, R.N., Yang, C.-S. & Chhabra, S.K. (1997) CYP2E1 genetic polymorphism and the risk of nasopharyngeal carcinoma in Taiwan. *J. Natl. Cancer Inst.* , 89, 1207-1212

Irvine, R.A., Yu, M.C., Ross, R.K. & Coetzee, G.A. (1995) The CAG and GGC microsatellites of the androgen receptor gene are in linkage disequilibrium in men with prostate cancer. *Cancer Res.*, 55, 1937-1940

Kalow, W. (1962) *Pharmacogenetics: heredity and response to drugs*. Philadelphia, W.B. Saunders

Kellerman, G., Shaw, C.R. & Luyten-Kellerman, M. (1973) Aryl hydrocarbon hydroxylase inducibility and bronchogenic carcinoma. *New Engl. J. Med.*, 289, 934-937

Kihara, M., Kihara, M. & Noda, K. (1995) Risk of smoking for squamous and small cell carcinomas of the lung modulated by combinations of CYP1A1 and GSTM1 gene polymorphisms in a Japanese population. *Carcinogenesis*, 16, 2331-2336

Kivisto, K.T., Griese, E.-U., Stuven, T., Fritz, P., Friedel, G., Kroemer, H.K. & Zanger, U.M. (1997) Analysis of CYP2D6 expression in human lung: implications for the association between CYP2D6 activity and susceptibility to lung cancer. *Pharmacogenetics*, 7, 295-302

Knowler, W.C., Williams, R.C., Pettitt, D.J. & Steinberg, A.G. (1988) Gm 3;5;13;14 and type 2 diabetes mellitus: an association in American Indians with genetic admixture. *Am. J. Hum. Genet.*, 43, 520-526

Krontiris, T.G., DiMartino, N.A., Colb, M. & Parkinson, D.R. (1985) Unique allelic restriction fragments of the human Ha-ras locus in leukocyte and tumour DNAs of cancer patients. *Nature*, 313, 369-374

Lander, E. & Kruglyak, L. (1995) Genetic dissection of complex traits: guidelines for interpreting and reporting linkage results. *Nature Genet.*, 11, 241-247

Lang, N.P., Butler, M.A., Massengill, J., Lawson, M., Stotta, R.C., Haver-Jensen, M. & Kadlubar, F.F. (1994) Rapid metabolic phenotypes for acetyl-transferase and cytochrome P4501A2 and putative exposure to food-borne heterocyclic amines increases risk for colorectal cancer or polyps. *Cancer Epidemiol. Biomarkers Prev.*, 3, 675-682

Lerman, C., Shields, P.G., Audrain, J., Main, D., Cobb, B., Boyd, N.R. & Caporaso, N. (1998) The role of the serotonin transporter gene in cigarette smoking. *Cancer Epidemiol. Biomarkers Prev.*, 7, 253-255

London, S.J., Sullivan-Klose, T., Daly, A.K. & Idle, J.R. (1997) Lung cancer risk in relation to the CYP2C9 genetic polymorphism among Caucasians in Los Angeles County. *Pharmacogenetics*, 7, 401-405

Lower, G.M., Nilsson, T., Nelson, C.E., Wolf, H., Gamsky, T.E. & Bryan, G.T. (1979) N-acetyl-transferase phenotype and risk in urinary bladder cancer: approaches in molecular epidemiology. Preliminary results in Sweden and Denmark. *Environ. Health Perspect.*, 29, 71-79

Maenpaa, J., Pelkonen, O., Cresteil, T. & Rane, A. (1993) The role of cytochrome p450 3A (CYP3A) isoforms in oxidative metabolism of testosterone and benzphetamine in human adult and fetal liver. *J. Steroid Biochem.*, 44, 61-67

Manenti, G., Binelli, G., Gariboldi, M., Canzian, F., DeGregorio, L., Falvella, F.S., Dragani, T.A. & Pierotti, M.A. (1994) Multiple loci affect genetic predisposition to hepatocarcinogenesis in mice. *Genomics*, 23, 118-124

McGlynn, K.A., Rosvold, E.A., Lustbader, E.D., Hu, Y., Clapper, M.L., Zhou, T., Wild, C.P., Xia, X.L., Baffoe-Bonnie, A., Ofori-Adjei, D., Chen, G.C., London, W.T., Shen, F.M. & Buetow, K.H. (1995) Susceptibility to hepatocellular carcinoma is associated with genetic variation in the enzymatic detoxification of aflatoxin B_1. *Proc. Natl. Acad. Sci. USA*, 92, 2384-2387

Micka, J., Milatovich, A., Menon, A., Grabowski, G.A., Puga, A. & Nebert, D.W. (1997) Human Ah receptor (AHR) gene: localization to 7p15 and suggestive correlation of polymorphism with CYP1A1 inducibility. *Pharmacogenetics*, 7, 95-102

Miyagawa, K. Genetic instability and cancer. (1998) *Int. J. Hematol.*, 67 (1), 3-14

Murata, M., Tagawa, M., Kimura, M., Kimura, H., Watanabe, S. & Saisho, H. (1996) Analysis of a germ line polymorphism of the p53 gene in lung cancer patients; discrete results with smoking history. *Carcinogenesis*, 17, 261-264

Nakachi, K., Imai, K., Hayashi, S. & Kawajiri, K. (1993) Polymorphism of the CYP1A1 and glutathione-S-transferase genes associated with susceptibility to lung cancer in relation to cigarette dose in a Japanese population. *Cancer Res.*, 53, 2994-2999

Nakajima, T., Elovaara, E., Anttila, S., Hirvonen, A., Camus, A.-M., Hayes, J.D., Ketterer, B. & Vainio, H. (1995) Expression and polymorphism of glutathione S-transferase in human lungs: risk factors in smoking-related lung cancer. *Carcinogenesis*, 16, 707-711

Nebert, D.W. & Duffy, J.J. (1997) How Knockout mice will be used to study the role of drug-metabolizing enzymes and their receptors during reproduction and development, and in environmental toxicity, cancer and oxidative stress. *Biochem. Pharmacol.*, 53, 249-254

Nowell, P.C. & Hungerford, D.A. (1960) A minute chromosome in human chronic granulocytic leukemia. *Science*, 132, 1497

Oda, Y., Tanaka, M. & Nakanishi, I. (1994) Relation between the occurrence of K-ras gene point mutations and genotypes of polymorphic N-acetyltransferase in human colorectal cancer carcinomas. *Carcinogenesis*, 15(7), 1365-1369

Paul, J.R., Melnick, J.L. & Riordan JT (1952) Comparative neutralizing antibody patterns to Lansing (type 2) poliomyelitis virus in different populations. *Am. J. Hygiene*, 56, 232-251

Pensotti, V., Radice, P., Presciuttini, S., Calistri, D., Gazzoli, I., Perez, A.P.G., Mondini, P., Buonsanti, G., Sala, P., Rossetti, C., Ranzani, G.N., Bertario, L. & Pierotti, M.A. (1997) Mean age of tumour in hereditary nonpolyposis colorectal cancer (HNPCC) families correlates with the presence of mutations in DNA mismatch repair genes. *Genes, Chromosomes and Cancer*, 19, 135-142

Phillips, J.A., Mehta, K., Fernandez, C. & Raveche, E.S. (1992) The NZB mouse as a model for chronic lymphocytic leukaemia. *Cancer Res.*, 52, 437-443

Reichardt, J.K.V., Makridakis, N., Henderson, B.E., Yu, M.C., Pike, M.C. & Ross, RK. (1995) Genetic variability of the human SRD5A2 gene: implications for prostate cancer risk. *Cancer Res.*, 55, 3973-3975

Risch, N. & Merikangas, K. (1996) The future of genetic studies of complex human diseases. *Science*, 273, 1516-1517

Scrivner, C.R., Beaudet, A., Valle, D. & Sly, W.S., eds. (1995) *The metabolic and molecular basis of inherited disease. Volumes I-III, 7th Ed.* New York, McGraw-Hill

Seidegard, J., Pero, R.W., Miller, D. & Beattie, E.J. (1986) A glutathione transferase in human leukocytes as a marker for susceptibility to lung cancer. *Carcinogenesis*, 7, 751-753

Schulz, W.A., Krummeck, A., Rosinger, I., Eickelmann, P., Neuhaus, C., Ebert, T., Schmitz-Drager, B.J. & Sies, H. (1997) Increased frequency of a null-allele for NAD(P)H: quinone oxidoreductase in patients with urological malignancies. *Pharmacogenetics*, 7, 235-239

Soini, Y., Chia, S.C., Bennett, W.P., Groopman, J.D., Wang, J.S., De Benedetti, V.M., Cawley, H., Welsh, J.A., Hansen, C., Bergasa, N.V., Jones, E.A., Di Bisceglie, A.M., Trivers, G.E., Sandoval, C.A., Calderon, I.E., Munoz Espinosa.L.E. & Harris, C.C. (1996) An aflatoxin-associated mutational hotspot at codon 249 in the p53 tumor-suppresser gene in HCC. *Cancer*, 17(5), 1007-1020

Spielman, R.S., McGinnis, R.E. & Ewens, W.J. (1993) Transmission test for linkage disequilibrium: the insulin gene region and insulin-dependent diabetes mellitus (IDDM). *Am. J. Hum. Genet.*, 32, 506-512

Spitz, M.R. & Hsu, T.C. (1994) Mutagen sensitivity as a marker of cancer risk. *Cancer Detect. Prev.*, 18, 299-303

Spitz, M.R., Hsu, T.C., Wu, X., Fueger, J.J., Amos, C.I. & Roth, J.A. (1995) Mutagen sensitivity as a biological marker of lung cancer risk in African Americans. *Cancer Epidemiol. Biomarkers Prev.*, 4, 99-103

Taylor, J.A., Hirvonen, A., Watson, M., Pittman, G., Mohler, J.L. & Bell, D.A. (1996) Association of prostate cancer with vitamin D receptor gene polymorphism. *Cancer Res.*, 56, 4108-4110

Tomatis, L. (1994) Transgenerational arcinogenesis: a review of the experimental and epidemiological literature. *Jpn. J. Cancer Res.*, 85, 443-454

Tuchman, M., Stoeckeler, J.S., Kiang, D.T., O'Dea, R.F., Ramnraine, M.L. & Mirkin, B.L. (1985) Familial pyrimidemia and pyrimidinuria associated with severe fluorouracil toxicity. *New Engl. J. Med.*, 313, 245-249

Uematsu, F., Kikuchi, H., Motomiya, M., Abe, T., Sagami, I., Ohmachi, T., Wakui, A., Kanamara, R. & Watanabe, M. (1991) Association between restriction fragment length polymorphism of human cytochrome P450IIE1 gene and susceptibility to lung cancer. *Jpn. J. Cancer Res.*, 82, 254-256

Wistuba, I.I., Lam, S., Behrens, C., Virmani, A.K., Fong, K.M., LeRiche, J., Samet, J.M., Srivastava, S., Minna, J.D. & Gazdar, A.F. (1997) Molecular damage in the bronchial epithelium of current and former smokers. *J. Natl. Cancer Inst.*, 89, 1366-1372

Vaury, C., Laine, R., Noguiez, P., de Coppet, P., Jaulin, C., Praz, F., Pompon, D. & Amor-Gueret, M. (1995) Human glutathione S- transferase M1 null genotype is associated with high inducibility of cytochrome p450 1A1 gene transcription. *Cancer Res.*, 55, 5520-5523

Neil Caporaso
Pharmacogenetic Section,
Genetic Epidemiology Branch,
National Cancer Institute,
EPN 439,
Rockville, MD 20892, USA

Metabolic Polymorphisms and Susceptibility to Cancer
W. Ryder
IARC Scientific Publications No. 148
International Agency for Research on Cancer, Lyon, 1999

Chapter 5. Somatic alterations and metabolic polymorphisms

Andrew N. Freedman

Cancer is a multistep process in which multiple genetic alterations occur, causing a cumulative adverse effect on the control of cell differentiation, cell division and growth control. Somatic alterations acquired at the level of the cell become fixed in the developing cancer as chromosomal translocations, deletions, inversions, amplifications or point mutations. Since the ultimate unit of susceptibility to carcinogens is at the level of the cell, somatic gene alterations play an important role in carcinogenesis, as all neoplastic tumours exhibit somatic alterations. The incorporation of somatic alterations, such as oncogenes and tumour-suppressor genes, into epidemiological research provides an opportunity to clarify the role of exposure, other genetic changes and prognosis in cancer pathogenesis. The manner in which environmental factors act to initiate, accelerate or retard neoplastic progression is currently being investigated using somatic gene mutational spectra to identify specific etiological carcinogens. Exploring the relationships between germline and somatic alterations may help to identify the timing of genetic events, important etiological exposures and gene-gene epistatic phenomena. Examining somatic alterations within the context of carcinogen-metabolizing enzymes may elucidate specific carcinogenic mechanisms. The use of somatic alterations to predict prognoses for patients with various malignancies may also help to enhance our ability to define subgroups of patients with different disease courses and treatment responses.

Genetic changes during neoplastic development support the view that cancer is a genetic disease. It is generally accepted that inherited susceptibility plays an important role in the risk of malignancy. Studies consistently show an increased risk of cancer in relatives of cancer cases, frequently of the same type of cancer. Inherited cancer syndromes due to highly penetrant germline alterations may cause several cancers within an affected family, but it is estimated that these genes account for less than 5% of all common cancers. While other susceptibility markers, including metabolic polymorphisms and DNA repair deficiencies, may also play a role in some cancers, all neoplastic tumours exhibit somatic alterations as a universal feature of neoplastic carcinogenesis.

Somatic alterations

Cancer is a multistep process in which multiple genetic alterations occur, causing a cumulative adverse effect on the control of cell differentiation, cell division and growth control (Foulds,

1958). Somatic alterations acquired at the level of the cell are found in all neoplasms and become fixed in the developing cancer as chromosomal translocations, deletions, inversions, amplifications or point mutations. These alterations are an integral component of genetic susceptibility to cancer and have been described as the determinate unit of susceptibility to carcinogens at the level of the cell (Albertini et al., 1996).

Theodor Boveri, many years before determining the exact chromosome number in normal human somatic cells, hypothesized in his book *On the Problem of the Origin of Malignant Tumours* (1914) that malignant tumours could develop from an abnormal chromosome constitution, possibly resulting from cell division enhancing or suppressing chromosomes, propagating from a single cell (Sandberg, 1979). Almost 60 years later, molecular biologists discovered that specific chromosome translocations were associated with cancers such as chronic myelogenous leukaemia and Burkitt's lymphoma (Rowley, 1973; Manolov & Manolova, 1973). Moreover, many of these chromosomal abnormalities contain cancer-related genes or protooncogenes activated in their new translocated regions.

Remarkable technological advances in molecular biology have now helped scientists to define cancer as a disease resulting from the clonal expansion of a single somatic cell following a genotoxic event. Somatic gene alterations play an important role in carcinogenesis and include oncogenes and tumour-suppressor genes that control the cell cycle and genomic stability, and mediate apoptosis or programmed cell death (Friend et al., 1988). Studies of successive histopathological stages that differentiate carcinogenic progression suggest that five or six mutations in protooncogenes and tumour-suppressor genes may be necessary to establish a fully neoplastic lesion (Vogelstein et al., 1988).

The adenoma-carcinoma genetic sequence

Malignant tumours of the colorectum provide an exceptional model to describe the process by which genetic mutations induce and modulate neoplastic tumour development. Fearon and Vogelstein (1990) proposed that colorectal carcinogenesis is a multi-step process involving mutations of both oncogenes and tumour-suppressor genes contributing to adenoma formation, and additional mutations allowing progression to a carcinoma (Fig. 1). In their model, mutation of the apc gene, located on chromosome 5q (Powell et al., 1993), and altered methylation processes lead to abnormal epithelial proliferation and micro-adenoma formation (Counts et al., 1995). Mutations of the K-ras gene located on the short arm of chromosome 12 induce an early adenoma to progress to an intermediate adenoma (Bos, 1988). Deletion and/or mutation of the dcc (deleted in colorectal carcinoma) gene on chromosome 18q is associated with the progression of an intermediate adenoma to a late adenoma (Hedrick et al., 1994), while deletion and mutation of the p53 gene on the short arm of chromosome 17 occur at the transition of an adenoma to a carcinoma (Fearon, 1993).

Molecular epidemiology

Recent advances in molecular biological techniques have led to the emergence of the term "molecular epidemiology" to describe the approach that incorporates molecular, cellular and other biological measurements into epidemiologi-

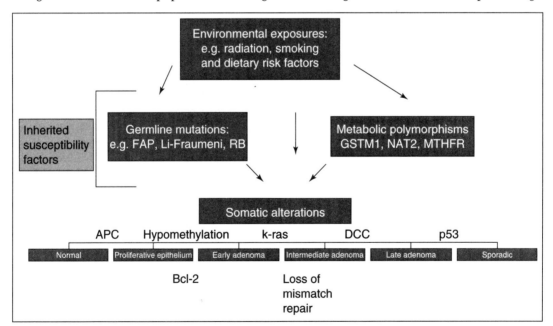

Figure1. Model of the relationship of environmental exposures to inherited susceptibility factors (i.e. germline mutations and metabolic polymorphisms) and somatic alterations.

cal research (*Molecular Epidemiology: Principles and Practices*. Edited by Schulte, P.A. & Perera F.P., Academic Press, Inc. Harcourt Brace and Company, 1993). The incorporation of somatic alterations into epidemiological research provides great promise for the elucidation of various aspects of cancer pathogenesis, including delineation of the continuum of events between an exposure and a malignant phenotype, enhancement of knowledge about the mechanisms by which exposure and disease are related, identification of early events in the natural history of tumour development, reduction of misclassification of both disease and exposure classifications, development of individual and group risk assessments, and improvement of prognostic capabilities. The present Chapter explores the relationship of somatic alterations to environmental exposure, other genetic changes (germline mutations and metabolic polymorphisms), and cancer progression.

Relationship to exposure

The role of somatic alterations is well documented but the precise manner in which environmental factors act to initiate, accelerate or retard neoplastic progression is a fundamental area of concern. To study this, investigations must be designed to examine both exposures (e.g. aflatoxin B1, tobacco) and molecular alterations (i.e. oncogene expression, mutational spectrum). As an example of this approach, we review investigations of the best-studied gene in this group, the p53 tumour-suppressor gene.

The p53 gene and etiology

The p53 gene is a tumour-suppressor gene of central importance because it is mutated in approximately 50% of all human cancers (Hollstein *et al.*, 1991; Greenblatt *et al.*, 1994). Tumour-suppressor genes are vulnerable sites of critical DNA damage, because they function normally in cells to control cell cycle regulation and inhibit clonal expansion and subsequent genotoxic events (Harris, 1996).

Loss of tumour-suppressor function can occur by damage to the genome through mutation, resulting in uncontrolled proliferation and neoplastic development. Recent molecular investigations have shown that the p53 tumour-suppressor gene is an ideal candidate to study the interplay between genes and environmental exposures, since carcinogens and mutagens leave characteristic alterations in the p53 genome (Hollstein *et al.*, 1991; Greenblatt *et al.*, 1994).

The type and location of mutations in a specific DNA sequence define a mutational spectrum (Dogliotti *et al.*, 1996). When p53 alterations are examined separately by cancer type, the frequencies of alteration, the codon position of the mutation and the type of mutation (transition or transversion) all vary (Greenblatt *et al.*, 1994). The variability in the mutational spectra observed among different tumours suggests that the etiologies of these mutations are distinct in different tumour types (Harris, 1991). For example, the induction of skin carcinoma by ultraviolet light is suggested by the occurrence of p53 mutations at dipyrimidine sites including CC to TT double base changes (Harris, 1991; Brash *et al.*, 1991; Dumaz *et al.*, 1994). This variability exhibited by the p53 mutational spectra may imply that specific physical and chemical agents produce representative genetic mutations in heterogenous tissues.

The evaluation of p53 gene alterations offers many advantages in the study of etiology besides its revealing mutational spectra. Alteration of the p53 gene is the most common genetic abnormality found in human cancer, and it can be investigated and differentiated among many common cancers. p53 mutational events are diverse, including specific missense changes (e.g. guanine (G) to adenine (A) vs. guanine (G) to thymine (T)), transversions vs. transitions, mutations at CpG DNA sites, and preferential DNA strand repair bias, allowing extensive inferences regarding mechanisms of DNA damage and mutation (Greenblatt *et al.*, 1994).[1] Laboratory assays for mutational analysis of the p53 gene are now rela-

---

[1] *Transitions* refer to mutations in which one purine base is substituted for the other (A for G or G for A) or one pyrimidine is substituted for the other (C for T or T for C).
Transversions are defined by a mutation in which either purine base is substituted for either pyrimidine or vice versa.
CpG dinucleotides refer to DNA methylation of cytosine to 5-methylcytosine at cytosine-phosphor-guanine dinucleotides. These nucleotides are estimated to have a tenfold to fortyfold higher mutation rate than other nucleotides largely due to spontaneous deamination of 5-methylcytosine.

tively uncomplicated and can be performed in tissue obtained from archival paraffin blocks (Bennett *et al.*, 1991). Moreover, its entire coding region is highly conserved in vertebrates, allowing the extrapolation of data from animal models (Greenblatt *et al.*, 1994).

The p53 gene and liver cancer

Many epidemiological investigations have shown that dietary aflatoxin exposure is a primary etiological factor in human hepatocellular carcinoma (HCC) (Wogan, 1992). Aflatoxins comprise a group of mycotoxins produced by the common fungus *Aspergillus flavis* which are food contaminants in many developing countries. Aflatoxins, and particularly aflatoxin B1 (AFB1) are highly mutagenic and carcinogenic, producing liver tumours in experimental animal studies (Busby, W.F. & Wogan, G.N. Aflatoxins. In: Searle, C.E., ed. *Chemical Carcinogens. Vol 2.* Washington DC, American Chemical Society, pp. 945-1136, 1984). However, the precise mechanisms by which AFB1 leads to hepatocarcinogenesis are not known. Because of the mutagenic effects of AFB1 in experimental systems there is great interest in identifying possible oncogenes, such as p53, which may serve as critical molecular targets in AFB1 carcinogenesis (Shen *et al.*, 1996).

Bressac *et al.* (1991) and Hsu *et al.* (1991) reported that AFB1 dietary exposure may be related to a specific type of p53 mutation in human HCC. They demonstrated that nearly half of all HCCs from areas of high AFB1 exposure (southern Africa and Qidong, China) contained transversions of guanine to thymine at codon 249 of the p53 tumour-suppressor gene. In subsequent molecular studies more than 1500 human HCC samples from diverse geographical regions with varying AFB1 exposure have been examined for p53 mutations (Shen *et al.*, 1996). In general, high levels of AFB1 are found in developing countries with tropical weather (i.e. southern Africa, parts of Asia) whereas low or negligible levels are found in developed areas such as Europe, Japan and the USA. More than 50% of HCC patients harbour a G to T transversion at codon 249 of the p53 gene in areas of high aflatoxin exposure. In contrast, less than 2% of cases with HCC in areas with low levels of AFB1 contain these same codon alterations, although a fifth of patients' tumours

exhibited some type of p53 alteration. Experimental *in vitro* evidence shows that AFB1 preferentially induces G to T transversions in codon 249, and forms AFB1-adducts at this codon (Puisieux *et al.*, 1991). The G to T mutation at codon 249 of the p53 tumour-suppressor gene is therefore believed to be a fingerprint left by AFB1 in the development of human HCC, and AFB1 may play a causative role in hepatocarcinogenesis in populations with high dietary exposure to AFB1.

While the role of AFB1 in p53-induced HCC is strong, many questions in these studies concerning methodology and confounding remain unanswered. Almost all the studies originate from only two regions of high AFB1 exposure, Qidong in China, and southern Africa (Shen *et al.*, 1996). Studies from other well-defined regions of high AFB1 exposure have not been reported. Whether this is due to a lack of investigations in these geographical areas or to a publication bias against negative findings is not clear. Furthermore, most studies rely on ecological data on AFB1 exposure and are unable to provide the actual level of an individual's AFB1 exposure. Hepatitis B virus (HBV) infection has also been identified as a major etiological factor in HCC (IARC Monographs on the Evaluation of Carcinogenic Risk to Humans. *Hepatits viruses, Vol. 59.* Lyon, IARC, 1994: pp. 45-255). Therefore HBV could be a strong confounder or effect modifier in studies of AFB1 and p53, since a high prevalence of HBV infection is always found in areas of high AFB1. There is also evidence of a synergistic effect of HBV infection with AFB1 (Ross *et al.*, 1992). Future studies should incorporate precise individual measures of AFB1 exposure and account for the potential confounding of HBV infection.

The p53 gene and lung cancer

Lung cancer is another well-studied tumour that provides a good example of the use of somatic alterations to uncover evidence of etiological agents. Tobacco smoking is the single most important risk factor for lung cancer and is the leading cause of cancer death in the USA (Miller *et al.*, 1993). Carcinogens in cigarette smoke, such as benzo[a]pyrene, are strongly implicated as causative agents in the development of lung cancer (Hecht *et al.*, 1993). About 60% of human lung cancers contain mutations in the p53 tumour-suppressor gene, which are believed to occur early in lung carcinogenesis (Hollstein *et al.*, 1991; Greenblatt *et al.*, 1994). Of these mutations, 40% are guanine (G) to thymine (T) transversions (Greenblatt *et al.*, 1994; Hollstein *et al.*, 1996) and are typical of mutagenesis involving certain types of polycyclic aromatic hydrocarbons present in cigarette smoke, including metabolites of benzo[a]pyrene (Chen *et al.*, 1990). The p53 lung cancer mutational spectrum differs markedly from the mutational spectrum of other tumour types with dissimilar etiological exposures, such as colon cancer. Several studies of p53 mutations in relation to smoking history report that G:C to T:A transversions are positively associated with lifetime cigarette smoking (Chiba *et al.*, 1990; Takahashi *et al.*, 1991; Nuorva *et al.*, 1994; Ryberg *et al.*, 1994; Kondo *et al.*, 1996; Takeshima *et al.*, 1993; Suzuki *et al.*, 1992). Previous studies in mice exposed to benzo[a]pyrene revealed a predominance of these G to T transversions in the ras gene, another common somatic alteration in lung carcinoma (You *et al.*, 1989). Moreover, the distribution of benzo[a]pyrene metabolite adducts along the p53 gene in bronchial cell lines preferentially occurs at guanine positions in codons that are the predominant mutational hot spots in human lung cancer (Denissenko *et al.*, 1996). The accumulation of these data allows one to suggest that lung cancer is caused by specific carcinogens present in cigarette smoke, constituting a direct etiological link between smoking and lung cancer.

While the case of the association between smoking exposure and the p53 gene in lung cancer is highly suggestive, these studies raise many questions: the interpretation of mutational spectra and environmental interactions is still controversial. While certain findings suggest that some mutagens have narrow mutational spectra and that each agent might leave a specific identifying fingerprint of the site and type of DNA damage (McMichael, 1994), the reality is more likely to be that mutational patterns are characteristic and instructive but not unique as fingerprints. These associations are further complicated since animal and experimental studies are traditionally used to describe baseline interactions of exposures and resulting DNA changes, and the results of these

studies may vary according to the conditions in which they are performed (Dogliotti *et al.*, 1996). For example, experimental studies have shown that the resulting mutational spectra vary greatly with the dose of the mutagen administered (Dogliotti *et al.*, 1996). Caution must therefore be exercised when interpreting mutational spectra studies in identifying the cause of a tumour.

Although 40% of lung tumours express G to T transversions in the p53 gene, these may occur at a variety of codons, as only a few hot spots have been identified (Greenblatt *et al.*, 1994). This may demonstrate a lack of specificity or alternatively a multiplicity of targets for these mutations if benzo[a]pyrene is the major carcinogenic exposure. Perhaps one of the many other carcinogens present in tobacco smoke contributes to these or other types of mutation at an array of p53 gene codons. Distinguishing which particular carcinogen among the thousands identified in tobacco smoke induces which p53 gene mutation is a daunting task. Even G to T transversions can be induced by other agents, including oxidative DNA damage or nitrosamines (Lindahl, 1993). Furthermore, epidemiological associations of p53 mutation and G to T transversions with smoking history have not been consistently found (Chiba *et al.*, 1990; Takahashi *et al.*, 1991; Nuorva *et al.*, 1994; Ryberg *et al.*, 1994; Kondo *et al.*, 1996; Takeshima *et al.*, 1993; Suzuki *et al.*, 1992), and no well-designed epidemiological studies have specifically investigated this apparent correlation. Another 20% of lung tumours do not express G-T transversions in p53 genes, and 40% of all tumours exhibit no mutations in these genes. Although G to T transversions in ras alterations are found in animals exposed to benzo[a]pyrene, p53 mutations are rarely seen in these animal models of lung cancer, making it difficult to extrapolate these results to humans (Greenblatt *et al.*, 1994). It is therefore vital to distinguish between mutations related to specific exposures (mutational spectra) and those that are simply a consequence of tumour progression (Vineis & Caporaso, 1995). It is possible that a bias of patient selection may occur in many studies. For example, heavy-smoking patients with late-stage tumours may have a higher prevalence of p53 mutations due to tumour progression, and therefore any relationship between smoking and p53 is merely a consequence of confounding by tumour differentiation. Alternatively, the tumours studied may be overrepresented by surgically resectable specimens, therefore reflecting the small proportion of early-stage resectable tumours. The study of the interaction of somatic molecular events with environmental exposures is extremely complex, and continued investigation of the p53 gene in large cohort investigations with good measures of environmental exposures may help towards understanding these complexities.

Although molecular biologists know that alterations in specific DNA sequences progress to cancer, the risk and protective factors that influence these alterations and exactly how they operate remain unknown. Therefore, studies of the characteristics of somatic alterations may aid epidemiologists in segregating the relative effects of various risk factors in the etiology and pathogenesis of cancer. In addition, monitoring somatic mutations in vivo may eventually be a useful biological marker for evaluating cancer risk from exposure to environmental mutagens (Perera & Whyatt, 1994; Suk et al., 1996). The analysis of somatic genetic alterations and their relationship to environmental exposures and endogenous molecular processes in human

tumours can be expected to prove an invaluable adjunct to the study of epidemiological risk factors in cancer.

Relationship to genetic changes
Germline mutations
For a small percentage of the population, the inheritance of a specific defective gene significantly increases the risk of developing cancer (Li, 1995). Individuals with inherited tumour-suppressor defects have an increased frequency of somatic mutations and cancers (Harris, 1996; Li, 1995; Knudson, 1994). The activation of several oncogenes and tumour-suppressor genes is necessary to initiate tumours, but for those individuals who inherit a tumor-suppressor gene defect, one less genetic event is necessary in the accumulation of mutations to induce a cancer. Table 1 presents several examples of tumour-suppressor genes involved in both autosomal dominant inheritance as well somatic mutations in human cancer.

Products of tumour-suppressor genes normally block abnormal growth and malignant transformation and contribute to malignancy only when the function of both alleles is lost. Knudson (1971) described his "two-hit" hypothesis based on the age distribution of retinoblastoma in

Tumour-suppressor gene	Locus	Somatic mutations		Inherited mutations	
		Major types	Neoplasms	Syndrome	Neoplasms
p53	17p	Missense	Most human cancer types	Li-Fraumeni	Sarcomas, and breast and brain carcinomas
RB1	13q	Deletion or nonsense	Retinoblastoma, osteosarcoma, carcinomas of the breast, prostate, bladder and lung	Retinoblastoma	Retinoblastoma, osteosarcoma
APC	5q	Deletion or nonsense	Carcinomas of the colon, stomach and pancreas	Familial adenomatous polyposis	Carcinomas of colon, thyroid and stomach
NF1	17q	Deletion	Schwannomas	Neurofibromatosis type 1	Neural tumours

Table 1. Examples of tumour-suppressor genes involved in both somatic and inherited human cancers

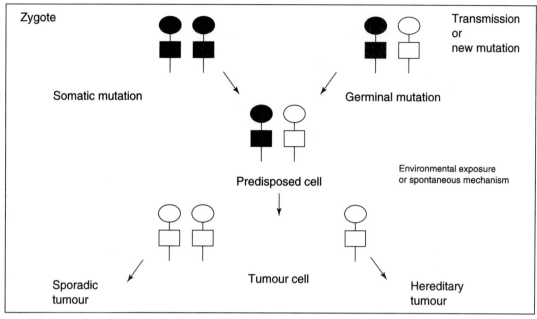

Figure 2. Knudson's two-hit hypothesis differentiating between hereditary and somatic tumours

hereditary and sporadic forms (Fig. 2). In the hereditary form, the first mutation of a tumour-suppressor gene is carried in the germline and a second mutation (due to environmental or spontaneous mechanisms) results in inactivation of tumour-suppressor function, giving rise to the tumour. Both mutations occur in the same somatic cell in the sporadic form.

Li-Fraumeni cancer syndrome (LFS)
In an analogous manner, germline mutations in the p53 tumour-suppressor gene are observed in approximately half of all families with Li-Fraumeni cancer syndrome (LFS) (Malkin et al., 1990). These rare cancer families have a striking history of a variety of forms of cancer at a very early age including several kinds of sarcoma, brain and breast cancer. p53 was considered a candidate for the gene responsible for LFS since this gene is inactivated in the sporadic forms of many cancers (Strong et al., 1992). LFS is an example of a collection of cancers that occur in both familial and sporadic form. In the familial form, one of the two mutations necessary to inactivate the p53 gene is present in the germline, but in the sporadic form both mutations are somatic events. Carriers of a mutated p53 gene in fami-

lies exhibiting Li-Fraumeni syndrome have a 50% chance of developing cancer by the age of 35, and their risk may increase to 90% by the age of 65 (Malkin et al., 1990; Strong et al., 1992).

LFS and somatic alterations
Although inherited p53 mutations are present in all somatic cells, malignant transformation is limited to certain organs and target cells. This knowledge can be used to explore both the timing of somatic p53 alterations and their etiology in sporadic cancers (Keihues et al., 1997). A comparison of the origin of tumours associated with p53 germline mutations with the incidence of somatic p53 mutations in respective sporadic tumours can designate organs in which p53 mutations are likely to initiate malignant transformation rather than being a late event in tumour progression. For example, the fractions of tumours in families with p53 germline mutation is highest for sarcomas (24% of tumours), breast cancer (24%) and brain tumours (13%) and is similar to the incidence of somatic p53 mutations in these sporadic tumours. These observations suggest that p53 mutations are capable of initiating the process of malignant transformation in these tumours. Various neoplasms also

show a high incidence of somatic p53 mutations but are rarely associated with p53 germline mutations. These include lung, colon, liver and gastric cancers. There could be a number of reasons for this discrepancy. One possibility is that p53 mutation is a late alteration in tumorigenesis of these tumour types and other earlier alterations must occur to initiate carcinogenesis, as in colon cancer (i.e. apc, Kras) (Fearon, 1993). Additionally, individuals with p53 germline mutations may not reach the age by which they would develop these cancer types, since these tumours typically occur in later years. A related possibility is that additional environmental influences are necessary for malignant transformation, such as smoking in lung carcinoma and AFB1 or HBV in liver cancer. It is interesting that familial clustering of gastric carcinoma in association with p53 germline mutation has only been observed in Japan (Horio et al., 1994). Epidemiological studies indicate that Japan's high incidence of gastric cancer is probably due to particular dietary exposures (Haenszel & Kurihara, 1968). Other host factors, such as a particular genetic background including specific metabolic polymorphic genes, may also be involved.

Hereditary nonpolyposis colorectal cancer (HNPCC)
A colorectal cancer syndrome that has recently been attributed to a deficiency in DNA repair may occur in 5-10% of individuals developing colorectal cancer (Lynch & Smyrk, 1996). Hereditary nonpolyposis colorectal cancer (HNPCC) is an autosomal dominant disorder characterized by the onset of colorectal cancer at an average age of 44 (Lynch et al., 1992). Phenotypically, HNPCC patients differ from familial adenomatous polyposis (FAP) patients as no polyposis is present. Therefore, until recently an extensive family history of colorectal cancer was the only way to identify HNPCC. Germline mutations for HNPCC have now been identified on chromosomes 2, 3 and 7 which cause DNA instability due to defective mismatch repair (or replication error repair, (RER)) mechanisms (Lynch & Smyrk, 1996). Patients with HPNCC have inherited one normal and one mutant mismatch repair gene allele. While normal cells from these patients do not display any genetic instability or mismatch

repair deficiency, tumour cells have lost or mutated the remaining normal allele, resulting in genomic instability.

HNPCC and somatic alterations
The significance of DNA repair deficiency in the carcinogenic process is that these abnormalities cause multiple and sequential somatic alterations in cells, promoting the evolution of genetic changes with a bearing on the development of cancer. It was recently reported that inactivation of the transforming growth factor β (TGF-β) receptor gene occurs almost uniformly among tumours with replication error repair phenotypes (Parsons et al., 1996). TGF-β II is a multifunction growth factor that regulates cell differentiation and the expression of extracelluar matrix protein, and inhibits the growth of many cells, including the epithelial cell type (Wrana et al., 1994). When these receptors are inactivated the cells lose their responsiveness to TGF-β. This loss of growth inhibition may be an important step in the tumorigenesis of some cancers. It is therefore believed that DNA mismatch repair defect targets microsatellite sequences of TGF-β gene and inactivates it through somatic mutation (Parsons et al., 1996).

Metabolic polymorphisms
As advances in molecular biology make it possible to examine genetic factors on a population level our knowledge of the interaction between genetic susceptibility to cancer and environmental exposures will be greatly increased. Due to cost and labour limitations, previous studies of gene-environment interaction have been confined to investigations of simply one metabolic polymorphism or somatic alteration. Technical advances can be expected to facilitate the study of critical interactions between gene and environment by investigating etiological exposures and their influence on several areas of host genetic susceptibility factors.

Metabolic polymorphisms and somatic alterations
One way to enhance the study of etiological pathways in carcinogenesis is to examine the association of somatic alterations at different steps of cancer progression. The study of specific markers, as in the Vogelstein model (Fearon & Vogelstein, 1990), in relation to exposure, may explain the

association between known risk factors and genetic alterations (Fig.1). Examining the hypothesis that a specific carcinogen or its metabolite is selectively metabolized by either detoxification or activation by specific drug/xenobiotic metabolizing enzymes can indicate a common susceptibility to cancer. Extending these studies, the specific carcinogens generated may subsequently interact with specific gene sequences to selectively induce mutations (Fig. 1). Therefore, the inheritance of a specific genotype (e.g. GSTM1 null, mutant BRCA1) may increase the probability of mutations occurring at etiological loci (e.g. p53, ras) with exposure to an environmental carcinogen (e.g. smoking).

p53, EPHX, GSTM1 and AFB1 in HCC

A study on the association of environmental exposures, their detoxification enzymes, and resulting somatic alterations was recently reported by McGlynn et al. (1995). Primary hepatocellular carcinoma, a tumour common in East Asia and southern Africa, has been attributed to risk factors of hepatitis B virus and exposure to a mycotoxin, AFB1, a contaminant found in various foods of these regions. In vitro experiments have demonstrated that AFB1 mutagenic metabolites bind to DNA and produce specific G to T transversions. Interestingly, in HCC endemic areas an unusual mutational hot spot has been reported on the p53 gene at codon 249 and G-to-T transversions. McGlynn et al. conducted a case-control study in Shanghai, China, of 52 individuals with HCC and 116 healthy controls, in order to investigate whether the specific polymorphisms of the metabolizing enzymes EPHX and GSTM1, which metabolize AFB1, were related to HCC and p53 codon 249 mutation. The results indicated that the GSTM1 null and mutant allele 2 of EPHX were significantly more common in cases than controls. p53 codon 249 mutations were detected in 10 of 52 tumour samples. All 10 of the mutations occurred in tumours from individuals with the mutant allele 2 EPHX alleles and 8 of them occurred in individuals with the GSTM1 null genotype. These investigators concluded that susceptibility to AFB1-induced hepatocellular carcinoma was associated with low activity of the detoxification enzymes epoxide hydratase and GSTM1 genotypes, resulting in increased p53 mutations.

p53, Ki-ras, CYP1A1, GSTM1 and smoking in lung cancer

Another good example of incorporating the study of metabolic polymorphism with somatic alterations has recently been reported by Kawajiri et al. (1996.). Primary tumour and normal lung tissues were obtained from 187 NSCLC patients undergoing surgery at Saitama Cancer Centre Hospital. Tumour tissue was analysed for p53 and Ki-ras mutations, while normal tissue was analysed for specific polymorphisms of the metabolizing CYP1A1 and GSTM1 genes. The results suggested that smokers showed a higher frequency of p53 gene mutation in a dose-response manner, although no association with Ki-ras was apparent. An increase in the mutational frequency of both p53 and Ki-ras was proportional to the number of susceptible alleles, including the MspI polymorphism of the CYP1A1 gene, which has been associated with smoking-induced lung cancer. The patients with the recessive homozygote (C or m2/m2) genotypes were at a fivefold higher risk of having a mutation in Ki-ras or p53 mutation than those with a homozygote genotype (A or m1/m1). The patients with the recessive homozygote (C or m2/m2) genotypes were at a fifteenfold higher risk of having simultaneous mutations in both p53 and Ki-ras genes than those with homozygote genotypes (A or m1/m1). A ninefold to elevenfold increased probability of having mutations of the p53 and Ki-ras genes was observed in combined recessive homozygote (C or m2/m2) CYP1A1 and GSTM1 null genotypes among smokers, although no specific type of p53 or ras mutations were detected. These findings suggest that the synergistic increase in the mutation frequency of the p53 gene among individuals with particular genotypes of CYP1A1 and GSTM1 is consistent with increased polycyclic aromatic hydrocarbon adduct formation, resulting in an increased probability of p53 mutations in smoking-induced lung cancer. A recent study of epithelial ovarian cancer also reported that p53 mutations in patients' tumours were significantly more common among individuals who were GSTM1 null (Sarhanis et al., 1996). These are a few of the first examples of how genetic differences in carcinogen metabolizing enzymes among individuals may be one of the important determinants of chemically induced damage to somatic alterations and therefore of cancer susceptibility.

Relationship to disease

Prognosis

The identification of specific pathological parameters which predict prognoses for patients with various malignancies may help to enhance our ability to define subgroups of patients with different disease courses and treatment responses. In particular, survival analysis of somatic alterations has been pursued in the hope of improving therapy for patients with particular tumour characteristics. During the past five years there has been an exponential growth in the number of studies on the value of the p53 tumour-suppressor gene in cancer prognosis because of its acknowledged importance in human cancer.

The p53 gene is the most common genetic abnormality in human malignancies, and mutant protein expression (overexpression), which is frequently associated with p53 mutation, can be simply detected using immunohistochemical techniques. Biologically, since p53 normal function induces apoptosis and preserves genetic stability, loss of function is likely to be associated with tumour progression. Both experiments on animals and in vitro investigations support the hypothesis that p53 is an important prognostic indicator.

Many investigations have been undertaken to examine whether p53 alterations may be associated with poor prognosis in cohorts of patients with particular neoplasms. One example of a typical investigation of this type is an immunohistochemical study of p53 protein overexpression in transitional cell carcinoma of the upper urinary tract (Nakanishi et al., 1996). The investigators examined 149 formalin-fixed paraffin-embedded tumour tissues from patients diagnosed as having transitional cell carcinoma of the upper urinary tract. Tumours were stained with an anti-p53 antibody, and were considered positive if 10% or more of tumour cells were positive for p53 overexpression, and negative if less than 10% of tumour cells were positive for p53 nuclear overexpression. Overall, 26.8% of samples were found to be positive for p53 overexpression. Expression of p53 was significantly associated with the estab-

lished clinicopathological indicators of stage and grade. A univariate analysis indicated that stage, grade and p53 overexpression were each significantly associated with overall survival. In the multivariate analysis only stage and p53 overexpression were independent prognostic indicators.

This study is just one example of the many prognostic investigations of p53 somatic alterations, and can be used to explore the many technical and epidemiological limitations that may distort results. Interpretation of this type of study is often difficult since studies may differ in the way p53 mutation is detected; some use sequencing, SSCP or other less sensitive techniques (Hall et al., 1994; Dowell & Hall, 1995). The majority of studies use immunohistochemistry to define protein overexpression, which is frequently but not always associated with p53 mutation. Immunohistochemistry adds additional problems since the choice of antibodies, antibody concentrations, and protocols including microwave antigen retrieval techniques, may vary considerably between studies. Furthermore, the assumed high correlation between p53 mutation and overexpression differs according to the tumour type. An arbitrary percentage of tumour cells (e.g. 10%) is often used to distinguish tumours considered to be p53 mutation positive from those considered to be p53 negative. While most studies define an arbitrary a priori cut-off, others examine the correlation between p53 mutation and immunohistochemistry by analysing a subset of their samples for p53 mutation. Other investigators choose the best separation of p53 categories with respect to clinical outcome. To further complicate interpretation, studies often differ with respect to patient selection criteria, tissue processing and interpretation of data.

Statistical analysis may also distort results and subsequent conclusions, particularly in the examination of the independence of p53 as a prognostic variable. Since p53 is often highly correlated with grade and stage it is frequently a prognostic indicator when examined by itself in univariate analysis. Evaluation of the data by multivariate methods is therefore a necessary step in assessing whether p53 is an independent prognostic indicator. Often only large studies can be used to evaluate certain markers using a multivariate analysis, particularly if there is only a modest association between the marker and survival. Future large studies examining survival parameters in relation to specific somatic alterations (e.g. mutant p53) and metabolic polymorphisms (e.g. GSTM1 null) may enhance our ability to predict prognosis and provide more individualized treatment.

Concluding remarks

Molecular epidemiology has the opportunity to confront disease at the molecular level and consider the complex interactions between somatic alterations, etiological exposures and inherent genetic differences. Current and newly available technology can be expected to simplify the analysis of a multitude of genetic polymorphisms, using small samples of genomic DNA which are easily accessible from archival paraffin blocks, hair follicles or buccal swabs. Improved analysis of somatic alterations should become possible by microdissection and comparative genome hybridization techniques. These advances in technology should augment the number of "genetic studies" undertaken and expand the number of hypotheses that may be pursued. Future studies can be expected to examine a number of etiological exposures, somatic alterations and perhaps several inherited susceptibility factors concurrently, including metabolic polymorphisms, germline cancer-predisposing mutations, and DNA repair capacities. A serious interdisciplinary approach will be needed to integrate information and technology from various biomedical fields into appropriate study designs for the examination of cancer susceptibility.

It is important to consider that although molecular epidemiological studies of somatic alteration or other genetic changes may have a large genetic component, they must be guided by good epidemiological principles. Careful consideration must be given to prevent bias in the design, analysis and interpretation of these studies. The interpretation of any associations should have a sound biological foundation in which the associations are assessed in terms of etiological mechanisms and disease progression within the context of the carcinogenic processes, and should not depend on statistical associations generated without appropriate prior evaluation of the biological basis. In addition to biological plausibility, other important factors in the interpretation of associations must include the strength of the association, possible dose-response effects, temporality, and the consistency of the associations in multiple studies.

References

Albertini, R.J., Nicklas, J.A. & O'Neill, J.P. (1996) Future research directions for evaluating human genetic and cancer risk from environmental exposures. *Environ.Health Perspect.*, 104, 503-510

Bennett, W.P., Hollstein, M.C., He, A., Zhu, S.M., Resau, J.H., Trump, B.F., Metcalf, R.A., Welsh, J.A., Midgley, C., Lane, D.P. & Harris, C.C. (1991) Archival analysis of p53 genetic and protein alterations in Chinese oesophageal cancer. *Oncogene*, 6, 1779-1784

Bos, J.L. (1988) The ras gene family and human carcinogenesis. *Mutat. Res.*, 195, 255-271

Brash, D.E., Rudolph, J.A., Simon, J.A., Lin, A., Mckenna, G.J., Baden, H.P., Halperin, A.J. & Ponten, J. (1991) A role for sunlight in skin cancer: UV-induced p53 mutations in squamous cell carcinoma. *Proc. Natl. Acad. Sci. USA*, 88, 10124-10128

Bressac, B., Kew, M., Wands, J. & Ozturk, M. (1991) Selective G to T mutations of p53 gene in hepatocellular carcinoma from southern Africa. *Nature*, 350, 429-431

Busby, W.F. & Wogan, G.N. (1984) Aflatoxins. In: Searle, C.E., ed, *Chemical Carcinogens. Volume 2.* Washington DC, American Chemical Society, pp. 945-1136

Chen, R.H., Maher, V.M. & McCormick, J.J. (1990) Effect of excision repair by diploid human fibroblasts on the kinds and locations of mutations induced by (+/-)-7 beta, 8 alpha-dihydroxy-9 alpha, 10 alpha-epoxy-7,8,9,10-tetrahydrobenzo[a]pyrene in the coding region of the HPRT gene. *Proc. Natl. Acad. Sci. USA*, 87, 8680-8684

Chiba, I., Takahashi, T., Nau, M.M., D'Amico, D., Curiel, D.T., Mitsudomi, T., Buchhagen, D.L., Carbone, D., Piantadosi, S. & Koga, H. (1990) Mutations in the p53 gene are frequent in primary, resected non-small cell lung cancer. *Oncogene*, 5, 1603-1610

Counts, J. & Goodman J. (1995) Alterations in DNA methylation may play a variety of roles in carcinogenesis. *Cell*, 83, 13-15

Denissenko, M.F., Pao, A., Tang, M. & Pfeifer, G.P. (1996) Preferential formation of benzo[a]pyrene adducts at lung cancer mutational hotspots in p53. *Science*, 274, 430-432

Dogliotti, E. (1996) Mutational spectra: from model systems to cancer-related genes. *Carcinogenesis*, 17, 2113-2118

Dowell, P. & Hall, P. (1995) The p53 tumour-suppressor gene and tumour prognosis: is there a relationship? *J. Pathol.*, 177, 221-224

Dumaz, N., Stary, A., Soussi, T., Daya-Grosjean, L. & Sarasin, A. (1994) Can we predict solar UV radiation as the causal event in human tumours by analysing the mutation spectra of the p53 gene? *Mutat. Res.*, 307, 375-386

Fearon, E.R. (1993) Molecular genetic studies of the adenoma-carcinoma sequence. *Adv. Intern. Med.*, 39, 123-147

Fearon, E.R. & Vogelstein, B.(1990) A genetic model for colorectal tumorigenesis. *Cell*, 61, 759-776

Foulds, L. (1958) The natural history of cancer. *J. Chron. Dis.*, 8, 2

Friend, S.H., Dryja, T.P. & Wienberg, R.A. (1988) Oncogenes and tumour-suppressing genes. *N. Engl. J. Med.*, 52, 1651-1659

Greenblatt, M.S., Bennett, W.P., Hollstein, M. & Harris C.C. (1994) Mutations in the p53 tumour suppressor gene: clues to cancer etiology and molecular pathogenesis. *Cancer Res.*, 54, 4855-4878

Haenszel, W. & Kurihara, M. (1968) Studies of Japanese migrants. I. Mortality from cancer and other diseases among Japanese in the United States. *J. Natl. Cancer Inst.*, 40, 43-68

Hall, P.A. & Lane, D.P. (1994) P53 in tumour pathology: can we trust immunohistochemistry?- revisited. *J. Pathol.*, 172, 1-4

Harris, C.C. (1991) Chemical and physical carcinogenesis: advances and perspectives for the 1990s. *Cancer Res.*, 51 (Suppl.), 5023s-5044s

Harris, C.C. (1996) p53 tumour-suppressor gene: at the crossroads of molecular carcinogenesis, molecular epidemiology, and cancer risk assessment. *Env. Health Perspect.*, 104, 435-439

Hecht, S.S., Carmella, S.G., Murphy, S.E., Foiles, P.G. & Chung F.L. (1993) Carcinogen biomarkers related to smoking and upper aerodigestive tract cancer. *J. Cell Biochem.* (Suppl. 17F), 27-35

Hedrick, L., Cho, K.R., Fearon, E.R., Wu, T.C., Kinzler, K.W. & Vogelstein, B. (1994) The DCC gene product in cellular differentiation and colorectal tumorigenesis. *Genes Dev.*, 8, 1174

Hollstein, M., Shomer, B., Greenblatt, M., Soussi, T., Hovig, E., Montesano, R. & Harris, C.C. (1996) Somatic point mutations in the p53 gene of human tumours and cell lines: updated compilation. *Nucleic Acids Res.*, 24, 141-146

Hollstein, M., Sidransky, D., Vogelstein, B. & Harris C.C. (1991) P53 mutations in human cancers. *Science*, 253, 49-53

Horio, Y., Suzuki, H., Ueda, R., Koshikawa, T., Sugiura, T., Ariyoshi, Y., Shimokata, K. & Takahashi T. (1994) Predominantly tumour-limited expression of a mutant allele in a Japanese family carrying a germline p53 mutation. *Oncogene*, 19, 1231-1235

Hsu, I.C., Metcalf, R.A., Sun, T., Welsh, J.A., Wang, N.J. & Harris, C.C. (1991) Mutational hotspot in the p53 gene in human hepatocellular carcinomas. *Nature*, 350, 427-428

International Agency for Research on Cancer. (1994) Hepatitis viruses. In: *IARC monographs on the evaluation of carcinogenic risk to humans, Vol. 59.* Lyon, IARC, pp. 45-255

Kawajiri, K., Eguchi, H., Nakachi, K., Sekiya, T. & Yamamoto, M. (1996) Association of CYP1A1 germ line polymorphisms with mutations of the p53 gene in lung cancer. *Cancer Res.*, 56, 72-76

Keihues, P., Schauble, B., Hausen, A.Z., Esteve, J. & Ohgaki, H. (1997) Tumours associated with p53 germline mutations: a synopsis of 91 families. *Am. J. Pathol.*, 150, 1-13

Knudson, A.G. (1971) Mutation and cancer: statistical study of retinoblastoma. *Proc. Natl. Acad. Sci. USA*, 68, 820-823

Knudson, A.G. (1994) Hereditary cancer, oncogenes, and anti-oncogenes. *Cancer Res.*, 45, 1437-1443

Kondo, K., Tsuzuki, H., Sasa, M., Sumitomo, M., Uyama, T. & Monden, Y. (1996) A dose-response relationship between the frequency of p53 mutations and tobacco consumption in lung cancer patients. *J. Surg. Oncol.*, 61, 20-26

Li, F.P. (1995) Inherited susceptibility to cancer: from epidemiology to interventional research. *Proc. Am. Assoc. Cancer Res.*, 36, 648

Lindahl, T. (1993) Instability and decay of the primary structure of DNA. *Nature*, 362, 709-715

Lynch, H.T. & Smyrk, T. (1996) Hereditary non-polyposis colorectal cancer (Lynch syndrome): an updated review. *Cancer*, 78, 1149-1167

Lynch, H.T., Watson, P., Smyrk, T.C., Lanspa, S.J., Bonan, B.M., Boland, C.R., Lynch, J.F., Cavalieri, R.J., Leppert, M., White, R., Sidransky, D. & Vogelstein, B. (1992) Colon cancer genetics. *Cancer Suppl.*, 70, 1300-1311

Malkin, F., Li, F.P., Strong, L.C., Fraumeni, J.F. Jr., Nelson, C.E., Kim, D.H., Kassel, J., Gryka, M.A., Bischoff, F.Z., Tainsky, M.A. & Friend, S.H. (1990) Germline p53 mutants in familial syndrome of breast cancer, sarcomas, and other neoplaasms. *Science*, 250, 1233-1238

Manolov, G. & Manolova, Y. (1973) Marker band in one chromosome 14 from Burkitt lymphoma. *Nature*, 237, 33-34

McGlynn, K.A., Rosvold, E.A., Lustbader, E.D., Hu, Y., Clapper, M.L., Zhou, T., Wild, C.P., Xia, X-L., Baffoe-Bonnie, A., Ofori-Adjei, D., Chen, G.C., London, W.T., Shen, F-U. & Buetow, K.H. (1995) Susceptibility to hepatocellular carcinoma is associated with genetic variation in the enzymatic detoxification of aflatoxin B_1. *Proc. Nat. Acad. Sci. USA*, 92, 2384-2387

McMichael, A.J. (1994) "Molecular epidemiology": new pathway or new travelling companion? *Am. J. Epidemiol.*, 140, 1-11

Miller, B.A., Ries, L.A.G., Hankey, B.F., Kosary, C.L., Harras, A., Devesa, S.S. & Edward, B.K., eds. (1993) *SEER cancer statistics review: 1973-1990.* National Cancer Institute. NIH Pub. No. 93-2789

Nakanishi, K., Kawai, T. & Torikata, C. (1996) Immunohistochemical evaluation of p53 oncoprotein in transitional cell carcinoma of the upper urinary tract. *Hum. Pathol.*, 27, 1336-1340

Nuorva, K., Makitaro, R., Huhti, E., Kamel, D., Vahakangas, K., Bloigu, R., Soini, Y. & Paakko, P. (1994) p53 protein accumulation in lung carcinomas of patients exposed to asbestos and tobacco smoke. *Am. J. Respir. Crit. Care Med.*, 150, 528-533

Parsons, R., Myeroff, L., Liu, B., Willson, J.K.V., Markowitz, S., Kinzler, K.W. & Vogelstein, B. (1996) Microsatellite instability and mutations of the transforming growth factor B type II receptor gene in colorectal cancer. *Cancer Res.*, 55, 5548-5550

Perera, F.P. & Whyatt, R.M. (1994) Biomarkers and molecular epidemiology in mutation/cancer research. *Mutat. Res.*, 313, 11-129

Powell, S.M., Zilz, N., Beazer-Barclay, Y., Bryan, T.M., Hamilton, S.R., Thibodeau, S.N., Vogelstein, B. & Kinzler, K.W. (1992) APC mutations occur early during colorectal tumorigenesis. *Nature*, 359, 235-237

Puisieux, A., Lim, S., Groopman, J. & Ozturk, M. (1991) Selective targeting of p53 gene mutational hotspots in human cancers by etiologically defined carcinogens, *Cancer Res.*, 51, 6185-6189

Ross, R., Yuan, J.M., Yu, M., Wogan, G.N., Qian, G.S., Tu, J.T., Groopman, J.D., Gao, Y.T. & Henderson, B.E. (1992) Urinary aflatoxin biomarkers and risk of hepatocellular carcinoma. *Lancet*, 339, 943-946

Rowley, J.D. (1973) A new consistent chromosome abnormality in chronic myelogenous leukaemia identified by quinacrine flourescene and Giemsa staining. *Nature*, 243, 290-293

Ryberg, D., Kure, E., Lystad, S., Skaug, V., Stangeland, L., Mercy, I., Borresen, A.L. & Haugen, A. (1994) p53 mutations in lung tumours: relationship to putative susceptibility markers for cancer. *Cancer Res.*, 54, 1551-1555

Sandberg, A.A. (1979) Before 1956: some historical background to study of the chromosomes in human cancer and leukaemia. *Cancer Genet. Cytogenet.*, 1, 87-94

Sarhanis, P., Redman, C., Perrett, C., Brannigan, K., Clayton, R.N., Hand, P., Musgrove, C., Suarez, V., Jones, P., Fryer, A.A., Farrell, W.E. & Strange, R.C. (1996) Epithelial ovarian cancer: influence of polymorphism at the glutathione-S-transferase GSTM1 and GSTT1 loci on p53 expression. *Br. J. Cancer*, 74, 1757-1761

Schulte, P.A. & Perera, F.P., eds. (1993) *Molecular Epidemiology: Principles and Practices*. San Diego, Academic Press, Harcourt Brace and Company

Shen, H.M. & Ong, C.N. (1996) Mutations of the p53 tumour-suppressor gene and ras oncogenes in aflatoxin hepatocarcinogenesis. *Mutat. Res.*, 366, 23-44

Strong, L.C., Williams, W.R. & Tainsky, M.A. (1992) The Li-Fraumeni syndrome: from clinical epidemiology to molecular genetics. *Am. J. Epidemiol.*, 135, 190-199

Suk, W.A., Collman, G. & Damstra, T. (1996) Human monitoring: research goals and needs. *Environ. Health Perspect.*,104, 479-483

Suzuki, H., Takahashi, T., Kuroishi, T., Suyama, M., Ariyoshi, Y. & Ueda, R. (1992) p53 mutations in non-small cell lung cancer in Japan: association between mutations and smoking. *Cancer Res.*, 52, 734-736

Takahashi, T., Suzuki, H., Hida, T., Sekido, Y., Ariyoshi, Y. & Ueda, R. (1991) The p53 gene is very frequently mutated in small-cell lung cancer with a distinct nucleotide substitution pattern. *Oncogene*, 6, 1775-1778

Takeshima, Y., Seyama, T., Bennett, W.P., Akiyama, M., Tokuoka, S., Inai, K., Mabuchi, K., Land, C.E. & Harris C.C. (1993) p53 mutations in lung cancers from non-smoking atomic-bomb survivors. *Lancet*, 342, 1520-1521

Vineis, P. & Caporaso, N. (1995) Tobacco and cancer: epidemiology and the laboratory. *Environ. Health Perspect.*, 103, 156-160

Vogelstein, B., Fearon, E.R., Hamilton, S.R., Kern, S.E., Preisinger, A.C., Leppert, M., Nakamura, Y., White, R., Smits, A.M.M. & Bos, J.L. (1988) Genetic alterations during colorectal tumour development. *N. Engl. J. Med.*, 319, 525-532

Wogan, G.N. (1992) Aflatoxins as risk factors for hepatocellular carcinoma in humans. *Cancer Res.*, 52, 2114s-2118s

Wrana, J.L., Attisano, L., Weiser, R., Ventura, F. & Massague, J. (1994) Mechanism of activation of the TGF-B receptor. *Nature*, 370, 341-347

You, M., Candrian, U., Maronpot, R.R., Stoner, G.D. & Anderson, M.W. (1989) Activation of the Ki-ras protooncogene in spontaneously occurring and chemically induced lung tumours of the strain A mouse. *Proc. Natl. Acad. Sci. USA*, 86, 3070-3074

Andrew N. Freedman
National Cancer Institute,
Genetic Epidemiology Branch,
Executive Plaza North, Rm. 313,
6130 Executive Blvd., MSC 7344,
Bethesda, MD 20892-7344, USA

Metabolic Polymorphisms and Susceptibility to Cancer
W. Ryder
IARC Scientific Publications No. 148
International Agency for Research on Cancer, Lyon, 1999

Chapter 6. Strategic issues in the design and interpretation of studies on metabolic polymorphisms and cancer

Paolo Vineis and Núria Malats

This Chapter describes in a simple way the most important issues of epidemiological design, with emphasis on studies on metabolic polymorphisms. Different options are offered to the researcher who approaches a molecular epidemiology study. Case-control studies and cohort studies have different and sometimes complementary advantages and disadvantages. The sources of bias and the choice of controls, with specific problems in the context of investigations on metabolic polymorphisms, are key issues. Confounding is an issue that needs further clarification in the field, partly because of the lack of complete biological knowledge on the complex relationships between exposure, markers of susceptibility, and cancer. Metabolic polymorphisms are correctly interpreted as effect modifiers of the exposure-disease relationship. This interpretation implies that studies should be planned in order to have sufficient statistical power and that an interactive term should be modelled in the statistical analysis.

A large number of genes coding for molecules (enzymes and receptors) involved in xenobiotic metabolism have been characterized in humans. Genetic polymorphisms of several phase I enzymes (CYP1A1, CYP1A2, CYP2A6, CYP2D6, CYP2E1), phase II enzymes (GSTM1, GSTM3, GSTs, NAT1, NAT2), and members of the nuclear receptor family (estrogen receptor, aryl hydroxylase receptor) have shown an association with an increased risk of cancer. For other metabolic enzymes the evidence of a relationship with cancer remains equivocal. Further research is needed that takes into account the combined effect of different polymorphisms, exposures, and co-factors on cancer etiology. One important issue, drawn from a recent review on this topic (d'Errico *et al.*, 1996) is the heterogeneity in the design, the conduct and, consequently, the findings of epidemiological studies on metabolic polymorphisms and cancer risk. The analysis of the effects of metabolic polymorphisms on cancer development raises a number of methodological issues that should be carefully addressed before extensive studies are conducted. Some of them are considered below.

Test validation: enzyme inducibility, genotype-phenotype correlation, and distribution of polymorphisms by ethnic group, gender and other covariates; reliability and accuracy of tests, sources of error

What is relevant to cancer is the metabolic status (phenotype) of the individual at the time when carcinogenesis begins, probably more than ten years before the diagnosis of the most common cancers. Because it is impossible to obtain this information except in the context of cohort studies (although such a design has not been applied to metabolic susceptibility studies until now), researchers use "surrogates" of former metabolism status such as "phenotype at present time" or genotype. Several matters have to be considered in respect of the use of such "surrogates". The most important is that phenotype is a very complex phenomenon in which multiple and unknown factors are suspected to be involved. Secondly, for some enzymes there is no definite evidence of phenotypic variation (CYP1A1, CYP1A2, CYP3A, GSTs). Thirdly, since the phenotype is not stable over time, the correlation between past and present phenotype may vary depending on numerous factors, both endogenous (i.e. hormone status, oxidative stress, age, previous and present diseases) and exogenous (i.e. drugs, diet, environmental exposures), that can induce or inhibit enzymatic activity. Finally, measurement of enzymatic activity is cumbersome, both *in vivo* and *in vitro*, and is not easily obtainable in target tissues. Although genotypes are much easier to determine with current techniques and are not influenced by other factors, they have not been always identified (CYP1A2, CYP2D6) and their association with phenotype has not been well elucidated for some enzymes (CYP2E1, NAT2, CYP2D6, CYP1A1). For instance, three main slow-acetylator alleles and a large number of minor rare alleles for the NAT2 enzyme which make the phenotype-genotype correlation more difficult to interpret have been identified (Nebert, 1997). Despite the complexity of this phenomenon, there is a need to study in greater depth the genotype-phenotype relationship for most of the enzymes before they can be used as markers of susceptibility in large epidemiological studies (see Chapter 8).

The geographical distribution of metabolic polymorphisms is highly variable *according to segregation rules*. Briefly, the NAT2 phenotype was classified as slow or rapid acetylator according to the isoniazid metabolism. The frequency of slow acetylators is 50% among Caucasians, 10% among Japanese, and >90% in African populations. Regarding CYP2D6, two phenotypes have been described, poor and extensive debrisoquine metabolizers. The frequency of poor metabolizers is 6-10% in Caucasians, 4-5% in Blacks, and <1% in Asians. For CYP1A1, two CYP1A1 genetic polymorphisms were described ten years ago (Msp I and Ile/Val) and the frequency of the rare allele is <1% in Caucasians and 5-20% in Asians. Recently, Taioli *et al.* (1995) described a new genetic polymorphism in CYP1A1 (MspI in intron 7) present in 15% of African-Americans but absent in Caucasians and Asians.

Nebert (1997) provides two possible explanations for the different allelic frequencies in populations: (1) they could reflect different dietary exposures over the course of evolution, i.e. some alleles conferred evolutionary advantage in people exposed to food toxins; or (2) they could represent the selection of more resistant individuals on the basis of their genetic make-up.

Regarding phenotypic analysis, enzyme activity can be tested *in vitro*, using cultured peripheral blood lymphocytes or other cell types, and *in vivo* by measuring the metabolite(s) of an enzyme-specific probe in urine or blood. Neither of these approaches allows the classification of cases in precise categories according to enzyme activity. The application of phenotyping in epidemiological studies raises other practical and ethical problems extensively discussed by Benhamou *et al.* in Chapter 7. For genotype analysis, genomic DNA can be obtained from a wide variety of sources (i.e. blood, hair, urine sediment, swab, and paraffin-embedded tissue), amplified by polymerase chain reaction (PCR), and analysed with a variety of molecular techniques (i.e. restriction fragment length polymorphisms, Southern blot analysis, single-strand conformation polymorphism). Blömeke and Shields discuss these aspects in more detail in Chapter 13.

Among potential sources of error in the determination of enzyme activity are variation in: subject compliance; the dose of the substance administered; sample collection and storage; and the measurement of metabolites (see Chapter 7). Factors that can introduce errors in the genotype analysis are DNA degradation because of inappropiate sample collection and storage procedures, contamination during sample handling, false priming in PCR, polymerase fidelity, pseudogene detection, and low gel resolution (see Chapter 13). In order to characterize the magnitude of error, scientists should provide estimates of the accuracy of the test used, i.e. sensitivity and specificity. This is of great importance since misclassification determines the size of the study sample and affects the validity of the results (Hulka & Margolin, 1992; Rothman *et al.*, 1993). In Chapter 9, Rothman *et al.* provide examples of the effect of inaccuracies in genotype measurement depending on the prevalence of different polymorphisms.

Study design and choice of controls

The main types of design in epidemiology are cohort studies and case-control (case-referent) studies, which may include incident or prevalent cases. In addition, case-case studies, nested case-control studies, case-cohort studies, transitional studies, and meta-analysis have been introduced more recently and their application depends on the hypothesis to be tested and the means available. In Chapter 10 this issue is dealt with in greater depth by Boffetta and Pearce.

Case-control design

In a case-control design, "subjects are selected on the basis of whether they do (cases) or do not (controls) have a particular disease under study. The groups are then compared with respect to the proportion having a history of an exposure or characteristic of interest" (Hennekens & Buring, 1987). For example, cases may be affected by lung cancer, controls may be a sample of the general population, and the exposure/characteristic may be tobacco smoking *or* the CYP1A1 polymorphism.

In case-control studies, ascertainment of exposures/characteristics is usually retrospective, i.e. information is collected about the past and recent history of the subjects. While such exposures as those to smoking or asbestos vary over time, other characteristics are stable. A cross-sectional ascertainment of present smoking habits or a specific metabolic enzyme phenotype among cases and controls is not a completely valid choice, because most cases have probably changed their habits as a consequence of the disease, or their metabolic status has probably changed for the same reason. Chronic diseases like cancer are attributable to cumulative exposure over a long time; for example, the risk of lung cancer increases with the second power of the daily dose and the fourth power of smoking duration (Doll and Peto, 1978). Conversely, stable variables like gender, blood group and metabolic genotype can be validly measured with a cross-sectional design (e.g. the genotype in lymphocyte DNA of cases and controls).

In addition to the timing issue, a major problem in case-control studies is the quality of information, particularly when this is collected by interview. A serious limitation may be differential recall of exposure information by cases and controls (recall bias). This issue, obviously, is not relevant when blood is taken and biochemical or molecular measurements are made. However, the cross-sectional design creates problems - including various forms of bias - when the phenotype is measured, for example by HPLC analysis of caf-

feine metabolites. As Chapters 7 and 8 describe, cross-sectional measurement of the phenotype in cases and controls can be affected by several pitfalls.

Choice of controls

In theory, controls should be a representative sample of the source population generating the cases; in practice, the choice of controls has been quite variable. In the case of debrisoquine the controls selected in different investigations were healthy controls, heterogeneous groups of hospital patients, chronic pulmonary disease (COPD) patients matched to lung cancer cases, or urological controls matched to bladder cancer patients. The use of a specific group of patients as controls, in particular, is questionable if the phenotype is measured. In fact, we cannot rule out that the association we observe (for example, a higher proportion of rapid debrisoquine metabolizers in lung cancer patients) is due to an inverse association with the control disease; for example, COPD could, for some reason, be more frequent among poor metabolizers. Thus, choice of healthy versus hospitalized controls is preferable. However, hospital controls are usually included in studies on metabolic polymorphisms because of their higher response rate and compliance to the protocol, among other reasons. In the case of the genotype, which is stable over time, it is reasonable to think that the measurements represent the actual status of the subjects. On the other hand, the phenotype may change as a consequence of changing exposures (which induce or inhibit the enzyme activity), or as a consequence of the disease process itself or its treatment. Cancer, for example, implies metabolic changes that may alter the phenotypic status of the subjects. Cross-sectional measurements in accordance with a case-control design may therefore be misleading if disease-related metabolic impairment is not considered.

Case-case design

This approach is used to estimate the association between exposure and a genetic characteristic of tumour in order to understand the natural history of the cancer. Only cases with the disease are included and subsequently divided into two or more groups depending on the presence or the absence of a given feature of the tumour at the morphological or the molecular level, i.e. a specific histology, a somatic mutation, or an inherited trait. No classical control group is required. This is an efficient and valid strategy when the association between the exposure and the disease under study is known. Enzyme polymorphisms can be modelled as an exposure or as an effect modifier factor. The odds ratio is used to estimate the association between exposure and genetic characteristic and also for the interaction term. This design is based on the assumption that genetic susceptibility to the disease is not associated with the probability of being exposed, a circumstance that can occur when genetic susceptibility varies according to race and, consequently, to social class (Begg & Zhang, 1994; Piegorsch *et al.*, 1994; Rothman *et al.*, 1995). A recent example of case-case design application is the study of Brockmöller *et al.* (1996) on the association of different genetic polymorphisms with p53 mutations in bladder cancer. Bladder cancer patients were categorized according to the presence or the absence of p53 mutations, and the distribution of GSTM1, GSTT1, NAT2, CYP2D6, CYP1A1, CYP2A6 and CYP2E1 polymorphisms was studied in the two groups.

Cohort design
In this design "a group or groups of individuals are defined on the basis of the presence or absence of exposure to a suspected risk factor for a disease. At the time exposure status is defined, all potential subjects must be free from the disease under investigation, and eligible participants are then followed over a period of time to assess the occurrence of the outcome" (Hennekens & Buring, 1987). While cohort studies such as Doll and Hill's investigation on British doctors have provided very important information on the causes of human cancer, there is no published example of a cohort study on metabolic polymorphism. In fact the limitation of cohort studies is that a very large number of exposed/unexposed subjects needs to be recruited in order to identify a suitable number of cases of disease if the disease is rare (as with most cancers). The advantage of cohort studies over the case-control design is the higher quality of exposure information/assessment. This advantage is not appreciable when a genotype is mea-

sured, and is largely nullified by the inefficiency of collecting a large cohort to study a small number of cancer cases.

However, if the phenotype is measured instead of the genotype there can be some advantages in adopting a cohort rather than a case-control approach: (a) the phenotype is unstable and is influenced by therapies or other changes that may have occurred differentially in cases and healthy subjects; (b) the main interest lies in the interaction between the phenotype and some exposure (e.g. smoking or dietary habits), so that a concurrent measurement of both exposure and the "effect modifier" represented by the phenotype is quite logical.

Nested case-control design
This model, used in large cohort studies, involves identifying all subjects who develop the disease during the follow-up period and drawing a *matched* sample of the healthy subjects. The advantage of this design is that with more efficient sampling we may have estimates that are as stable as those obtained by analysing the whole cohort; this is particularly useful when we measure biochemical/molecular markers. Let us suppose that we collect blood from all the subjects belonging to a cohort (e.g. in the multicentric European Prospective Investigation into Cancer and Nutrition) and store them in liquid nitrogen at -196°C. When a case of cancer is diagnosed we take the patient's serum or buffy coat and, say, the serum/buffy coat of two participants who are still healthy (usually cases and controls are matched for the time lag between sample collection and sample analysis, to take analite degradation into account: see Chapters 7 and 8). We can then measure all the variables of interest, like biomarkers of dietary intake and the phenotype/genotype for relevant polymorphisms. To all intents and purposes such measurement provides estimates of the relevant parameters which are as accurate and precise as would be obtained from the whole cohort, at a cost several times lower.

One problem that can occur with this design and bias the results is related to the degradation of analites when biological samples are stored for a long time. Degradation may be so significant as to impede detection of the chemical. In addition, if the samples from the cases affected by the disease of interest and, respectively, those from controls (within a cohort design) are analysed at different times, bias can arise from differential degradation in the two series. For example, the researcher may decide, incorrectly, to analyse samples from cases as soon as these arise in the cohort, while controls are analysed at the end of the study. Since the levels of, say, vitamin C decrease rapidly with time, serious bias may arise from differential timing of measurement in the two series. The same can happen with metabolites of caffeine for phenotyping purposes. For this reason biochemical analyses should be performed after cases and controls have been matched with respect to the time elapsed since sample collection.

Assessment of outcomes of interest, relevant exposures and potential confounding variables

Outcome assessment

The choice of the outcome is variable in studies on metabolic polymorphisms: in the case of glutathione-S-transferase mu1, the outcomes that have been considered include micronuclei (van Poppel *et al.*, 1993), sister chromatid exchange (van Poppel *et al.*, 1993), urinary mutagenicity (Jorgensen *et al.*, 1987; Bartsch *et al.*, 1991), DNA adducts (Bartsch *et al.*, 1991), haemoglobin adducts (Yu *et al.*, 1994) and p53 mutations (Hollstein *et al.*, 1993; Brockmöller *et al.*, 1996), in addition to cancers of the bladder (Zhong *et al.*, 1993; Bell *et al.*, 1993; Okkels *et al.*, 1996), lung (Nakachi *et al.*, 1993; Nakajima *et al.*, 1995), colon (Chenevix-Trench *et al.*, 1995), breast (Zhong *et al.*, 1993; Ambrosone *et al.*, 1995), larynx (Jahnke *et al.*, 1996) and skin (Heagerty *et al.*, 1994). The relationship between a specific polymorphism and a specific outcome is not necessarily predictable. In fact there is some evidence that different outcomes may show a quite different, even opposite, association pattern with metabolic phenotypes. For example, the slow acetylator phenotype seems to be a risk factor for bladder cancer but a protective factor for colon cancer (d'Errico *et al.*, 1996). The biological explanation seems to reside in the different role that N-acetyltransferase has in the activation of aromatic amines, i.e. it activates aromatic amines from diet in the colon mucosa but deactivates them in the bladder.

Exposure assessment

The association between metabolic polymorphism and disease is usually considered in the light of at least one relevant exposure. In fact, metabolic polymorphism is interpreted as an effect modifier of the main exposure-disease relationship model. Sometimes, however, a polymorphism is considered as an exposure itself or as an outcome. The clearest example is represented by the N-acetyltransferase phenotype: its role seems to be strictly exposure-specific and *is expected* to be null if the relevant exposure to aromatic amines is not present. For example, among the group of workers studied by Cartwright (1982) (who were apparently exposed to 2-naphthylamine) and in smokers exposed to 4-aminobiphenyl, a role of the N-acetyltransferase (NAT) phenotype was clearly suggested, while it was completely absent in a cohort of Chinese workers exposed to benzidine (Hayes *et al.*, 1993). This discrepancy is now interpreted as a consequence of the fact that NAT is involved in the detoxification of 2-naphthylamine and 4-aminobiphenyl, while acetylation of benzidine occurs so frequently (95% of urinary metabolites) that any difference between slow and rapid acetylators is irrelevant for cancer risk (Rothman, personal communication).

An important point to consider regarding exposure is the dose-response relationship. Two modalities of dose-response relationship have been described when metabolic polymorphisms are taken into account: direct and inverse. In the former, the effect of the polymorphism is more evident at high levels of dose; in the latter, the opposite occurs. For example, high dose exposure saturates the enzyme activity both in slow and rapid acetylators, so that no effect of genotype is apparent. Consequently, in some cases the greater susceptibility of the slow metabolizers can be identified only upon low dose exposures (Vineis & Martone, 1995; Garte *et al.*, 1997). This effect has been described for CYP1A1 in relation to smoking and lung cancer (Nakachi *et al.*, 1993; Taioli *et al.*, 1995), for NAT2 in relation to nicotine and cotinine urine levels and Hb adducts (Vineis, 1994) and for GSTM1 in relation to asbestos and lung cancer (Smith 1994). In other instances the polymorphism may show an effect only at high doses, and the issue needs further clarification.

Accurate assessment of exposure is essential for estimation of the role of metabolic polymorphisms in a reliable way. Unfortunately, exposure assessment is rather poor in many studies, thus limiting the interpretability of results. Misclassification of exposure (independent of the disease and metabolic status) may imply a blurring of the relationship with metabolic polymorphism (see Chapters 9 and 10).

Covariate assessment

Intersubject variability in the measurement of metabolic polymorphism may arise at both the genotype and phenotype levels due to factors such as race, age, gender, tumour grade and stage, diet, other environmental exposures causing enzyme induction, and metabolic impairment due to disease processes. Some of these factors are potential confounders.

If we consider the metabolic phenotype for CYP1A2 we should also take into account that the enzyme is inducible by tobacco smoke, cruciferous vegetables, dietary heterocyclic aromatic amines and probably other exposures. Changes in these factors can therefore explain intersubject and intrasubject variation. Such factors may represent confounders of the association between the metabolic phenotype and a relevant exposure. For example, several studies suggest that the carcinogenic effect of heterocyclic aromatic amines on the colon mucosa might be modulated by CYP1A2. However, confounding would arise if,

for any reason, the control group included a higher proportion of subjects with the rapid CYP1A2 phenotype because they consume high levels of cruciferous vegetables that induce CYP1A2.

Confounding is formally defined as a spurious association between the exposure/characteristic under study (in this case the CYP1A2 phenotype) and the disease at issue (i.e. colon cancer), due to an extraneous exposure (the confounder) which is both a risk factor for the disease and a correlate of the exposure/characteristic under study. Cuzick deals with this subject in greater depth in Chapter 11.

Covariates should always be considered in studies on metabolic susceptibility. The distribution of phenotypes varies according to race, as for many other genetic traits (Rothman *et al*, 1993). For example (Table 1.), the slow acetylator phenotype frequency is as low as 6-15% among Asians whereas it is 50-60% among Caucasians. If race is a risk factor for the relevant disease (in the example, $OR_{Caucasians} = 5.76$), then it is a confounder of the association with the metabolic phenotype, as the theoretical association in Table 1. shows.

The example shows that an apparent association (OR = 2.25) almost disappears after stratification by race, which is clearly a confounder, being both a risk factor for disease and a correlate of metabolic polymorphism.

Other confounders may go undetected if they are unknown or unmeasured. In the case of the genotype we cannot exclude that the association

Table 1. Theoretical example of confounding by race of the association between metabolic polymorphisms and cancer		
	Metabolic polymorphism	
	Slow	**Rapid**	
ENTIRE POPULATION			
Cancer cases	450	50	OR = 2.25
Controls	400	100	
CAUCASIANS			
Cancer cases	375	25	OR = 1.30
Controls	230	20	
ASIANS			
Cancer cases	75	25	OR = 1.41
Controls	170	80	

(Mantel-Haenszel overall estimate = 1.36)

between disease and a metabolic polymorphism such as CYP2D6 may be due to a strong genetic linkage between the CYP2D6 gene and another trait that is the actual predisposing factor for lung cancer (Harris, 1989).

Identification of sources of bias: observation and selection of subjects

Bias is systematic error. "If the way in which participants are selected into the study is different for cases and controls, and that difference is related to their exposure status, then the possibility of bias exists in assessment of the association between the exposure and disease" (Hennekens & Buring, 1987). This particular form of bias, related to the selection of participants, is called selection bias. The following example refers to a specific type of selection bias named Berkson's bias. Let us suppose that a test is being conducted for the N-acetyl-transferase phenotype in a hospital-based case-control study. One can hypothesize that subjects who are slow acetylators have adverse reactions to drugs more easily than rapid acetylators (this was the case, for example, with isoniazide and the occurrence of peripheral neuritis). Among hospital controls it will then be found that a larger proportion of subjects are slow acetylators because they have been hospitalized for an adverse reaction to a particular drug or they suffer more severe disease as a consequence of the lower dosage of treatments, in comparison with non-hospitalized subjects.

"A second general type of bias may arise whenever non-comparable information is obtained from the different study groups (observation bias)" (Hennekens & Buring, 1987). A common example of observation bias occurs when the data collection or laboratory analyses are not blind as to the case or control status or are not equally accurate in the two series. In a population-based case-control study, for example, it may be easy to obtain timed urine samples (after administration of caffeine) from hospitalized cases, and much more difficult to do so from volunteers belonging to the general population. The consequences can be of two types: (a) selection bias, related to low response rate among population controls (although there is no reason to believe that slow or rapid metabolizers respond differently); (b) observation bias, if all the procedures are respected in the hospital setting but not in the population setting. The collection of

timed urine samples after the administration of a drug requires particular care; this is not necessarily the case when population volunteers are recruited. For example, for logistical reasons the time lag between collection and storage of samples can be longer for controls than for cases. Differential accuracy in collection, storage and laboratory analysis between cases and controls results in the distortion of estimates (Rothman et al., 1993).

Measures of association; interaction between polymorphism and chemical exposure and between different polymorphisms (epistasis); sample size and statistical power; subgroup analysis and multiple comparisons

The choice of the study design determines how the association between phenotype/genotype and disease can be measured. The measure of association used in cohort studies is the ratio of the incidence of the disease among the exposed to the incidence of the disease among the unexposed. This relative effect is usually called risk ratio (RR) (Rothman, 1986). In Chapter 10, Boffetta and Pearce differentiate risk ratio (cumulative incidence ratio) from rate ratio (incidence rate ratio). In short periods of time the two relative effects are similar. The usual measure of association in case-control studies, the odds ratio (OR), is meaningful under some assumptions concerning the methods of sampling. A first possibility is that the cases represent newly diagnosed incident cases occurring within a defined population, while the controls are sampled from the entire base population (i.e. those at risk at the beginning of follow-up). Under these assumptions, the OR is directly interpretable as a risk ratio. If the controls are selected longitudinally throughout the course of the study (sampling from the study base, or density sampling), then the OR is interpretable as an incidence rate ratio (Pearce, 1993). A third option is to sample controls from those who did not get the relevant disease at the end of the follow-up period (i.e. within the survivors); in this case, the OR is not easily interpretable, in particular if the disease is frequent. Therefore, if the first two designs are adopted (sampling from the population at start of follow-up or sampling from the study base throughout the course of the study) the OR will be a meaningful measure; otherwise it can be distorted. Further complications arise when the outcome at issue (disease status or other outcomes) is not a new occurrence (incident event), but a long-lasting state (prevalent event). In this case, the OR may be a distorted estimate of the prevalence ratio (Axelson *et al.*, 1994).

Phase I and phase II enzymes jointly regulate metabolism of carcinogens. Epistasis occurs when "the combined effect of two or more genes on a phenotype could not have been predicted as the sum of their separate effects" (Frankel & Schork, 1996). The study of Nakachi *et al.* (1993) represents an example of epistasis between two metabolic genes: they described the simultaneous effect of CYP1A1 rare allele and GSTM1 null allele on lung cancer risk. In addition to epistasis, interaction between a genetic trait (metabolic polymorphism) and an exposure is commonly described in metabolism studies. Cuzick (Chapter 11) discusses in detail different types of qualitative and quantitative interactions.

Because of the lower prevalence of some of these polymorphisms among the exposure categories and of the reduced possibility of analysing large numbers of samples, studies of molecular epidemiology may lack sufficient numbers to be conclusive. A recent review of the literature on four metabolic polymorphisms and cancer risk (d'Errico *et al.*, 1996) shows that most of the studies on this topic have a low statistical power: only 30% of them reached a power greater than 80% given a two-tailed test, an OR equal to or greater than 2, and an α = 0.05. This problem is even more important in susceptibility studies because their analysis requires modelling an interaction term with more stringent requirements as to the number of cases (Frankel & Schork, 1996).

Statistical complexities become more evident when multiple risk factors and endpoints are analysed (Cuzick, 1995). The assessment of multiple associations has become more frequent in epidemiology since the introduction of biomarkers in addition to classical exposures. When multiple comparisons are made, statistical significance at the p = 0.05 level is highly likely to occur by chance. Some examples of this problem can be drawn from the recent literature (van Poppel *et al.*, 1993). Further considerations should be raised when interaction is analysed in a large number of subgroups. Although this approach presents advantages in terms of statis-

tical power, the risk of finding a false positive result in subgroup analysis is higher. In a recent study by Ambrosone *et al.* (1996), tobacco was found to be a risk factor for breast cancer only in postmenopausal women who were slow acetylators. The biological significance of this result remains unclear. The statistical methods available and the evaluation of interactions and subgroup-specific results are not totally adequate in some studies. Cuzick discusses these matters extensively in Chapter 11 and suggests that there should be clear differentiation between "hypothesis-testing" and "hypothesis-generating" studies and that the statistical significance level should be raised in order to avoid potential false positive results.

Conclusions

Large-scale and carefully designed studies with a validated laboratory strategy are essential to conclusively determine the role of metabolic polymorphisms and their interaction in the etiology of cancer.

Ethical issues concerning the use of susceptibility markers in human populations are particularly sensitive. As usual in research on human subjects a detailed informed consent should be collected, specifying the meaning and the purposes of the analyses that will be performed. Information should be stored so as to respect confidentiality. The misuse of information on genetic susceptibility could create problems for individuals, for example with insurance companies or at work. Genetic susceptibility information should not be used to select non-susceptible persons for work in hazardous places. At present, genetically-based metabolic susceptibility is a subject relevant to research only, and not to applications for public health purposes.

Acknowledgements

This work has been partially funded by the Associazione Italiana per le Ricerche sul Cancro, the Italian National Research Council (Progetto Finalizzato ACRO, Grant No. 93.04716.CT04), a Special Training Award from the International Agency for Research on Cancer, a fellowship of the Direcció General de Recerca, Generalitat de Catalunya (CIRIT 1996BEAI300015), and the Fondo de Investigación Sanitaria (FIS 97/1138), Spain.

References

Ambrosone, C.B., Freudenheim, J.L., Graham, S., Marshall, J.R., Vena, J.E., Brasure, J.R., Laughlin, R., Nemoto, T., Michalek, A.M., Harrington, A.M., Ford, T.D. & Shields, P.G. (1995) Cytochrome P4501A1 and glutathione S-transferase (M1) genetic polymorphisms and postmenopausal breast cancer risk. *Cancer Res.*, 55, 3483-3485

Ambrosone C.B., Freudenheim J.L., Graham S., Marshall, J.R., Vena, J.E., Brasure, J.R., Laughlin, R., Nemoto, T., Gillenwater, K.A., Michalek, A.M., Harrington, A.M., Ford, T.D. & Shields, P.G. (1996) Cigarette smoking, N-acetyltransferase 2 genetic polymorphisms, and breast cancer. *JAMA*, 276, 1494-1501

Axelson, O., Fredriksson, M. & Ekberg K. (1994) Use of the prevalence ratio vs. the prevalence odds ratio as a measure of risk in cross-sectional studies. *Occup. Environ. Med.*, 51, 574 (letter)

Bartsch, H., Petruzzelli, S., De Flora, S., Hietanen, E., Camus, A.M., Castegnaro, M., Geneste, O., Camoirano, A., Saracci, R. & Giuntini C. (1991) Carcinogen metabolism and DNA adducts in human lung tissues as affected by tobacco smoking or metabolic phenotype: a case-control study on lung cancer patients. *Mutat. Res.*, 250, 103-114

Begg, C.B. & Zhang, Z.F. (1994) Statistical analysis of molecular epidemiology studies employing case-series. *Cancer Epidemiol. Biomarkers Prev.*, 3, 173-175

Bell, D.A., Taylor, J.A., Paulson, D.F., Robertson, C.N., Mohler, J.L., & Lucier G.W. (1993) Genetic risk and carcinogen exposure: a common inherited defect of the carcinogen-metabolism gene glutathione S-transferase M1 (GSTM1) that increases susceptibility to bladder cancer. *J. Natl. Cancer. Inst.*, 85, 1159-1164

Brockmöller, J., Kaiser, R., Kerb, R., Cascorbi, I., Jaeger, V. & Roots, I. (1996) Polymorphic enzymes of xenobiotic metabolism as modulators of acquired p53 mutations in bladder cancer. *Pharmacogenetics*, 6, 534-545

Cartwright, R., Ahmad, R.A., Barham-Hall, D., Glashan, R.W., Rogers, H.J., Higgins, E. & Kahn, M.A. (1982) Role of N-acetyltransferase phenotypes in bladder carcinogenesis: a pharmacogenetic epidemiological approach to bladder cancer. *Lancet*, 2, 842-845

Chenevix-Trench, G., Young, J., Coggan, M. & Board, P. (1995) Glutathione S-transferase M1 and T1 polymorphisms: susceptibility to colon cancer and age of onset. *Carcinogenesis*, 16, 1655-1657

Cuzick, J. (1995) Molecular epidemiology: carcinogens, DNA adducts, and cancer - still a long way to go. *J. Natl. Cancer. Inst.*, 87, 861-862

d'Errico, A., Taioli, E., Chen, X. & Vineis, P. (1996) Genetic metabolic polymorphisms and risk of cancer: a review of the literature. *Biomarkers*, 1, 149-173

Doll, R. & Peto, R. (1978) Cigarette smoking and bronchial carcinoma among regular cigarette smokers and lifelong non-smokers. *J. Epidemiol. Community Health*, 32, 303-313

Frankel, W.N. & Schork N.J. (1996) Who's afraid of epistasis? *Nature Genet.*, 14, 371-373

Garte, S., Zocchetti, C. & Taioli E. (1997) Gene-environmental interactions in the application of biomarkers of cancer susceptibility in epidemiology. In: Toniolo, P., Boffetta, P., Shuker D.E.G., Rothman, N., Hulka, B. & Pearce, N., eds. *Application of Biomarkers in Cancer Epidemiology*. Lyon, IARC Scientific Publication, pp. 251-264

Harris, C.C. (1989) Interindividual variation among humans in carcinogen metabolism DNA adduct formation and DNA repair. *Carcinogenesis*, 10, 1563-1566

Hayes, R.B., Bi, W., Rothman, N., Broly, F., Caporaso, N., Feng, P., You, X., Yin, S., Woosley, R. & Meyer, U. (1993) N-acetylation phenotype and genotype and risk of bladder cancer in benzidine-exposed workers. *Carcinogenesis*, 14, 675-678

Heagerty, A.H., Fitzgerald, D., Smith, A., Bowers, B., Jones, P., Fryer, A.A., Zhao, L., Alldersea, J. &

Strange, R.C. (1994) Glutathione S-transferase GSTM1 phenotypes and protection against cutaneous tumours. *Lancet*, 343, 266-268

Hennekens, C.H. & Buring, J.E. (1987) *Epidemiology in Medicine*. Boston; Little, Brown and Co.

Hollstein, M.C., Wild, C.P., Bleicher, F., Chutimataewin, S., Harris, C.C., Srivatanakul, P. & Montesano, R. (1993) p53 mutations and aflatoxin B1 exposure in hepatocellular carcinoma patients from Thailand. *Int. J. Cancer*, 53, 51-55

Hulka, B.S. & Margolin, B.H. (1992) Methodological issues in epidemiologic studies using biologic markers. *Am. J. Epidemiol.*, 135, 200-209

Jorgensen, K.V., Clayton, J.W. & Price, R.L. (1987) Evaluation of aflatoxin B1 mutagenesis: addition of glutathione and glutathione-S-transferase to the Salmonella mutagenicity assay. *Environ. Mutagen.*, 9, 411-419

Nakachi, K., Imai, K., Hayashi, S. & Kawajiri K. (1993) Polymorphisms of the CYP1A1 and glutathione S-transferase genes associated with susceptibility to lung cancer in relation to cigarette dose in a Japanese population. *Cancer Res.*, 53, 2994-2999

Nakajima, T., Elovaara, E., Anttila, S., Hirvonen, A., Camus, A.M., Hayes, J.D., Ketterer, B. & Vainio, H. (1995) Expression and polymorphism of glutathione S-transferase in human lungs: risk factors in smoking-related lung cancer. *Carcinogenesis*, 16, 707-711

Nebert, D.W. (1997) Polymorphisms in drug-metabolizing enzymes: what is their clinical relevance and why do they exist? *Am. J. Hum. Genet.*, 60, 265-271

Okkels, H., Sigsgaard, T., Wolf, H. & Autrup, H. (1996) Glutathione S-transferase mu as a risk factor in bladder tumours. *Pharmacogenetics*, 6, 251-256

Pearce, N. (1993) What does the odds ratio estimate in a case-control study? *Int. J. Epidemiol.*, 22, 1189-1192

Piegorsch, W.W., Weinberg, C.R. & Taylor, J.A. (1994) Non-hierarchical logistic models and case-only designs for assessing susceptibility in population-based case-control studies. *Stat. Med.*, 13, 153-162

Rothman, K.J. (1986) *Modern Epidemiology*. Boston; Little, Brown and Co.

Rothman, N., Stewart, W.F., Caporaso, N.E. & Hayes, R.B. (1993) Misclassification of genetic susceptibility biomarkers: implications for case-control studies and cross-population comparisons. *Cancer Epidemiol. Biomarkers Prev.*, 2, 299-303

Rothman, N., Stewart, W.F. & Schulte, P.A. (1995) Incorporating biomarkers into cancer epidemiology: a matrix of biomarker and study design categories. *Cancer Epidemiol. Biomarkers Prev.*, 4, 301-311

Smith, C.M., Kelsey, K.T., Wiencke, J.K., Leyden, K., Levin, S. & Christiani, D.C. (1994) Inherited glutathione-S-transferase deficiency is a risk factor for pulmonary asbestosis. *Cancer Epidemiol. Biomarkers Prev.*, 3, 471-477

Taioli, E., Crofts, F., Trachman, J., Demopoulos, R., Toniolo, P. & Garte, S.J. (1995) An African American specific CYP1A1 polymorphism is associated with adenocarcinoma of the lung. *Cancer Res.*, 55, 472-473

van Poppel, G., Verhagen, H., van't Veer, P. & van Bladeren, P.J. (1993) Markers for cytogenetic damage in smokers: associations with plasma antioxidants and glutathione S-transferase μ. *Cancer Epidemiol. Biomarkers Prev.*, 2, 441-447

Vineis, P., Bartsch, H., Caporaso, N., Harrington, A.M., Kadlubar, F.F., Landi, M.T., Malaveille, C., Shields, P.G., Skipper, P., Talaska, G. & Tannenbaum, S.R. (1994) Genetically based N-acetyltransferase metabolic polymorphism and low level environmental exposure to carcinogens. *Nature*, 369, 154-156

Vineis, P. & Martone, T. (1995) Genetic-environmental interactions and low-level exposure to carcinogens. *Epidemiology*, 6, 455-457

Yu, M.C., Ross, R.K., Chan, K.K., Henderson, B.E., Skipper, P.L., Tannenbaum, S.R. & Coetzee, G.A. (1995) Glutathione S-transferase M1 genotype affects aminobiphenyl-hemoglobin adduct levels in White, Black, and Asian smokers and non-smokers. *Cancer Epidemiol. Biomarkers Prev.*, 4, 861-864

Zhong, S., Wyllie, A.H., Barnes, D., Wolf, C.R. & Spurr, N.K. (1993) Relationship between the GSTM1 genetic polymorphism and susceptibility to bladder, breast and colon cancer. *Carcinogenesis*, 14, 1821-1824

Corresponding author
Paolo Vineis
Unit of Cancer Epidemiology,
S. Giovanni Battista Hospital and University of Torino,
Italy

Metabolic Polymorphisms and Susceptibility to Cancer
W. Ryder
IARC Scientific Publications No. 148
International Agency for Research on Cancer, Lyon, 1999

Chapter 7. Inherent difficulties in epidemiological studies involving phenotyping

Simone Benhamou, Christine Bouchardy and Evelyne Jacqz-Aigrain

Phenotyping studies on a possible association between genetic polymorphisms and cancer raise specific problems that are mostly related to accurate determination of enzymatic activity in individuals. These difficulties are addressed on the basis of investigations into the relationship between the CYP2D6 phenotype and lung cancer. Only the problems concerning the design and analysis of epidemiological studies and which are specifically related to the genetic polymorphism are discussed. In particular, factors likely to modify enzymatic activity are potential sources of error when assessing the relationship between cancer and genetic polymorphism. These factors are mainly related to the study population (ethnicity, co-administered drugs, underlying diseases, etc.) or to the phenotyping protocol (probe drugs, urine collection, techniques). These aspects of phenotyping-related difficulties are the key issues in the design of phenotyping studies.

Several genes encoding for enzymes involved in the metabolism of carcinogens are known to be polymorphically expressed in humans (Wolf *et al.*, 1994). Individual susceptibility to cancer might therefore partly depend on a genetically determined ability to metabolize carcinogens. It has been suggested that polymorphisms in a number of enzyme systems, including cytochrome P450s (CYPs), glutathione S-transferases (GSTs) and N-acetyltransferases (NATs) are involved in a wide range of human cancers (reviewed in d'Errico *et al.*, 1996). Epidemiological studies on the relationship between these host factors and cancers raise specific problems mostly connected with accurate determination of enzymatic activity in individuals.

General considerations on phenotyping tests
Several enzymes that are possibly involved in the metabolism of carcinogens exhibit extensive interindividual variability in their activity. This may be due to genetic factors, constitutional factors and environmental factors. So far, polymorphisms in genes encoding for the cytochrome P450s CYP1A1, CYP2A6, CYP2D6, CYP2C19, CYP2C9 and CYP2E1, GSTM1 and GSTT1, and

NAT1 and NAT2, are well characterized. Epidemiological studies have attempted to relate differences in the activity of these enzymes to cancer susceptibility. Advances in molecular techniques have allowed many allelic variants of several human genes to be characterized at a genetic level, and standardized genotyping tests have been developed. Until relatively recently the determination of an individual's enzymatic capacity was only possible by phenotypic assessment. Enzymatic activity should in theory be directly measured in the tissue of interest. A systematic collection of tissue samples in epidemiological studies is, however, usually impossible, mainly for ethical reasons. *In vitro* phenotyping is nevertheless essential for phenotype/genotype correlations. Other phenotyping methods, more readily applicable to large numbers of individuals, can be used to determine enzyme activities indirectly. Phenotypic expression can be determined using surrogate tissues (i.e. blood lymphocytes or monocytes) or *in vivo*, using probe drugs, in particular when the expression of the enzyme of interest is predominantly extrahepatic (e.g. CYP1A1) or when no appropriate probe is available (e.g. GSTM1). However, these phenotyping methods cause some difficulties, mainly related to factors interfering with enzyme activity and to technical problems in the measurement of this activity. The present paper focuses on the phenotyping with probes.

Phenotype determination using surrogate tissue

The lymphocyte assay, a method used to phenotype individuals, is briefly presented with the CYP1A1 enzyme as an example. This enzyme is inducible by polycyclic aromatic hydrocarbons (PAHs). The induced activity of CYP1A1 can be determined from the aryl hydrocarbon hydroxylase (AHH) or the ethoxyresorufin-O-deethylase (EROD) activity measured in lymphocytes after induction by PAHs. The procedure most widely used has been to expose human peripheral blood lymphocytes following mitogen stimulation to PAH and to compare the activities before and after induction (Kellermann et al., 1973a,b). Conflicting results have been reported concerning the variability in CYP1A1 induction levels (Kellermann et al., 1973a; Paigen et al., 1981; Trell et al., 1985). These discrepancies may be due to the methods used to assess enzymatic activity. It is well known that different initial lymphocyte concentrations and differences in human serum can greatly influence induced activity (Kouri et al., 1979). A standardized assay has been developed using cryopreserved lymphocytes allowing cell culture, activation and an enzymatic assay to be carried out for all blood samples simultaneously (Kouri et al., 1982). Moreover, induced enzyme activity is not quantified in a uniform manner and this could account also for the different conclusions drawn in the various studies. As CYP1A1 activity is very low in uninduced cells, small variations in uninduced values can greatly influence the final results when ratios between induced and uninduced values are considered. A PCR method to quantitate CYP1A1 mRNA levels could be an additional way of examining CYP1A1 expression (Heuvel et al., 1993).

Phenotype determination using probe drugs

Accurate measurement of phenotypic expression is only possible if probe drugs are enzyme-specific. As these drugs are mainly metabolized by the enzymes of interest, the phenotype, i.e. the genetic interindividual variations in enzyme activity, can be determined. Phenotyping tests are therefore based on the measurement of pharmacokinetic

parameters (e.g. elimination half-life, clearance, plasma concentration, constant rate of elimination) of the drug and/or a metabolite. Phenotyping may prove inapplicable to epidemiological studies if the collection of biological material, e.g. numerous blood and/or urinary samples, becomes cumbersome (Chapron et al., 1986). Easy, innocuous, precise, validated and reliable phenotyping tests are therefore required for epidemiological evaluation in populations.

The metabolic ratio (MR), which is the ratio of the excreted unmetabolized drug to its metabolite, is a very sensitive pharmacological parameter and is now generally used. The phenotyping tests currently employed make it possible to separate individuals into subpopulations (e.g. NAT2 "rapid" versus "slow" acetylators) but they can rarely discriminate, for instance, between homozygous extensive metabolizers and heterozygous intermediate metabolizers (e.g. CYP2D6 « extensive » versus « intermediate » metabolizers).

Several polymorphisms can be studied concomitantly by co-administering enzyme-specific probes (the so-called « cocktail approach ») mediated by distinct enzymatic systems and without metabolic interaction. For instance, CYP2D6, CYP2C19 and NAT2 polymorphisms can be studied using debrisoquine, mephenytoin and caffeine as probe drugs respectively. Conversely, only one probe that is metabolized into several metabolites, each produced by a specific enzyme, can be used to evaluate the activity of several enzymes. For instance, caffeine has been used as a probe for both CYP1A2 and NAT2 enzymes. However, while some phenotyping tests are validated, others would merit further validation. The existence of distinct metabolic CYP1A2 phenotypes using caffeine is controversial. The metabolic pathways of caffeine are, in fact, very complex. Several urinary metabolite ratios have been proposed for in vivo CYP1A2 activity. Poor correlations have been reported for some of these ratios (Notarianni et al., 1995), indicating that all of them cannot determine distinct CYP1A2 phenotypes, if any (see Chapter 16 by Landi et al.).

Administering probe drugs raises some practical and ethical difficulties since they are contraindicated in some individuals (e.g. children, pregnant women, subjects with a proven allergy to the drugs or structurally related compounds) or may exert some undesirable pharmacological effects. For example, using the probe drug debrisoquine at high doses may induce severe hypotension in CYP2D6 poor metabolizers when prolonged drug action occurs due to reduced metabolic clearance (Eichelbaum & Gross, 1990). A clinical protocol has been developed to administer debrisoquine to hospitalized patients thought to be susceptible to the deleterious effects of this drug (Green-Gallo *et al.*, 1991).

Other problems include, most importantly, the concomitant administration of other drugs metabolized via the same metabolic pathway as the probe drug, competing with it for the enzyme under study. Drug metabolism can also be influenced by physiopathological factors (e.g. renal, hepatic and cardiovascular functions, obesity), or environmental factors (e.g. tobacco, alcohol, coffee, stress). In addition there may be differences between ethnically different populations in respect of the use of probe drugs for phenotyping, which must first be validated in a population of the same ethnic origin as the one under study.

Several aspects of phenotyping-related difficulties raised in epidemiological studies are addressed here on the basis of investigations into the relationship between CYP2D6 activity and lung cancer, perhaps the site most extensively studied in relation to functional polymorphisms.

General considerations on CYP2D6 genetic polymorphism

It is now clear that CYP2D6 may catalyse the activation of a tobacco-specific pulmonary carcinogen, 4-(methylnitrosamino)-1-(3-pyridyl)-1-butanone (NNK), although to a lesser extent than other P450 cytochromes (Hecht, 1996). The CYP2D6 polymorphism, responsible for the metabolism of the antihypertensive drug debrisoquine, is inherited as an autosomal recessive trait (Price-Evans *et al.*, 1980). Two distinct phenotypes can be defined, the extensive metabolizer (EM) and the poor metabolizer (PM). Individuals who metabolize the drug at a reduced rate and predominantly excrete the unmetabolized compound are assumed to be homozygous poor metabolizers. The PM phenotype,

Table 1. Exclusion criteria in CYP2D6 phenotyping studies on lung cancer

Authors	Lung cancer patients		Controls
	Medication exclusions	Cancer therapy exclusions	Medication exclusions
Ayesh et al., 1984	Drugs known to interfere with DBQ No drugs after 9.30 pm the day before the test, nor for 2 hours after the start	Chemotherapy or radiotherapy	No drugs after 9.30 pm the day before the test, nor for 2 hours after the start
Roots et al., 1988	Drugs known to interfere with DBQ	Any therapy	
Law et al., 1989	Drugs known to interfere with DBQ		
Caporaso et al., 1990	Quinidine treatment	Chemotherapy or radiotherapy	Quinidine treatment
Benitez et al.,1991	Drugs known to interfere with DBQ	Surgery,chemotherapy or radiotherapy	Any drug
Horsmans et al., 1991	Drugs known to interfere with DBQ		Any drug
Duché et al., 1991	----		Any drug for healthy controls
Puchetti et al.,1994	Any drug	Surgery	Quinidine or neuroleptics
Shaw et al., 1995	Drugs known to interfere with DBQ	Any therapy	Drugs known to interfere with DBQ
Bouchardy et al., 1996	Drugs known to interfere with DMP		Drugs known to interfere with DMP

DBQ: debrisoquine; DMP: dextromethorphan

accounting for 5-10% in Caucasian populations (Price-Evans et al., 1980), results from the absence of a CYP2D6 protein (Gonzalez et al., 1988) or from an altered protein (Broly & Meyer, 1993). To determine CYP2D6 enzyme activity it was necessary to administer a probe drug, such as debrisoquine, sparteine or dextromethorphan (Schmid et al., 1985) and then measure the urinary excretion of metabolized and unmetabolized drug over a set period of time. Numerous studies in European populations have shown similar phenotype frequencies using these probes (Alvan et al., 1990). When debrisoquine is used, enzyme activity is determined by calculating the metabolic ratio, which is the percentage dose of excreted debrisoquine divided by the percentage dose of its metabolite 4-hydroxydebrisoquine.

Phenotyping has been performed in at least ten case-control studies on lung cancer (see Table 1). These studies have produced conflicting results and form a basis for discussing problems associated with both methodological issues and phenotype assessment.

Potential sources of error in studies on lung cancer involving CYP2D6 phenotyping

Issues of the design and analysis of epidemiological studies involving genetic polymorphisms are not markedly different from those in other epidemiological studies. We shall focus on sources of error specifically related to the genetic polymorphism.

Exclusion criteria

Special attention must be paid to potential confounding or effect modifier factors before attempting to link the CYP2D6 polymorphism to disease susceptibility. Apart from medical contraindications to the phenotyping test, exclusion criteria concern all the situations in which CYP2D6 activity could be modified. These criteria often limit enrolment in epidemiological studies. Indeed, in one of the two studies reporting participation rates (Caporaso et al., 1990; Shaw et al., 1995) a low accrual rate was observed in both cases (33%) and controls (22%) (Caporaso et al., 1990).

Ethnicity

The capacity to hydroxylate debrisoquine has now been determined in a number of different populations, and considerable interethnic variations have

been reported in PM frequency (5-10% among Caucasians, 2% among American Blacks and less than 1% among Orientals). Moreover, in the Chinese population no clear bimodality has been found in debrisoquine metabolic ratios and the distribution among extensive metabolizers shifts to the right towards higher values in Chinese people versus Caucasians (Bertilsson et al., 1992). It is therefore crucial that ethnicity be considered a potential confounding factor because of variation in phenotypic frequencies and possibly in exposure to carcinogens.

Medication

The drugs identified as being affected by the CYP2D6 polymorphism include lipophilic β-blocking agents, tricyclic antidepressants, neuroleptics, and miscellaneous drugs such as dextromethorphan and codeine. The concomitant administration of these drugs known or suspected to interfere with the phenotyping test is of major importance in phenotyping studies. The intake of drugs that inhibit or induce enzyme activity leads to misclassification into a metabolic phenotype. For instance, CYP2D6 activity in extensive metabolizers can be partially or totally monopolized by quinidine treatment. In this case, genetic extensive metabolizers may be reversibly "transformed" into phenotypic poor metabolizers (Leemann et al., 1986). To circumvent potential false phenotyping results, medication known to affect the phenotyping test should be withheld to permit patient inclusion in epidemiological studies. However, this is usually not feasible, particularly with neuroleptics or cardiovascular drugs, and in practice all subjects (both cancer patients and controls) taking such medication should not be included in studies or should be excluded from subsequent analysis. This exclusion criterion makes epidemiological studies far more difficult to organize and often restricts their size. In one study (Caporaso et al., 1990), more than 23% of potentially eligible patients were not enrolled because of possible drug interference with phenotyping. Moreover, because some drugs have a long elimination half-time they can interfere with the phenotyping test several days after the last intake. Information on the date and hour of intake should therefore be collected for all medication administered at least during the week preceding the phenotyping test. Interviewers should pay attention to possible patient self-medication or administration by night staff of drugs such as tranquillizers without a formal medical prescription. The recording of medication cannot be correctly achieved without the collaboration of both patients and nurses.

The number of drugs known to interfere with phenotyping tests depends on pharmacological knowledge, which is advancing rapidly. For instance, a list of contraindications to CYP2D6 phenotyping using dextromethorphan (Bouchardy et al., 1996), compiled in 1988, was extended to include more than three drugs before the end of the accrual in 1992. Such lists, used for patient recruitment, should be based on the trademarks, not only on active chemical components. Compiling these lists is time-consuming, especially in view of the increasing number of drug associations.

Moreover, as any drug is likely to be a potential inhibitor or inducer of the activity of the enzyme under study and of secondary metabolic routes, all medication has to be accurately and exhaustively recorded.

Different exclusion criteria for interference of co-administered drugs were applied between the studies, and, within the studies, between cases and controls (Table 1). For example, the criteria applied to lung cancer patients were: no exclusion (Duché et al., 1991), exclusion of subjects with quinidine treatment (Caporaso et al., 1990), taking specific medications known to be metabolized by CYP2D6 (Ayesh et al., 1984; Roots et al., 1988; Law et al, 1989; Benitez et al., 1991; Horsmans et al., 1991; Shaw et al., 1995, Bouchardy et al., 1996), and taking any drug (Puchetti et al., 1994). Some studies excluded all medication use among controls (Benitez et al., 1991; Horsmans et al., 1991, Duché et al., 1991), and in one study medication was withheld for 9.5 hours prior to debrisoquine phenotyping (Ayesh et al., 1984). Only three studies applied the same exclusion criteria for both cases and controls: quinidine treatment (Caporaso et al., 1990) and any drug known to interfere with the phenotyping test (Shaw et al., 1995; Bouchardy et al., 1996). Different exclusion criteria between cases and controls could potentially introduce biases in the phenotyping results. For instance, according to the intake of drugs inhibiting or inducing

enzyme activity, the number of poor metabolizers among cases could be erroneously increased or decreased if these medications were more frequently used by cases than by controls.

Other factors

Numerous environmental factors or underlying diseases could, in theory, modify phenotypic expression. Of them, severe hepatic, renal or cardiac failure could interfere with phenotyping results. These exclusion criteria have not always been reported in epidemiological studies. A weak influence of many environmental factors on debrisoquine metabolism has been suggested (Steiner et al., 1985). A modest association has been found between coffee consumption and debrisoquine polymorphism, but smoking and various other factors such as alcohol or body weight did not influence the metabolic ratio (Steiner et al., 1985). Likewise, no significant differences were found among phenotypic groups in relation to age, sex or smoking habits in the urinary excretion of dextromethorphan and its metabolite dextrorphan (Puchetti et al., 1994). However, some of the preliminary results of our study show that the dextromethorphan metabolic ratio is not influenced by the extent of tobacco exposure in extensive metabolizers but is significantly correlated with the mean daily consumption in poor metabolizers without a change in phenotype attribution (Piguet et al., 1997). The shift in the PM metabolic ratio suggests that heavy smoking induces some CYP2D6-like activity either due to another P450 isoform or an enzyme with overlapping substrate selectivity.

Studied population

Ideally, only newly diagnosed (incident) cases of the cancer of interest should be enrolled as different survival rates are observed among cases according to the phenotype. The reproducibility of phenotype assignment after surgical resection of lung tumour or after therapy has been assessed in several studies. The metabolic phenotype did not change following tumour resection (Roots et al., 1988; Duché et al., 1991; Shaw et al., 1994) or cancer therapy (Roots et al., 1988; Horsmans et al., 1991), suggesting that neither the tumour itself nor cancer therapy modifies metabolism and that prevalent cases are likely to have had the same metabolic phenotype at diagnosis.

Any pathology capable of modifying enzyme activity produces epidemiological results that are extremely difficult to interpret. Several recent studies have attempted to link the CYP2D6 PM phenotype/genotype with various diseases. CYP2D6 poor metabolizers were suggested to be at increased risk for Parkinson disease (Smith *et al.*, 1992), and it has also been reported that personality characteristics are related to the CYP2D6 PM phenotype (Llerena *et al.*, 1993). In hospital-based case-control studies, inclusion of diseases suspected to be associated with CYP2D6 polymorphism in the control group can modify the estimation of lung cancer risk. To avoid such selection bias in the control group a large variety of medical diagnoses for controls should be included and the distribution of metabolic phenotypes should be examined for each medical diagnosis. In phenotyping studies on lung cancer, control individuals were usually healthy volunteers or patients with nonmalignant pulmonary diseases. The metabolizing capacity of debrisoquine could potentially differ between controls with or without pulmonary diseases. The frequency of PMs among controls with pulmonary diseases was comparable to that observed among other control subjects (Shaw *et al.*, 1995). However, because of the potential effect of genetic polymorphism on the progression of disease and associations with different diseases, it would be preferable to select incident cases and population controls in case-control studies.

Conducting epidemiological studies using *in vivo* phenotyping tests is generally laborious and time-consuming. The participation of individuals in phenotyping studies is conditioned by the administration of a probe drug and urine collection. In one study, 26% of subjects were not enrolled because it was impossible to schedule protocol requirements and 15% because of refusal (Caporaso *et al.*, 1990). Variation in factors which influence willingness to participate between cases and controls could bias results. PMs may be less willing to participate in studies on drug metabolism if they have experienced previous adverse drug reactions related to a deficient metabolizing capacity (Shaw *et al.*, 1995). If PMs recently diagnosed with lung cancer are less likely to volunteer than PM controls, then a differential bias will distort the findings.

Phenotype assessment

Since phenotyping studies attempt to relate differences in enzyme activities to cancer susceptibility, errors in the measurement of these activities could produce false estimates of cancer risk. Sources of error in the assessment of metabolic activity may lie in the phenotyping protocol (e.g. type and dose of substance administered, urine collection, and techniques used).

— Probe drug

The schedule phenotyping protocols used in the case-control studies on lung cancer are described in Table 2. In most previous studies the sympathicolytic antihypertensive drug debrisoquine was administered as a prototypical substrate to determine CYP2D6 polymorphic activity. Dextromethorphan, a readily available non-prescription cough suppressant presenting no danger of hypotension, was used in two recent studies. The metabolic ratio of the urinary concentration of the probe drug to that of its metabolite was assumed to reflect CYP2D6 enzyme activity. The accuracy of the phenotyping test is of major concern in epidemiological studies. Assay accuracy is defined by its sensitivity (proportion of susceptible subjects correctly classified) and its specificity (proportion of non-susceptible subjects correctly classified). The prevalence of a genetic polymorphism should be considered to assess the bias caused by risk factor misclassification; e.g. poor metabolizers classified as extensive metabolizers and *vice versa* (Rothman *et al.*, 1993). Given the high prevalence of the CYP2D6 extensive phenotype (90-95% in Caucasians), assay sensitivity is important, since decreased sensitivity markedly increases bias while poor specificity produces a slight bias (Rothman *et al.*, 1993). Based on the comparison of the respective metabolic ratios, a complete correlation was reported between deficient dextromethorphan O-demethylation and poor debrisoquine 4-hydroxylation capacities, and a close correlation was reported between the O-demethylation of dextromethorphan and the 4-hydroxylation of debrisoquine (Schmid *et al.*, 1985). Two phenotyping studies in the French population have confirmed the value of *in vivo* phenotyping with dextromethorphan (Larrey *et al.*, 1987; Jacqz *et al.*, 1988). Dextromethorphan now appears to be more suitable than debrisoquine in studies on genetic differences in oxidative metabolism. Dextromethorphan is recommended as the most appropriate probe drug since it is highly selective for CYP2D6, thus reducing misclassification in oxidative level assignment (Schmid *et al.*, 1985; Dayer *et al.*, 1990). Moreover, due to its high affinity for the polymorphic enzyme (nearly a tenfold factor compared to debrisoquine and twentyfold compared to sparteine) it is less sensitive to inhibition by other drugs. Lastly, dextromethorphan is available worldwide and is innocuous, whereas adverse drug reactions related to a deficient metabolizing capacity could occur with debrisoquine.

— Dose administered

The dose of debrisoquine administered was 10 mg in all the studies except for one in which doses were based on age and body weight, and the dose of dextromethorphan base administered was around 20 mg (Table 2). Since the metabolic ratio is the ratio of the proportion of the dose excreted as unmetab-

Table 2. Characteristics of phenotyping protocol in studies on lung cancer						
Authors	**Drug**	**Dose**	**Start of the test**	**Urine collection**	**Phenotyping technique**	**Cut-off points for phenotype classification**
Ayesh *et al.*,1984	DBQ	10mg	7 am	8 h	Electron-capture GC	PM (MR>12.6); IM (MR: 1-12.6); EM (MR<1)
Roots *et al.*, 1988	DBQ	5.0, 7.5 or 10 mg in relation to age and body weight	Morning	5 h	GC	PM (MR>12); EM (MR≤12)
Law *et al.*,1989	DBQ	10mg	7 am	8 h	Electron-capture GC	PM (MR>12.6); EM (MR≤12.6)
Caporaso *et al.*, 1990	DBQ	10 mg	Morning/	8 h	Electron-capture GC	Blacks: PM (MR>26.4); IM (MR: 4.2-26.4); EM (MR< 4.2) Whites: PM (MR>11.7); IM (MR: 4.8-11.7); EM (MR<4.8)
Benitez *et al.*, 1991	DBQ	10 mg	10 pm	8 h	Flame ionization GC	PM (MR>12.6); IM (MR: 1-12.6); EM (MR<1)
Horsmans *et al.*, 1991	DBQ	10 mg	Evening	8 h	GLC	PM (MR>12.6); EM (MR≤12.6)
Duché *et al.*, 1991	DBQ	10 mg	8 am	8 h	Flame ionization GC	PM (MR>13.18); EM (MR≤13.18)
Puchetti *et al.*, 1994	DMP	17.4 mg	Evening	8 h	GC	PM (MR>0.669); IM (MR: 0.176-0.669); EM (MR<0.176)
Shaw *et al.*, 1995	DBQ	10 mg	10 pm	8 h	HPLC	PM (MR>7.39); EM (MR≤7.39) PM (MR>12.6); IM (MR: 1-12.6); EM (MR<1) PM (MR>20.8); IM (MR: 1.93-20.8); EM (MR<1.93) Five levels according to the control distribution of log(MR)
Bouchardy *et al.*, 1996	DMP	19.3 mg	Evening	8-12 h	HPLC	Continuous log(MR), Three levels according to the control distribution of log(MR) PM (MR>0.3); EM (MR≤0.3)

DBQ: debrisoquine; DMP: dextromethorphan base
GC: gas chromatography; GLC: gas-liquid chromatography; HPLC: high-performance liquid chromatography
MR: metabolic ratio; PM: poor metabolizers; IM: intermediate metabolizers; EM: extensive metabolizers

olized drug to that excreted as metabolized drug, it is sensitive to slight changes in metabolite concentration. Small doses may lead to underestimation of the metabolizing capacity if the metabolite is present at a very low concentration (Shaw *et al.*, 1995).

— Sample collection

In general, urine collection for less than 8 hours may not yield an accurate representation of metabolizing capacity. However, with CYP2D6, the time during which urine is collected may only constitute a minor source of error. Indeed, the metabolic ratio remains stable after the first hour and over the next 12 hours. In epidemiological studies, urine was collected as from 5 hours (Roots *et al.*, 1988) until 12 hours had elapsed (Bouchardy *et al.*, 1996). Moreover, a high correlation between metabolic ratios from daytime and overnight phenotyping has been demonstrated (Shaw *et al.*, 1990). Daytime or overnight urine collection was performed in all studies except one in which the two were combined (Caporaso *et al.*, 1990).

— Compliance

For practical reasons, drug intake and urine collection are generally completed by the participants in epidemiological studies. Errors in phenotyping results can be due to variation in subject compliance with the phenotype protocol. It is therefore essential to control for effective drug intake and adequacy of urine collection.

— Laboratory assays

Regarding laboratory techniques, it has been shown that electron-capture gas chromatography (GC) exhibits excess variability in comparison with high-performance liquid chromatography (HPLC), and that HPLC is more sensitive in phenotyping studies with debrisoquine (Fox *et al.*, 1993). However, GC was most frequently used in the epidemiological studies and HPLC was used in only two recent studies (Table 2). The validity of phenotypic expression should be investigated within and between laboratories, and in any case an individual's enzymatic activity should be determined blindly in the same laboratory for both cases and controls.

Lung cancer and CYP2D6 phenotype

The debrisoquine phenotyping test cannot distinguish CYP2D6 homozygous extensive metabolizers

from heterozygous metabolizers. A metabolic ratio of 12.6 generally depicts the antimode between CYP2D6 EM and PM in Caucasian populations. Different metabolic ratios have been used as thresholds between phenotype categories (Table 2). A two-way classification into the EM or PM phenotype was considered in four of the ten phenotyping case-control studies on lung cancer. The major limitation of this classification is that the very small numbers of PM individuals result in a low statistical power. If an "intermediate" group is not identified, trends in lung cancer risks with increasing levels of CYP2D6 enzyme activity are not demonstrated. In some studies, increased statistical power was achieved for comparisons by combining poor and intermediate metabolizers (Caporaso *et al.*, 1990) or by studying enzymatic activity with arbitrary categories based on tertile distribution (Bouchardy *et al.*, 1996). However, comparable estimates of lung cancer risk can only be produced by using the classification into PM and EM phenotypes shared by all the phenotyping studies. Crude estimates of the risk for poor metabolizers, using other subjects as the reference category, are given in Table 3. In one study the lung cancer risk associated with the PM phenotype was increased (Shaw *et al.*, 1995) and in another it was close to 1 (Bouchardy *et al.*, 1996), but a decreased risk was observed in the remaining eight studies. The decrease in risk for PMs was marked in four studies (OR ≤ 0.2) but of borderline significance in two (Law *et al.*, 1989; Puchetti *et al.*, 1994). However, given the very strong association between tobacco and lung cancer, the effect of smoking should be strictly controlled when estimating the lung cancer risk associated with enzyme activity. Without such adjustment, associations observed between lung cancer and enzyme activity could be artefactual.

It has been suggested that differences in the distribution of histological types and in smoking exposure could partly account for the heterogeneity between studies (Caporaso, 1995). The risk due to the CYP2D6 polymorphism could be more pronounced for the histological types most strongly associated with tobacco smoking (in particular, squamous and small-cell types) and may only be apparent in subgroups of smokers. The CYP2D6 phenotype was reported in six studies according to histological types and only in two studies according to the levels of smoking. The crude estimates of

Table 3. CYP2D6 phenotyping studies on lung cancer

Authors	Population[a]	Controls	Numbers of		OR (95% CI) for PM	Smokers	
			PM[b]	EM		%	Pack-years
Ayesh et al.,1984	Lung cancer		4	241	0.17 (0.05-0.53)	100	60
	Squamous & small cell		na	na	---		
	Controls	COPD	21	213		100	59
Roots et al.,1988	Lung cancer		19	251	0.61 (0.32-1.15)	94	45
	Squamous & small cell		13	140	0.74 (0.35-1.54)		
	Controls	No cancer	30	240		65	30
Law et al.,1989	Lung cancer		2	102	0.21 (0.03-1.06)	100	55
	Squamous & small cell		na	na	---		
	Controls	22 no cancer 82 healthy	9	95		100	54
Caporaso et al., 1990	Lung cancer		1	88	0.08 (0.01-0.58)	100	57
	Squamous & small cell		0	56	0.00		
	Controls	55 COPD 37 cancers	12	80		100	67
						na	36
Benitez et al.,1991	Lung cancer		4	80	0.67 (0.17-2.41)	98	na
	Squamous & small cell		1	72	0.18 (0.01-1.45)		
	Controls	Healthy	10	133		100	na
Horsmans et al., 1991	Lung cancer		5	86	0.75 (0.22-2.40)	97	na
	Squamous & small cell		4	69	0.75 (0.20-2.62)		
	Controls	Healthy	12	155		na	na
Duché et al., 1991	Lung cancer		10	143	0.82 (0.35-1.90)	100	48
	Squamous & small cell		na	na	---		
	Controls	135 COPD 115 healthy	20	234		100	49
						na	na
Puchetti et al., 1994	Lung cancer		1	115	0.16 (0.01-1.07)	na	na
	Squamous & small cell		na	na	---		
	Controls	Healthy	45	809		na	na
Shaw et al.,1995	Lung cancer		29	306	1.21 (0.68-2.17)	97	61
	Squamous & small cell		12	148	1.04 (0.48-2.21)		
	Controls	No cancer	27	346		71	37
Bouchardy et al., 1996	Lung cancer		10	118	1.02 (0.39-2.65)	100	48
	Squamous & small cell		10	118	1.02 (0.39-2.65)		
	Controls	No cancer	12	145		100	42

[a] Caucasian population in all studies, except for that of Caporaso et al. (1990), in which both Caucasians and African-Americans were considered.

[b] The cut-off points for phenotype classification using debrisoquine were 7.39 (Shaw et al., 1995), 11.7 (Caporaso et al., 1990), 12 (Roots et al., 1988), 13.18 (Duché et al., 1991), and 12.6 in other studies; using dextromethorphan they were 0.669 (Puchetti et al., 1994) and 0.3 (Bouchardy et al., 1996).

COPD: chronic obstructive pulmonary disease; PM: poor metabolizers; EM: extensive metabolizers; OR: odds ratio; CI: confidence interval

na: not available

squamous and small-cell lung cancer risk associated with the PM phenotype were not significantly heterogeneous within the studies (Table 3) and a summary risk of 0.70 (95% CI: 0.47-1.03) was found, giving support to the hypothesis of a protective effect of the PM phenotype on smoking-related lung cancer. Inconsistent results were reported regarding the extent to which tobacco exposure might modulate the effect of the CYP2D6 phenotype on lung cancer risk. Interactive effects of CYP2D6 activity and daily tobacco consumption have been reported for lung (Bouchardy *et al.*, 1996) and, to a less extent, for larynx cancer (Benhamou *et al.*, 1996). Increasing levels of CYP2D6 activity increase the lung cancer risk only among heavy smokers. This association limited to heavy smokers was not found in two other studies (Caporaso *et al.*, 1990; Shaw *et al.*, 1995), although an increased risk at elevated levels of pack-years of smoking was suggested (Caporaso *et al.*, 1990; Caporaso, 1995). The complexity of the mechanisms of the modifier effect of tobacco in the association between lung cancer and genetic polymorphisms is worth considering. For example, CYP1A1 was related to a remarkably elevated risk mainly among the lightest smokers in Japan (Nakachi *et al.*, 1993), supporting the hypothesis that genetic variation in the ability to metabolize a particular carcinogen may be irrelevant at a very high exposure level (Vineis *et al.*, 1994). In contrast, it was suggested that GSTM1 deficiency and combined GSTM1/GSTT1 null genotype modulated the lung cancer risk among the heaviest smokers (Kihara *et al.*, 1994; Jourenkova *et al.*, 1997). Well-designed studies on such complex gene-environment interactions should provide a better understanding of the modulating role of these enzymes in lung carcinogenesis.

Phenotype versus genotype

Phenotyping and genotyping approaches can be used to relate levels of enzyme expression to cancer susceptibility. These two methods are complementary (Caporaso, 1996).

Recent advances in molecular biology have allowed easy detection of allelic variants on polymorphic DNA sequences and have made it possible to standardize DNA assays on a large scale. Genotyping, which can be performed at any time in an individual's life, requires a small sample of

any kind of tissue or the practical blood sample. It also allows the detection of heterozygotic individuals as well as rare genotypes. The consequences of changes in DNA sequences have to be clearly identified in terms of gene expression. This means that each polymorphic sequence has to be studied in cell cultures or tissue biopsies in order to determine its functional significance on enzymatic activity. Without these results it would be hazardous to interpret any modification in disease susceptibility by a given genotype.

In addition to genotyping, phenotypic expression can be determined as a possible marker of cancer susceptibility. In theory this approach should be better than that of genotyping as it measures enzyme expression directly inside the cell during « normal » metabolism. Furthermore, phenotyping is the only approach capable of assessing how environmental factors can modify enzymatic activities. Nevertheless, phenotyping determination is technically less accurate than genotyping. Enzymatic activity can be modified by environmental factors, age or health conditions and may not be suitable for measuring what happened 10-20 years previously. In addition, phenotypic expression is often not easy to measure in the target tissue (e.g. lung or colon) and has to be investigated in other cells (e.g. lymphocytes) or organs (e.g. liver) using probe drugs. The ideal situation would be to have several measurements of enzyme activity throughout life and to use these values in prospective studies.

Thus it appears that both genotyping and phenotyping assays offer advantages and disadvantages.

Conclusions

Epidemiological studies involving *in vivo* phenotyping are generally laborious, mainly because of exclusion criteria and phenotyping protocol requirements. Since phenotyping studies attempt to relate differences in enzyme activities to cancer susceptibility, factors modifying enzyme activities or errors in the measurement of these activities produce epidemiological results that are extremely difficult to interpret. These aspects of phenotyping-related difficulties are the key issues in the design of phenotyping studies.

DNA-based assays are increasingly used in epidemiological studies. This approach has advantages over phenotyping, particularly because it cannot be influenced by confounding (e.g. medication and environmental factors). However, phenotyping is the only way to understand the action of the gene in the organism and remains essential for investigating the functional implications of genomic DNA changes.

References

Alvan, G., Bechtel, P., Iselius, L. & Gundert-Remy, U. (1990) Hydroxylation polymorphisms of debrisoquine and mephenytoin in European populations. *Eur. J. Clin. Pharmacol.*, 39, 533-537

Ayesh, R., Idle, J.R., Ritchie, J.C., Crothers, M.J. & Hetzel, M.R. (1984) Metabolic oxidation phenotypes as markers for susceptibility to lung cancer. *Nature*, 312, 169-170

Benhamou, S., Bouchardy, C., Paoletti, C. & Dayer, P. (1996) Effects of CYP2D6 activity and tobacco on larynx cancer risk. *Cancer Epidemiol. Biomarkers Prev.*, 5, 683-686

Benitez, J., Ladero, J.M., Jara, C., Carillo, J.A., Cobaleda, J., Llerena, A., Vargas, E. & Munoz, J.J. (1991) Polymorphic oxidation of debrisoquine in lung cancer patients. *Eur. J. Cancer*, 27, 158-161

Bertilsson, L., Lou, Y.Q., Du, Y.L., Liu, Y., Liao, X.M., Wang, K.Y., Reviriego, J., Iselius, L. & Sjöqvist, F. (1992) Pronounced differences between native Chinese and Swedish populations in the polymorphic hydroxylations of debrisoquine and *S*-mephenytoin. *Clin. Pharmacol. Ther.*, 51, 388-397

Bouchardy, C., Benhamou, S. & Dayer, P. (1996) The effect of tobacco on lung cancer risk depends on CYP2D6 activity. *Cancer Res.*, 56, 251-253

Broly, F. & Meyer, U.A. (1993) Debrisoquine oxidation polymorphism: phenotypic consequences of a 3-base-pair deletion in exon 5 of the CYP2D6 gene. *Pharmacogenetics*, 3, 123-130

Caporaso, N.E., Tucker, M.A., Hoover, R.N., Hayes, R.B., Pickle, L.W., Issaq, H.J., Muschik, G.M., Green-Gallo, L., Buivys, D., Aisner, S., Resau, J.H., Trump, B.F., Tollerud, D., Weston, A. & Harris, C.C. (1990) Lung cancer and the debrisoquine metabolic phenotype. *J. Natl. Cancer Inst.*, 82, 1264-1272

Caporaso, N., DeBaun, M.R. & Rothman, N. (1995) Lung cancer and CYP2D6 (the debrisoquine polymorphism): sources of hererogeneity in the proposed association. *Pharmacogenetics*, 5, S129-S134

Caporaso, N. (1996) Genetic susceptibility and the common cancers. *Biomarkers*, 1, 174-177

Chapron, D.J., Kramer, P.A. & Mercik, S.A. (1996) Effect of concomitant isoniazid administration on determination of acetylator phenotype by sulphadimidine. *Eur. J. Pharmacol.*, 30, 463-466

Dayer, P. (1990) Advantages and drawbacks of probe drugs for the assessment of phenotypic expression of cytochrome P450db1 (P450D6). In: Alvan, G., Balant, L.P., Bechtel, P.R., Gram, L.F. & Pithan, K., eds, *European Cooperation in the Field of Scientific and Technical Research: European Consensus Conference on Pharmacogenetics*. Brussels; pp. 33-42

d'Errico, A., Taioli, E., Chen, X. & Vineis, P. (1996) Genetic metabolic polymorphisms and the risk of cancer: a review of the literature. *Biomarkers*, 1, 149-173

Duché, J.C., Joanne, C., Barre, J., de Cremoux, H., Dalphin, J.C., Depierre, A., Brochard, P., Tillement, J.P. & Bechtel, P. (1991) Lack of a relationship between the polymorphism of debrisoquine oxidation and lung cancer. *Br. J. Clin. Pharmacol.*, 31, 533-536

Eichelbaum, M. & Gross, A.S. (1990) The genetic polymorphism of debrisoquine/sparteine metabolism - clinical aspects. *Pharmacol. Ther.*, 46, 377-394

Fox, S.D., Shaw, G.L., Caporaso, N.E., Welsh, S.E., Mellini, D.W., Falk, R.T. & Issaq, H.J. (1993) The determination of debrisoquine and its 4-hydroxy metabolite in urine by capillary gas chromatography and high performance liquid chromatography. *J. Liq. Chromatogr.*, 16, 1315-1327

Gonzalez, F.J., Skoda, R.C., Kimura, S., Umeno, M., Zanger, U.M., Nebert, D.W., Gelboin, H.V., Hardwick, J.P. & Meyer, U.A. (1988) Characterization of the common genetic defect in humans deficient in debrisoquine metabolism. *Nature*, 331, 442-446

Green-Gallo, L.A., Buivys, D.M., Fisher, K.L., Caporaso, N., Slawson, R.G., Elias, G., Didolkar, M.S., Ivusich, W.J. & Resau, J.H. (1991) A protocol for the safe administration of debrisoquine in biochemical epidemiologic research protocols for hospitalized patients. *Cancer*, 68, 206-210

Hecht, S.S. (1996) Recent studies on mechanisms of bioactivation and detoxification of 4-(methylnitrosamino)-1-(3-pyridyl)-1-butanone (NNK), a tobacco-specific lung carcinogen. *Crit. Rev. Toxicol.*, 26, 163-181

Heuvel, J.P.V., Clark, G.C., Thompson, C.L., McCoy, Z., Miller, C.R., Lucier, G.W. & Bell, D.A. (1993) CYP1A1 mRNA levels as a human exposure biomarker: use of quantitative polymerase chain reaction to measure CYP1A1 expression in human peripheral blood lymphocytes. *Carcinogenesis*, 14, 2003-2006

Horsmans, Y., Desager, J.P. & Harvengt, C. (1991) Is there a link between debrisoquine oxidation phenotype and lung cancer susceptibility? *Biomed. Pharmacother.*, 45, 359-362

Jacqz, E., Dulac, H. & Mathieu, H. (1988) A phenotyping study of polymorphic drug metabolism in the French Caucasian population. *Eur. J. Clin. Pharmacol.*, 35, 167-171

Jourenkova, N., Reinikanen, M., Bouchardy, C., Husgafvel-Pursiainen, K., Dayer, P., Benhamou, S. & Hirvonen, A. (1997) Effects of glutathione *S*-transferases *GSTM1* and *GSTT1* genotypes on lung cancer risk among smokers. *Pharmacogenetics*, 7, 515-518

Kellermann, G., Cantrell, E. & Shaw, C.R. (1973a) Variations in extent of aryl hydrocarbon hydroxylase induction in cultured human lymphocytes. *Cancer Res.*, 33, 1654-1656

Kellermann, G., Luyten-Kellermann, M. & Shaw, C.R. (1973b) Genetic variation of aryl hydrocarbon hydroxylase in human lymphocytes. *Am. J. Hum. Genet.*, 25, 327-331

Kouri, R.E., Imblum, R.L., Sosnowski, R.G., Slomiany, D.J. & McKinney, C.E. (1979)

Parameters influencing quantitation of 3-methylcholanthrene-induced aryl hydrocarbon hydroxylase activity in cultured human lymphocytes. *J. Environ. Pathol. Toxicol.*, 2, 1079-1098

Kouri, R.E., McKinney, C.E., Slomiany, D.J., Snodgrass, D.R., Wray, N.P. & McLemore, T.L. (1982) Positive correlation between high aryl hydrocarbon hydroxylase activity and primary lung cancer as analysed in cryopreserved lymphocytes. *Cancer Res.*, 42, 5030-5037

Larrey, D., Amoutel, G., Tinel, M., Letteron, P., Berson, A., Labbe, G. & Pessayre, D. (1987) Polymorphism of dextromethorphan oxidation in a French population. *Br. J. Clin. Pharmacol.*, 24, 676-679

Law, M.R., Hetzel, M.R. & Idle, J.R. (1989) Debrisoquine metabolism and genetic predisposition to lung cancer. *Br. J. Cancer*, 59, 686-687

Leemann, T., Dayer, P. & Meyer, U.A. (1986) Single-dose quinidine treatment inhibits metoprolol oxidation in extensive metabolizers. *Eur. J. Clin. Pharmacol.*, 29, 739-741

Llerena, A., Edman, G., Cobaleda, J., Benitez, J., Schalling, D. & Bertilsson, L. (1993) Relationship between personality and debrisoquine hydroxylation activity. *Acta Psychiatr. Scand.*, 87, 23-28

Nakachi, K., Imai, K., Hayashi, S. & Kawajiri, K. (1993) Polymorphisms of the *CYP1A1* and glutathione *S*-transferase genes associated with susceptibility to lung cancer in relation to cigarette dose in a Japanese population. *Cancer Res.*, 53, 2994-2999

Notarianni, L.J., Oliver, S.E., Dobrocky, P., Bennett, P.N. & Silverman, B.W. (1995) Caffeine as a metabolic probe: a comparison of the metabolic ratios used to assess CYP1A2 activity. *Br. J. Clin. Pharmacol.*, 39, 65-69

Paigen, B., Ward, E., Reilly, A., Gurtoo, H.L., Minowada, J., Steeland, K., Havens, M.B. & Sartori, P. (1981) Seasonal variation of aryl hydrocarbon hydroxylase in human lymphocytes. *Cancer Res.*, 41, 2757-2761

Piguet, V., Bouchardy, C., Benhamou, S. & Dayer, P. (1997) CYP2D6 status in tobacco smokers. *Proceedings of the American Society for Clinical Pharmacology and Therapeutics.* San Diego, March 5-8, 1997

Price-Evans, D.A.P., Maghoub, A., Sloan, T.P., Idle, J.R. & Smith, R.L. (1980) A family and population study of the genetic polymorphism of debrisoquine oxidation in a white British population. *J. Med. Genet.*, 17, 102-105

Puchetti, V., Faccini, G.B., Micciolo, R., Ghimenton, F., Bertrand, C. & Zatti, N. (1994) Dextromethorphan test for evaluation of congenital predisposition to lung cancer. *Chest*, 105, 449-453

Roots, I., Drakoulis, N., Ploch, M., Heinemeyer, G., Loddenkemper, R., Minks, T., Nitz, M., Otte, F. & Koch, M. (1988) Debrisoquine hydroxylation phenotype, acetylation phenotype, and ABO blood groups as genetic host factors of lung cancer risk. *Klin. Wochenschr.*, 66, 87-97

Rothman, N., Stewart, W.F., Caporaso, N.E. & Hayes, RB. (1993) Misclassification of genetic susceptibility biomarkers: implications for case-control studies and cross-population comparisons. *Cancer Epidemiol. Biomarkers Prev.*, 2, 299-303

Schmid, B., Bircher, J., Preisig, R. & Küpfer, A. (1985) Polymorphic dextromethorphan metabolism: co-segregation of oxidative O-demethylation with debrisoquine hydroxylation. *Clin. Pharmacol. Ther.*, 38, 618-624

Shaw, G.L., Falk, R.T., Caporaso, N.E., Issaq, H.J., Kase, R.G., Fox, S.D. & Tucker, M.A. (1990) Effect of diurnal variation on debrisoquine metabolic phenotyping. *J. Natl. Cancer Inst.*, 82, 1573-1575

Shaw, G.L., Falk, R.T., Deslauriers, J., Nesbitt, J.C., McKneally, M.F., Frame, J.N., Feld, R., Issaq, H.J., Ruckdeschel, J.C. & Hoover, R.N. (1994) Lung tumour resection does not affect debrisoquine metabolism. *Cancer Epidemiol. Biomarkers Prev.*, 3, 141-144

Shaw, G.L., Falk, R.T., Deslauriers, J., Frame, J.N., Nesbitt, J.C., Pass, H.I., Issaq, H.J., Hoover, R.N. & Tucker, M. (1995) Debrisoquine metabolism and lung cancer. *Cancer Epidemiol. Biomarkers Prev.*, 4, 41-48

Smith, C.A.D., Gough, A.C., Leigh, P.N., Summers, B.A., Harding, A.E., Maranganore, D.M., Sturman, S.G., Schapira, A.H.V., Williams, A.C., Spurr, N.K. & Wolf, C.R. (1992) Debrisoquine hydroxylase gene polymorphism and susceptibility to Parkinson's disease. *Lancet*, 339, 1375-1377

Steiner, E., Iselius, L., Alvan, G., Lindsten, J. & Sjöqvist, F. (1985) A family study of genetic and environmental factors determining polymorphic hydroxylation of debrisoquine. *Clin. Pharmacol. Ther.*, 38, 394-401

Trell, L., Kosgaard, R., Janzon, L. & Trell, E. (1985) Distribution and reproducibility of aryl hydrocarbon hydroxylase inducibility in a prospective population study of middle age male smokers and non-smokers. *Cancer*, 56, 1988-1994

Vineis, P., Bartsch, H., Caporaso, N., Harrington, A.M., Kadlubar, F.F., Landi, M.T., Malaveille, C., Shields, P.G., Skipper, P., Talaska, G. & Tannenbaum, S. (1994) Genetically based N-acetyltransferase metabolic polymorphism and low-level environmental exposure to carcinogens. *Nature*, 369, 154-1456

Wolf, C., Smith, C. & Forman, D. (1994) Metabolic polymorphisms in carcinogen metabolizing enzymes and cancer susceptibility. *Br. Med. Bull.*, 50, 718-731

Corresponding author
Simone Benhamou
INSERM U521, Unit of Cancer Epidemiology, Institut Gustave-Roussy, 39 rue Camille, Desmoulins, 94805 Villejuif cedex, France

Metabolic Polymorphisms and Susceptibility to Cancer
W. Ryder
IARC Scientific Publications No. 148
International Agency for Research on Cancer, Lyon, 1999

Chapter 8. Xenobiotic-metabolizing enzymes and cancer risk: correspondence between genotype and phenotype

Olavi Pelkonen, Hannu Raunio, Arja Rautio and Matti Lang

Metabolic activation and/or inactivation of a carcinogen is usually studied in appropriate *in vitro* systems but ultimately needs confirmation from *in vivo* studies, i.e. phenotype studies. It determines what initially happens to a carcinogen to which an organism is exposed. Consequently, it is of major importance to investigate the correspondence between any particular genotype of a carcinogen-metabolizing enzyme and its phenotypic expression, if any. The need to elucidate the relationship between genotype and phenotype is particularly important now, when methods for uncovering changes in genomic DNA are rather easy, even routine. There are several examples where the correspondence between a variant allele and an altered phenotype, measured by a probe drug or by some other means, has been elucidated (e.g. several alleles of CYP2D6). However, there are also cases where this correspondence has either not been studied (sometimes because of a lack of suitable probe substances) or has remained unclear (e.g. CYP1A1 or CYP2E1), despite case-control studies demonstrating an association between a variant allele and cancer risk. In the end one has to address the basic question as to how the genotype determines the phenotype and whether there is any biologically plausible link between the genotypic differences and cancer susceptibility. A knowledge of the complete sequence of events, from the gene to the outcome, would be helpful in unravelling the implications and possible preventive and treatment strategies to be employed in cases where clear associations between carcinogen-metabolizing enzymes and cancer susceptibility have been uncovered.

When considering the significance of phenotype and genotype in relation to cancer it is necessary to stress that it is the phenotype that is of importance to any possible outcome resulting from exposure to chemicals. This being recognized, the first task should be to investigate whether a genotypic change is actually "carried over" to the phenotype, i.e. what we can observe *in vivo* as a consequence of chemical exposure. The need to elucidate the relationship between genotype and phenotype is becoming particularly important nowadays when methods to uncover changes in genomic DNA are rather easy, even routine. Modern molecular biological methods allow the rapid determination of allelic variants, be they changes in single base pairs or in longer stretches of DNA. However, an increasing problem is that associations of allelic differences to cancer susceptibility are being explored without specific knowledge as to whether the alleles under study are actually causing changes in the phenotype and whether the phenotype even has a theoretical association with the studied outcome.

Genes coding for carcinogen-metabolizing enzymes are typical in that they consist of a structural gene with variable numbers of exons and introns and regulatory sequences in both 5' and 3' areas of the structural genes. The regulation of many of these genes is rather complex, with various environmental, host and genetic factors affecting expression. It is therefore possible that in addition to mutations in the structural gene, ones relevant to the phenotype occur in both 5'- and 3'-flanking regulatory sequences and in other genes coding for transacting factors (e.g. regulatory proteins). Furthermore, gene deletion or multiplication may affect enzymatic activity (Ingelman-Sundberg & Johansson, 1995). For each of these categories there are well known or suspected examples: a number of single base-pair mutations in almost all the genes of carcinogen-metabolizing enzymes; a null allele of GSTM1 gene as an example of structural gene deletion; a putative CYP1A1 regulatory gene (AHR gene) mutation affecting the inducibility of the CYP1A1 enzyme (a thoroughly studied example is the induction of CYP1A1 in the inbred strains of mice); and CYP2D6 gene multiplication (Meyer et al., 1990; Raunio et al.,1995; Kroemer & Eichelbaum, 1995; Fujii-Kuriyama et al., 1995). It thus appears that several types of change at the genomic level may influence the phenotype: 1) catalytic properties of an enzyme may be changed because protein structure is altered due to mutations in exons; 2) protein may be completely absent due to mutations leading to truncated mRNA that is not capable of directing translation, or due to complete or partial deletion of the gene; 3) protein may be expressed at variable levels because of changes in transcription or because of gene multiplication.

Different scenarios can be envisaged, ranging from the simple to the complex. The simplest case is that of "one gene, one protein", which solely catalyses the reaction of interest, and in which a single mutation leads to a complete inactivation of the gene product. The CYP2D6A or GSTM1 null alleles are examples of this. If the gene is not inducible or otherwise under remarkable environmental control the correlation between genotype and phenotype should be, at least in principle, straightforward and simple. The situation is more complex when the reaction under study ("phenotype") is catalysed by a number of enzymes with variable catalytic properties and expressions and where the gene is under the influence of several environmental and host factors. In this situation the elucidation of the relationship between phenotype and genotype is extremely difficult. Unfortunately, the situation often seems to be of the latter type, i.e. the genotype-phenotype relationship is very complex.

In our view, therefore, a reliable elucidation of the genotype-phenotype relationship is possible in only a few cases where gene regulation is simple and the probe substances that can be used are particularly informative about the catalytic properties of a single enzyme.

The extent of exposure may be very important for the outcome and for its dependence on genotypic/phenotypic traits (Vineis et al., 1994). It is quite possible that under exceptional exposure conditions, i.e. very high levels of exposure, interindividual differences in susceptibility are irrelevant, whereas they are of significance under low-level exposures typical for most human exposures. Thus the extent of exposure might be a modifying factor that determines whether the role of a genotype/phenotype can be unravelled in a particular study.

Determination of genotype

It is clear that genotyping, if technically impeccable, has some considerable advantages over phenotyping, such as unequivocal determination of the genetic background and lack of confounding by most host and environmental factors (Caporaso et al., 1995). There are, however, some problems with genotyping studies. As mentioned above the basic problem is to understand which phenotype is created by an allele. As recently as five years ago this was often difficult. With multiple alleles the task was even more daunting, at least when in vivo approaches were used, and results were commonly obtained from opportunistic studies (for example, availability of suitable individuals) rather than from well-defined experiments. At present there are some indirect methods for tackling this basic problem. With the aid of a variety of heterologous expression systems it is possible, although sometimes technically demanding, to express variant alleles and measure the activities of the expressed proteins (Gonzalez & Korzekwa, 1995). If the activity in the in vitro system is known it should be possible to design appropriate in vivo studies with suitable probe substances and thus obtain basic information about genotype-phenotype correlation. This information should be the basic building block in the validation of both genotyping and phenotyping assays.

Another, perhaps more theoretical, problem concerns genotype stability in the light of mutation pressure from, e.g. oxygen radicals. Does this affect an individual's expression of xenobiotic metabolizing enzymes?

Determination of phenotype

The biological rationale in considering the activity and expression of xenobiotic metabolizing enzymes as possible cancer susceptibility factors is that by activating or inactivating carcinogenic substances the enzymes change the levels of carcinogens in the tissues and cells, thus contributing to the multistage process of carcinogenesis at one or more stages.

In the past, interindividual metabolic variations have been determined by *in vivo* metabolism or combined *in vivo/in vitro* assays. Accordingly the phenotype has been determined in various ways, including direct measurements of enzyme activities in tissue samples (e.g. liver biopsies), *ex vivo* methods for measuring inducibility in cultured lymphocytes, and the use of so-called probe drugs *in vivo* (Pelkonen & Breimer, 1994). The interpretation and reproducibility of these studies has often been difficult due to many confounding factors (Caporaso et al.,1995) and therefore all these phenotyping methods raise serious questions.

In vivo approaches: probe drugs

A number of more or less suitable probe drugs have been employed for the determination of metabolic polymorphisms (Gonzalez, 1992; Pelkonen et al., 1995). Ideally, the parameter to be determined, whether a metabolite, metabolic ratio or rate of elimination, should reflect quantitatively the expression of the allele being probed for. In the simplest case the metabolism of the probe drug is exclusively catalysed by only one enzyme encoded by one allele, and hence the polymorphism under study should basically be a differentiation between an active and an inactive allele, the latter resulting from mutation or deletion. In this case the use of a probe drug should give straightforward information about the genotype. Such a situation may exist, e.g. with some CYP2D6 alleles, which, in a homozygous individual, may result in a lack of active enzyme and no debrisoquine 4-hydroxylase activity. If differences in the catalytic properties of enzymes encoded by the polymorphic alleles are only quantitative, the characteristics of the probe drug and the assay become crucial. In this case the ability to differentiate between two alleles giving rise to enzymes of different activities (or to differentiate between

heterozygotes and homozygotes) becomes dependent on, e.g. the pharmacokinetic properties of the drug, the parameter to be measured and the exact time of blood or urine collection. For validation of the methodology in such situations the employment of theoretical calculations should be considered (Tucker et al., 1995).

In addition to these principal problems a number of practical issues should be addressed when probe drugs are used. Most of these issues are related to the administration of drugs or other chemicals to individuals: compliance with oral drugs taken without close supervision, possible risks due to potential side-effects and toxicity, inconvenience to both the researcher and the volunteer if a compound has to be given parenterally; the selection of route and dose; and so on (Pelkonen et al.,1995).

Determination of phenotype: ex vivo approaches

Sometimes the enzyme of interest is not significantly expressed in the tissue relevant to pharmacokinetics - normally liver - (e.g. CYP1A1) or there are no appropriate *in vivo* probes available (e.g. for some GST enzymes). In these cases *in vivo* studies cannot be performed and the phenotype has to be characterized otherwise. One solution has been to use blood lymphocytes or monocytes as material for enzymatic determinations (Raunio, 1995b). These types of *ex vivo* assay may, however, add further complications in that the process of isolation and culturing cells may change the expression and activity of the enzyme to be measured. If the polymorphism of interest relates to "all or none" enzyme activity this approach is possible, but it becomes difficult to use if quantitative differences ought to be analysed, as is the case when inducibility is being measured.

Determination of phenotype: in vitro approaches

In humans, ethical considerations limit the availability of tissue samples, making it problematic to plan and execute systematic studies. In addition there are several practical problems. Target tissues are available only occasionally and the conditions in which they are obtainable may not be optimal for the preservation of enzyme activities, or the samples may not be adequately representative of the population relevant to the study. Because of these limitations, *in vitro* studies using tissue samples are useful mainly for basic investigations on phenotype-genotype correlations. In addition, liver biopsies may be very useful for the validation of *in vivo* probes, since pharmacokinetic parameters of a majority of probe drugs are determined by hepatic activities (Pelkonen & Breimer, 1994).

General problems of phenotyping
— Confounding factors
It is well documented that a number of host and environmental factors may influence and act as confounders of the drug metabolism phenotype. These include age, hormonal status, disease, drug-drug interactions and dietary habits (Kalow, 1993, Caporaso *et al.*, 1995). While the studies have provided interesting information on the regulation of various enzyme activities and in some cases also on how enzymatic activity could be associated with cancer risk, it is difficult to judge from them which is the "real phenotype" that should be compared to the genotype. Since it is the gene that eventually dictates how the enzyme is expressed, even under the most complicated influence of endogenous and exogenous factors, it should theoretically be possible always to understand the relationship between the genotype and the phenotype. For this, a complete understanding of gene regulation is, however, necessary and, except for very few, simple cases, we are a long way from this goal.

— Timing of phenotype determination
Another problem, partly related to the confounding factors, is the timing of phenotype determination. For example, in practice it is very difficult to perform prospective studies where the phenotype is analysed in the same period as the exposure to a carcinogen or carcinogens. Usually we have to perform phenotyping in a case-control setting, i.e. in situations where the critical exposure could have taken place as long as tens of years previously. In addition, an important problem is the stability of the phenotype over time. At the time of measurement the phenotype may not be the same as the phenotype at the onset of the disease, if, for example, the subject under investigation gives up smoking or changes her/his diet.

— Tissue specific expression of carcinogen-metabolizing enzymes and use of surrogate tissue to predict phenotype of target tissue
One of the most challenging problems in the characterization of the human drug metabolism phenotype stems from the fact that most of the catalysing enzymes are expressed in a tissue-specific manner leading to great differences between tissues in the activation and inactivation of carcinogens. Therefore the phenotype of interest should, in principle, be determined in the tissue of interest. Because of the limited availability of human samples this, however, may be possible only rarely, for example occasionally in relation to surgery, and therefore it is difficult to design systematic studies on the assumption that tissue samples are available.

These problems have led to various attempts to estimate the enzymatic activities in tissues of interest by alternative methods. One approach is to make indirect measurements, for instance by using surrogate tissues or probe drugs *in vivo* to extrapolate the activity in the tissue of interest. Ideally, a surrogate tissue should represent the target tissue in such a way that the behaviour of a carcinogen of importance for the final outcome, i.e. manifest cancer, is faithfully reproduced in (or is in a meaningful correlation with) the surrogate tissue. Unfortunately, in most instances the use of surrogate tissue is out of the question because of limited information on the expression of relevant enzymes in the target tissue.

It is obvious, therefore, that ideal target tissues are difficult to obtain. Nevertheless, because of the difficulties in obtaining human material, surrogate tissues have been chosen for many studies in a more or less opportunistic way. For example, blood lymphocytes, hair follicles, surface epithelia from skin or buccal mucosa or "surplus" tissue from surgery have been used (Raunio *et al.*, 1995). When using these tissues one should always keep in mind that they may not reflect well activities in the target tissue and, e.g. in *ex vivo* regulation studies their inducibility may be different from that of the target tissue.

In any case, human tissue samples are extremely valuable for basic studies when information is required on tissue specificity, catalytic properties and the mode of regulation of human carcinogen-metabolizing enzymes.

Critical appraisal of correspondence between genotype and phenotype of some carcinogen-metabolizing enzymes

We consider below what is known about genotype-phenotype relationships of some of the most important carcinogen-metabolizing enzymes and indicate some critical research needs.

CYP1A1

On the basis of variable enzyme (AHH) activity and/or variable inducibility of the enzyme in peripheral lymphocytes it has been suggested that polymorphism exists at the phenotypic level. However, universal agreement on this matter is lacking. Discrepant results have been obtained in studies that have tried to link CYP1A1 polymorphisms with cancer susceptibility (Raunio et al., 1995a; Nebert et al., 1996). Recently, several polymorphic alleles of the CYP1A1 gene have been uncovered. MspI RFLP reflects a point mutation at a site downstream of the last exon, and this mutation is in a linkage disequilibrium with an AT to GC transition (Ile462Val mutation) in exon 7 (Kawajiri et al., 1993). A number of studies have addressed the relationship between these variant alleles and activity and/or inducibility, and found either modest or no differences in CYP1A1-catalysed activities among the different alleles (Jacquet et al.,1996; Crofts et al., 1994; Landi et al., 1994; Wedlund et al., 1994). Expression of the CYP1A1-Val462 allele in E. coli showed that its catalytic properties did not differ significantly from the wild-type CYP1A1-Ile462 (Zhang et al.,1996), suggesting that the observed association between the variant allele and lung cancer incidence in Japanese (Kawajiri et al., 1993) may not be due to altered rates of procarcinogen activation. Two other variant alleles, a T→C transition downstream of exon 7 specific for African-Americans (Crofts et al., 1994), and a C→A transversion (Thr461Asp mutation) in exon 7 (Cascorbi et al., 1996) have been characterized, but their significance for the phenotype is not known.

CYP1A1 is predominantly an extrahepatic enzyme and therefore it has been difficult to find an in vivo probe to determine its level of expression. In several studies, surrogate tissues have therefore been used, which in most cases have been lymphocytes and monocytes, although hair follicles and some other easily available tissues have also been suggested for this purpose (Raunio et al., 1995b). Critical research is needed in order to better define the genotype/phenotype relationships and also to determine whether the activity and inducibility of CYP1A1 are critical for carcinogenicity.

CYP1A2

This enzyme is one of the major P450s in human liver, representing on average about 15 % of the total P450 content (Guengerich, 1995). The metabolism of caffeine (and its N3-demethylated products) and theophylline is mainly catalysed by CYP1A2 and they can therefore be used as in vivo probes (Pelkonen & Breimer, 1994; Kalow & Tang, 1993). Caffeine clearance determinations have indicated widely variable activity and inducibility of CYP1A2 by, e.g. cigarette smoking. Although even a trimodal distribution of CYP1A2 activity in human populations has been claimed on the basis of various caffeine metabolite ratios, widely discrepant results exist (Tucker et al., 1995). To our knowledge no corresponding polymorphisms have yet been observed at genotypic level. There is some evidence for an association between phenotype as determined by caffeine and susceptibility to cancer (Kadlubar, 1994). Research is vitally necessary in order to answer the following questions. Is phenotypic variability in the elimination of caffeine (or other probe drugs) based on genotypic differences affecting metabolism and/or inducibility? What is critical in cancer susceptibility: activity or inducibility?

CYP2A6

CYP2A6 mediates the metabolism of several human carcinogens, including aflatoxins and nitrosamines (see Chapter 17). There appears to be a wide phenotypic interindividual and interethnic variability in CYP2A6 activity when it is measured as in vivo urinary excretion of 7-hydroxycoumarin or as coumarin 7-hydroxylation activity in liver samples (Pelkonen et al.,1993; Shimada et al.,1996). However, the properties of the only available probe drug, coumarin, are less than ideal for a precise estimation of interindividual variability (Pelkonen & Raunio, 1995). Two variant alleles of the CYP2A6 gene have recently been demonstrated

(Fernandez-Salguero et al.,1995) but their effects on activity and/or inducibility are not known (Fernandez-Salguero & Gonzalez, 1995). For future research the elucidation of genotype-phenotype relationships is the most critical task.

CYP2C9 and CYP2C19

These enzymes are members of one of the most complex CYP families and both play a role in drug metabolism. By using S-mephenytoin as a probe drug it was shown that CYP2C19 exhibited a polymorphic phenotype. The genetic basis for the deficiency in CYP2C19-mediated S-mephenytoin hydroxylation was elucidated first (Goldstein & de Morais, 1994) and the principal defect proved to be a single base pair mutation in exon 5 of the CYP2C19 gene, creating an aberrant splice site (de Morais et al., 1994b). Another variant allele with a point mutation in exon 4 was also identified (de Morais et al., 1994a). The two variant alleles, originally named as m1 and m2, have been redesignated as CYP2C19*2 and CYP2C19*3 respectively, CYP2C19*1 being the wild-type allele (Daly et al., 1996). CYP2C19*2 is much more common in Caucasians and CYP2C19*3 accounts for approximately 20% of the poor metabolizers in Orientals (de Morais et al., 1994a). In addition to impaired S-mephenytoin metabolism, CYP2C19*2 homozygosity leads to reduced omeprazole 5-hydroxylation (Ieiri et al., 1996).

The CYP2C9 gene also exhibits polymorphism. Three CYP2C9 alleles have been identified (Daly et al.,1996), and expression studies of the variant alleles suggest that at least impaired warfarin and tolbutamide metabolism can be ascribed to these genetic variations (Haining et al., 1996; Sullivan-Klose et al., 1996).

Curiously, no procarcinogenic substrates are currently known for the CYP2C enzymes, but in view of the wide array of xenobiotics metabolized by members of this subfamily (Goldstein & de Morais, 1994; Gonzalez & Gelboin, 1994) the possibility of procarcinogenic substrates should not be ruled out. Very recently, two preliminary studies have tried to link the CYP2C polymorphisms to cancer risk (London et al., 1996; Tsuneoka et al., 1996).

CYP2D6

This enzyme is discussed in detail in Chapter 18. Several reliable in vivo probes (debrisoquine, sparteine, dextromethorphan, metoprolol) are available and variant alleles or genomic changes leading to null, reduced or increased enzymatic activity have been extensively characterized (Daly et al., 1996; Caporaso et al., 1995). Nevertheless, some critical research needs remain: relationships between genotype/phenotype and carcinogen metabolism are not well defined in humans (or just not reported because of negative findings) and reliable biological explanations are needed for suggested associations with cancer susceptibility and CYP2D6 polymorphism, supported by experimental results.

CYP2E1

A few studies have been carried out suggesting that chlorzoxazone 6-hydroxylation is a fair indicator of hepatic CYP2E1 activity (Dreisbach et al., 1995; Peter et al.,1990). At the genotypic level, several RFLP alleles (RsaI in the 5'-flanking region, DraI in intron 6 and TaqI in intron 7) have been uncovered (Ingelman-Sundberg & Johansson, 1995). Several studies have addressed the question of whether chlorzoxazone metabolism in vivo is associated with the CYP2E1 variant alleles. No associations have yet been found in either Caucasians or Japanese (Kim et al., 1995, 1996; Carriere et al., 1996; Lucas et al.,1995), indicating that the variant alleles found to date do not affect CYP2E1 activity in vivo.

The elucidation of relationships between genotype and phenotype is therefore a critical research area. Because CYP2E1 is regulated by several environmental factors (e.g. induction by ethanol), the question of whether activity or inducibility is critical for possible cancer risk needs to be addressed. Another important point to be considered is the relatively high expression of CYP2E1 in several extrahepatic tissues (Ingelman-Sundberg, 1993). Is expression in the target tissue critical for toxicity, and how can extrahepatic expression of CYP2E1 be measured?

CYP3A

Useful in vivo probes are available for the determination of CYP3A activity (midazolam, dapsone, eryhromycin) (Wrighton & Stevens, 1992), and several important carcinogens are known to be metabolized and activated by the CYP3A enzymes. Nevertheless, to our knowledge no studies have been published to date about the relationship between these enzymes and cancer susceptibility. The probable reason for this is that there are no polymorphisms or other hereditary conditions convincingly ascribed to CYP3A enzymes.

N-acetyltransferases (NATs)

Acetylation polymorphism (what is currently known as NAT2 polymorphism) was the first pharmacogenetic condition extensively studied (Weber & Hein, 1985). Several well-characterized in vivo probes (sulfadimidine, isoniazide, caffeine) are currently available for phenotyping slow and rapid acetylators, although some controversy exists as to whether heterozygotes can be detected by these probes. At the genotypic level a large number of variant alleles have been characterized and PCR-based methods are available for the analysis of most of them (Vatsis et al., 1995). However, more research is needed for better definition of the genotype/phenotype relationships with respect to critical carcinogens in humans.

NAT1 variant alleles have also been uncovered recently and employed in cancer susceptibility studies (Vatsis et al., 1995). Little is known about the contribution of these variants to the phenotype.

Glutathione S-transferases (GSTs)

Among several GST enzymes, at least GSTM1 and GSTT1 exhibit genetic polymorphisms (Pemble et al.,1994; Ketterer et al., 1992). No in vivo probes are available for these polymorphic enzymes. Therefore the polymorphic phenotype of, e.g. GSTM1 has to be studied ex vivo in peripheral lymphocytes, using styrene oxide as a substrate. For the genotype, PCR-based methods for the detection of variant alleles of both GSTM1 and GSTT1 are well established. Because GSTM1 polymorphism is actually a gene deletion, it represents a "simple" case in cancer susceptibility studies. Future studies are desirable on the expression of the enzymes in target tissues and on the association between the genetic polymorphism and the detoxification of relevant carcinogens.

Other enzymes

Thiopurine S-methyltransferase (TPMT) is a cytosolic enzyme that preferentially catalyses the S-methylation of aromatic and heterocyclic sulfhydryl compounds, including the commonly used cancer therapeutic agents mercaptopurine and thioguanine (Weinshilboum, 1992). PCR-based methods have been developed to detect the two variant alleles (TPMT*2 and TPMT*3), permitting diagnosis of heterozygous and homozygous individuals who would develop severe side-effects if treated with standard doses of purine analogues (Krynetski et al., 1996).

Dihydropyrimidine dehydrogenase (DPD) is the first and rate-limiting enzyme in the catabolism of thymine and uracil. By virtue of its ability to degrade pyrimidines, DPD is responsible for the metabolism of fluoropyrimidine drugs, such as the extensively used cancer drug 5-fluorouracil (Gonzalez & Fernandez-Salguero, 1995). DPD deficiency is associated with toxic effects after 5-fluorouracil treatment. An individual with a complete lack of DPD activity and his family were found to possess mRNA with a deletion, resulting in a non-functional DPD enzyme (Meisma et al., 1995). The reason for the deletion proved to be a G to A point mutation that leads to skipping of an entire exon during pre-RNA transcription (Wei et al., 1996). A genotyping test for this mutation is now available to detect individuals who would be at high risk of developing 5-fluorouracil toxicity during cancer chemotherapy (Wei et al., 1996).

Regulatory genes

The induction of CYP1A1 and, partially, that of CYP1A2, is regulated by two gene products, the Ah receptor (AHR) and the aryl hydrocarbon nuclear translocator (ARNT). Polymorphic forms of the AHR gene were first found in inbred strains of mice, and this explained the differences between C57BL/6 and DBA/2 mice in the affinities of their AHRs to TCDD (Fujii-Kuriyama et al., 1995). Two variant alleles of the human AHR gene have subsequently been reported (Kawajiri et al., 1995); both contain a point mutation but only one leads to an amino acid change (Arg554-Lys554). This germline polymorphism of the AHR gene was not associated with AHH inducibility or with lung cancer incidence (Kawajiri et al., 1995).

An MspI RFLP has been reported in the human ARNT gene (Johnson *et al.*, 1992) but this finding has not been verified by other laboratories, and its significance for the regulation of the CYP1A genes is unknown. There is a clear need for more detailed analysis of variations in the AHR and ARNT genes, and of how these variations might be reflected at the phenotype level.

Concluding remarks

It seems clear that we are still far from an adequate elucidation of the correspondence between phenotype and genotype in respect of most carcinogen-metabolizing enzymes. With the help of current molecular biological techniques it is much easier to discover and characterize new variant alleles and genetic changes and to employ them in straightforward genetic epidemiological studies than to proceed in the first place to more cumbersome studies on the basic question as to how the genotype is determining the phenotype and whether any biologically plausible link can be expected between genotypic differences and cancer susceptibility. Eventually, however, it is necessary to understand the complete sequence of events from gene to outcome, so that we can confidently see the implications and possibly arrive at preventive and treatment

Table 1. Major allelic variants and polymorphisms of human CYP genes and their phenotypic expressions			
Gene	Variant allele	*In vitro* activity	*In vivo*
CYP1A1	M1: 3'-Msp1-RFLP m2: Ile462Val	No change No change	No probe drugs known; lymphocytes, etc., as surrogates
CYP1A2	Not known	Very variable	Two to three phenotypes with probe drugs (caffeine)?
CYP2A6	V1: Leu160His V2: several changes	0 0	Phenotype unclear Null phenotype
CYP2B6	Not known	Variable (80 % zero expression?)	No probe drugs known
CYP2C9	Ile359Leu	Decreased	Retarded elimination of probe drugs (tolbutamide, warfarin)
CYP2C19	M1: exon 5 cryptic splice site M2: exon 4 stop codon	0 0	Retarded elimination or changed enantiomeric ratios of probe drugs (mephenytoin, omeprazole)
CYP2D6	About 25 variant alleles identified	Zero, increased, decreased	Several useful probe drugs available (e.g. dextromethorphan)
CYP2E1	5'-,3'-, intron-	No change?	Probe drug chlorzoxazone
CYP2F1	Not known	?	Expression in lung
CYP3A4	Not known	Very variable	Several probe drugs available (may measure also other CYP3A enzymes)
CYP3A5	Not known	Very variable	No specific probe drugs available
CYP3A7	Not known	Fetus-specific, very low in adults	No specific probe drugs available
CYP4B1	Not known	?	Expression in lung

strategies for cases where clear associations between carcinogen-metabolizing enzymes and cancer susceptibility have been uncovered.

Acknowledgements

The authors have been supported by the Academy of Finland Council for Health Research (grant numbers 1051029 and 34555). The present review is a contribution towards the achievement of the goals of Action COST B1 and EU-Biomed 2 project EUROCYP.

References

Caporaso, N., DeBaun, M.R. & Rothman, N. (1995) Lung cancer and CYP2D6 (the debrisoquine polymorphism): sources of heterogeneity in the proposed association. *Pharmacogenetics*, 5, s129-s134

Carriere, V., Berthou, F., Baird, S., Belloc, C., Beaune, P. & de Waziers, I. (1996) Human cytochrome P450 2E1 (CYP2E1): from genotype to phenotype. *Pharmacogenetics*, 6, 203-211

Cascorbi, I., Brockmöller, J. & Roots, I. (1996) A C4887A polymorphism in exon 7 of human CYP1A1: population frequency, mutation linkages, and impact on lung cancer susceptibility. *Cancer Res.*, 56, 4965-4969

Crofts, F., Taioli, E., Trachman., J, Cosma, G.N., Currie, D., Toniolo, P. & Garte, S.J. (1994) Functional significance of different human CYP1A1 genotypes. *Carcinogenesis*, 15, 2961-2963

Daly, A.K., Brockmöller, J., Broly, F., Eichelbaum, M., Evans, W.E., Gonzalez, F.J., Huang, J.-D., Idle, J.R., Ingelman-Sundberg, M., Ishizaki,T., Jacqz-Aigrain, E., Meyer, U.A., Nebert, D.W., Steen, V.M., Wolf, C.R. & Zanger, U.M. (1996) Nomenclature for human CYP2D6 alleles. *Pharmacogenetics*, 6, 193-201

de Morais, S.M.F., Wilkinson, G.R., Blaisdell, J., Meyer, U.A., Nakamura, K. & Goldstein, J.A. (1994a) Identification of a new genetic defect responsible for the polymorphism of (S)-mephenytoin metabolism in Japanese. *Mol. Pharmacol.*, 46, 594-598

de Morais, S.M.F., Wilkinson, G.R., Blaisdell, J., Nakamura, K., Meyer, U.A. & Goldstein, J.A. (1994b) The major genetic defect responsible for the polymorphism of S-mephenytoin metabolism in humans. *J. Biol. Chem.*, 269, 15419-15422

Dreisbach, A.W., Ferencz, N., Hopkins, N.E., Fuentes, M.G., Rege, A.B., George, W.J. & Lertora, J.J.L. (1995) Urinary excretion of 6-hydroxychlorzoxazone as an index of CYP2E1 activity. *Clin. Pharmacol. Ther.*, 58, 498-505

Fernandez-Salguero, P., Hoffman, S.M.G., Cholerton, S., Mohrenweiser, H.,Raunio, H., Rautio, A., Pelkonen, O., Huang, J., Evans, W.E., Idle, J.R. & Gonzalez, F.J. (1995) A genetic polymorphism in coumarin 7-hydroxylation: sequence of the human CYP2A genes and identification of variant CYP2A6 alleles. *Am. J. Hum. Genet.*, 57, 651-660

Fernandez-Salguero, P. & Gonzalez, F.J. (1995) The CYP2A gene subfamily species differences, regulation, catalytic activities and role in chemical carcinogenesis. *Pharmacogenetics*, 5, S123-S128

Fujii-Kuriyama, Y., Ema, M., Mimura, J., Matsushita, N. & Sogawa, K. (1995) Polymorphic forms of the Ah receptor and induction of the CYP1A1 gene. *Pharmacogenetics*, 5, S149-S153

Goldstein, J.A. & de Morais, S.M.F. (1994) Biochemistry and molecular biology of the human CYP2C subfamily. *Pharmacogenetics*, 4, 285-299

Gonzalez, F.J. (1992) Human cytochromes P450: problems and prospects. Trends *Pharmacol. Sci.*, 13, 346-352

Gonzalez, F.J. & Fernandez-Salguero, P. (1995) Diagnostic analysis, clinical importance and molecular basis of dihydropyrimidine dehydrogenase deficiency. *Trends Pharmacol. Sci.*, 16, 325-327

Gonzalez, F.J. & Gelboin, H.V. (1994) Role of human cytochromes P450 in the metabolic activation of chemical carcinogens and toxins. *Drug Metab. Rev.*, 26, 165-183

Gonzalez, F.J. & Korzekwa, K.R. (1995) Cytochromes P450 expression systems. *Annu. Rev. Pharmacol. Toxicol.*, 35, 369-390

Guengerich, F.P. (1995) Cytochromes P450 of human liver. Classification and activity profiles of the major enzymes. In: Pacifici, G.M. & Fracchia, G.N., eds, *Advances in Drug Metabolism in Man*. Luxembourg, Office for the Official Publications of the European Communities, pp.179-231

Haining, R.L., Hunter, A.P., Veronese, M.E., Trager, W.F. & Rettie, A.E. (1996) Allelic variants of human cytochrome P450 2C9: baculovirus-mediated expression, purification, structural characterization, substrate stereoselectivity, and prochiral selectivity of the wild-type and I359L mutant forms. *Arch. Biochem. Biophys.*, 333, 447-458

Ieiri, I., Kubota, T., Urae, A., Kimura, M., Wada, Y., Mamiya, K., Yoshioka, S., Irie, S., Amamoto, T., Nakamura, K., Nakano, S. & Higuchi, S. (1996) Pharmacokinetics of omeprazole (a substrate of 2C19) and comparison with two mutant alleles, CYP2C19m1 in exon 5 and CYP2C19m2 in exon 4, in Japanese subjects. *Clin. Pharmacol. Ther.*, 59, 647-653

Ingelman-Sundberg, M. (1993) Ethanol-inducible cytochrome P450 2E1. Regulation, radical formation and toxicological importance. In: Poli, G., Albano, E. & Dianzani, M.U., eds, *Free Radicals: from Basic Science to Medicine*. Basel, Birkhäuser, pp. 287-301

Ingelman-Sundberg, M. & Johansson, I. (1995) The molecular genetics of the human drug metabolizing cytochrome P450s. In: Pacifici, G.M. & Fracchia, G.N., eds, *Advances in Drug Metabolism in Man*. Luxembourg, Office for the Official Publications of the European Communities, pp. 534-585

Jacquet, M., Lambert, V., Baudoux, E., Muller, M., Kremers, P. & Gielen, J. (1996) Correlation between P450 CYP1A1 inducibility, MspI genotype and lung cancer incidence. *Eur. J. Cancer*, 32A: 1701-1706

Johnson, B.S., Brooks, B.A., Reyes, H., Hoffman, E.C. & Hankinson, O. (1992) An MspI RFLP in the human ARNT gene, encoding a subunit of the nuclear form of the Ah (dioxin) receptor. *Hum. Mol. Genet.*, 1, 35

Kadlubar, F.F. (1994) Biochemical individuality and its implications for drug and carcinogen metabolism: recent insights from acetyltransferase and cytochrome P4501A2 phenotyping and genotyping in humans. *Drug Metab. Rev.*, 26, 37-46

Kalow, W. (1993) Pharmacogenetics: its biologic roots and the medical challenge. *Clin. Pharmacol. Ther.*, 54, 235-241

Kalow, W. & Tang, B.-K. (1993) The use of caffeine for enzyme assays: a critical appraisal. *Clin. Pharmacol. Ther.*, 53, 503-514

Kawajiri, K., Nakachi, K., Imai, K., Watanabe, J. & Hayashi, S. (1993) The CYP1A1 gene and cancer susceptibility. *CRC Crit. Rev. Oncol. Hematol.*, 14, 77-87

Kawajiri, K., Watanabe, J., Hidetaka, E., Nakachi, K., Kiyohara, C. & Hayashi, S. (1995) Polymorphisms of human Ah receptor gene are not involved in lung cancer. *Pharmacogenetics*, 5, 151-158

Ketterer, B., Harris, J.M., Talaska, G., Meyer, D.J., Pemble, S.E., Taylor, J.B., Lang, N.P. & Kadlubar, F.F. (1992) The glutathione S-transferase supergene family, its polymorphism, and its effects on susceptibility to lung cancer. *Environ. Health Perspect.*, 98, 87-94

Kim, R.B., O'Shea, D. & Wilkinson, G.R. (1995) Interindividual variability of chlorzoxazone 6-hydroxylation in men and women and its relationship to CYP2E1 genetic polymorphisms. *Clin. Pharmacol. Ther.*, 57, 645-655

Kim, R.B., Yamazaki, H., Chiba, K., Oshea, D., Mimura, M., Guengerich, F.P., Ishizaki, T., Shimada, T. & Wilkinson, G.R. (1996) *In vivo* and *in vitro* characterization of CYP2E1 activity in Japanese and Caucasians. *J. Pharmacol. Exp. Ther.*, 279, 4-11

Kroemer, H.K. & Eichelbaum, M. (1995) Molecular bases and clinical consequences of genetic cytochrome P450 2D6 polymorphism. *Life Sci.*, 56, 2285-2298

Krynetski, E.Y., Tai, H.-L., Yates, C.R., Fessing, M.Y., Loennechen, T., Schuetz, J.D., Relling, M.V. & Evans, W.E. (1996) Genetic polymorphism of thiopurine S-methyltransferase: clinical importance and molecular mechanisms. *Pharmacogenetics*, 6, 279-290

Landi, M.T., Bertazzi, P.A., Shields, P.G., Clark, G., Lucier, G.W., Garte, S.J., Cosma, G. & Caporaso, N.E. (1994) Association between CYP1A1 genotype, mRNA expression and enzymatic activity in humans. *Pharmacogenetics*, 4, 242-246

London, .S.J, Daly, A.K., Leathart. J.B.S., Navidi. W.C. & Idle, J.R. (1996) Lung cancer risk in relation to the CYP2C9*1/CYP2C9*2 genetic polymorphism among African Americans and Caucasians in Los Angeles County, California. *Pharmacogenetics*, 6, 527-533

Lucas, D., Menez, C., Girre, C., Berthou, F., Bodenez, P., Joannet, I., Hispard, E., Bardou, L.-G. & Menez, J.-F. (1995) Cytochrome P450 2E1 genotype and chlorzoxazone metabolism in healthy and alcoholic Caucasian subjects. *Pharmacogenetics*, 5, 298-304

Meisma, R., Fernandez-Salguero, P., van Kuilenburg, A.B.P., van Gennip, A.H. & Gonzalez, F.J. (1995) Human polymorphism in drug metabolism: mutation in the dihydropyrimidine dehydrogenase gene results in exon skipping and thymine uracilurea. *DNA Cell Biol.*, 14, 1-6

Meyer, U.A., Skoda, R.C. & Zanger, U.M. (1990) The general polymorphism of debrisoquine/sparteine metabolism-molecular mechanisms. *Pharmacol. Ther.*, 46, 297-308

Nebert, D.W., McKinnon, R.A. & Puga, A. (1996) Human drug-metabolizing enzyme polymorphisms: effects on risk of toxicity and cancer. *DNA Cell Biol.*, 15, 273-280

Pelkonen, O., Raunio, H., Rautio, A., Mäenpää, J. & Lang, M.A. (1993) Coumarin 7-hydroxylase: characteristics and regulation in mouse and man. *J. Irish Coll. Phys. Surg.*, 22, 24-28

Pelkonen, O., Rautio, A. & Raunio, H. (1995) Specificity and applicability of probes for drug metabolizing enzymes. In: Alvan, G., Balant, L.P., Bechtel, P.R., Boobis, A.R., Gram, L.F., Paintaud, G. & Pithan, K., eds, *European Cooperation in the Field of Scientific and Technical Research - COST B1 Conference on the Variability and Specificity in Drug Metabolism*. Luxembourg, European Commission, pp. 147-158

Pelkonen, O. & Breimer, D.D. (1994) Role of environmental factors in the pharmacokinetics of drugs - considerations with respect to animal models. In: Welling, P.G. & Balant, L.P., eds, *Handbook of Experimental Pharmacology*. Basel, Karger, pp. 289-332

Pelkonen, O. & Raunio, H. (1995) Individual expression of carcinogen-metabolizing enzymes: cytochrome P4502A. *J. Occup. Environ. Med.*, 37, 19-24

Pemble, S.E., Schroeder, K.R., Spencer, S.R., Meyer, D.J., Hallier, E., Bolt, H.M., Ketterer, B. & Taylor, J.B. (1994) Human glutathione S-transferase theta (GSTT1): cDNA cloning and the characterization of a genetic polymorphism. *Biochem. J.*, 300, 271-276

Peter, R., Böcker, R.G., Beaune, P.H., Iwasaki, M., Guengerich, F.P. & Yang, C.-S. (1990) Hydroxylation of chlorzoxazone as a specific probe for human liver cytochrome P-450 IIE1. *Chem. Res. Toxicol.*, 3, 566-573

Raunio, H., Husgafvel-Pursiainen, K., Anttila, S., Hietanen, E., Hirvonen, A. & Pelkonen, O. (1995a) Diagnosis of polymorphisms in carcinogen-activating and inactivating enzymes and cancer susceptibility - review. *Gene*, 159, 113-121

Raunio, H., Pasanen, M., Mäenpää, J., Hakkola, J. & Pelkonen, O. (1995b) Expression of extrahepatic cytochrome P450 in humans. In: Pacifici, G.M. & Fracchia, G.N., eds, *Advances in Drug Metabolism in Man*. Luxembourg, European Commission, Office for Official Publications of the European Communities, pp. 234-287

Shimada, T., Yamazaki, H. & Guengerich, F.P. (1996) Ethnic-related differences in coumarin 7-hydroxylation activity catalysed by cytochrome P2402A6 in liver microsomes of Japanese and Caucasian populations. *Xenobiotica*, 26, 395-403

Sullivan-Klose, T.H., Ghanayem, B.I., Bell, D.A., Zhang, Z.-Y., Kaminsky, L.S., Shenfield, G.M., Miners, J.O., Birkett, D.J. & Goldstein, J.A. (1996) The role of the CYP2C9-Leu359 allelic variant in the tolbutamide polymorphism. *Pharmacogenetics*, 6, 341-349

Tsuneoka, Y., Fukushima, K., Matsuo, Y., Ichikawa, Y. & Watanabe, Y. (1996) Genotype analysis of the CYP2C19 gene in the Japanese population. *Life Sci.*, 59, 1711-1715

Tucker, G.T., Rostami-Hodjegan, A., Nurminen, S. & Jackson, P.R. (1995) Phenotyping populations: pharmacokinetic and statistical issues. In: Alvan, G., Balant, L.P., Bechtel, P.R., Boobis, A.R., Gram, L.F., Paintaud, G. & Pithan, K., eds, *European Cooperation in the Field of Scientific and Technical Research - COST B1 Conference on the Variability and Specificity in Drug Metabolism*. Luxembourg, European Commission, pp. 191-203

Vatsis, K.P., Weber, W.W., Bell, D.A., Dupret, J.-M., Evans, D.A.P., Grant, D.M., Hein, D.W., Lin, H.J., Meyer, U.A., Relling, M.V., Sim, E., Suzuki, T. & Yamazoe, Y. (1995) Nomenclature for N-acetyltransferases. *Pharmacogenetics*, 5, 1-17

Vineis, P., Bartsch, H., Caporaso, N., Harrington, A.M., Kadlubar, F.F., Landi, M.T., Malaveille, C., Shields, P.G., Skipper, P., Talaska, G. & Tannenbaum, S.R. (1994) Genetically based N-acetyltransferase metabolic polymorphism and low-level environmental exposure to carcinogens. *Nature*, 369, 154-156

Weber, W.W. & Hein, D.W. (1985) N-acetylation pharmacogenetics. *Pharmacol. Rev.* 37, 25-79

Wedlund, P.J., Kimura, S., Gonzalez, F.J. & Nebert, D.W. (1994) 1462V mutation in the human CYP1A1 gene: lack of correlation with either the Msp I 1.9 kb (M2) allele of CYP1A1 inducibility in a three-generation family of East Mediterranean descent. *Pharmacogenetics*, 4, 21-26

Wei, X., McLeod, H.L., McMurrough, J., Gonzalez, F.J. & Fernandez-Salguero, P. (1996) Molecular basis of the human dihydropyrimidine dehydrogenase deficiency and 5-fluorouracil toxicity. *J. Clin. Invest.*, 98, 610-615

Weinshilboum, R.M. (1992) Methylation pharmacogenetics: thiopurine methyltransferase as a model system. *Xenobiotica*, 22, 1055-1071

Wrighton, S.A. & Stevens, J.C. (1992) The human hepatic cytochromes P450 involved in in drug metabolism. *Crit. Rev. Toxicol.*, 22, 1-21

Zhang, Z.-Y., Fasco, M.J., Huang, L., Guengerich, F.P. & Kaminsky, L.S. (1996) Characterization of purified human recombinant cytochrome P4501A1-Ile462 and -Val462: assessment of a role for the rare allele in carcinogenesis. *Cancer Res.*, 56, 3926-3933

Corresponding author
Olavi Pelkonen
University of Oulu,
Department of Pharmacology and Toxicology,
Kajaanintie 52 D,
FIN-90220 Oulu, Finland

Metabolic Polymorphisms and Susceptibility to Cancer
W. Ryder
IARC Scientific Publications No. 148
International Agency for Research on Cancer, Lyon, 1999

Chapter 9. The impact of misclassification in case-control studies of gene-environment interactions

Nathaniel Rothman, Montserrat Garcia-Closas, Walter T. Stewart and Jay Lubin

In this Chapter we describe the impact of risk factor misclassification in case-control studies designed to estimate gene-environment interactions. We show that under certain scenarios even small amounts of exposure or genotype misclassification can substantially attenuate the interaction effect and, as a consequence, dramatically increase the sample size required to study these interactions. A consideration of how sample size is affected by exposure and genotype misclassification in the study design phase should help to identify situations where obtaining better risk factor information is crucial for the feasibility of studies.

The misclassification of risk factor information is a common problem in epidemiological studies. Sources of exposure misclassification have been extensively described (Armstrong et al., 1992) and misclassification errors of genetic polymorphisms, which can occur in phenotype or genotype assays, are discussed in the current volume by Vineis and Malats (Chapter 6), Benhamou et al. (Chapter 7), Pelkonen et al. (Chapter 8) and Blömeke and Shields (Chapter 13). We first consider the effects of misclassification in studies of a single risk factor (e.g. genotypes or environmental exposures, broadly defined as exogenous or endogenous carcinogenic agents), and then examine the effects of misclassification in studies of multiplicative interactions between factors. In each section we review the effects of misclassification on the estimated odds ratio (OR) and required sample size, and then illustrate the effects with examples.

Misclassification in studies of one risk factor

The impact of the misclassification of risk factors on estimates of risk and sample size has been extensively addressed (Bross, 1954; Lilienfeld, 1962; Copeland et al., 1977; Shy et al., 1978; Gladen & Rogan, 1979; Greenland, 1980; Flegal et al., 1986; Rothman et al., 1993). In the present Chapter we focus on the effect of misclassifica-

tion of a dichotomous exposure or genotype (i.e. exposed versus unexposed or susceptible versus non-susceptible) on the estimation of the odds ratio measuring the association between the risk factor and disease and on the required sample size to study this association. The true odds ratio is denoted as OR_T and the observed or estimated odds ratio as OR_O. The evaluation of the effects of misclassifying variables with more than two categories or which are continuous measures is beyond the scope of this Chapter.

Misclassification of a dichotomous risk factor is defined by two probabilities: sensitivity (the probability of correctly classifying risk factor positive subjects) and specificity (the probability of correctly classifying risk factor negative subjects). When misclassification is non-differential with regard to disease status, that is, the sensitivity and specificity do not depend on case or control status, the OR_O is generally biased towards the null value of no association (Copeland et al., 1977; Flegal et al., 1986). As a consequence, for a given level of statistical power, a larger sample size is required to detect the attenuated OR_O (Armstrong et al., 1992). The impact of misclassification depends on (1) the prevalence of the risk factor among the controls and (2) the magnitude of the OR_T. Reduced sensitivity tends to have a stronger impact on the magnitude of bias in the OR_O

when the prevalence of the risk factor is high rather than low, and reduced specificity tends to have a stronger impact on the magnitude of the bias when the prevalence is low (Flegal *et al.*, 1986). For a given prevalence of the risk factor the bias in the OR_O increases with the magnitude of the OR_T (Flegal *et al.*, 1986).

As pointed out by Flegal *et al.* (1986), the effects of exposure misclassification on measures of relative risk are complex and not easily generalized, and the potential degree of bias should therefore be evaluated in each particular situation. We illustrate below the effects of misclassification in particular examples which may be of interest in studies of genetic susceptibility to cancer.

Examples

The examples below illustrate the outlined principles in the study of an exposure or genetic factor associated with a fourfold increase in risk of disease ($OR_T = 4$). The OR_O in the presence of misclassification is a function of the OR_T, the true

prevalence of the risk factor in the controls, and the sensitivity and specificity of the risk factor classification (Kleinbaum *et al.*, 1982; Flegal *et al.*, 1986). To illustrate the effects of misclassification we calculated the expected OR_O for a range of values for prevalence, sensitivity and specificity using previously published formulae (Kleinbaum *et al.*, 1982; Flegal *et al.*, 1986). We then estimated the number of subjects necessary to achieve 80% power to detect the expected OR_O, using a two-sided test at the 5% level as described by Schlesselman (1974).

Figs. 1a and 1b show how the OR_O and sample size requirement change as risk factor sensitivity ranges from 0.5 to 1.0 and as the prevalence of the risk factor varies over 0.1, 0.5, and 0.8 (given $OR_T = 4$, a 1:1 case to control ratio, non-differential misclassification, perfect specificity and a desired 80% power). The three lines represent three different risk factor prevalences. Under these conditions, sensitivity has the greatest impact on the OR_O and sample size requirements at medium to high prevalences of the risk factor

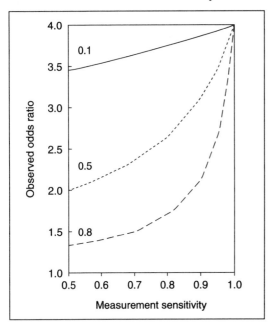

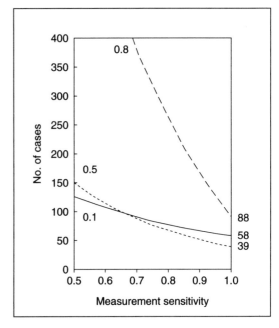

Figure 1a. Observed odds ratio as a function of measurement sensitivity for different prevalences of the risk factor (____ 0.1 prevalence, ... 0.5 prevalence, - - - 0.8 prevalence). True odds ratio equals 4.0.

Figure 1b. Number of cases required to have 80% power to detect an odds ratio of 4.0 using a two-sided test at the 5% level, as a function of measurement sensitivity for different prevalences of the risk factor (____ 0.1 prevalence, ... 0.5 prevalence, - - - 0.8 prevalence). Case:control ratio is 1:1.

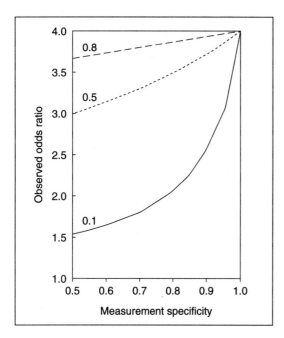

Figure 2a. Observed odds ratio as a function of measurement specificity for different prevalences of the risk factor (____ 0.1 prevalence, ... 0.5 prevalence, - - - 0.8 prevalence). True odds ratio equals 4.0.

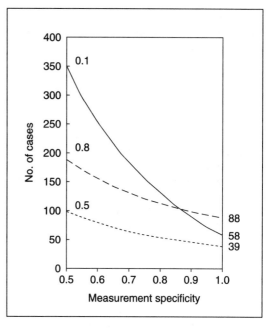

Figure 2b. Number of cases required to have 80% power to detect an odds ratio of 4.0 using a two-sided test at 5% level, as a function of measurement specificity for different prevalences of the risk factor (____ 0.1 prevalence, ... 0.5 prevalence, - - - 0.8 prevalence). Case:control ratio is 1:1.

and this impact decreases as the prevalence becomes lower. For example, when the prevalence is 0.5, a sensitivity of 0.9 results in an OR_O of 3.1 and requires 52 cases and 52 controls, while a sensitivity of 0.7 results in an OR_O of 2.4 and requires 88 cases and 88 controls.

Figs. 2a and 2b illustrate the same scenario except that sensitivity is perfect (1.0) and specificity varies from 0.5 to 1.0. Under these conditions, specificity has the greatest impact on the OR_O and sample size requirements at low prevalences. For example, when the risk factor prevalence is 0.1, a specificity of 0.9 results in an OR_O of 2.6 and requires 90 cases and 90 controls, while a specificity of 0.7 results in an OR_O of 1.8 and requires 183 cases and 183 controls.

The knowledge that risk factor prevalence determines the relative importance of sensitivity and specificity of exposure assessment or genetic analysis can assist investigators to select techniques that minimize the impact of misclassification in their studies. For example, a genotype assay with essentially perfect specificity but with slightly less than perfect sensitivity (e.g. due to alleles not detected by the assay) would have a minimal impact on the OR_O for a relatively low prevalence allele but could have a more substantial impact for a high prevalence allele.

Misclassification in studies of a multiplicative interaction between two risk factors

This section illustrates the effects of misclassification in case-control studies which seek to determine if a disease-exposure association, as measured by the OR, varies for subjects with and without a hypothesized at-risk genotype. A multiplicative interaction implies that the OR for people exposed to both the at-risk genotype and the exposure (i.e. the joint OR) is greater than the product of the OR for the genotype and exposure alone. The interaction effect is the factor by which the joint OR is different from the multiplication of the genetic and exposure effects individually. We focus on the study of multiplicative interaction. However, studies of departures from additive models may also be of interest (Pearce, 1989), especially when the goal is to estimate disease frequency reduction (Kleinbaum *et al.*, 1982).

In studies where the aim is to investigate the presence of a multiplicative interaction between two risk factors and disease, the sample size required is generally much larger than if the aim is to detect a single risk factor effect (Smith & Day, 1984; Lubin & Gail, 1990). The required sample size depends on the true magnitude of association with disease and the true prevalences of the two risk factors, as well as on the sensitivity and specificity for each risk factor (Greenland, 1983).

The effect of misclassification in the assessment of interactions has received only limited attention (Greenland, 1980; Flegal *et al.*, 1986; Cox & Elwood, 1991). If the genotype and environmental exposure are independent in the population and misclassification of either is non-differential with regard to both disease status and each other, the interaction effect tends to be biased towards the null value (Greenland, 1980). Moreover, in general when misclassification of exposure is differential with regard to disease status, which may occur in case-control studies, but is non-differential with regard to genotype, the interaction effect is also biased towards the null (Garcia-Closas *et al.*, 1997).

Examples

Here we illustrate the impact of misclassification on the study sample size and the bias of both the interaction effect and the joint OR. To simplify matters the genotype and environmental exposures are defined as dichotomous variables and are assumed to be independent of each other in the population. Furthermore, misclassification of exposure and genotype are assumed to be independent of each ·other and disease status. The observed ORs in the presence of misclassification were calculated using previously published formulae which express the expected cell counts from a 2 x 2 x 2 table cross-classifying disease, exposure and genotype as a function of the true cell counts and the classification probabilities (i.e. sensitivity and specificity) (Kleinbaum *et al.*, 1982). Sample size calculations were performed as described by Lubin & Gail (1990).

For the examples presented here, genotype prevalence is fixed at 0.5, whereas exposure

Table 1. True odds ratios used in an example of gene-environment interaction

		Odds ratios	
		Genotype	
		–	+ (at-risk allele)
Exposure	–	1.0	2.0
	+	2.0	12.0

prevalence takes values of 0.1, 0.5 and 0.8. As shown in Table 1, the effect of the at-risk genotype in the absence of the environmental exposure and the effect of the exposure in the absence of the at-risk genotype have been arbitrarily set at 2.0, the joint effect (or joint OR) of the genotype and exposure has been set at 12.0, and the interaction effect has been set to 3.0 (i.e. 12.0/(2.0 x 2.0)). The gene-specific exposure ORs are 6.0 (genotype (+) = 12.0/2.0) and 2.0 (genotype (-) = 2.0/1.0). The numbers shown in Table 1 are true and expected parameters that do not depend on the number of cases and controls.

Perfect sensitivity and specificity are rarely attained in the measurement of environmental exposures. An environmental exposure assessment method that resulted in 0.8 sensitivity would generally be considered excellent. Table 2 shows the OR_T and OR_O for genotype and exposure when the prevalence of each is 0.5,

Table 2. True odds ratios and observed odds ratios (shown in parentheses) when exposure sensitivity is 0.8[1]

		True (observed) odds ratios	
		Genotype	
		–	+ (at-risk allele)
Exposure	–	1.0	2.0 (3.1)
	+	2.0 (1.7)	12.0 (10.3)

[1] Prevalence of both exposure and at-risk allele among controls = 50%; exposure specificity, genotype sensitivity and genotype specificity = 100%.

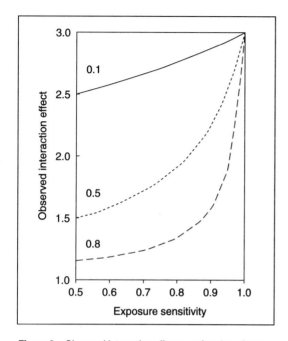

Figure 3a. Observed interaction effect as a function of exposure sensitivity for different exposure prevalences (___ 0.1 prevalence, ... 0.5 prevalence, - - - 0.8 prevalence). True interaction effect is 3.0, the true ORs of disease given exposure among non-susceptibles and given genotype among unexposed are both 2.0, and the genotype prevalence is 0.5.

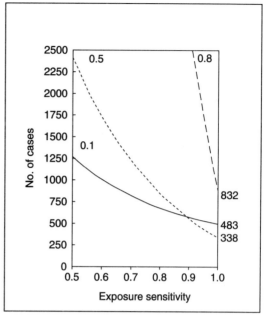

Figure 3b. Number of cases required to have 80% power to detect a threefold interaction using a two-sided test at 5% level, as a function of exposure sensitivity for different exposure prevalences (___ 0.1 prevalence, ... 0.5 prevalence, - - - 0.8 prevalence). The true ORs of disease given that exposure among non-susceptibles and genotype among unexposed are both 2.0, and the genotype prevalence is 0.5. Case:control ratio is 1:1.

exposure sensitivity is 0.8 and exposure specificity is 1.0. As we would expect from the non-differential nature of the misclassification, the gene-specific exposure ORs (genotype (+) = 10.3/3.1; genotype (-) = 1.7/1.0) are biased towards the null value. On the other hand, the genotype OR among unexposed subjects is biased away from the null (from 2.0 to 3.1). This reflects the fact that although the genotype is perfectly measured in this example, the observed genotype OR among the unexposed in the presence of exposure misclassification is a weighted average of the genotype OR among truly unexposed subjects and truly exposed subjects who were classified as unexposed. The interaction effect is attenuated from 3.0 to 1.95 (10.3/(1.7 x 3.1)), and the sample size required to have 80% power increases from 338 cases and 338 controls with perfect exposure assessment to 847 cases and 847 controls with 0.8 sensitivity.

Figs. 3a and 3b illustrate the impact on the interaction effect of varying exposure sensitivity from 0.5 to 1.0 while holding exposure specificity at 1.0. Again, the three lines represent three different exposure prevalences. The impact of sensitivity on the observed interaction effect is much greater for common exposures than for rare exposures (Fig. 3a). The attenuation in the observed interaction effect translates into an increased required sample size (Fig. 3b). For example, for an exposure prevalence of 0.5, lowering exposure sensitivity from 0.9 to 0.7 more than doubles the required sample size (from 560 to 1223 cases). At an exposure prevalence of 0.8, the sample size is dramatically increased even by small amounts of exposure inaccuracy, calling into question the feasibility of the study.

Figs. 4a and 4b illustrate results obtained when exposure sensitivity is held at 1.0 and exposure specificity is varied from 0.5 to 1.0.

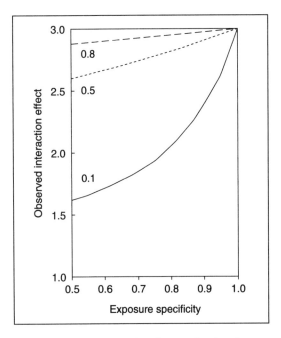

Figure 4a. Observed interaction effect as a function of exposure specificity for different exposure prevalences (___ 0.1 prevalence, ... 0.5 prevalence, - - - 0.8 prevalence). The true interaction effect is 3.0, the true ORs of disease given that exposure among non-susceptibles and genotype among unexposed are both 2.0, and genotype prevalence is 0.5.

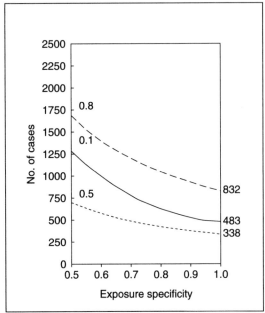

Figure 4b. Number of cases required to have 80% power for detection of a threefold interaction using a two-sided test at 5% level, as a function of exposure specificity for different exposure prevalences (___ 0.1 prevalence, ... 0.5 prevalence, - - - 0.8 prevalence). The true ORs of disease given that exposure among non-susceptibles and genotype among unexposed are both 2.0. Case:control ratio is 1:1.

They show that, under our assumptions, the effect of exposure specificity is greater for rare than for common exposures. For an exposure prevalence of 0.1, lowering exposure specificity from 0.9 to 0.7 increases the required sample size by about 50% (from 523 to 784 cases), whereas the effect is smaller for exposure prevalences of 0.5 and 0.8.

Figs. 5a and 5b illustrate the effect of exposure sensitivity and specificity on the observed joint

Table 3. Impact of exposure and genotype misclassification on sample size requirements to detect gene-environment interaction[1]			
Example	Exposure accuracy	Genotype accuracy	# cases needed for 80% power to detect interaction
	Sensitivity	Sensitivity	
1	1.0	1.0	338
2	1.0	0.95	442
3	0.8	1.0	847
4	0.8	0.95	1156

[1] Interaction model described in Table 1; prevalence of both at-risk genotype and exposure = 0.5 among controls; genotype and exposure specificity = 1.0; 1:1 case to control ratio.

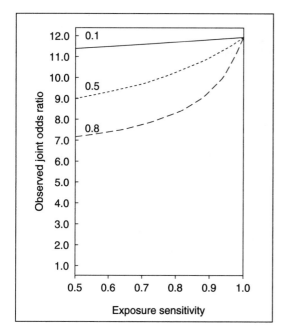

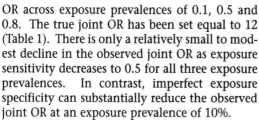

Figure 5a. Observed joint odds ratio as a function of exposure sensitivity for different exposure prevalences (____ 0.1 prevalence, ... 0.5 prevalence, - - - 0.8 prevalence). The true joint odds ratio is 12.0, the true odds ratios of disease given that exposure among non-susceptibles and genotype among unexposed are both 2.0, and the genotype prevalence is 0.5.

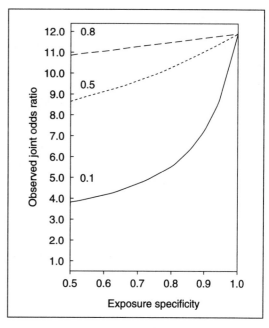

Figure 5b. Observed joint odds ratio as a function of exposure specificity for different exposure prevalences (____ 0.1 prevalence, ... 0.5 prevalence, - - - 0.8 prevalence). The true joint odds ratio is 12.0, the true ORs of disease given that exposure among non-susceptibles and genotype among unexposed are both 2.0, and the genotype prevalence is 0.5.

OR across exposure prevalences of 0.1, 0.5 and 0.8. The true joint OR has been set equal to 12 (Table 1). There is only a relatively small to modest decline in the observed joint OR as exposure sensitivity decreases to 0.5 for all three exposure prevalences. In contrast, imperfect exposure specificity can substantially reduce the observed joint OR at an exposure prevalence of 10%.

In exploring the effects of exposure misclassification we have assumed that the genotype was perfectly measured. However, misclassification of genetic status can occur (Cascorbi *et al.*, 1995; Blömeke & Shields, Chapter 13) and has an additional influence on sample size requirements. Table 3 illustrates the impact of changing genotype sensitivity from 1.0 to 0.95 on sample size, both in the absence and presence of non-differential exposure misclassification. In the absence of exposure misclassification, a genotype sensitivity of 0.95 increases the sample size by about 30% (from 338 to 442 cases). When exposure sensitiv-

ity is 0.8 rather than 1.0, the increase due to the genotype error is 36% (from 847 to 1156). Thus, even small genotype errors can substantially increase the required sample size to detect a gene-environment interaction, and this increase is greater when the exposure is also misclassified.

Concluding remarks

These examples show that, in certain scenarios, even small amounts of exposure misclassification can substantially attenuate the interaction effect, and therefore substantially increase the already large sample size required to study gene-environment interactions. Errors in genotype determination further increase the required sample size. Considering how sample size is affected by exposure misclassification in the study design phase helps to identify situations where obtaining better exposure information is crucial for the feasibility of the study.

References

Armstrong, B.K., White, E. & Saracci R. (1992) *Principles of Exposure Measurement in Epidemiology.* Oxford, Oxford University Press, pp. 49-136

Bross, I. (1954) Misclassification in 2 X 2 tables. *Biometrics,* 10, 478-486

Cascorbi, I., Drakoulis, N., Brockmöller, J., Maurer, A., Sperling, K. & Roots, I. (1995) Arylamine N-acetyltransferase (*NAT2*) mutations and their allelic linkage in unrelated Caucasian individuals: correlation with phenotypic activity. *Am. J. Hum. Genet.,* 57, 581-592

Copeland, K.T., Checkoway, H., McMichael A.J. & Holbrook, R.H. (1977) Bias due to misclassification in the estimation of relative risk. *Am. J. Epidemiol.,* 105, 488-495

Cox, B. & Elwood, M.J. (1991) The effect on the stratum-specific odds ratios of non-differential misclassification of a dichotomous covariate. *Am. J. Epidemiol.,* 15, 202-207

Diamond, E. & Lilienfeld, A.M. (1962) Effects of errors in classification and diagnosis in various types of epidemiological studies. *Am. J. Public Health,* 52(11), 37-44

Flegal, K.M., Brownie, C. & Haas, J.D. (1986) The effects of exposure misclassification on estimates of relative risk. *Am. J. Epidemiol.,* 123, 736-751

Garcia-Closas, M., Thompson, D.W. & Robins, J.M. (1998) Differential misclassification and the assessment of gene-environment interactions in case-control studies. *Am. J. Epidemiol.,* 147, 426-433

Gladen, B. & Rogan, W.J. (1979) Misclassification and the design of environmental studies. *Am. J. Epidemiol.,* 109, 607-616

Goldstein, A.M., Falk, R.T., Korczak, J.F. & Lubin, J.H. (1997) Detecting gene-environment interactions using a case-control design. *Am. J. Hum. Genet.,* 14, 1085-1089

Greenland, S. (1980) The effect of misclassification in the presence of covariates. *Am. J. Epidemiol.,* 112, 564-569

Greenland, S. (1983) Tests for interaction in epidemiologic studies: a review and a study of power. *Stat. Med.,* 2, 243-251

Kleinbaum, D.G., Kupper, L.L. & Morgenstern, H. (1982) *Epidemiologic Research: Principles and Quantitative Methods.* New York, Van Nostrand Reinhold

Lubin, J.H. & Gail, M.H. (1990) On power and sample size for studying features of the relative odds of disease. *Am. J. Epidemiol.,* 131, 552-566

Pearce, N. (1989) Analytic implications of epidemiological concepts of interaction. *Int. J. Epidemiol.,* 18, 976-980

Rothman, N., Stewart, W.F., Caporaso, N.E. & Hayes, R.B. (1993) Misclassification of genetic susceptibility biomarkers: implications for case-control studies and cross-population comparisons. *Cancer Epidemiol. Biomarkers Prev.,* 2, 299-303

Schlesselman J.J. (1974) Sample size requirements in cohort and case-control studies of disease. *Am. J. Epidemiol.,* 99, 381-384

Shy, C.M., Kleinbaum, D.G. & Morgenstern, H. (1978) The effect of misclassification of exposure in epidemiologic studies of air pollution health effects. *Bull. NY Acad. Med.,* 54, 1155-1156

Smith, P.G. & Day, N.E. The design of case-control studies: the influence of confounding and interaction effects. *Int. J. Epidemiol.,* 13, 356-365

Corresponding author
Nathaniel Rothman
NIH/NCI EPS 8116,
Bethesda, MD 20892,
USA

Metabolic Polymorphisms and Susceptibility to Cancer
W. Ryder
IARC Scientific Publications No. 148
International Agency for Research on Cancer, Lyon, 1999

Chapter 10. Epidemiological studies on genetic polymorphism: study design issues and measures of occurrence and association

Paolo Boffetta and Neil Pearce

As with other epidemiological studies, the design and analysis of a study including genetic polymorphisms generally involve relating a particular disease or health outcome to a particular exposure or genetic trait, while assessing the presence of systematic error, controlling random error and assessing effect modification (interaction) with other exposures or traits. In studies of determinants and mechanisms of disease, markers of genetic polymorphism are generally treated either as exposure variables or as effect modifiers. In epidemiological studies the study base can be completely enumerated, and the cases can be identified as either incident or prevalent cases (incidence and prevalence studies). Alternatively, the study may involve cases of the disease (or condition) under investigation and a control group sampled from the study base that generated the cases (incidence and prevalence case-control studies). Most available studies on metabolic polymorphism and cancer risk are incidence case-control studies. Their major methodological problem is the selection of controls, which may be an important source of bias. Another important limitation of many available studies is the small sample size, which may be inadequate for assessing statistical interaction when the metabolic polymorphism is treated as an effect modifier.

In general, etiological epidemiological research on cancer involves studying the external, modifiable causes of diseases in populations (McMichael, 1995) with the intention of developing preventive interventions. In addition, genetically determined risk factors are studied with the intention of identifying high-risk individuals and increasing the efficacy of prevention (Caporaso & Goldstein, 1997). Using biomarkers to obtain better measurements of internal exposure (dose), disease or individual susceptibility can enhance the study of both external causes of cancer and genetic traits. The present book explains the use of markers of genetic polymorphisms, which are a specific type of biomarkers of susceptibility. Issues of design and analysis in studies using markers of genetic polymorphisms are not markedly different from those involved in studies using other types of biomarkers, or in other epidemiological studies (McMichael, 1994; Pearce et al.,

1995). When both genetic polymorphisms and external exposures are studied, the analysis of interaction is of particular interest (Rothman, 1995; Pearce & Boffetta, 1997) (Fig. 1A). However, if the relevant carcinogen is unknown or if exposure cannot be measured the existence of effect modification will be unknown, but it will be observed that persons with a given polymorphism have a higher cancer risk than persons without it. In this case, genetic polymorphism is studied as an independent risk factor for cancer (Fig. 1B).

As in other epidemiological studies the design and analysis of a study including genetic polymorphisms involve in general relating a particular disease (or health outcome, such as a marker of early effect) to a particular exposure or genetic trait, while assessing the possibility of systematic error, controlling random error, and assessing effect modification (interaction) with other exposures or traits. We shall consid-

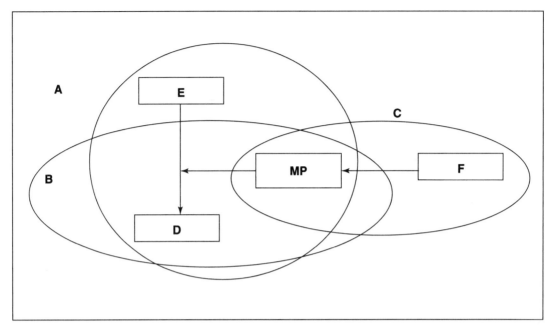

Figure 1. Examples of different epidemiological approaches to the study of metabolic polymorphism. Exposure E is causally related to disease D; and the effect of E on D is modified by the metabolic polymorphism MP, which in turn is determined by factor F.
In study A the E-D relationship is addressed: MP is studied as effect modifier.
In study B, E is unknown and only the MP-D relationship is addressed: MP is studied as disease risk factor.
In study C, only the F-MP relationship is addressed (e.g. transitional study): MP is studied as outcome.

er each of these aspects of study design and analysis in turn. In studies of determinants and mechanisms of disease, markers of genetic polymorphism are treated as exposure variables. However, markers of polymorphism, and in particular phenotypic markers, can be influenced by additional factors, and studies can be conducted in which the marker is treated as outcome variable (Fig. 1C). These studies are sometimes included in the category of transitional studies (Hulka et al., 1990).

A major problem in studies of genetic polymorphisms is the difference between genotype and phenotype. This distinction is crucial because, although markers of genotype are very unlikely to change over time (if they are measured accurately), markers of phenotype (which is usually more etiologically relevant) may change over time as the phenotype is affected by other environmental exposures and by disease progression. In addition, there may be considerable problems in measuring pheno-type accurately at one particular point in time.

These problems of measurement of phenotypic expression, and of changes in phenotypic expression over time, are the key issues in the design of epidemiological studies of genetic polymorphisms.

Types of epidemiological studies and measures of occurrence and association

As a general model, epidemiological studies are based on the experience of a particular population during a particular period of time. Miettinen (1985) has termed this study population the "base population" and its experience over time the "study base". Epidemiological study designs differ only in how the study base is defined and how information is drawn from it (Checkoway et al., 1989). Thus, epidemiological studies may involve measuring either the incidence or prevalence of disease. This distinction is important in studies involving genetic polymorphisms. In genotype-based studies both incidence and prevalence studies provide the same information if genotype does not influence survival. In phenotype-based studies, on the other hand, it is usually preferable to measure incidence rather than prevalence since cases could change their phenotype with disease progression. In addition, prevalence is influenced by survival, which may affect both genotype- and phenotype-based studies.

Incidence studies

Incidence studies measure the incidence of disease in one or more study populations, which are completely enumerated. Cohort studies are the best known of studies of this kind, but incidence studies also include national or regional cancer incidence statistics (e.g. annual cancer incidence rates) based on routinely collected cancer registry information. Three measures of disease incidence are commonly used in incidence studies (Fig. 2).The (person-time) *incidence rate* (or incidence density (Miettinen, 1985)) is a measure of disease occurrence per unit time. A second measure of disease occurrence is the *incidence proportion* (cumulative incidence (Miettinen, 1985)) or *risk*, which is the proportion of study subjects who experience the outcome of interest at any time during the follow-up period. A third possible measure of disease occurrence is the *incidence odds*

(Greenland, 1987), which is the ratio of the number of subjects who experience the outcome to the number of subjects who do not.

Corresponding to these measures of disease occurrence are three principal ratio measures of effect which can be used in incidence studies involving comparison of two or more populations or groups (e.g. those with and those without a particular genetic polymorphism). The measure of primary interest is often the *rate ratio* (incidence density ratio), which is the ratio of the incidence rate in the exposed group to that in the non-exposed group. A second commonly used effect measure is the *risk ratio* (incidence proportion ratio), which is the ratio of the incidence proportion in the exposed group to that in the non-exposed group. When the outcome is rare over the follow-up period the risk ratio is approximately equal to the rate ratio. A third possible effect measure is the incidence *odds ratio*, which is the ratio of the incidence odds in the exposed group to that in the non-exposed group. An analogous approach can be used to calculate measures of effect based on differences rather than ratios, in particular the *rate difference* and the *risk difference*. It should, however, be pointed out that when the disease is rare the difference between the different measures of effect is small.

Incidence case-control studies

If obtaining exposure information is costly or difficult (which may be the situation in a study of genetic polymorphisms) it may be more efficient to conduct an incidence case-control study by obtaining exposure information on all of the incident cases of the disease under study and a sample of controls selected at random from the study base. The relative risk measure is the incidence *odds ratio*; the effect measure which this estimates depends on the manner in which controls are selected. Again there are three main options (Pearce, 1993).

One option is to select controls from those who do not experience the outcome during the follow-up period, i.e. the *survivors* (those not developing the outcome at any time during the follow-up period). In this instance a sample of controls chosen by *cumulative incidence sampling* estimates the exposure odds of the survivors,

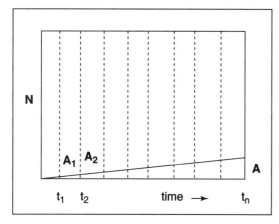

Figure 2. Measures of disease incidence in incidence studies. During the study of duration of n unit time intervals, a total of A cases arise out of N study subjects.
During each time interval, a total of A_i cases arise out of N_i study subjects.
Cumulative incidence = A/N
Incidence odds = A/(N-A)
Incidence rate = $(\Sigma A_i / N_i)/n$

and the odds ratio obtained in the case-control study therefore estimates the incidence odds ratio in the *base population*. Controls can also be sampled from the entire base population (those at risk at the beginning of follow-up), rather than just from the survivors (those at risk at the end of follow-up). In such *case-base sampling* the controls estimate the exposure odds in the base population of persons at risk at the start of follow-up, and the odds ratio obtained in the case-control study therefore estimates the risk ratio in the base population. The third approach is to select controls longitudinally throughout the course of the study (Miettinen, 1976); this is sometimes described as "risk-set sampling" (Robins *et al.*, 1986), "sampling from the study base" (the person-time experience) (Miettinen, 1985), or "*density sampling*" (Kleinbaum *et al.*, 1982). In this instance, the controls estimate the exposure odds in the study base, and the odds ratio obtained in the case-control study therefore estimates the rate ratio in the study base. Most of the epidemiological studies available in the literature on metabolic polymorphism and cancer risk can be defined as incidence case-control studies. In this type of study the choice of the controls represents the most problematic aspect of design and is particularly subject to selection bias.

Although in many case-control studies the study base is not explicitly identified, it is necessary for the investigator to conceptualize it in order to assess the appropriateness of the choice of controls. This is particularly difficult in clinic-based studies, in which the study base is defined not only in terms of relatively simple characteristics such as age, gender and residence, but also in terms of access to a given department of a given hospital.

Prevalence studies

The term *prevalence* denotes the number of cases of disease existing in a population at the time a study is conducted. If we denote the prevalence of a disease in the study population by P and assume that the incidence rate is constant over time (and that migration into and out of the study base is not related to "exposure" status), then it can be shown (Rothman, 1986) that the prevalence odds (P/(1 - P)) is equal to the incidence rate (I) multiplied by the average disease duration (D):

$$\frac{P}{(1-P)} = ID$$

Thus, the *prevalence odds* is directly proportional to the disease incidence, and the *prevalence odds ratio* estimates:

$$OR = \frac{I_1 \times D_1}{I_0 \times D_0}$$

An increased prevalence odds ratio may thus reflect the influence of factors which increase the disease incidence and/or factors which increase disease duration. The different mechanisms involved in increasing disease incidence or disease duration are likely to involve different time patterns of exposure, genetic factors and disease. For example, suppose that a particular genetic polymorphism has no effect on cancer incidence but is associated with poorer survival in people who develop cancer. A cancer prevalence study would then show a lower prevalence of cancer in those with the polymorphism, whereas a cancer incidence study would show no association with the polymorphism, and a study of the incidence of cancer mortality would show a greater mortality rate in those with the polymorphism.

Prevalence case-control studies

Just as an incidence case-control study can be used to obtain the same findings as a full cohort study, a prevalence case-control study can be used to obtain the same findings as a full prevalence study in a more efficient manner. A sample of controls estimates the "exposure" (to an external agent or genetic trait) odds of the non-cases, and the odds ratio obtained in the prevalence case-control study therefore estimates the prevalence odds ratio in the base population, which in turn estimates the incidence rate ratio if the average duration of disease is the same in the exposed and non-exposed groups.

Other types of epidemiological studies

The four types of epidemiological studies described above cover the various approaches in terms of the strategy of sampling from the study base and identifying the cases of disease occurring in the study base (incident or prevalent cases). Alternative designs in studies of metabolic polymorphism and cancer risk (e.g. comparisons between series of cases of cancer, such as cases of lung cancer with differing histology) should be avoided in studies aimed at assessing the risk of cancer linked to metabolic polymorphisms.

Transitional studies may not fall into the scheme presented here. These are studies designed to bridge the gap between laboratory experiments and population-based epidemiology (Hulka et al., 1990; Schulte & Perera, 1997). The goal of transitional studies is to characterize and validate the biomarker of susceptibility and to optimize its condition of use. Generally, transitional studies involve healthy individuals or groups of patients and are based on samples of convenience. Transitional studies have been particularly useful for developing assays of phenotypic polymorphisms based on the administration of drugs such as debrisoquine and sulfamethazine: an example is the study by Green-Gallo et al. (1991) aimed at developing a protocol for the safe administration of debrisoquine in hospitalized patients who may undergo hypotensive episodes after the drug has been given. While transitional studies are of great importance for determining the validity of markers of susceptibility, they should be considered as distinct from epidemiological studies. In all cases the distinction between transitional and applied studies should be clearly maintained.

Exposure

As noted above, a genetic polymorphism may be considered in epidemiological studies both as an effect modifier and as an independent risk factor. In either situation, markers of the genotype are unlikely to change over time, provided that they are measured accurately (organ transplant is an example of change in genotype), but their phenotypic expression may do so. It is therefore important to measure the phenotypic expression at the etiologically relevant period (Pearce et al., 1986, 1995). In general, phenotypic expression depends on the combination of genes and environment. For example, the CYP1A2 phenotype is influenced by the gene and an array of external factors, such as tobacco smoking and meat consumption. An

additional important problem is that the phenotype may change as a result of the disease process or due to the drugs administered because of the disease. One example is the phenotypic assay based on debrisoquine metabolism, which is used to measure CYP2D6 polymorphism and can be altered by concomitant administration of other medicaments (Caporaso et al., 1992). This may affect the measurement of phenotype in cancer case-control studies. However, there may be other important changes in phenotypic expression over time as a result of other exposures unrelated to the disease process. If it is not possible to take repeated biological samples over time, and if phenotypic expression is likely to have changed over time, then it is essential that the samples taken relate to the etiologically relevant time period. In particular, stored biological samples may not validly measure long-term patterns of exposure, unless the samples have been taken repeatedly over the course of the study (Armstrong et al., 1992).

Systematic error

The major possible types of systematic error (bias) are the same in studies involving genetic polymorphisms and in traditional epidemiology (Boffetta, 1995). The various types of bias can be grouped into three major classes: selection bias, information bias and confounding (Rothman, 1986).

Selection bias

Selection bias arises from the procedures whereby study participants are chosen from the study base. Selection bias can be avoided by including all the study base (i.e. a cohort study), or by selecting controls as a random sample of the study base (in a case-control study) and obtaining a response rate of 100%. This is often impracticable, however, particularly if phenotyping requires the administration of drugs with possible adverse reactions. In some situations selection bias can be controlled in the analysis by identifying factors that are related to subject selection and controlling for them as confounders. The statistical issues involved in controlling for selection bias in the analysis are essentially the same as those involved in controlling for sources of confounding.

Selection bias is of particular concern in case-control studies where controls are not chosen as a random sample of the study base, e.g. if they are chosen from persons with other diseases (Pearce & Checkoway, 1988). The choice of hospital controls may be particularly problematic since a given polymorphism may be associated with an increased - or decreased - probability of developing a disease included among those from which controls are drawn. For example, among nine studies conducted in Caucasian populations on the phenotypic expression of the CYP2D6 polymorphism, assessed by response after debrisoquine administration, and lung cancer risk, the prevalence of poor metabolizers in controls varied between 6% (Hirvonen et al., 1993) and 13% (Caporaso et al., 1990). If controls are selected from a pool of patients with different diseases, it is unlikely that the polymorphism under study affects the risk of hospitalization of a large proportion of them. Care should therefore be taken in hospital-based studies to avoid selecting controls with a narrow series of diseases (Pearce & Checkoway, 1988). An additional concern arises from the observation that polymorphism may affect participation in epidemiological studies: for example, the fact that poor metabolizers of CYP2D6 were overrepresented among healthy volunteers enrolled in a clinical trial (Llerena et al., 1989) may be explained by effect of the CYP2D6 on brain function (Caporaso et al., 1995).

Information bias
Information bias involves misclassification of the study participants with respect to disease or exposure status. Thus, the concept of information bias refers to those people actually included in the study, whereas selection bias refers to the selection of the study participants from the study base while confounding generally refers to non-comparability of subgroups within the study base. The various methodological issues of validity, reproducibility and stability of markers of genetic polymorphisms are part of the more general problem of information bias. Errors can occur in phenotyping due to variation in subject compliance, doses administered, differing methods of sample collection, and exposure to factors that inhibit or induce enzyme activity (Brosen et al., 1987; d'Errico et al., 1996). Errors can occur in genotyping due to errors in DNA techniques (Heim & Mayer, 1991).

Rothman et al. (1993) noted that the prevalence of a polymorphism must be considered when evaluating the likely extent of misclassification. When a polymorphism is common (close to 50%), sensitivity is important, as a small decrease in sensitivity may cause the misclassification of many subjects, whereas a corresponding decrease in specificity produces little bias. The converse applies when a polymorphism is rare.

Non-differential information bias occurs when the likelihood of misclassification of exposure is the same for cases and non-cases of disease (or when the likelihood of misclassification of disease is the same for exposed and non-exposed persons). Non-differential misclassification of exposure generally biases the relative risk estimate towards the null value of 1.0 (Copeland et al., 1977). Hence, non-differential information bias tends to produce "false negative" findings and is of particular concern in studies that find no association between exposure and disease.

Differential information bias occurs when the likelihood of misclassification of exposure is different in cases and non-cases (or the likelihood of misclassification of disease is different in exposed and non-exposed persons). This can bias the observed effect estimate in either direction, either towards or away from the null value.

Information bias can drastically affect the validity of a study. As a general principle it is important to ensure that the misclassification is non-differential by ensuring that "exposure" information is collected in an identical manner in cases and non-cases (or that disease information is collected in an identical manner in the exposed and non-exposed groups). In this situation the bias is in a known direction (towards the null) and, although there may be concern that not finding a significant association (between exposure and disease) may be due to non-differential information bias, at least one can be confident that any positive findings are not a consequence of information bias. Thus, the aim of data collection is not to obtain perfect information but to acquire comparable information in a similar manner from the groups being compared, even if this means ignoring more detailed exposure information where this is not available for both groups. However, it is clearly important to collect information that is as detailed and accurate as possible. When it is not possible to collect perfect information on all subjects it is vital that information from cases and controls be collected in a similar manner.

As noted above, the major concern in studies involving genetic polymorphisms is that the phenotypic expression may be influenced by the disease itself. In addition to cases, this issue applies to controls enrolled in hospital-based case-control studies. This situation is different from the problem of selection bias due to the influence of polymorphism on the disease of the controls (i.e. when the polymorphism increases the risk of some of the control diseases occurring); the problem is rather that unspecific pathological processes, such as chronic inflammation and altered lipid metabolism, may lead to changes in the expression of, or biases in the measurement of, a phenotypic polymorphism in large subsets of hospital-based controls. This problem is particularly relevant since phenotype measurements are usually more feasible in hospital-based studies. It is less so in incidence cohort studies (or nested incidence case-control studies) in which the marker is measured on biological material collected before the onset of disease, provided that cases diagnosed within a short interval after sample collection are excluded and the validity of the measurement of the polymorphism is not influenced by storage (although in this case differential bias may be avoided by matching according to time of sample storage). The fact that the relationships between exposure, marker and disease are in most cases obscure limits the interpretation of the findings of biomarker-based studies with respect to the presence or absence of information bias.

Confounding

Confounding occurs when the exposed and non-exposed groups in the study base are not comparable because of inherent differences in background disease risk (Greenland & Robins, 1986) attributable to exposure to other risk factors. The concept of confounding thus generally refers to the study base, although, as noted above, confounding can also be introduced (or removed) by the manner in which study participants are selected from the study base. If no other biases are present, three conditions are necessary for a factor to be a confounder (Rothman, 1986). First, a con-

founder is a factor that is predictive of disease (in the absence of the exposure under study). Second, a confounder is associated with exposure or genetic trait in the study base. Third, a variable that is intermediate in the causal pathway between exposure and disease is *not* a confounder. The latter condition may be hard to assess since it is difficult to determine causal pathways empirically.

The potential for confounding is of major concern in all epidemiological studies, including those involving genetic polymorphisms. The availability of accurate measures of genetic polymorphisms does not reduce the need to control for confounding, since genetic polymorphisms may not only vary by demographic factors (d'Errico *et al.*, 1996) but may also be coincidentally associated with other risk factors for disease. In other words, the marker is independent of the exposure-disease relationship but is determined by the exposure, which is a risk factor of the disease. For example, smoking seems to influence phenotypic assays for polymorphisms of CYP1A2 and UDP-glucuronosyltransferase, as measured by the metabolic ratios of caffeine metabolism and paracetamol metabolism: both glucuronidation capacity, as assessed by the metabolic ratio of urinary paracetamol and paracetamol glucuronide, and CYP1A2 activity, as assessed by the analysis of caffeine metabolites, are increased in smokers and in comparison with non-smokers (Bock *et al.*, 1994).

The most straightforward method of controlling confounding in the analysis of both an exposure and an effect modifier involves stratifying the data into subgroups according to the levels of the confounder(s) and calculating a summary effect estimate which summarizes the information across strata. However, it is usually not possible to control simultaneously for more than two or three confounders when using stratified analysis. This problem can be mitigated to some extent by the use of mathematical modelling, but this may in turn produce problems of multicollinearity when variables that are highly correlated are entered simultaneously into the model.

In general, control for confounding requires careful use of *a priori* knowledge, together with assessment of the extent to which the effect estimate changes when the factor is controlled in the analysis. Most epidemiologists prefer to make a decision based on the latter criterion, although it can be misleading, particularly if misclassification is occurring (Greenland & Robins, 1985). The problem with markers of genetic polymorphism, however, is that previous knowledge of their associations with exposures is very limited. The decision to control for a presumed confounder can certainly be made with more confidence if there is supporting prior knowledge that the factor is predictive of disease. It is therefore important that studies are conducted in close collaboration with scientists with a deep knowledge of the mechanisms in which the enzymes under investigation are involved.

Misclassification of a confounder leads to a loss of ability to control confounding, although control may still be useful provided that misclassification of the confounder is unbiased (Greenland, 1980).

When appropriate information is not available to control confounding directly it remains desirable to assess its potential strength and direction. For example, it may be possible to obtain information on a surrogate for the confounder of interest. Even though confounder control is imperfect in this situation, it is still possible to examine whether the main effect estimate changes when the surrogate is controlled in the analysis, and to assess the strength and direction of the change. Alternatively, it may be possible to obtain accurate confounder information for a subgroup of participants (cases and non-cases) in the study, and to assess the effects of confounder control in this subgroup.

A related approach involves obtaining confounder information for a sample of the study base (or a sample of the controls in a case-control study).

Random error

Random error occurs in any epidemiological study, just as it occurs in experimental studies. It is often referred to as "chance", although it can perhaps more reasonably be regarded as "ignorance", at least at the macroscopic level (Checkoway et al., 1989). Even in an experimental study, in which participants are randomized into "exposed" and "non-exposed" groups, there are "random" differences in background risk

between the compared groups, but these diminish in importance (i.e. the random differences "even out") as the size of the study grows. In epidemiological studies there is no guarantee that differences in baseline (background) risk will "even out" between the exposure groups as the study size grows, but it is necessary to make this assumption in order to proceed (Greenland & Robins, 1986). An adequate study size may therefore control random error (formulae to calculate the required sample size are available in Breslow & Day, 1987) but, in practice, the study size depends on the number of available participants and the available resources. Within these limitations it is desirable to make the study as large as possible, taking into account the trade-off between including more participants and gathering more detailed information about a smaller number of participants (Greenland, 1988).

As for other epidemiology studies, in those involving genetic polymorphisms statistical power is a function of the prevalence of exposure and the magnitude of risk; a polymorphism with high prevalence and high relative risk can be evaluated in small populations, whereas a polymorphism with low prevalence and low relative risk requires a larger population. One example of this problem is the study of the MspI restriction fragment length polymorphism of the CYP1A1 gene. While the prevalence of homozygotic mutants in controls is of the order of 20% in Japanese populations (Kawajiri et al., 1990; Nakachi et al., 1991, 1993), the value is much lower in other populations, especially among Caucasians in Europe and North America, where it has been found to range from 0.5% to 4% (Tefre et al., 1991; Shields et al., 1993; Alexandrie et al., 1994; Ambrosone et al., 1995). It should be noted that the number of cases required in a case-control study to reach a statistical power of 80% for the detection of a statistically significant relative risk of 1.8, which is close to that observed in some Japanese studies, is 210 with a prevalence of 20% among controls and over 1500 with a prevalence of 2% (assuming in both circumstances one control per case and no confounding). The optimal balance between precision and validity depends on a number of considerations, including the relative costs of the various exposure measurement techniques (Greenland, 1988).

In general, however, small study size is a drawback of many available studies on metabolic polymorphism and cancer risk. Even for a polymorphism with relatively high prevalence, such as N-acetyl transferase, showing a prevalence of slow acetylators of the order of 40-60% in most populations, only 7 of the 26 studies in the literature have power above 70% to detect a relative risk of 2. This represents the average size of the effect of slow acetylation polymorphism (d'Errico et al., 1996). A proper consideration of study size should be a required feature of the design of any study on metabolic polymorphism and cancer.

Interaction

Effect modification (interaction) occurs when the estimate of effect of exposure depends on the level of another factor in the study base (Miettinen, 1974). The term statistical interaction denotes a similar phenomenon in the observed data. The former term will generally be used here. Effect modification is distinct from confounding (or selection or information bias) in that it does not represent a bias that should be removed or controlled but rather a real difference in the effect of exposure in various subgroups, and this may be of considerable interest. The clearest example of interaction is that of a factor being hazardous in one group and protective in another. More generally the risk may be elevated in both groups but the strength of the effect may vary. A typical example of effect modification in studies involving genetic polymorphisms is the estimate of the risk of disease due to an external agent in subgroups of the population with a different genetic susceptibility marker, such as the polymorphism for an enzyme implicated in the activation or detoxification of the agent (Caporaso & Goldstein, 1997). In this situation, effect modification should be interpreted with considerable care, since the presence of statistical interaction may depend on the statistical methods used. In fact, all secondary risk factors modify either the rate ratio or the rate difference, as uniformity over one measure implies non-uniformity over the other. If the assessment of the joint effects of two factors is a fundamental goal of the study then calculating stratum-specific effect estimates can do this. It is less clear how to proceed if statistical interaction is occurring, but assessment of joint effects is not an analytical goal. Some authors (e.g.

Kleinbaum et al., 1982) argue that it is not appropriate in this situation to calculate an overall estimate of effect summarized across levels of the effect modifier. However, it is common to ignore this stipulation if the difference in effect estimates is not too great (Pearce, 1989). In fact, valid analytical methods (e.g. standardized rate ratios) have been specifically developed for this situation (Rothman, 1986). Cuzick tackles this topic in Chapter 11.

Conclusions

The methodological considerations involved in classical epidemiological studies on issues such as measurement of disease, measurement of exposure, selection bias, confounding, precision and interaction also apply to studies involving genetic polymorphisms, and in most cases the methodological problems of this type of study do not require solutions different from those used in classical studies. Cohort studies are in general more suitable for investigating phenotypes that may be significantly modified by exposure or disease, while case-control studies are more efficient for genotype-based investigations. In some cases the focus on effect modification (statistical interaction) may require a substantial increase in study size and study costs.

Acknowledgements

The Wellington Asthma Research Group is supported by a core programme grant from the Health Research Council of New Zealand.

References

Alexandrie, A.-K., Ingelman-Sundberg, M., Seidegard, J., Tornling, G., and Rannug, A. (1994) Genetic susceptibility to lung cancer with special emphasis on CYP1A1 and GSTM1: a study on host factors in relation to age at onset, gender and histological cancer types. Carcinogenesis, 15, 1785-1790

Ambrosone, C.B., Freudenheim, J.L., Graham, S., Marshall, J.R., Vena, J.E., Brasure, J.R., Laughlin, R., Nemoto, T., Michalek, A.M., Harrington, A., Ford, T.D., & Shields, P.G. (1995) Cytochrome P4501A1 and glutathione S-transferase (M1) genetic polymorphisms and postmenopausal breast cancer risk. Cancer Res. 55, 3483-3485

Armstrong, B.K., White, E. & Saracci, R. (1992) *Principles of Exposure Measurement in Epidemiology*. New York, Oxford University Press

Bock, K.W., Schrenk, D., Fortser, A., Griese, E.U., Morike, K., Brockmeier, D. & Eichelbaum, M. (1994) The influence of environmental and genetic factors on CYP2D6, CYP1A2 and UDP-glucuronosyltransferase in man using sparteine, caffeine, and paracetamol as probes. *Pharmacogenetics*, 4, 209-218

Boffetta, P. (1995) Sources of bias, effect of confounding in the application of biomarkers to epidemiological studies. *Toxicol. Lett.*, 77, 235-238

Breslow, N.E. & Day, N.E. (1987) *Statistical Methods in Cancer Research, Vol. II: The Design and Analysis of Cohort Studies* (IARC Sci. Publ. No. 82). Lyon, IARC

Brosen, K., Gram, L.F., Haghfelt, T.T. & Bertlisson, L. (1987) Extensive metabolizers of debrisoquine become poor metabolizers during quinidine treatment. *Pharmacol. Toxicol.*, 60, 312-314

Caporaso, N. & Goldstein, A. (1997) Issues involving biomarkers in the study of genetics of human cancer. In: Toniolo, P., Boffetta, P., Shuker, D.E.G., Rothman, N., Hulka, B. & Pearce, N., eds. *Application of Biomarkers in Cancer Epidemiology* (IARC Sci. Publ. No. 142). Lyon, IARC, pp. 237-250

Caporaso, N.E., DeBaun, M.R. & Rothman, N. (1995) Lung cancer and CYP2D6 (the debrisoquine polymorphism): sources of heterogeneity in the proposed association. *Pharmacogenetics*, 5 (Suppl.), S129-S134

Caporaso, N.E., Shields, P.G., Landi, M.T., Shaw, G.L., Tucker, M.A., Hoover, R., Sugimura, H., Weston, A. & Harris, C.C. (1992) The debrisoquine metabolic phenotype and DNA-based assays: implications of misclassification for the association of lung cancer and the debrisoquine metabolic phenotype. *Environ. Health Perspect.*, 98, 101-105

Caporaso, N.E., Tucker, M.A., Hoover, R.N., Hayes, R.B., Pickle, L.W., Issaq, H.J., Muschik, G.M., Green Gallo, L., Buivys, D., Aisner, S., Resau, J.H., Trump, B.F., Tollerud, D., Weston, A. & Harris, C.C. (1990) Lung cancer and debrisoquine metabolic phenotype. *J. Natl. Cancer Inst.*, 82, 1264-1272

Checkoway, H., Pearce, N. & Crawford-Brown, D. (1989) *Research Methods in Occupational Epidemiology*. New York, Oxford University Press

Copeland, K.T., Checkoway, H., McMichael, A.J. & Holbrook, R.H. (1977) Bias due to misclassification in the estimation of relative risk. *Am. J. Epidemiol.*, 105, 488-495

d'Errico, A., Taioli, E., Xiang, C. & Vineis, P. (1996) Genetic metabolic polymorphisms and the risk of cancer: a review of the literature. *Biomarkers*, 1, 149-173

Green-Gallo, L.A., Buivys, D.M., Fisher, K.L., Caporaso, N., Slawson, R.G., Elias, G., Didolkar, M.S., Ivusich, W.J. & Resau, J.H. (1991) A protocol for the safe administration of debrisoquine in biochemical epidemiologic research protocols for hospitalized patients. *Cancer*, 68, 206-210

Greenland, S. (1980) The effect of misclassification in the presence of covariates. *Am. J. Epidemiol.*, 112, 564-569

Greenland, S. (1987) Interpretation and choice of effect measures in epidemiologic analyses. *Am. J. Epidemiol.*, 125, 761-768

Greenland, S. (1988) Statistical uncertainty due to misclassification: implications for validation substudies. *J. Clin. Epidemiol.*, 41, 1167-1174

Greenland, S. & Robins, J.M. (1985) Confounding and misclassification. *Am. J. Epidemiol.*, 122, 495-506

Greenland, S. & Robins, J.M. (1986) Identifiability, exchangeability and epidemiological confounding. *Int. J. Epidemiol.*, 15, 413-419

Heim, M.H. & Mayer, U.A. (1991) Genetic polymorphism of debrisoquine oxidation: restriction fragment analysis and allele-specific amplification of mutant alleles of CYP2D6. *Meth. Enzymol.*, 206, 173-183

Hirvonen, A., Husgafvel-Pursiainen, K., Anttila, S., Karjalainen, A., Pelkonen, O. & Vainio, H. (1993) PCR-based CYP2D6 genotyping for Finnish lung cancer patients. *Pharmacogenetics*, 3, 19-27

Hulka, B.S., Wilcosky, T.C. & Griffith, J.D. (1990) *Biological Markers in Epidemiology*. New York, Oxford University Press

Kawajiri, K., Nakachi, K., Imai, K., Yoshii, A., Shinoda, N. & Watanabe, J. (1990) Identification of genetically high risk individuals to lung cancer by DNA polymorphism of the cytochrome P450IA1 gene. *FEBS Lett.*, 263, 131-133

Kleinbaum, D.G., Kupper, L.L. & Morgenstern, H. (1982) *Epidemiologic Research: Principles and Quantitative Methods*. Belmont, Lifetime Learning Publications

Llerena, A., Cobaleda, J. & Benitez, J. (1989) Debrisoquine hydroxylation phenotypes in healthy volunteers. *Lancet*, i, 1398

McMichael, A.J. (1994) Invited commentary - 'Molecular epidemiology': new pathway or new travelling companion? *Am. J. Epidemiol.*, 140, 1-11

McMichael, A.J. (1995) Re: Invited commentary - 'Molecular epidemiology': new pathway or new travelling companion? Author replies *Am. J. Epidemiol.*, 142, 225

Miettinen, O.S. (1974) Confounding and effect modification. *Am. J. Epidemiol.*, 100, 350-353

Miettinen, O.S. (1976) Estimability and estimation in case-referent studies. *Am. J. Epidemiol.*, 103, 226-235

Miettinen, O.S. (1985) *Theoretical Epidemiology*. New York, Wiley and Sons

Nakachi, K., Imai, K., Hayashi, S., Watanabe, J. & Kawajiri, K. (1991) Genetic susceptibility to squamous cell carcinoma of the lung in relation to cigarette smoking dose. *Cancer Res.*, 51, 5177-5180

Nakachi, K., Imai, K., Hayashi, S. & Kawajiri, K. (1993) Polymorphisms of the CYP1A1 and glutathione S-transferase genes associated with susceptibility to lung cancer in relation to cigarette dose in a Japanese population. *Cancer Res.*, 53, 2994-2999

Pearce, N.E. (1989) Analytic implications of epidemiological concepts of interaction. *Int. J. Epidemiol.*, 18, 976-980

Pearce, N.E. (1993) What does the odds ratio estimate in a case-control study? *Int. J. Epidemiol.*, 22, 1189-1192

Pearce, N. & Boffetta, P. (1997) General issues of study design and analysis in the use of biomarkers in cancer epidemiology. In: Toniolo, P., Boffetta, P., Shuker, D.E.G., Rothman, N., Hulka, B. & Pearce, N., eds, *Application of Biomarkers in Cancer Epidemiology* (IARC Sci. Publ. No. 142). Lyon, IARC, pp. 47-57

Pearce, N.E. & Checkoway, H.A. (1988) Case-control studies using other diseases as controls: problems of excluding exposure-related diseases. *Am. J. Epidemiol.*, 127, 851-856

Pearce, N.E., Checkoway, H. & Shy, C.M. (1986) Time-related factors as potential confounders and effect modifiers in studies based on an occupational cohort. *Scand. J. Work Environ. Health*, 12, 97-107

Pearce, N., de Sanjosé, S., Boffetta, P., Saracci, R., Kogevinas, M. & Savitz, D. (1995) Limitations of biomarkers of exposure in cancer epidemiology. *Epidemiology*, 6, 190-194

Robins, J.M., Gail, M.H. & Lubin, J.H. (1986) More on biased selection of controls for case-control analyses of cohort studies. *Biometrics*, 42, 1293-1299

Rothman, K.J. (1986) *Modern Epidemiology*. Boston; Little, Brown

Rothman, N. (1995) Genetic susceptibility bio-markers in studies of occupational and environmental cancer: methodologic issues. *Toxicol. Lett.*, 77, 221-225

Rothman, N., Stewart, W.F., Caporaso, N.E. & Hayes, R.B. (1993) Misclassification of genetic susceptibility biomarkers: implications for case-control studies and cross-population comparisons. *Cancer Epidemiol. Biomarkers Prev.*, 2, 299-303

Schulte. P.A. & Perera, F.P. Transitional studies. In: Toniolo, P., Boffetta, P., Shuker, D.E.G., Rothman, N., Hulka, B. & Pearce, N., eds, *Application of Biomarkers in Cancer Epidemiology* (IARC Sci. Publ. No. 142). Lyon, IARC, pp. 19- 29

Shields, P.G., Caporaso, N.E., Falk, R.T., Sugimura, H., Trivers, G.E., Trump, B.F., Hoover, R.N., Weston, A. & Harris, C.C. (1993) Lung cancer, race, and a CYP1A1 genetic polymorphism. *Cancer Epidemiol. Biomarkers Prev.*, 2, 481-485

Tefre, T., Ryberg, D., Haugen, A., Nebert, D.W., Skaug, V., Brogger, A. & Borresen, A.L. (1991) Human CYP1A1 (cytochrome P(1)450) gene: lack of association between the Msp I restriction fragment length polymorphism and incidence of lung cancer in a Norwegian population. *Pharmacogenetics*, 1, 20-25

Corresponding author
Paolo Boffetta
Unit of Environmental Cancer Epidemiology,
International Agency for Research on Cancer,
150 cours Albert-Thomas,
69372 Lyon cedex 08, France

Metabolic Polymorphisms and Susceptibility to Cancer
W. Ryder
IARC Scientific Publications No. 148
International Agency for Research on Cancer, Lyon, 1999

Chapter 11. Interaction, subgroup analysis and sample size

Jack Cuzick

The term "interaction" has both statistical and scientific connotations that do not always coincide. Multistage models are used as a bridge between these two viewpoints and as a way of illustrating the different types of qualitative interaction. The most important type of interaction for metabolic polymorphisms is between a genetic trait and an environmental or lifestyle exposure. In some cases these factors act multiplicatively on the risk ratios and so do not interact in the statistical sense. Nevertheless, the risk can be much higher when both are present. Interactions present severe problems of interpretation, as naive comparisons in subgroups can be very misleading and can produce false positive results because of the large number of comparisons. Methods for combating this are discussed. The main requirement, however, is for a substantially larger sample size than would be required for estimating the main effects.

Interaction

It is important to consider interaction in terms of both statistical models and biological mechanisms. In both usages the concept is used to describe effect modification, in the sense that the effect or strength of one predictor variable cannot be fully described without reference to the value (or level) of one or more modifying variables. In statistical terms the simplest model comes from linear regression, in which an outcome variable (y) depends on the value of factors (x, z) both separately and through an additional term related to the product of the two. In symbols

$$(1) \quad y = \alpha_0 + \alpha x + \beta z + \gamma xz + error$$

where α_0 is the constant term, x and z are the independent variables or main effects (usually centred at their means) with regression coefficients (α, β) and xz is the interaction term with coefficient γ. When $\gamma = 0$, there is no interaction. In general there is no reason why the interaction term should take a simple multiplicative form, and more complicated expression can also be considered. Indeed the same can be said for the main effects, which need not be linear in the independent variable. In general any relationship for which the outcome cannot be expressed on some scale (e.g. logarithmic) as an additive function of the independent variables is said to contain interaction.

For disease-exposure relationships, risks (or odds ratios of disease) are more often considered on a multiplicative scale so that they become additive on a log scale. If p denotes the probability of disease, the commonly used logistic model relates p to risk factors via the logit or log odds ratio. When there are two factors with an interaction, this takes the following form:

$$(2) \quad logit \; p \equiv \log \left(\frac{p}{1-p} \right) = \alpha_0 + \alpha x + \beta z + \gamma xz$$

Again when $\gamma = 0$, the model is said to have no interaction. This example illustrates another point, namely that interaction depends on the form of the model chosen. For example, if $\gamma = 0$ in (2) and an attempt were made to fit the linear model (1), in general an interaction term would be needed. When x and z are categorical variables (e.g. absence/presence of exposure, sex, genotype, age group) a more general model can be considered which attaches a coefficient (log-odds ratio) to each category (except the baseline or reference group) and, when interaction is present, to each (x, z) pair of categories. In symbols:

$$(3) \quad logit \; (p) = \alpha_0 + \sum \alpha_i x_i + \sum \beta_j z_j + \sum\sum \gamma_{ij} x_i z_j$$

where $\{x_i\}$ denotes the (non-baseline) categories for x and $\{z_j\}$ those for z. It should be noted that the number of coefficients for interaction is the product of the number of non-base categories for each variable, which rapidly becomes very large if each variable has more than a few levels. This basic problem, known as the "curse of dimensionality", has important implications to which we shall return later.

Multi-stage models

The widespread use of the logistic model for disease studies is partly due to its mathematical convenience, but for cancer it also has a basis in the multi-stage model of carcinogenesis. In general it is believed that cancer results from a series of events, occurring at the DNA level, usually thought to be between two and six. If the events occur independently the probability of all events occurring by a particular time is the product of their individual probabilities. Thus if an exposure or host-factor increases the probability of a particular event by a certain multiple it increases the probability of cancer by the same multiple. Furthermore, if two exposures or host factors increase the probability of *different* events by given multiples, then the probability of cancer is increased by the *product* of these factors. Thus the logarithm of the probability of cancer is related additively to the two factors. When the disease probability p itself is small $1-p$ is near unity so that logit $(p) \cong \log (p)$ and model (2) or (3) is appropriate. In this case there would be said to be no interaction between the factors.

However, when two factors affect the *same* stage this may not be true. In this case the factors may interact in a variety of different ways. For example, if both factors lead to the same mutation in a linear dose-dependent manner the combined effect may be equivalent to the cumulative dose and the excess risk associated with each variable can be added on a linear scale. Alternatively, where possible, the cumulative dose arising from the two exposures can be used as a new variable. This may be appropriate, for example, when different alcoholic beverages or sources of ionizing radiation are being considered. However, if either factor is likely to cause the event with high probability by itself the cumulative effect may be similar to the effect of either factor alone, in which case there would be a **negative** interaction.

The multi-stage model of carcinogenesis has a number of other implications for the development of cancer, including the shape of age-incidence curves, the relationship with dose and

duration of exposure, and the age of starting or stopping an exposure (Armitage & Doll, 1961; Doll, 1971; Moolgavkar, 1978, 1981; Peto, 1982).

Qualitative versus quantitative interactions

The multi-stage models considered above relate to the situation in which there is no interaction. Thus for log-linear models the risks associated with different factors are multiplicative, as illustrated by the hypothetical example shown in Table 1.

Table 1. Hypothetical examples of relative odds of disease arising from two non-interacting factors

| | | Factor B | |
		Absent	Present
	Absent	1.0	2.5
Factor A			
	Present	4.0	10.0

In this example the risk (odds) of disease is increased fourfold when factor A is present and 2.5-fold when factor B is present. When they are both present the risk is increased tenfold. In absolute terms the risk is far greater when both factors are present but they are said not to interact because each factor multiplies the risk related to the other by a constant amount. Thus factor B increases the relative odds from 1 to 2.5 when factor A is absent and from 4 to 10 when it is present.

The above situation contrasts with the following one.

Table 2. Relative odds of disease associated with a positive quantitative interaction

| | | Factor B | |
		Absent	Present
	Absent	1.0	2.5
Factor A			
	Present	4.0	20.0

In this case the effect of the factors is as above when they occur individually, but when both are present the combined effect is twice as large as before. Thus factor A increases the risk fourfold when factor B is absent but eightfold when it is present. Similarly factor B increases the risk 2.5 times when factor A is absent but fivefold when it is present. This is an example of a **positive quantitative interaction**. The effect of each factor increases the risk regardless of whether the other factor is present, but the *degree* of the effect may not be the same. Thus factor B is an effect modifier of factor A (and vice versa), but the modification is quantitative in the sense that the direction of the effect is unchanged. We also call this a positive interaction because the combined effect of the two factors is larger than the product of their individual effects.

The situation can be compared to the following one.

Table 3. Relative odds of disease associated with a negative quantitative interaction

		Factor B	
		Absent	Present
Factor A	Absent	1.0	2.5
	Present	4.0	5.0

Here the interaction is still quantitative in that both factors increase the risk regardless of the value of the other factor, but the combined effect is less than the product of the two, although greater than that of either factor alone, giving a **negative quantitative interaction.**

In some cases two factors may be influencing the same disease mechanism but to a different degree. Consider the following situation.

Table 4. Relative odds of disease associated with a negative qualitative interaction indicating the effect of factor B only in a subgroup of the population

		Factor B	
		Absent	Present
Factor A	Absent	1.0	2.5
	Present	4.0	4.0

In this case both factors increase risk but when factor A is present there is no additional effect of factor B, and adding factor A to factor B only increases the risk to the degree found for factor A alone, leading to a **negative qualitative interaction**. This outcome is not uncommon in drug trials (except that risks are replaced by benefits) where two drugs affect the same mechanism in such a way that the combination is no better than the better drug alone. A similar pattern may occur in exposure-gene interactions, where one factor may have a dominant effect on a stage of the carcinogenic process but when it is absent other factors play a role. For example, the risk of breast cancer may be so strong for a particular gene that factors influencing hormonal levels (age at childbirth or menarche) may be unimportant when it is present but are risk factors in its absence. Conversely, exposure effects could be sufficiently strong to render a metabolic polymorphism unimportant for a heavily exposed individual (e.g. a current smoker) but could affect risk in a lightly exposed person (e.g. passive smoke recipients).

The following table illustrates a form of **positive qualitative interaction.**

Table 5. Relative odds of disease illustrating a positive qualitative interaction

		Factor B	
		Absent	Present
Factor A	Absent	1.0	1.0
	Present	1.0	4.0

In this case, factor B is only associated with increased risk in the subset of individuals who also possess factor A. If factor A is a host factor (genotype/phenotype) and factor B is an exposure, the interpretation is that only the subgroup possessing factor A is susceptible to exposure factor B. There are great statistical dangers in making this sort of statement, as discussed below. In practice it can be very difficult to distinguish this case from the weak positive quantitative interaction illustrated in Table 2. In fact even non-interacting factors can mimic this form if the individual effects are weak, since the multiplicative effect of non-interacting factors can make the risk much clearer when both are present. As a general principle it is important to establish the existence of a main effect for each factor separately before attempting to look for interactions. However, there are a few examples where this sort of interaction may be occurring (Wei *et al.*, 1993; Kato *et al.*, 1995), and more are likely to arise as gene-environment interactions are more fully explored.

A less likely scenario is illustrated in Table 6.

Table 6. Relative odds of disease illustrating an antagonistic qualitative interaction

| | | Factor B | |
		Absent	Present
	Absent	1.0	1.0
Factor A			
	Present	0.5	2.0

Here factor A is protective when factor B is absent but increases the risk when it is present. This is hard to justify on mechanistic grounds and has been clearly demonstrated only very rarely in studies on humans. If factor B were present in about half the population there would be little overall effect of factor A when considered alone. Table 6 illustrates an *a priori* unlikely situation of a qualitative interaction of an exposure having little overall effect but an opposite effect in different subgroups. Scepticism about the reliability of such an interaction when there are no significant main effects should be very high and very strong evidence is needed. An example where such an interaction has been suggested is the role of metabolic polymorphisms on the relationship of smoking to breast cancer (Ambrosone *et al.*, 1996).

Biological types of interaction
All interactions are treated the same way mathematically. It is useful, however, to consider the different types of biological interaction separately because their interpretations differ.

1. Interaction between two exposures.
Because cancer epidemiology has primarily focused on external causes there are a number of examples of disease related to two or more expo-

sures. Examples include the role of tobacco and alcohol on oesophageal cancer, hepatitis B infection and aflatoxin exposure in liver cancer, radon and cigarette smoking in lung cancer, asbestos and smoking in lung cancer, and, more contentiously, exposure to human papilloma virus (often measured as a sexual behaviour variable) and smoking in cervical cancer. They all possess an important requisite for studying interaction, namely that each factor individually is clearly associated with disease. Yet even here it is rare for there to be evidence suggesting risk differing from that obtained by multiplying individual risks. This is probably because the exposures affect different stages and would not be expected to interact. Even in the case of alcohol and tobacco in oesophageal cancer, where both main effects are large, a careful analysis of one large study has shown no evidence for interaction (Breslow & Day, 1980).

2. Host factor - exposure interactions.
This is a situation where interactions are most likely to occur and relates directly to the theme of this book. In this case it is more likely that an exposure and a host factor related to susceptibility pertain to the same stage in the carcinogenic process, and thus a larger range of behaviour for their joint effect might be expected. This increased complexity places greater demands on statistical methods and also heightens the possibility of misinterpretation of data. Simple examples relate to effect modifications of exposure by age and sex, such as the greater impact of radiation on a variety of cancers in children and adolescents (BEIR V, 1990) or the interaction of sex and race with Epstein-Barr virus in nasopharyngeal cancer in Asia (Hirayama, 1978).

However the greatest interest is in interactions between exposures and specific genes that regulate metabolic pathways or immunological mechanisms. For highly penetrant genes with relative risks in excess of ten, such as BRCA1, there may be little need for specific external exposures, although they may conceivably bring forward the age at diagnosis by effectively removing a stage in the carcinogenic process. However, for less penetrant genes, where the risk ratio is twofold to threefold or smaller overall, there is much greater scope for interaction with specific exposures. The metabolic polymorphisms considered in this book fall into this class and their interaction with specific exposures and each other warrants careful study.

A standard logistic model without an interaction term (as in Table 1) reflects a multiplicative effect of exposure and genotype on risk. Even though the relative risk associated with exposure is similar to that found in individuals not possessing the high-risk genotype, the absolute magnitude of the risk associated with high exposures is much larger and more easily detectable in individuals possessing the gene, and is likely to be more highly statistically significant, because of the greater proportion of cases. A good example of this is the role of smoking and the NAT gene in bladder cancer. Most studies show no interaction between the two (Cartwright et al., 1982; Hein, 1988), but the risk associated with the NAT gene is much greater in smokers.

Most metabolic polymorphisms probably affect carcinogenesis by modifying the effective dose of carcinogen which reaches DNA. When the effect is proportional to dose a model including a dose level term and a main effect for the gene, but no interaction term, is appropriate.

A positive interaction occurs when the effect of the exposure is disproportionately greater in those carrying a specific gene compared to those who do not. The simplest situation occurs when the exposure only increases risk in susceptible individuals, as in Table 5. This is not the only possibility, and an example fitting the same scenario, illustrated in Table 2, has been described by Wu et al. (1995), involving a positive association of smoking and bleomycin-induced breaks in chromosomes 2, 4 and 5 with lung cancer incidence. However, even in this case a formal test for statistical significance of the interaction term was non-significant.

At the other extreme is a model in which saturation of some normal detoxifying mechanism occurs at high exposures, leading to increased risk, whereas low exposures only increase risk in individuals who have a defective or inefficient detoxifying mechanism as in Table 4 (with factor A as high exposure and factor B as genotype). This has been suggested as a possible mechanism for the effect of the GSTM1-null allele on the smoking and lung cancer relationship (Alexandrie et al., 1995), but the situation is still unclear (d'Errico et al., 1996). Another example where this mecha-

nism may be relevant is in the role of sunlight and DNA repair in basal cell skin cancer (Wei et al., 1993).

3. Gene-gene interactions.

The multi-stage model implies that several genes must be damaged before cancer occurs. In addition to genes influencing metabolism, which influences the effective dose of carcinogen, there are at least three classes of genes thought to be involved in human carcinogenesis: proto-oncogenes (e.g. ras), tumour suppressor genes (p16), and genes involved in apoptosis (bcl2). Although experimental systems have demonstrated the cooperation of oncogenes in producing cancer (Teich, 1997), and consistent changes at multiple genes have been demonstrated for naturally occurring human cancers, most notably colon cancer (Fearon & Vogelstein, 1990), the establishment of risk associated with more than one mutation or polymorphism is not well documented. This is not surprising in respect of rare highly penetrant genes (also the location and age at onset of colon cancer associated with mutation in the apc may be an example) where a single event is rate-limiting, but might be expected in lower-risk genotypes. The scarcity of such reports probably reflects the infancy of this field, where clearly documented effects for even single genes are only just beginning to emerge. However, a few reports of interaction between phase I and phase II detoxifying enzyme have been reported in Japanese populations (Hayashi et al., 1992; Nakachi et al., 1993; Kihara & Noda, 1995). (See Chapter 22 for further details.)

When genes affect different stages the multi-stage model suggests they should not interact. An exception to this is when a mutation in one gene (e.g. p53 or the mismatch repair genes) increases the risk of a subsequent mutation, in which case a positive interaction might be expected in some circumstances. When two genes affect the same stage, such that a mutation in only one is needed to facilitate carcinogenesis, a negative interaction would be expected.

Confounding

In its most general sense, confounding occurs when the unadjusted or crude odds ratio (OR) for a variable A differs from the odds ratio conditional on the value of another variable B. In this case variable A is said to be confounded by B, or B is a confounder for A. In this general sense, confounding exists whenever there is an interaction between A and B, but it can also exist in the absence of an interaction because of unequal distributions in the different strata. The most striking example of this kind of confounding is illustrated by Simpson's paradox, in which the direction of an association can even be reversed. This is most easily explained by the following example.

| | | Exposure | |
		Present	Absent
Disease	Present	100	20
	Absent	200	100

Males

| | | Exposure | |
		Present	Absent
Disease	Present	25	200
	Absent	10	200

Females

In this example the odds ratio for exposure is 2.5 in both males and females, but because the exposure was so much more common in males a table not adjusting for sex gives the **opposite** odds ratio:

| | | Exposure | |
		Present	Absent
Disease	Present	125	220
	Absent	210	300

$$OR = \frac{(300)(125)}{(220)(215)} = 0.81$$

In this case sex is a confounding factor for exposure. Age is another common confounding factor, and can create or distort relationships

between exposure and disease in case-control (and other) studies when the age distribution differs between cases and controls.

In general a confounding factor is associated with (i.e. has an odds ratio not always equal to unity) both the exposure of interest and disease status. Many authors restrict the use of the term "confounding" to the case where the conditional odds ratio between disease and exposure does not depend on the value of the confounder (but differs from the crude odds ratio). This is an attempt to restrict the use of the term "confounding" to cases where disturbances in the odds ratio are related to imbalances in the case/control ratio in different strata, and not to a true interaction between the variables.

In the more general case where the OR is affected by the value of the confounder, the term **effect modifier** is often used. In this case an adjusted summary odds ratio is inadequate and it is necessary to specify the risk associated with different levels of the confounder. This is the circumstance most often encountered with metabolic polymorphisms, when the presence or absence of a gene may influence the association between an exposure and development of disease.

A number of problems arise in attempting to adjust for confounders. There is little doubt about the importance of adjusting for age and sex, but other variables are not so easily dismissed as confounding factors. One case is when two similar variables are highly correlated, for instance when they are essentially different measures of the same exposure. Adjusting for either will negate the risk associated with the another, as with pack-years of cigarettes smoked and duration of smoking. In such cases it is appropriate either not to adjust or firstly to create a summary exposure measure combining all relevant variables. Methods for doing this via principal components or partial least squares have been described by Stone & Brooks (1990). Another problem arises when both variables are on the same causal pathway. The emergence of good biomarkers for exposure or early disease states has made this more problematic.

A good example is the number of sexual partners and positivity for human papilloma virus (HPV) DNA in the development of cervical neoplasia. In general, many more (high-risk) sexual partners increase the risk of having HPV, which is thought to be the direct link to the disease. Often, adjusting for HPV causes the relationship with the number of sexual partners to be greatly weakened or to disappear, but to say that the number of sexual partners is confounded by HPV infection is inappropriate to what is understood to be the meaning of confounding. In this case it is useful to study the link between sexual behaviour and HPV and that between HPV and cervical neoplasia separately and to see the extent to which a direct pathway explains the overall relationship. A similar example is that of the current number of cigarettes smoked and salivary cotinine levels and the risk of lung cancer, although in this case cotinine is a much more direct measure of exposure. However, it is not helpful to say that current tobacco consumption is confounded by cotinine levels.

Lastly, it should be noted that it is often only possible to adjust incompletely for confounding, principally as a consequence of the confounder being inaccurately specified because either it measures the exposure of interest indirectly, or the categories are too broad, or there is substantial misclassification. A good example is the possible role of sexual behaviour in the relationship between cigarette smoking and cervical cancer (Szarewski & Cuzick, 1996).

Subgroup analysis

Although interactions between metabolic polymorphisms and exposures are more biologically plausible than many other possible types of interaction, the curse of dimensionality means that there is a large number of subgroups to consider and that at the most only a small proportion of these is biologically relevant. Consequently, stringent statistical procedures and careful interpretation are required before a putative interaction can be confidently accepted. In particular, much caution is needed to avoid the over-interpretation of nominal P values.

The problem is well appreciated in the area of HLA-disease associations, where the number of alleles is very large, creating a large number of subgroups even in the absence of interactions with exposure. A similar problem of interaction-induced subgroups occurs for this system when studying haplotypes, where the number of relevant subgroups can be a sizeable fraction of the product of the number of alleles at the different loci. As the number of relevant loci examined increases the problems in assessing metabolic polymorphisms are similar but become even more extreme if interactions with different exposures are also considered.

Various statistical procedures have been devised to deal with this problem but none are entirely satisfactory.

Tests for interaction

One approach is to test for interaction in models (1), (2) or (3). For models (1) and (2) this involves a single interaction term. For model (3) the standard test is an overall test for the set of all interaction terms, and generally this has low power if the number of levels is large. Even for a 2 x 2 table, where there is only one interaction term, the power of this test can be quite low. Consider the following table of events associated with two factors A and B for individuals with a disease of interest.

		Factor B		
		Absent	Present	Total
Factor A	Absent	44	56	100
	Present	56	144	200
	Total	100	200	300

Let us assume that each factor is present in 50% of the population and that they are independent so that each cell represents 25% of the population. Let us also assume that the number of unaffected individuals observed (controls) in each cell is large (say 1000). Then each of the main effects (factor A present or factor B present) is associated with a risk ratio of 2 (200/100) and the variance of the estimator for the logarithm of the odds ratio is approximately $1/100 + 1/200 = 0.015$. By contrast the interaction odds ratio is $(144/56)/(56/44) = 2.02 \cong 2$ and the variance of the logarithm of this is estimator $1/44 + 1/56 + 1/56 + 1/144 \cong 0.065$, which is more than four times as large. Thus, for this hypothetical example, the sample size needed to estimate the interaction term or to demonstrate its statistical significance at any given power is more than four times as large as for the main effect. This is typical of the increase in sample size required to adequately detect an interaction of the same size as the main effect. Note that if we had focused on the subgroup in which factor B was present, the odds ratio associated with factor A would have been 2.57 and the variance of the log odds would have been 0.0248, giving an increase in efficiency of $(\log 2.57/\log 2)^2 (0.065/0.0248) = 4.30$ for the subgroup analysis. Thus if one had only studied individuals where factor B was present an effect of factor A could have been demonstrated with a sample size only 23% of that needed to detect the interaction. Even if data were collected on all individuals but only the subgroup where factor B was present were considered, the required sample size for any given power would be only 89% of that needed to detect the main effect, even though a positive effect was still apparent in the subgroup ignored. The advantages in terms of power are obvious, but the chances of overinterpreting subgroup-specific results must not be overlooked. Thus there is a real danger of finding false positive results.

A good example of this can be found in the literature on cardiovascular clinical trials. Lee *et al.* (1980) demonstrated the hazards of uncritical examination of subgroups more clearly than would be possible by theoretical discussion. In this example, 1073 patients treated for coronary artery disease and recorded in a data bank were given fictitious randomizations to mock treatment A or mock treatment B. The patients had already been treated and their outcome was known so that the differences between the two groups were truly determined only by the flip of a coin. A number of prognostically important factors were recorded, including:

sex
age
history of previous myocardial infarction
history of congestive heart failure
cardiomegaly on X-ray
diagnostic Q-waves
resting ST-T-wave abnormalities
left ventricular end-diastolic pressure
arteriovenous oxygen difference
single-vessel disease
three-vessel disease
abnormal left ventricular contraction
signficant mitral insufficiency
left main stenosis.

Not surprisingly there were no overall differences in survival between the two groups, either before or after stratification for prognosic factors, and the prognostic factors appeared to be well balanced between the two groups. However, on close examination it was found that among the group of patients with three-vessel disease and an abnormal left ventricular contraction pattern, those patients given treatment A fared significantly better. This subgroup comprised 397 patients and a logrank test for a survival difference gave $\chi^2 = 5.4$, $P = 0.02$. This difference, however, could be partly explained by an imbalance of prognostic factors in the subgroup, after correction for which the difference was not statistically significant ($\chi^2 = 2.4$, $P = 0.12$). However, further investigation revealed that treatment A showed even greater superiority in the subgroups of 298 patients with three-vessel disease, an abnormal left ventricular contraction pattern and a history of congestive heart failure. Here the difference was quite striking ($\chi^2 = 10.0$, $P = 0.0016$) and was not appreciably diminished after correcting for other prognostic factors ($\chi^2 = 9.3$, $P = 0.0024$).

After having spent many years coordinating entry and follow-up for such a large trial, an investigator would be only too willing to dwell upon these results and no doubt would be able to find a convincing explanation as to why treatment A was more effective in this high-risk group of patients. Further examples of this problem in the clinical trial context can be found in EBCTCG (1990).

Similar scenarios could be imagined for observational studies of gene-environment interactions. Given the amount of work required to amass a cohort, collect material, and perform the assays, there is considerable pressure to produce a positive result. The surest way to do this is to dredge through subgroups until something emerges. The fact that exposures and genetic factors are both under study increases the number of possible subgroups, and if different end points (for example based on biomarkers) are considered, the number of possible subgroups becomes very large.

Case-only studies
When the only interest is in the interaction between two factors it is possible to dispense with controls altogether if certain assumptions are

made. A recent discussion of the issues has been provided by Khoury & Flanders (1996). Various designs exist based on 1) cases only, 2) cases and parents, 3) affected relative (sib) pairs. The simplest situation is a case-only study with a dichotomous exposure and genotype. In the usual case-control study the interaction odds ratio is the ratio of the OR for exposure in those with and without the gene of interest. Under the assumption that the exposure is unrelated to the gene in controls, a little algebra shows that this is the same as the OR between the gene and exposure in cases. The assumption that exposure is independent of genotype in the general population is crucial and may not always be fulfilled, especially if exposure leads to unpleasant side-effects (e.g. alcohol exposure and alcohol dehydrogenase polymorphisms). Another limitation is the inability to look at the effects of exposure or genetic polymorphisms alone. However, the gain in accuracy and the reduction in cost brought about by not having to test controls (Piegorsch *et al.*, 1994) make this a useful design in some circumstances.

Corrections for multiple comparisons

Multiple comparisons arising from the examination of separate subgroups can be adjusted for directly. The simplest approach is to use a Bonferroni correction in which the nominal P value obtained is multiplied by the number of subgroups examined. Thus if 20 subgroups were examined a nominal P value of less than 0.0025 would be required to claim a significant result at the 5% level. This is a very conservative approach and can often lead to the downplaying of real differences. A somewhat less conservative approach was proposed by Simes (1986). For this method the tests in each subgroup are ordered in terms of decreasing significance (increasing P values). If n tests are performed and the ordered P values are $p_1 \leq p_2 \leq ... \leq p_n$, Simes suggested that:

$$P = \max (np_i/i)$$

$$i \leq n$$

and showed that this gave correct significant levels when the tests were independent. P appears to be approximately correct or slightly conserva-

tive much more generally. However, when large numbers of tests are performed the chances of missing a real effect are still large. In practice it can be difficult to determine how many subgroups exist and how many potential tests might be performed, as interesting subgroups are usually identified interactively as the analysis progresses.

A more reasonable approach is to put some structure on the hierarchy of tests considered (Cuzick, 1982). This depends to some extent on which subgroups are expected to show a difference. Where possible a list of the subgroup interactions of interest should be specified in advance and, ideally, lodged with a third party along with the study protocol. Results in pre-specified subgroups should be given greater credence than those found by a *post hoc* examination of the data.

Another useful guideline is that one should be more suspicious of results in subgroups when there is not a significant difference for each main effect involved. Because antagonistic qualitative interactions are so much less plausible, greater weight can be ascribed to a stronger effect in a specific subgroup when each factor itself is clearly related to disease. Thus for gene-exposure interactions one would like to see an overall effect for the gene alone without considering the specific exposure, and vice versa.

Empirical Bayes approaches

Given the difficulty of assessing significant levels associated with variables in studies that consider many factors, one approach has been to view them only as exploratory studies, in which any observed association must be verified in a more focused confirmatory investigation. Thomas *et al.* (1985) considered this approach and concluded that neither statistical significance nor estimated relative risk were appropriate measures on which to rank putative risk factors. They also showed that splitting any individual study into hypothesis generating and hypothesis verification halves was inefficient. An empirical Bayes approach was recommended in which the data are used to estimate a prior likelihood of a real association, and this is then used to produce posterior estimates (likelihoods) of the relative risk of association with each exposure. These relative risks are the mean or mode of the posterior distribution of the relative risk (odds ratio) and are used to rank the exposures. The rankings are then used to determine the priority of further evaluation in new confirmatory studies. The effect of this is to downweight maximum likelihood estimates of risks, and the degree of downweighting depends on the amount of information available about the size of the risk. Variables with a lot of information are thus downweighted less than those with less information, so that a moderate but better established risk (usually based on more exposed individuals) may be ranked higher than an apparently larger risk which is so rare that there is a wider confidence interval for its true magnitude. Similar methodology has been used to adjust estimated relative risks in small geographical areas or temporal windows. More details can be found in Thomas *et al.* (1985).

Use of biomarkers
Biomarkers can help to clarify the relationship between exposures, genes and disease (Vineis, 1992; Rothman & Hayes, 1995). They are probably most useful when the direct relationships are statistically significant but still weak. In this case the greater power available from mechanistically more direct relationships with biomarkers can help to clarify relationships within subgroups or other fine details. However, because mechanistic relationships should be more clearly established than the more difficult connections with disease, a higher level of statistical significance should be demanded. In this case a level of P < 0.001 is more appropriate than the conventional P < 0.05. Further details are developed in Cuzick (1995).

In the end a two-stage procedure is probably most useful for assessing an interaction or an effect found only in one subgroup. The first stage, consisting of hypothesis generation, need not be unduly concerned with the problems of subgroup analysis. However, any putative results have to be verified in a separate confirmatory study in which they are clearly identified as the test hypothesis at the outset, and adjustment for multiple comparisons should be made if there is more than one hypothesis. The guidelines suggested above can be helpful in making tentative judgements about subgroup-specific results, but if applied too vigorously they can lead to the dis-

missal of real effects. However, if results in subgroups are accepted at face value a large number of false association will be suggested. If one separates hypothesis generation from hypothesis testing an intermediate category of tentative but promising results is needed. The replication of findings in other groups of patients then gives credence to the results in a way that could never be achieved in one study, and ultimately provides the degree of evidence necessary before the results are applied in public health measures and elsewhere.

Sample size
A full discussion of sample size calculations for the interaction term is very complicated and beyond the scope of this paper. They depend on the model chosen, the type of test used and other variables involved in stratification or adjustment. Some further details can be found in Smith & Day (1984). However, many of the main points can be made by considering a simple model employing two factors that are either absent or present and using simple ratio estimators for odds ratios. Consider the simple case shown in Table 5, where the risk is only apparent when both exposure and genotype are present. We consider this model in greater detail by letting the risk be R, the proportion of cases exposed α, and the proportion of cases with the gene β. This is illustrated in Table 7.

Table 7. Odds ratios for two factors when an effect is seen only if both are present

		Factor B Exposure		
		Absent	Present	Proportion of Total
Factor A Gene	Absent	1	1	$1-\alpha$
	Present	1	R	α
	Proportion of Total	$(1-\beta)$	β	1

The risk (R) for the susceptibility subgroup is attenuated to $1 + \alpha\,(R - 1)$ for the main effect associated with the gene and to $1 + \beta\,(R - 1)$ for the exposure comparison. Thus if only 20% of the population possess the susceptibility gene a fourfold risk is attenuated to 1.6 and the sample size required in order to detect this is ($\log 4/\log 1.6)^2 = 8.7$ times larger than if the exposure effect applied to the whole population.

If it is desired to consider the ability to detect the interaction itself, the calculations are more tedious and require consideration of the number of cases and controls in each of the four cells. Let n_{00}, n_{01}, n_{10}, n_{11} denote the number of cases in the four cells corresponding to factor A (gene effect) and factor B (exposure) being (absent, absent), (absent, present), (present, absent), or (present, present); and let N_{00}, N_{01}, N_{10}, N_{11} denote the corresponding numbers for controls.

If R is defined as the interaction odds ratio (i.e. the ratio of the OR for exposure in those with and without the gene), then the odds ratio estimator for R is

$$\hat{R} = \left(\frac{n_{11}N_{10}}{n_{10}N_{11}} \bigg/ \frac{n_{01}N_{00}}{n_{01}N_{00}} \right)$$

The log of the interaction odds ratio is $\log R$ and the variance of $\log \hat{R}$ is approximately

$$\text{Var}(\log \hat{R}) \cong \sum_{j=0}^{1} \sum_{i=0}^{1} \left(\frac{1}{n_{ij}} + \frac{1}{N_{ij}} \right)$$

To have 90% power to detect an interaction of size R, when 5% 2-sided significance levels are used, one requires that

$$\frac{(\log R)^2}{\text{Var}(\log \hat{R})} \geq (Z_{\alpha/2}+Z_{1-\beta})^2 = (1.96+1.28)^2 = 10.5$$

When the number of controls is large compared to cases, the terms involving $1/N_{ij}$ can be ignored when computing the variance. Also when exposure and susceptible genotype are both rare, the dominant term in the variance is $1/n_{11}$. In this limiting case, one requires that $n_{11} > 10.5/(\log R)^2$. When R = 4 for example, $n_{11} > 5.46$, which, if exposed individuals and susceptible genotypes are each found in only 10% of the cases (and the true OR= 4), leads to a requirement of more than 200 cases, and an even larger number of controls. Here the advantages of considering only exposed individuals when looking for genotype effects are obvious.

By making the assumption that exposure and genotype are independent in controls a case-only design effectively removes the control component from the variance, and achieves the same power as a study with a larger number of controls per case.

Extensions to stratified models, involving the use of a Mantel-Haenszel estimate of the interaction odds ratio, can be obtained as indicated by Smith and Day (1984). Sample size estimates for maximum likelihood estimators for a logistic model can be derived from asymptotic theory for MLEs, but no simple expressions arise and computer evaluation is necessary.

Acknowledgements

Gratitude is expressed to Drs M. Bacchi, G. Ronco and P. Sasieni for their helpful comments.

References

Alexandrie, A. K., Sundberg, M. I., Seidegard, J., Tornling, G. & Rannug, A. (1995) In: *Proceedings of the ISSX Workshop on Glutathione S-transferases*. Taylor Francis

Ambrosone, C.B., Freudenheim, J.L., Graham, S., Marshall, J.R., Vena, J.E., Brasure, J.R., Mickalek, A.M., Laughlin, R., Nemoto, T., Gillenwater, K.A. & Shields, P.G. . (1996) Cigarette smoking, N-acetyltransferase 2 genetic polymorphisms, and breast cancer risk. *JAMA*, 276, 1494-1501

Armitage, P. & Doll, R. (1961) Stochastic models for carcinogenesis. In: Neyman, J., ed, *Proceedings of the Fourth Berkeley Symposium on Mathematical Statistics and Probability*. Berkeley, University of California Press, pp. 19-38

BEIR V (Committee on the Biological Effects of Ionizing Radiation). (1990) *Health Effects of Exposure to Low Levels of Ionizing Radiation*. Washington, National Academy of Sciences

Breslow, N.E. & Day, N.E. (1980) *Statistical Methods in Cancer Research, Volume 1 - The Analysis of Case-control Studies*. Lyon, IARC (Scientific Publication No. 32)

Cartwright, R.A., Glashan, R.W., Rogers, H.J., Ahmad, R.A., Barham-Hall, D., Higgins, E. &

Kahn, M.A. (1982) Role of *N*-acetyltransferase phenotypes in bladder carcinogenesis: a pharmacogenetic epidemiological approach to bladder cancer. *Lancet*, ii, 842-845

Cuzick, J. (1982) The assessment of subgroups in clinical trials. *Experientia* [Suppl.], 41, 224-235

Cuzick, J. (1995) Molecular epidemiology: carcinogens, DNA adducts, and cancer - still a long way to go. *J. Natl. Cancer Inst.*, 87, 861-862

d'Errico, A., Taioli, E., Chen, X. & Vinei, P. (1996) Genetic metabolic polymorphisms and the risk of cancer: a review of the literature. *Biomarkers*, 1, 149-173

Doll, R. (1971) The age distribution of cancer: implications for models of carcinogenesis. *J. R. Stat. Soc. (A)*, 134, 133-166

EBCTCG. (1990) *Treatment of Early Breast Cancer: Worldwide Evidence 1985-1990.* Oxford, Oxford University Press

Fearon, E.R. & Vogelstein, B. (1990) A genetic model for colorectal tumorigenesis. *Cell*, 61, 759-767

Hayashi, S., Watanabe, J. & Kawajiri, K. (1992) High susceptibility to lung cancer analysed in terms of combined genotypes of CYP1A1 and mu-class glutathione S-transferase genes. *Jpn. J. Cancer. Res.*, 83, 866-870

Hein, D.W. (1988) Acetylator genotype and arylamine-induced carcinogenesis. *Biochem. Biophys. Acta*, 948, 37-66

Hirayama, T. (1978) Descriptive and analytical epidemiology of nasopharyngeal cancer. In: de-Thé, G., Ito, Y. &. Davis, W., eds, *Nasopharyngeal Carcinoma: Etiology and Control.* Lyon, IARC, pp. 167-189

Kato, S., Bowman, E.D., Harrington, A.M., Blömeke, B. & Shields, P.G. (1995) Human lung carcinogen-DNA adduct levels mediated by genetic polymorphisms *in vivo. J. Natl. Cancer Inst.*, 87, 902-907

Khoury, M.J. & Flanders, W.D. (1996) Nontraditional epidemiologic approaches in the analysis of gene-environment interaction: case-control studies with no controls! *Am. J. Epidemiol.*, 144, 207-213

Kihara, M. & Noda, K. (1995) Risk of smoking for squamous and small-cell carcinomas of the lung modulated by combinations of CYP1A1 gene polymorphisms in a Japanese population. *Carcinogenesis*, 16, 2331-2336

Lee, K.L., McNeer, J.F., Starmer, C.F., Harris, P.J. & Rosati, R.A. (1980) Clinical judgement and statistics: lessons from a simulation randomized trial in coronary artery disease. *Circulation*, 61, 508-515

Moolgavkar, S.H. (1978) The multistage theory of carcinogenesis and the age distribution of cancer in man. *J. Natl. Cancer Inst.*, 61, 49-52

Moolgavkar, S.H. & Knudson, A.G. Jr. (1981) Mutation and cancer: a model for human carcinogenesis. *J. Natl. Cancer Inst.*, 66, 1037-1052

Nakachi, K., Imai, K., Hayashi, S. & Kawajiri, K. (1993) Polymorphisms of the CYP1A1 and glutathione S-transferase genes associated with susceptibility to lung cancer in relation to cigarette dose in a Japanese population. *Cancer Res.*, 53, 2994-2999

Peto, J., Seidman, H. & Selikoff, I.J. (1982a) Mesothelioma mortality in asbestos workers: implications for models of carcinogenesis and risk assessment. *Br. J. Cancer*, 45, 124-135

Peto, R. (1982b) Statistical aspects of cancer trials. In: Halnan, K.E. *et al.*, eds, *Treatment of Cancer.* London, Chapman and Hall

Piegorsch, W., Weinberg, C.R. & Taylor, J.A. (1994) Non-heirarchical logistic models and case-only designs for assessing susceptibility in population-based case-control studies. *Stat. Med.*, 13, 153-162

Rothman, N. & Hayes, R.B. (1995) Using biomarkers of genetic susceptibility to enhance the study of cancer etiology. *Environ. Health Perspect.*, 103 (Suppl. 8), 291-295

Simes, R.J. (1986) An improved Bonferroni procedure for multiple tests of significance. *Biometrica*, 73, 751-754

Smith, P.G. & Day, N.E. (1984) The design of case-control studies: the influence of confounding and interaction effects. *Int. J. Epidemiol.*, 13, 356-365

Stone, M. & Brooks, R.J. (1990) Continuum regression. Cross-validated sequentially constructed prediction embracing ordinary least squares, partial least squares and principal components regression. *J. R. Stat. Soc. (B)*, 52, 237-269

Szarewski, A. & Cuzick, J. (1996) Effect of smoking cessation on cervical lesion size. *Lancet*, 347, 1619-1620

Teich, N.M. (1997) Oncogenes and cancer. In: Franks, L.M. & Teich, N.M., eds, *Introduction to the Cellular and Molecular Biology of Cancer*. Third Edition. Oxford, Oxford University Press, pp. 169-207

Thomas, D.C., Siemiatycki, J., Dewar, R., Robins, J., Goldberg, M. & Armstrong, B.G. (1985) The problem of multiple inference in studies designed to generate hypothesis. *Am. J. Epidemiol.*, 122, 1080-1095

Vineis, P. (1992) The use of biomarkers in epidemiology: the example of bladder cancer. *Toxicol. Lett.*, 64/65, 463-467

Wei, Q., Matanoski, G.M., Farmer, E.R., Hedayati, M.A. & Grossman, L. (1993) DNA repair and aging in basal cell carcinoma: a molecular epidemiology study. *Proc. Natl. Acad. Sci. USA*, 90, 1614-1618

Wu, X., Hsu, T.C., Annegers, J.F., Amos, C.I., Fueger, J.J. & Spitz, M.R. (1995) A case-control study of nonrandom distribution of bleomycin-induced chromatid breaks in lymphocytes of lung cancer cases. *Cancer Res.*, 55, 557-561

Jack Cuzick
Department of Mathematics, Statistics and Epidemiology,
Imperial Cancer Research Fund,
PO Box 123,
61 Lincoln 's Inn Fields,
London, WC2A 3PX

Metabolic Polymorphisms and Susceptibility to Cancer
W. Ryder
IARC Scientific Publications No. 148
International Agency for Research on Cancer, Lyon, 1999

Chapter 12. Design and analysis issues in case-control studies addressing genetic susceptibility

Paul Brennan

Case-control studies are among the main study designs for investigating the effect of environmental exposures on disease etiology and are now becoming more frequently used to examine the influence of genetic susceptibility. Incorporating a case-control design to examine genetic exposure would seem appropriate as the main problems of case-control studies, those of bias and confounding, are more easily avoided. However, they do not have a strong image and are thought to provide too many spurious findings as a result of chance, bias or confounding. This criticism has often been valid, especially for many early studies based on small numbers of poorly defined cases that were compared to convenient groups of local controls. New family-based study designs that account for these problems have been suggested, including the transmission disequilibrium test. However, the traditional format of case-control studies may be improved by incorporating methodological refinements developed over the past 30 years in environmental epidemiology. The present Chapter attempts to outline these issues and to provide guidelines for the selection of cases and controls and for the analysis of genetic data from case-control studies. Alternative, family-based study designs will also be discussed. Finally, a comprehensive analysis approach to gene-environment and gene-gene interaction is proposed.

The case-control study

The basic design of a case-control study involves comparing a group of individuals with a disease (the cases) to a group of individuals representative of the underlying population (the controls). Under some appropriate assumptions the odds ratio of exposure in the cases and controls gives an estimate of how much more likely the disease is in someone exposed compared with someone unexposed, i.e. the risk ratio. How close the odds ratio is to the true underlying risk ratio will depend on the extent of three contaminating factors: bias, confounding and chance (Rothman, 1986). These factors have to be assessed in a slightly different context when the exposure variable is genetic as opposed to environmental.

Selection of cases and controls: avoiding bias

Bias arises from two main sources: the selection of study subjects from the underlying study population and the accuracy with which information is obtained from them. Regarding the former, the selection of cases in a case-control study should be

based on all individuals within a population who develop a disease, or on a representative sample of them (Wacholder *et al.*, 1992). While this is the ideal situation, practical constraints often mean that more convenient groups are identified. The main choice is whether to select incident or prevalent cases. Incident cases, defined as cases with recent onset disease, have a strong advantage over prevalent cases that may have had the disease for some years by the time of recruitment: prevalent cases tend to be biased towards those with a longer disease duration. If an association with a particular gene is observed it is difficult to separate whether there is an effect of the gene on susceptibility or on survival. In a recent case-control study of glutathione S-transferase M1 (GSTM1) and the development of bladder cancer (Brockmöller *et al.*, 1994), 296 bladder cancer cases with prevalent disease were identified and compared to 400 controls for the presence of the GSTM1 null genotype. GSTM1 is a phase II carcinogen-detoxifying enzyme with a low activity considered to be a possible risk factor. The results indicated an increased risk of 40% associated with possessing the null genotype, GSTM1*0/0 (Table 1a). An alternative plausible explanation consistent with these results is that the null genotype does not represent an increased risk for developing bladder cancer but instead is associated favorably with survival. It would therefore be overrepresented in a group of prevalent cases when compared to the background population. As GSTM1*0/0 was considered *a priori* as a strong potential risk factor on the basis of phenotypic data the alternative hypothesis that it may be related to increased survival is weak. However, given the data set alone it would not be possible to separate these two competing explanations, thus highlighting the necessity to recruit incident cases when available. When a mixture of incident and prevalent cases is recruited an alternative is to present the results separately for the two groups.

In what has been termed the "study base principle" the selection of controls should ensure that they form a representative sample of the population from which the cases arose (Wacholder *et al.*, 1992). Obtaining a representative control group is one of the most difficult tasks in many case-control studies because factors related to inclusion, such as social class, education and lifestyle, may be related to the exposure variables under consideration. For example, if controls with a healthy lifestyle were more likely to participate in a study, subsequent comparisons of cases and controls would be biased. When the exposure variables are genetic these problems would seem to be less severe as lifestyle and demographic variables are unlikely to be associated strongly with genetic factors, although mild associations cannot be ruled out. In the past many genetic case-control studies have used control groups of convenience, e.g. laboratory workers or groups of blood donors. Again it is impossible to determine whether any difference between case and control genotypes is due to the disease or to a selection methodology such that cases and controls are of slightly different ethnic groups or different age structure. This problem has been called confounding due to population stratification. However, as it is a feature of the study and not of the disease relationship it can also be defined as a selection bias. An appropriate study design to reduce the possibility of this bias requires the control group to be of similar age and

ethnic background to the case group. This can be achieved by the following methods: (i) matching individual controls for each case by ethnic background and other demographic factors; (ii) obtaining information on these factors and stratifying the analysis; or (iii) restricting the cases and controls to one particular population. Brockmöller *et al.* (1994) reduced the possibility of this selection bias by using the last two strategies, including only cases and controls of German origin and stratifying the analysis by age and sex.

Another important principle for ensuring a lack of bias is the "comparable accuracy principle" (Wacholder *et al.*, 1992). This states that the accuracy of measuring exposure should be similarly high for both cases and controls. Little attention has been paid to the sensitivity and specificity of different genotyping methods, and problems can occur when gene frequencies of cases are compared to those of control groups that were typed in the past by inferior methods. This problem can also arise when cases and controls are typed in different laboratories, or even within the same laboratory by different individuals. As an assessment of misclassification is usually not a routine part of a laboratory's work the extent of bias introduced when comparing results obtained from different methods is usually unknown. Avoiding this form of bias is essentially a matter of study design such that genetic information from cases and controls is obtained using equivalent protocols.

It is also difficult to ensure comparable accuracy between cases and controls when exposure is based on phenotype data instead of the actual genotype. Most early studies of genetic susceptibility and cancer were based on phenotype data, e.g. administering a drug and measuring the relative concentration of unchanged drug and its metabolites in urine. Phenotype information is attractive because it provides a measure of the relevant biological dose. It is, however, subject to various sources of misclassification including the distorting effect of underlying disease, which differs between cases and controls. Phenotype measurements may also be influenced by lifestyle factors such as alcohol and cigarette consumption. If these factors are also related to the disease a case-control comparison based on phenotypes may be severely biased. The general problem of the phenotype being related to risk factors of disease and not to the disease itself is one of confounding, and is dealt with in more detail by Boffetta and Pearce in Chapter 10. While phenotypic data can be seen as complementary to genotype information, on their own they provide a weaker measure of genetic susceptibility than the actual genotype.

Confounding and linkage disequilibrium

Confounding is a major problem when environmental risk factors are being investigated, as many lifestyle exposures correlate strongly with each other and their individual effects need to be identified and separated. This requires knowledge of what factors are correlated and accurate measurement of them. A similar situation exists in case-control studies with genetic data because of linkage disequilibrium (LD), the phenomenon whereby alleles on one gene are inherited with particular alleles on neighbouring genes. For some families of genes situated close to one another on the same chromosome, e.g. class II HLA genes, this has led to haplotypes, (groups of alleles from different genes), which tend to be inherited together. For example, two common HLA haplotypes are the A1-B1-DR3 haplotype and the A2-B44-DR4 haplotype. An observed association between a disease and HLA B1 could occur because of a true association with HLA A1 or HLA DR3. A rigorous test of LD therefore requires knowledge of which alleles are correlated or tend to be inherited together. This is still difficult because of the incomplete understanding of the human genome. Also, even when most of the neighbouring alleles have been identified and their function is at least partially understood, as is the case with the HLA region, knowledge of which alleles are inherited together as haplotypes usually requires information on which alleles were inherited from each parent. It should be borne in mind that LD is only a possibility between alleles of genes situated very close to each other on the same chromosome, generally less than one centimorgan apart. This corresponds, very roughly, to about 1500 kilobases. Unless sustained by favourable selection, LD tends to weaken over generations as a result of recombination and should finally disappear. From what is understood of the GST family of genes, LD between GSTM1 and other GST genes would not appear possible. Whereas GSTM is situated on chromosome 1, GSTA is situated on chromosome 6 and GSTP on chromosome 11 (Smith *et al.*, 1995). The position of GSTT is not known. For another common gene family of genetic polymorphisms, the n-acetyltransferase genes NAT1 and NAT2, it is possible that disease associations with either could arise as a result of LD. Both genes are situated close together on the short arm of chromosome 8 (8p22) and both are functionally polymorphic (Smith *et al.*, 1995). The presence of an important tumour-suppressor gene in this region has also been suggested (Kelemen *et al.*, 1994). More detailed discussion of GST and NAT genes appears in Chapter 19 (Strange & Fryer) and Chapter 20 (Hirvonen).

An alternative to the case-control study design is a family-based design that involves typing not only the affected individuals but their parents as well. If an individual has genotype A1A2 and the parents have genotypes A1A3 and A2A4, the genotype which the individual does not inherit (A3A4) provides a virtual control that is perfectly matched for ethnic group and removes the possibility of bias from this source (Fig. 1). A comparison of genotype frequencies between cases and controls may be used to calculate genotype relative risks. This method may also be extended to cases in which there is information on only one parent (Curtis & Sham, 1995). Cases should be considered as individually matched to their virtual control and the analysis should reflect this by being similar to that of a matched case-control study (Breslow & Day, 1980). A specific instance of a

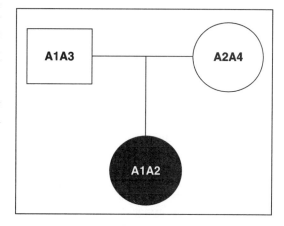

Figure 1. Transmitted alleles, non-transmitted alleles and the transmission disequilibrium test.
Transmitted alleles: A1, A2
Non-transmitted alleles: A3, A4

family-based study is the transmission disequilibrium test (TDT), which identifies parents who are heterozygous for a putative risk allele (Spielman *et al.*, 1993). This may be analysed as a matched case-control study, and the odds ratio associated with the risk allele is simply the number of times the affected offspring inherits the risk allele from a heterozygous parent divided by the number of times the affected offspring inherits the alternative allele. Parents who are not heterozygous for the risk allele offer no information for this comparison. This method was first used to test the association between insulin-dependent diabetes mellitus and the 5'FP class 1 susceptibility allele (Spielman *et al.*, 1993). Of 124 heterozygote parents of diabetic offspring, 78 transmitted the class 1 allele and 46 the non-susceptibility allele. This results in a matched odds ratio of 1.70 with a 95% confidence interval (1.16, 2.50).

TDT tests involve considerable extra effort in obtaining parental genetic information, and whether this is a worthwhile use of resources is questionable. Similar information can be obtained from a well-conducted matched case-control study with a minimal possibility of ethnic differences between cases and controls biasing the results. For most planned studies of chronic disease the question is academic because, frequently, both parents of a case have died. However, in family-based studies where the information is available the TDT test does provide an attractive study design for testing association.

The role of chance
Traditionally, an analysis of the role of chance in genetic association studies has generally relied on the calculation of significance tests and correction for the number of comparisons, for example by incorporating Bonferroni's correction factor (Svejgaard & Ryder, 1994). Thus a 5% significance level may be adequate if one genetic site is tested, whereas a significance level of 0.0005 is necessary if 100 genes are tested. This is done to ensure that the overall probability of identifying one false positive result remains at 5%. The penalty for this imposition of more stringent significance criteria is that a true positive result is more likely to go undetected. This reasoning therefore assumes that a false positive result has a more serious consequence than a false negative result. The limita-

tions of significance testing have been well documented in the epidemiological literature and most studies are now based on an estimation approach involving confidence intervals (Rothman, 1990). However, many reviewers and editors of genetics journals still prefer significance levels and correction factors (Svejgaard & Ryder, 1994), although little attention is paid to studies which are of such weak power that a true effect is unlikely to be found even when it exists. For example, a recent meta-analysis of ten studies of NAT2 genotype or phenotype and bladder cancer indicated that none had a power of 90% to detect an odds ratio of at least 2.0, and four had a power of less than 50% (d'Errico *et al.*, 1996). The present author's position is that false positive results can be identified in subsequent studies and therefore have less serious consequences than a series of false negative results occurring in studies of low power.

The use of significance tests and of correction for multiple comparisons in genetic studies is especially concerning as technological advances are allowing a greater number of genetic tests to be conducted in a relatively short time. This means that even more stringent statistical criteria are required to ensure against false positive results as more and more genes are tested. If the previous TDT analysis of diabetes had analysed 50 candidate genes instead of just one the observed association with 5'FP class 1 would have been classified as negative. More frequent use of likelihood methods to assess the strength of results, as is seen in other areas of genetic epidemiology, would also be a welcome development (Goodman & Royall, 1988; Poole, 1987). Alternative approaches, including empirical Bayes procedures, are discussed by Cuzick in Chapter 11.

Issues of analysis
Case-control analysis of genetic data can be based on the presence or absence of at least one functional allele, the presence or absence of 0, 1 or 2 alleles, or on specific genotypes. For example, the GSTM1 polymorphism is based on three main alleles, GSTM1*0, GSTM1*A and GSTM1*B, (a rare allele, GSTM1*3, has also been detected but will not be considered here). In GSTM1*0 the gene is deleted and homozygotes for this allele, GSTM1*0/0, express no protein (Smith *et al.*, 1995). This is the null polymorphism for which an increased risk of

Table 1a. Bladder cancer and GSTM1 deficiency

GSTM1	Cases	Controls	OR	95% CI
Null	175	203	1	
Positive	121	197	1.40	(1.40, 1.90)
	296	400		

Data from Brockmöller *et al.* (1994)

Table 1b. Stratified by genotype group

GSTM1	Case	Control	OR	95% CI
Null	175	203	1	
A/O or A/A	69	134	1.67	(1.18, 2.38)
B/O or B/B	45	53	1.02	(0.65, 1.58)
A/B	7	10	1.23	(0.47, 3.19)

various cancer types has been postulated. Most analyses assume that the active alleles GSTM1*A and GSTM1*B are equally protective and that possessing two alleles confers no extra protective effect over possessing one allele. While such assumptions are reasonable if based on phenotypic data, an analysis of trends in risk associated with different genotypes is still valuable when the information is available. In Table 1b, the results of the study of bladder cancer by Brockmöller *et al.* (1994) are extended. As well as the crude increase in risk of 40% associated with possessing two null alleles as

Table 2. Basal cell carcinoma of the skin and *GSTM1* genotypes

	Case	Control	OR	95% CI
GSTM1 Null	231	79	1	
Positive	204	74	1.06	(0.74, 1.53)
A/O or A/A	126	40	0.93	(0.60, 1.44)
B/O or B/B	71	25	1.03	(0.61, 1.73)
A/B	7	9	3.76	(1.40, 10.08)

Data from Heagerty *et al.* (1994)

compared with an A or B allele, the authors were able to estimate the evidence for increased risk for GSTM1*0/0 separately when compared to those with just the A allele (*A/0 and A/A) as well as those with just the B allele (*B/0 and *B/B). This indicated that the increased risk for *0/0 was restricted to comparison of those who possessed the A allele (OR = 1.67) but not the B allele (OR = 1.02). These results suggest that any protective effect from the GSTM1 polymorphism is due to possession of the A allele. It was not possible to identify A/A and B/B homozygotes although the A/B group provided intermediate results. These results need to be interpreted in the light of phenotype data suggesting a similar effect of A and B alleles, and further studies based on genotype data are necessary to clarify the association.

In a similar study of basal cell carcinoma (BCC) of the skin, no protective effect was observed for various groups of genotypes including any A or B allele, just the A allele, or just the B allele (Table 2) (Heagerty *et al.*, 1994). However, a strong protective effect was observed with possession of the A/B genotype (OR = 3.76), suggesting that two expressed alleles confer a stronger effect than just one. Although it was not possible to identify the A/A and B/B homozygotes, these results illustrate the value of utilizing all available genotype information in trying to understand the mechanism of the polymorphism.

A problem with conducting an analysis based on genotype data is that it will inevitably lead to small numbers of cases and controls with some genotypes. For example, the final OR of 3.76 for GSTM1*A/B was based on seven positive cases and nine positive controls. This association could have been observed because of a real 'double dose' effect among the cases with two alleles being required to exert a protective effect, or simply because a high number of controls with this genotype occurred as a result of chance. Both of these possibilities can be examined by estimating the gene frequencies of specific alleles in the case and control groups and calculating the expected number of the GSTM1*A/B genotype based on the law of Hardy-Weinberg equilibrium, which states that for two alleles, A and B, with gene frequencies $g(A)$ and $g(B)$, the expected frequencies of genotypes AA, AB and BB are $g(A)g(A)$, $2g(A)g(B)$, and $g(B)g(B)$ respectively.

Table 3. Observed and expected GSTM1 genotype frequencies in study of basal cell carcinoma, assuming Hardy-Weinberg equilibrium (Heagerty *et al.*)						
				GSTM1* (Observed/Expected)		
	g(0)	g(A)	g(B)	0/0	A/0+A/A+B/0+B/B	A/B
Controls	0.71	0.18	0.12	79/76.2	65/70.4	9/6.4
Cases	0.74	0.17	0.09	231/237.6	197/183.8	7/13.6

In Table 3 the estimated gene frequencies g(A) and g(B) of alleles A and B in the same study of BCC are estimated from the observed number of individuals either heterozygous or homozygous for A and B (the phenotype frequencies), along with the three groups of genotypes. Gene frequencies are obtained by recognizing that the phenotype frequency of an allele 'x' is $2g(x) - \{g(x)\}^2$ (Matsuura & Eguchi, 1990). This equation is solved using the standard formula for quadratic equations. The results are not conclusive in indicating whether the protective effect associated with GSTM1*A/B is due to a deficit of this genotype in the cases rather than a random excess observed in the controls, as both a small case deficit and a small control excess is seen. Indeed, it is possible that the large observed odds ratio could be explained by these two chance occurrences.

The frequencies of case genotypes might depart from Hardy-Weinberg equilibrium because of an etiological 'double dose' effect of possessing two alleles. However, there is usually no reason to suspect why the control genotypes should not obey Hardy-Weinberg equilibrium. One possibility, suggested by Lathrop (1983), is to use the expect-

ed genotype frequencies among the controls in the calculation of the odds ratio. This effectively removes an element of variation from the calculation of the odds ratios, and the confidence intervals, calculated using Woolf's estimates, reflect this by being smaller. The association between BCC of the skin and GSTM1*A/B in the study of Heagerty *et. al.* (1994) was recalculated using the expected control frequencies of the genotypes GSTM1*A/B and *0/0. This resulted in an odds ratio of 2.75 with a 95% confidence interval (1.12, 6.76) (Table 4). While this odds ratio is slightly lower than the original one, as part of the excess observed in the controls is assumed to be due to chance, the confidence interval is narrower, reflecting the increased precision. Using Lathrop's estimates, se(InOR) is 0.45. Woolf's estimate of the original standard error is 0.52, representing a relative gain in efficiency of 16%, (0.52/0.45).

Gene-environment interaction and gene-gene interaction

That no chronic disease can be considered as being either of purely genetic or purely environmental etiology is becoming increasingly clear. Also, as MacMahon (1969) postulated, environmental factors often exert their influence through the genetic mechanism of mutation while genetic mechanisms have the potential to change the environment. This has led to the old debate of "nature versus nurture" being replaced by one of "nature and nurture" in a study of gene-environment interaction. Interaction between two agents may be defined as coparticipation in the same causal mechanism leading to disease development (Yang & Khoury, 1997). Identification of interaction is therefore important when attempting to understand a disease process. However, there is some confusion over the appropriate measure for assessing the presence or absence of

Table 4. Basal cell carcinoma and GSTM1* A/B. Calculation of odds ratio using expected control genotype frequencies based on data from Heagerty *et al.*		
GSTM1*		
	Case	Control
0/0	231	76.2
A/B	7	6.36
OR = 2.75	95%CI (1.12, 6.76)	

an interaction effect. The primary reason for this confusion is that the statistical models commonly used to assess the joint effect of two factors generally assume a multiplicative effect between them. However, if a biological understanding of the disease process is invoked it appears that the joint effect of two independent risk factors will be closer to the sum of their individual effects if no interaction is present between them (Yang & Khoury, 1997; Rothman, 1986). Consider the multistage theory of carcinogenesis which maintains that a cell becomes cancerous after undergoing a series of mutations, and for a specific neoplasm assumes that a simple two-stage model holds, the first an initiating event and the second a promoting event. Furthermore, there are two distinct initiating mutations (I_1 and I_2) which occur with a spontaneous background rate of 1×10^{-3} for a specific time unit, and two promoting events (P_1 and P_2) which both occur with a background rate of 1×10^{-2} for the same arbitrary time. The incidence rate of both events $I_1 \to P_1$

and $I_2 \to P_2$ is therefore 1×10^{-5}. Now consider two exposures, a genetic susceptibility (G) which causes 5×10^{-3} I_1 mutations and an environmental exposure (E) which causes 9×10^{-2} P_2 mutations. If we assume that a cancerous cell occurs only after the joint events $I_1 \to P_1$ or $I_2 \to P_2$ then G and E act independently as they affect different causal pathways, i.e. there is no biological interaction between them. This is reflected in the incidence of disease in the four exposure groups (Table 5a). The overall risk is the sum of the individual risks minus the background risk. Similarly, the risk ratio for the two exposures is the sum of the individual risk ratios minus 1. Thus the expected relative risk under a model of no interaction is RR(GE) = RR(G)+RR(E)-1. This suggests a further measure, the relative excess risk due to interaction (RERI), which may be calculated as: RERI = RR(GE)-RR(E)-RR(G)+1. Whereas a RERI of 0 indicates no biological interaction between G and E, positive values indicate synergistic action and negative values indicate antagonistic action.

Table 5a. Hypothetical incidence of cancerous cell outcome under two causal pathways, $I_1 \to P_1$ and $I_2 \to P_2$

Exposure	$I_1 \to P_1$	$I_2 \to P_2$	Rate	Rate ratio
None	1×10^{-5}	1×10^{-5}	2×10^{-5}	1
G	6×10^{-5}	1×10^{-5}	7×10^{-5}	3.5
E	1×10^{-5}	10×10^{-5}	11×10^{-5}	5.5
GE	6×10^{-5}	10×10^{-5}	16×10^{-5}	8

Table 5b. Hypothetical incidence of cancerous cell outcome including two further causal pathways, $I_1 \to P_2$ and $I_2 \to P_1$

Exposure	$I_1 \to P_2$	$I_2 \to P_1$	Overall rate (incl. $I_1 \to P_1$ and $I_2 \to P_2$)	Rate ratio
None	1×10^{-5}	1×10^{-5}	4×10^{-5}	1
G	6×10^{-5}	1×10^{-5}	14×10^{-5}	3.5
E	10×10^{-5}	1×10^{-5}	22×10^{-5}	5.5
GE	61×10^{-5}	1×10^{-5}	77×10^{-5}	19.25

Two further disease pathways, $I_1 \rightarrow P_2$ and $I_2 \rightarrow P_1$, were assumed not to occur. If these two causal pathways are assumed to exist the greatest rate of cancerous cells occurs in the group $I_1 \rightarrow P_2$, as a large number of cells are initiated by the genetic susceptibility and promoted by the environmental exposure, an example of biological interaction (Table 5b). The overall RR incorporating all four causal pathways is the same for the presence of G or E only, but increased to 19.25 for the joint presence of E and G. In this example there is multiplicative interaction between the two components and RR(EG) = RR(E)*RR(G). The RERI is 11.25, indicating that the interaction between the two components is the most important contributing factor to the incidence of cancerous cells. A statistical analysis of interaction based on a multiplicative model (such as logistic regression) would indicate an absence of interaction, as multiplicative models assume that RR(EG) = RR(E)*RR(G). An inference regarding biological interaction based on an analysis of such statistical interaction would be erroneous.

The hypothetical data in Table 5a present an absence of any interaction and those in Table 5b allows for an interaction between two different factors occurring at different stages. Under these two situations the joint risk ratio is predicted on the basis of the individual risk ratios. However, various other models of interaction are possible, including interaction between factors acting at the same stage and possibly having unknown antagonistic or enhancing effects. These other models of interaction would result in different predicted estimates of combined risk ratios (Siemiatycki & Thomas, 1981; Ottman, 1996).

The usefulness of investigating gene-environment interaction is illustrated in Table 6. These data are from a population-based case-control study of lung cancer and occupational exposure comprising 159 cases and 153 controls (Caporaso et al., 1989). One of the main occupational outcomes was asbestos exposure and occupational histories indicated "likely" asbestos exposure in 17 cases and 6 controls, giving OR = 2.93 with a 95% confidence interval (1.16, 7.42). When stratified by debrisoquine metabolic phenotype information, a strong interaction was observed between likely asbestos exposure, extensive metabolization of debrisoquine, and lung cancer. The RERI associated with the interaction effect is 15.08.

As well as assessing interaction between genetic and environmental exposures it is important to consider that the effects of different polymorphisms may interact with each and that these should be analysed in a similar fashion. For example, interactive effects between GSTM1 and cytochrome CYP1A1 genotypes have previously been postulated, as have joint effects between the GSTM1 and GSTT1 polymorphisms and smoking-related cancers (Smith et al., 1995).

A major problem in studies attempting to obtain an accurate measure of interaction is that the sample size required increases sharply. Even under the most favourable conditions of a common exposure and common genotype, and a moderately strong interaction, the number of cases and

Table 6. Lung cancer risk, asbestos exposure and debrisoquine metabolic phenoype (Caporaso et al.)					
Asbestos exposure	Debrisoquine EM	Controls	Cases	OR	95%CI
–	–	65	16	1	–
+	–	3	1	1.35	(0.1, 10.3)
–	+	82	126	6.24	(3.4, 11.5)
+	+	3	16	21.67	(5.92-77.73)

EM = Extensive metabolism
RERI = 21.67-6.24-1.35+1 = 15.08

controls required to achieve a power of 80% is at least 200 of each (Hwang *et al.*, 1994). A recently proposed study design which aims to be more efficient for assessing gene-environment interaction is the case-only study (Khoury & Flanders, 1996). A group of cases is stratified into a 2x2 table on the basis of two exposure variables and, provided that these exposures are unrelated in the population, the case-only odds ratio calculated from the table is related to the individual odds ratios for each exposure separately by the following formula:

$$OR_{ca} = OR_{ge}/(OR_g * OR_e)$$

where OR_{ca} is the case-only odds ratio.

For example, an environmental and a genetic risk factor for rheumatoid arthritis (RA) occurring postpartum are breast-feeding and possession of the HLA DR4 allele respectively. Both of these factors have been estimated to increase the risk of RA approximately fourfold. A separate study investigating the presence of interaction among a group of cases estimated a case-only OR of 6.3 (Table 7) (Brennan *et al.*, 1996). This indicates that OR_{ge} is over six times greater than the product of the individual effects ($OR_g * OR_e$), implying substantial interaction.

The basic assumption of the case-only study design of independence between environmental exposure and genotype is likely to be satisfied in most cases. In the absence of genes associated by linkage disequilibrium this assumption also holds for the assessment of gene-gene interaction. The number of cases required is substantially smaller than the number that would be required for a traditional case-control study for the same power to detect interaction (Yang *et al.*, 1997). However, there are also several limitations. First, it is not possible to assess the individual effects of exposure or genotype. Second, the basis is a statistical model measuring departures from multiplicative interaction, and a case-only odds ratio of 1.0 does not necessarily indicate an absence of biological interaction. Third, the assumption of independence between the exposure and the genotype cannot be evaluated.

In summary, early genetic case-control studies tended to be characterized by small sample size, low power and poorly defined case and control groups. Although these studies provided some valuable information it will be necessary for future studies to be more rigorously designed in order to ensure valid results. Such considerations are especially important now as the conduct of large case-control studies involving various genetic markers is likely to become more common with the advent of new technology. These studies will not replace previous epidemiological research of environmental and lifestyle exposures but will complement it, allowing an examination of gene-environment interaction and subsequently a greater understanding of disease processes.

References

Brennan, P., Ollier, B., Worthington, J., Hajeer, A. & Silman, A. (1996) Are both genetic and reproductive associations with rheumatoid arthritis linked to prolactin? *Lancet*, 348, 106-109

Breslow, N.E. & Day, N.E. (1980) *Statistical Methods in Cancer Research. Volume 1. The Analysis of Case-control Studies.* Lyon, IARC (Scientific Publications, No. 32)

Brockmöller, J., Kerb, R., Drakaulis, N., Staffeldt, B. & Roots, I. (1994) Glutathione *S*-transferase M1 and its variants A and B as host factors of bladder cancer susceptibility: a case-control study. *Cancer Res.*, 54, 4103-4111

Caporaso, N., Hayes, R.B., Dosemeci, M., Hoover, R., Ayesh, R., Hetzel, M. & Idle, J. (1989) Lung cancer risk, occupational exposure, and the debrisoquine metabolic phenotype. *Cancer Res.*, 49, 3675-3679

Table 7. Case-only study of breast-feeding, HLA DR 4 and rheumatoid arthritis (Brennan *et al.*)		
HLA DR 4		
Breast-feeding history		
	Y	N
+	52	19
–	7	16
	59	35
OR_{ca} = 6.3	95% CI (2.3, 17.2)	

Curtis, D. & Sham, P.C. (1995) A note on the application of the transmission disequilibrium test when a parent is missing. *Am. J. Hum. Genet.*, 56, 811-812

d'Errico, A., Taioli, E., Chen, X. & Vineis, P. (1996) Genetic metabolic polymorphisms and the risk of cancer: a review of the literature. *Biomarkers*, 1, 149-173

Goodman, S.N. & Royall, R. (1988) Evidence and scientific research. *Am. J. Public Health*, 78, 1568-1574

Heagerty, A.H.M., Fitzgerald, D., Smith, A., Blowers, B., Jones, P., Fryer, A.A., Zhao, L., Alldersea, J. & Strange, R.C. (1994) Glutathione S-transferase GSTM1 phenotypes and protection against cutaneous tumours. *Lancet*, 343, 266-268

Hwang, S.-J., Beaty, T.H., Liang, K.-Y., Coresh, J. & Khoury,M.J. (1994) *Am. J. Epidemiol.*, 140, 1029-1037

Kelemen, P.R., Yaremko, M.L. & Kim, A.H. (1994) Loss of heterozygosity in b9 is associated with microinvasion in colorectal cancer. *Genes Chromosomes Cancer*, 11, 195-198

Khoury, M.J. & Flanders, D. (1996). Nontraditional epidemiologic approaches in the analysis of gene-environment interaction: case-control studies with no controls! *Am. J. Epidemiol.*, 144, 207-213

Lathrop, G.M. Estimating genotype relative risks. (1983) *Tissue Antigens*, 22, 160-166

MacMahon, B. (1968) Gene-environment interaction in human disease. *J. Psychiatr. Res.*, 6 (Suppl. 7), 393-402

Matsuura, M. & Eguchi, S. (1990) Estimation of gene frequency and test for Hardy-Weinberg equilibrium in the HLA system. *Environ. Health Perspect.*, 87, 149-155

Ottman, R. (1996) Theoretical epidemiology. Gene-environment interaction: definition and study designs. *Prev. Med.*, 25, 764-770

Poole, C. (1987) Beyond the confidence interval. *Am. J. Public Health*, 77, 195-199

Rothman, K.J., ed. (1986) *Modern Epidemiology*. Boston, Little Brown & Co.

Rothman, K.J. (1990) No adjustments are needed for multiple comparisons. *Epidemiol.*, 1, 43-46

Siemiatycki, J. & Thomas, D.C. (1981) Biological models and statistical interactions: an example from multistage carcinogenesis. *Int. J. Epidemiol.*, 10, 383-387

Smith, G., Satnley, L.A., Sim, E., Strange, R.C. & Wolf, C.R. (1995) Metabolic polymorphisms and cancer susceptibility. In: *Cancer Surveys. Volume 25: Genetics and Cancer: a Second Look*. Cold Spring Harbor Laboratory Press

Spielman, R.S., McGinnis, R.E. & Ewens, W.J. (1993) Transmission test for linkage disequilibrium: the insulin gene region and insulin-dependent diabetes mellitus (IDDM). *Am. J. Hum. Genet.*, 52, 506-516

Svejgaard, A. & Ryder, L.P. (1994) HLA and disease associations: detecting the strongest association. *Tissue Antigens*, 43, 18-27

Wacholder, S., McLaughlin, J.K., Silverman, D.T. & Mandel, J.S. (1992) Selection in case-control studies. *Am. J. Epidemiol.*,135, 1019-1028

Yang, Q. & Khoury, M.J. (1997) Evolving methods in genetic epidemiology. III. Gene-environment interaction in epidemiologic research. *Epidemiol. Rev.*, 19, 33-43

Yang, Q., Khoury, M.J. & Flanders, D.W. (1997) Sample size requirement in case-only designs to detect gene-environment interaction. *Am. J. Epidemiol.*, 146, 713-720

Paul Brennan
Environmental Cancer Epidemiology Unit,
International Agency for Research on Cancer,
150, Cours Albert-Thomas,
69372 Lyon Cedex 08, France

Metabolic Polymorphisms and Susceptibility to Cancer
W. Ryder
IARC Scientific Publications No. 148
International Agency for Research on Cancer, Lyon, 1999

Chapter 13. Laboratory methods for the determination of genetic polymorphisms in humans

B. Blömeke and P. G. Shields

The determination of genetic polymorphisms for susceptibility to human disease has been rapidly increasing since the introduction of the polymerase chain reaction (PCR). In most laboratories the ability exists to conduct studies on more than 10 000 persons, and the prospect of even larger investigations is approaching. Many methods can be used for genotyping individuals but some are more common and less expensive than others. Newer methods will allow for automation. As the number of studies on genetic polymorphisms increases it is to be expected that more pitfalls will be encountered. While larger studies will reduce the importance of misclassification, quality control methods will have to be applied to the processing of large numbers of samples.

Sources of DNA and DNA extraction

The most critical element in the successful analysis of genetic polymorphism is the quality of DNA. When the quality is poor, so is the result. Quality depends on the method of collection, the way in which cells or tissues are stored (e.g. method of freezing, storage temperature, media [paraffin blocks, dried blood dots]), DNA storage, duration of storage, the type of extraction, and the experience of the person performing it. DNA can be extracted from fresh, archival and ancient sources. For each, the number of possible sources has been steadily increasing as new methodologies have emerged (Table 1). For example, forensic analysis using the polymerase chain reaction (PCR) may use a single hair (Han *et al.*, 1992), sperm (Sajantila *et al.*, 1992), dried blood on a blotter (Jinks *et al.*, 1989), urine (Gasparini *et al.*, 1989), and even saliva on cigarette butts (Hochmeister *et al.*, 1991).

One of the most useful tissues for storage is whole blood because it requires little processing time and cost before archiving. Cell separation is avoided and the risk of contamination is reduced when large epidemiological studies are being conducted. Whole blood is typically stored in anticoagulants such as heparin or EDTA, although with heparin some problems in the PCR have occasionally been reported. It is believed that heparin and porphyrin compounds inhibit PCRs,

but purified haemoglobin or iron added to a PCR were not inhibitory (Cosma *et al.*, 1993), and there have been many successful studies. Whole blood storage might be particularly useful if Tth polymerases are used (Erlich *et al.*, 1991). This is a more robust enzyme than Taq™ polymerase (Panaccio *et al.*, 1993; Sparkman, 1992), and reduced temperature (FoLT = formamide low temperature) allows direct DNA amplification from blood without extraction. (Note, low temperatures [80°C-85°C for initial melting and annealing temperatures of 40°C or less] could increase non-specific priming and should therefore be tested). A common method for DNA extraction from whole blood is a Chelex™ 100 protocol (Bio-Rad Laboratory, Richmond, CA) (De Lamballerie *et al.*, 1992). Here, the blood is boiled in the presence of Chelex™ 100 resin. DNA recovery is reproducible, and is useful for small volumes (2-10 µl). Chelex™ 100 resin is routinely used for bloodstains, seminal stains, buccal swabs, hair and postcoital samples. A different approach for extracting DNA from small amounts (5 µl) of whole blood is immuno-PCR (Lew & Kelly, 1991). Using anti-histone antibodies in a capture assay or a microtitre tray, chromosomal DNA can be selectively bound and the PCR can then be performed in the same tube. If high molecular weight is needed, as with Southern blot

Table 1. Sources of DNA for genetic polymorphism analysis		
DNA source	**Method**	**Reference**
Whole blood	FoLT PCR (formamide low temperature) Boiling with Chelex™ 100 Immuno-PCR Rapid chemical extraction of high quality DNA	(Panaccio & Lew, 1991) (Panaccio et al., 1993) (De Lamballerie et al., 1992) (Lew & Kelly, 1991) (Jeanpierre, 1987) (Gustincich et al., 1991)
Leukocytes	Proteinase K/chemical extraction	(Sugimura et al., 1990) (Jeanpierre, 1987)
Hairs	Proteinase K/chemical extraction	(Higuchi et al., 1988) (Han et al., 1992) (Westwood & Werrett, 1990)
Sperm	Proteinase K/chemical extraction	(Sajantila et al., 1992)
DNA from dried blood on blotter and cotton cloth	Chelex™ 100 Proteinase K/chemical extraction	(Jinks et al., 1989) (Walsh et al., 1991) (Lin et al., 1994)
Urine	Proteinase K/chemical extraction	(Gasparini et al., 1989)
Saliva on cigarette butts	Proteinase K/chemical extraction	(Hochmeister et al., 1991)
Fresh tissues and biopsies	Proteinase K/chemical extraction	(Smith et al., 1987) (Shibata, 1992)
DNA swabs (cervical, vulvar, penile, buccal cells, nostril)	Cell lysis DNA adsorption to glass matrices Proteinase K/chemical extraction	(Nickerson et al., 1990) (Nikiforov et al., 1994) (Bertilsson et al., 1989) (Smits et al., 1992)
DNA from ethanol-fixed samples	Proteinase K/chemical extraction	(Broly et al., 1995)
Formaldehyde and paraffin- embedded tissues	Proteinase K/chemical extraction Sonication with glass beads/Proteinase K Boiling	(Goelz et al., 1985) (Greer et al., 1994) (Heller et al., 1992) (Kallio et al., 1991)
Museum specimens	Proteinase K/chemical extraction Centrifugation on Centricon 30 filters	(Higuchi et al., 1984; Paabo, 1985) (Paabo, 1989)

analyses, the method of Gustincich et al. (1991) can be used. Typical phenol-based extraction methods can also be employed (Sambrook et al., 1989). Initially, it is optimal to store whole blood by freezing (-70°C). The samples can be stored on ice and shipped, but freezing should occur within 24 hours at the most. However, when whole blood is frozen it is only useful for DNA recovery, as cell membranes are cracked and intact cells are unrecoverable. Plasma is mixed with cell contents.

Air-dried blood smears are another potential source of DNA, for example from smears on a microscope slide (Fey et al., 1987) or from dots blotted on to cards or cloth (Jinks et al., 1989; Lin et al., 1994; Walsh et al., 1991). These DNA sources allow easy and prolonged conservation of samples, especially for the amplification of PCR fragments of less than 200 bp (Jinks et al., 1989; Lagarde et al., 1995). For microscope slides, samples are air-dried without fixing, or they can be fixed with ethanol or methanol. For bloodstains on paper (Jinks *et al.*, 1989; Lin *et al.*, 1994) or cotton cloth (Walsh *et al.*, 1991), small areas of the original samples are cut (3 x 3 mm pieces), resuspended, and extracted using Chelex™ 100 or methods involving the use of phenol. In our laboratory we found only a 50% success rate for bloodstains on blotter using fragment sizes greater than 250 bp and a phenol-based extraction method, while Walsh et *al.* (1991) reported that 100% of their samples could be amplified using a Chelex™ 100 extraction method. These samples, while on cards, are optimally stored by freezing at -70°C, although storage at room temperature for periods of less than six months may be acceptable.

Individual blood components frequently serve as DNA sources, the most comonly used being white blood cells. Serum and plasma also provide DNA for genotyping (Lau *et al.*, 1995; Chan *et al.*, 1995; Stein *et al.*, 1995; Martin *et al.*, 1992; Secchiero *et al.*, 1995; Kato *et al.*, 1990; Leon *et al.*, 1977; Shapiro *et al.*, 1983; Vasioukhin *et al.*, 1994; Sorenson *et al.*, 1994), where the DNA comes from lysed cells or is released from lymphocytes (Anker *et al.*, 1975; Leon *et al.*, 1977). For DNA extraction, samples are concentrated by centrifugation (Kato *et al.*, 1990) or are directly digested with proteinase K. Digests are extracted with organic solvents or are used immediately for PCR amplification (Kato *et al.*, 1990). Some investigators isolated DNA using a phenol/chloroform/ether extraction followed by Cs_2SO_4 gradient (Vasioukhin *et al.*, 1994). Recently, we have shown that serum can be routinely used for PCR/RFLP genotyping of cancer susceptibility genes. The isolated DNA was intact to amplify a region of at least 529 base pairs, yields were between 162 and 1,060 ng DNA using 250 µl serum (n = 18). Based on our average usage of 20 ng per PCR, the extractable DNA could be used for 10 to 53 PCR-based genotyping assays. The possibility of genotyping using serum (or plasma) opens the field to many archived settings where conventional DNA sources are unavailable. After separation, the blood components should be frozen at -70°C.

DNA can be obtained non-invasively from the head. Hair bulb DNA can be obtained by washing the bulb in ethanol, digesting with Proteinase K and extracting by means of phenol-based methods (Higuchi *et al.*, 1988; Han *et al.*, 1992), or fixed in methanol and directly used for the PCR (Han *et al.*, 1992). The latter protocol was successfully used for two to six bulbs from freshly plucked hairs for each PCR (Westwood & Werrett, 1990). DNA can be obtained from the oral cavity (buccal membrane) or a nostril by swabbing with a cytobrush or cotton swab (Nikiforov *et al.*, 1994) or taking oral rinses (Nickerson *et al.*, 1990). The cell density of a single swab varies between 5 x 10^3 and 3 x 10^5 cells, and this is sufficient for PCR-based methods. Oral rinses with saline, preceded by swabbing, also yield acceptable DNA.

Tissue from pathology departments is an important source of archived material, in the form of preserved microscope slides, frozen tissues or paraffin-embedded tissue blocks. The type of fixative can greatly influence the quality of extracted DNA. The best fixative is 50% ethanol; formaldehyde and other fixatives are less satisfactory. Formaldehyde (4% aqueous solution) is the most commonly used fixative, and while it is good for proteins, reduced DNA yields are obtained because DNA leaks into the fixative solution (Jackson *et al.*, 1990). Extracting DNA from samples fixed in other agents is also possible, such as neutral-buffered formalin, paraformaldehyde, formol sublimate, and even Bouin's reagent, a fixative based on picric acid (Greer *et al.*, 1994)). As a rule of thumb, the smaller the fragment to be amplified by PCR (<200 bp), the greater the likelihood of success. Most protocols involve complete digestion of a dewaxed sample with Proteinase K (sometimes taking up to five days for larger pieces of tissue). Faster methods such as sonication (Heller *et al.*, 1992) and boiling (Kallio *et al.*, 1991) are available, but may be less efficient than the use of Proteinase K (Forsthoefel *et al.*, 1992). Phenol-based methods can also be used (Sambrook *et al.*, 1989). Using proteinase K digestion, we obtained DNA yields of between 1 µg and 11.7 µg from 5-µm and 20-µm sections.

Various methods have been described for DNA extraction from fresh tissues and biopsies. For cryopreserved material it is usual to begin by grinding up to 100 mg of tissue in liquid nitrogen to produce a fine powder. The resulting homogenate is used for the DNA extraction procedure. In the case of small fresh and frozen biop-

135

sies even crude lysates have been used for PCR amplifications (Shibata, 1992).

DNA from ancient organic remains has been used in several anthropological and evolutionary studies (Kato *et al.*, 1994; Paabo, 1989) and in forensic science (Higuchi *et al.*, 1984). The tissue can either be crushed or minced before Proteinase K digestion (for up to five days). The digest is then extracted with phenol/chloroform, or the DNA is recovered by centrifugation on Centricon 30 filters (Amicon, Beverly, MA) (Paabo, 1989). DNA yields vary between 200 ng and 20 µg per gram of dried tissue, approaching 0.005% and 5% respectively of the amount expected from fresh tissue. Because nuclear DNA is degraded after death by endogenous hydrolytic processes (Rebrov *et al.*, 1983) it seems likely that the rapidity with which the body is desiccated immediately after death is the major factor that determines the yield and suitability of DNA. Oxidation products of pyrimidines, AP sites, damaged sugar residues, as well as intra- and intermolecule cross-links are potential problems. Because of post-mortem changes in DNA, caution has to be exercised in the use of these samples. Several microsatellite repeats can be feasibly analysed in DNA from bones and teeth up to 5000 years of age. However, Ramos *et al.* (1995) found that the repeated analysis of each marker produced different genotypes in as many as 97% of samples. Alleles differing from the originals consisted of additions or deletions of 1-39 dinucleotides.

Once extracted, DNA should be stored at temperatures appropriate to its intended use. For long-term storage, -70°C is optimal. However, multiple aliquots are preferable in order to avoid repetitive freezing and thawing, which could result in DNA degradation. In our laboratory we try to store samples in aliquots useful for several months of assays, so that once thawing has occurred the samples can be left at 4°C. However, if the samples are not going to be used for at least four months we freeze them again. We have also stored samples at room temperature for over six months in aliquots useful for one PCR, without problems. The samples typically become dry but amplification is successful. Whenever working with stored DNA it is important to use a sterile technique so as to avoid microbial contamination. Furthermore, we try to manipulate samples as little as possible. Multiple pipetting seems to be a greater factor in DNA degradation than length of storage.

Genetic polymorphism analysis by the polymerase chain reaction (PCR)

The PCR is an *in vitro* method for enzymatically synthesizing defined sequences of DNA. The reaction uses two oligonucleotide primers that hybridize to opposite strands and flank the target DNA sequence of interest. The elongation of the primers to amplify the gene is catalysed by a thermostable polymerase, the one most often used being Taq™ DNA polymerase, which is derived from the thermophilic eubacterium *Thermus aquaticus*. Usually, all the reagents (deoxynucleotide triphosphates (dNTPs), primers, reaction buffer, target DNA and Taq™ polymerase) are mixed and a repetitive series of cycles involving template denaturation, primer annealing, and extension of the primers by the enzyme results in exponential accumulation of a specific DNA fragment. Special procedures to improve the PCR include the hot-start procedure, which is a prolonged step of denaturation administered before Taq™ polymerase addition, and a two-round amplification with nested priming (using two separate PCR assays, where the product of the first serves as the template for the second). Recently, the long PCR has been used, in which the thermostable DNA polymerases are employed (e.g. Vent, Deep Vent, Pwo or Pfu polymerase) to amplify fragments as long as 42 000 bp (see below). This assay, while useful, requires better quality DNA and success is more difficult to achieve.

An important component of a successful PCR lies in the selection of primers (Table 2). Ideally, the primers should have the same annealing temperature, resulting in high amplification efficiency. In the case of multiplex PCR amplification (amplifying more than one gene locus in a single reaction using more than one primer pair), the T_m values for all primer sets should be within the range of ±5°C. Similar annealing temperatures can be achieved by designing primers that are the same length and display not only a similar G/C base content but also similar percentage of G and C bases within the primer. A G plus C base percentage near 50% is optimal, allowing for effi-

Table 2. Optimum PCR primer designs	
Parameter	**Optimum values**
Oligonucleotide sequence	Unique
No self-complementarity	≤3 contiguous bases
No complementarity to another (especially at the 3' end)	≤3 contiguous bases
Match primer melting temperatures (T_m [°C] = 2AT+4GC)	Less than 5°C if possible
Base composition	G/C content near 50%
Base distribution	Random or 1-2 G/C nucleotides at the 3' end
Primer length	20-25 bases
Distance of intraprimer sequence 1. Fresh tissue, blood, cells, alcohol-fixed samples 2. Plasma, serum, formaldehyde-fixed and paraffin- embedded tissues 3. Museum specimens	 100-2000 bases apart 100-600 bases apart 100-150 bases apart

cient melting during the PCR. Primers that anneal with sequences displaying lower G/C contents can be compensated for by an increase in length, and primers of at least 17 bases are recommended as being statistically unique in the human genome (Thein & Wallace, 1986). The 3'-end of a primer is important for determining the annealing temperature. However, most of the rules for primer design are empirical and there is no guarantee of success. Computer programs are available to help in the selection of unique primers (Hillier & Green, 1991).

DNA polymerases can make errors at a low rate, which varies depending on the type of polymerase, the substrate and the reaction conditions. During the PCR, amplification products serve as a template for subsequent cycles. Polymerase errors are consequently inherited and these changes can accumulate. The errors produced by Taq™ polymerase, the most widely used for *in vitro* DNA amplification methods, can be higher than 10^{-3} per nucleotide at high dNTP and Mg^{2+} ion concentrations, and as low as 10^{-6} under other conditions. Other enzymes, such as polymerases from *Pyrococcus furiosus* (Pfu™) and *P. woesei*, (Pwo™) have an associated $3' \rightarrow 5'$ exonuclease activity, which selectively removes misincorporated nucleotides to generate a correctly base-paired primer terminus (proofreading), resulting in much higher fidelity. When the errors during PCR are distributed evenly throughout the fragment, no particular mutated sequence constitutes a major subpopulation. Here, the predominant species at each nucleotide position is that of the initial sequence. Therefore, for the detection of genetic polymorphisms where a homogeneous DNA population is analysed, PCR mistakes are of little concern. However, parameters increasing the error rate and the known context-dependent effects on the fidelity of polymerases (Goodman *et al.*, 1993) are to be avoided.

The ability to amplify as much as 25 kilobases of DNA using PCR (long PCR) has recently provided new opportunities. The combination of thermostable DNA polymerases with proofreading activity (e.g. Vent, Deep Vent, Pwo or Pfu polymerase) and ones lacking such activity (e.g. rTth polymerase) together with improved buffer and cycling conditions (longer extension times) (Cheng *et al.*, 1994a; Barnes, 1994; Cheng *et al.*, 1994b) can achieve longer amplification. Typical primers for long PCR amplifications have been 21-34 bp with melting temperatures near 65-70°C. The specificity of the primers is critical, as the amplification of long targets is compromised by preferential amplification of shorter nonspecific products. The product must be verified as the full-length target. Misamplification can be avoided by repeated reactions, use of different primer pairs or product digestion with specific restriction enzymes. This method allows the amplification of genes long enough to include several polymorphic sites and multiple adjacent genes (e.g. GSTM1 and GSTM3), and can be used to amplify across polymorphically deleted genes. The deletion is thereby seen conclusively. It also reduces the risk of amplifying pseudogenes (Steen et al., 1995; Broly et al., 1995).

Detection of genetic polymorphisms

The study of genetic polymorphisms in humans is playing an important role in the diagnosis of genetic and malignant diseases (Kerem et al., 1989; Fearon & Vogelstein, 1990), forensic sciences (Nakamura et al., 1987; Lander, 1989), and in gene mapping projects (Donis-Keller et al., 1987). Each of these applications involves the analysis of many samples and requires rapid, inexpensive, automated methods. Usually, methods that can be used to discover new mutations can be applied to typing those that are already known, as with Southern blot analysis (Southern, 1975), restriction fragment length polymorphism analysis (Botstein et al., 1980), allele-specific oligonucleotide hybridization (Conner et al., 1983), denaturing gradient gel electrophoresis (Myers et al., 1987), heteroduplex analysis (Keen et al., 1991), single-strand conformation polymorphism (Hayashi, 1991), allele-specific PCR (Chehab & Kan, 1989; Wu et al., 1989; Newton et al., 1989), allele-specific oligonucleotide probes (Saiki et al., 1986), and the detection of amplified products by oligomer hybridization (Kwok et al. 1989). Some detection methods do not rely on electrophoresis, for instance the oligonucleotide ligation assay (Landegren et al., 1988; Nickerson et al., 1990) and the primer-guided incorporation techniques, e.g. genetic bit analysis (Nikiforov et al., 1994).

Restriction length fragment polymorphisms (RFLP) have been frequently used (Goodfellow, 1992) for genetic linkage maps (Botstein et al., 1980), to identify individuals in forensic science (Nakamura et al., 1987), and for the detection of diseases (Chehab et al., 1987). RFLPs can be used for genetic polymorphism analysis where the

polymorphic site is within a palindromic run of nucleotides susceptible to cleavage by a known restriction endonuclease. The resulting fragment size pattern can be detected by Southern analysis (Budowle & Baechtel, 1990) or PCR followed by restriction digestion, and gel electrophoresis with ethidium bromide staining (Day & Humphries, 1994). It should be noted that restriction enzyme cleavage may be inefficient when the palindromic site is found near the end of the DNA fragment (for specifics see manufacturer's instructions). This is important if misclassification by incomplete digestion is to be avoided. Primers may be designed to include a non-polymorphic site susceptible to cleavage within the PCR fragment, in order to show completeness of digestion and enhance quality control. When the polymorphic site of interest is not contained within a restriction site it may be possible to introduce a palindrome artificially into a primer by modifying one or two bases so that a restriction site is created and the restriction enzyme cleaves off the primer.

The allele-specific PCR is commonly used when a polymorphic site of interest is not found within a palindromic sequence susceptible to restriction enzymatic digestion. This method is based on the principle that mismatches of the base at the 3' end of a primer do not amplify by PCR, or amplify at very low rates. The Taq^{TM} polymerase is especially useful for this because it lacks 3'-5' exonuclease activity. In its simplest form, two PCR assays are performed in parallel, using a common primer in both and unique allele-specific primers in each, the latter primers being matched to one polymorphic variant or the other. Perfect matches can then amplify, revealing which sequence is present. However, this method has the limitation that the lack of amplification may suggest a failed PCR attempt (multiplex PCR, amplifying an additional gene as an internal control, eliminates this possibility). Alternatively, the presence of a band might indicate false amplification, as occurs under suboptimal conditions (low annealing temperatures or magnesium concentrations). In fact this method is qualitative, not quantitative, and false amplification can therefore easily occur under the wrong conditions. It is thus important to optimize the conditions and to compare the intensity of bands for the matched and mismatched primers on the same gel. This method is frequently used as a two-step assay, the first step amplifying the gene of interest by PCR, and the second PCR using oligospecific probes in two simultaneous reactions. The advantage of this is that it increases the specificity by increasing the number of templates. However, the most critical step is the first one; a lack of successful amplification or inconsistent results in the second step are frequently due to a suboptimal first step.

PCR coupled with the oligonucleotide ligation assay (OLA) uses DNA ligases to join two adjacent oligonucleotides when hybridized to a DNA template under optimized conditions. Ligations occur only when the oligonucleotides are perfectly complementary to the template (Landegren *et al.*, 1988; Nickerson *et al.*, 1990). Two ligation reactions are run in parallel, corresponding to the oligonucleotides matching in sequence either of the polymorphic variants (allele-specific probes). For this method the allele-specific probes are biotinylated and the common primer is labelled at its 3' end with digoxigenin. The common primer is ligated to the allele-specific probe when matched to the DNA sequence. After ligation, the 5' biotinylated probes are captured on strepavidin-coated microtitre plates. If ligation has occurred the presence of the digoxigenin reporter is detected in an ELISA-based format. The advantage of this method is that the complete procedure can be performed on microtitre plates, allowing the automation (robotic workstations are available) and rapid processing of samples. Its disadvantage is that there is no control for successful amplification and no internal control in each reaction well.

Genetic bit analysis (GBA) belongs to the group of primer-guided nucleotide incorporation assays (Syvanen *et al.*, 1990, 1993; Kuppuswamy *et al.*, 1991). In this method (Nikiforov *et al.*, 1994), specific fragments of genomic DNA containing the polymorphic site(s) are amplified by PCR with one regular and one phosphorothioate-modified primer. The double-stranded DNA is rendered single-stranded and captured on microtitre plates by hybridization to an immobilized oligonucleotide primer, which is designed to hybridize to the DNA sequence immediately adjacent to the polymorphic site. A DNA polymerase

extends the 3' end of the oligonucleotide by just one base, using a mixture of one biotin-labelled and one fluorescein-labelled dideoxynucleotide triphosphate (ddNTP), corresponding to the bases of the two polymorphic alleles. Antibody conjugates of alkaline phosphatase and horseradish peroxidase are used to determine the nature of the extended base in an ELISA format. The method is highly flexible but has no internal control for successful PCR amplifications. The use of two labelled ddNTPs, allowing the determination of both alleles in the same well, increases throughput, reduces the amount of PCR targets required and, more importantly, serves as a powerful internal control for all post-PCR steps.

Dot or slot blot and reverse dot blot hybridizations are non-isotopic methods that use allele-specific oligonucleotide probes (Saiki *et al.*, 1986; Saiki *et al.*, 1989). Dot blots are performed following PCR in the region of interest, and the PCR product is blotted on to a membrane. The allele-specific probes are then hybridized to the blots, and under optimal conditions only the matched probes bind. The allele-specific probes are approximately 19 bp in length and the polymorphic base is located at the centre of the probe. For the reverse dot blot, allele-specific probes are fixed to a membrane strip and the amplified PCR fragments are hybridized to the immobilized probes. Binding to the complementary polymorphic site is detected via a biotin tag on the 5' end of the primer, followed by addition of a strepavidin-horseradish peroxidase complex that oxidizes tetramethylbenzidine, yielding a blue dot (Garcia-Pacheco *et al.*, 1995). The advantage of this method is that a panel of oligonucleotide probes can be used to type multiple alleles. The sensitivity is increased by the reverse dot blot because the amplified material is hybridized against several allelic probes in a single hybridization assay. Dot blots are ideal for polymorphisms that are not included in a palindromic restriction site, especially when only small amounts of starting material or degraded DNA are available for typing. The technique is at least ten times more sensitive then PCR-RFLP. Maekawa *et al.* (1995) compared the feasibility of this method with PCR-RFLP for the three common apolipoprotein E (apo E) genotypes using DNA from leukocytes. They found complete agreement for each sample (n = 93) but concluded that the RFLP was simpler to perform and more suitable for large-scale studies.

Conformational changes in single-stranded DNA caused by mutation can be exploited to detect polymorphic sites using single-stranded conformation polymorphism (SSCP) analysis (Orita et al., 1989). Since its inception, SSCP has been used very extensively in connection with PCR amplification (PCR-SSCP) for the detection of point mutations (for example p53, reviewed by Hayashi, 1991). It is a highly sensitive method, but its specificity and sensitivity vary with the technique employed. PCR-SSCP is a simple alternative to other genotyping procedures and allows for the simultaneous detection of both known and unknown mutations. In this analysis the target sequence is amplified by PCR, at which time the product is end-labelled by radioactive primers (Hayashi et al., 1989) or fluorescent primers (Broly et al., 1995), or the product is labelled during PCR by the addition of radioactive deoxynucleotide triphosphates to the PCR mixture (Petersen et al., 1990). The amplified product is then heated to dissociate the strands and is subjected to non-denaturing polyacrylamide gel electrophoresis. Polymorphism variants are detected as shifts in the mobility of bands using autoradiography or flourography. The latter method is suitable for an automated analysis. Although detection of alterations in electrophoretic mobility is strongly dependent on the size of the fragment (maximum 300-400 nucleotides per gel), this limitation can be avoided by enzymatic digestion of a large PCR fragment to smaller fragments (Peinado et al., 1993) or by SSCP analysis on smaller secondary fragments generated with a set of nested primers (Broly et al., 1995).

Quality control

The analysis of samples for epidemiology or the diagnosis of disease in the individual requires specific and consistent quality control measures. In clinical pathology laboratories, standards and protocols have been established by organizations such as the College of American Pathologists and The National Committee for Clinical Laboratory Standards. Their interests include forensic and paternity testing, beyond diagnostic assays, so that most of their criteria apply to the research laboratory performing genetic polymorphism analysis. There are standards for proficiency testing, quality improvement and control, use of standards, methods of interpretation, specimen handling, labelling and processing, and reporting of results. There are also criteria for facilities and the maintenance of equipment.

While studies in research settings may not demand the rigour of those in commercial laboratories it is nevertheless important to check continuously that results are reliable and that misclassification is avoided. Quality control methods are therefore needed as from initial sampling to the reporting of results.

The verification of sample collection obviously depends on the method of collection. New methods should be pilot-tested; those requiring a procedure to be effected by the study subject are difficult to verify. Protocols should be in place to ensure that materials (i.e. preservatives) have not been held beyond their expiry date. The times of sample collection, shipment and processing should be recorded in a logbook. A formal chain of custody may be helpful. One potential difficulty during sample collection is that of improper labelling. A unique identification number should be given to each subject at the time of enrolment, identifying both the subject and the study. Preprinted labels can be placed on the sample containers and the questionnaire to ensure that there are no errors. Labels should be tested before use to ensure that they remain fastened at freezer temperatures.

The enhanced sensitivity provided by a method such as PCR amplification demands rigorous attention to possible sample-to-sample contamination, contamination with inhibitors or organisms that can degrade DNA, and cross-contamination of DNA with PCR products or control DNA. During DNA extraction by phenol-based methods the organic and aqueous phases must be adequately separated to reduce contamination with RNA, haemoglobin and proteins. For Chelex™ 100 and other commercially distributed extraction methods the manufacturer's instructions should be followed closely and the methods should be tested before use in studies. The probability of contamination from organisms and of the cross-contamination of samples is reduced if gloves are changed frequently and if unnecessary manipulation in avoided. It is preferable to use screw-cap tubes rather than flip-top tubes to avoid contaminating the fingers when tubes are opened (openers, similar in style to can-openers, greatly reduce this problem). Absolute sterile technique is required because moulds can easily grow in samples and either inhibit the PCR or degrade the DNA. When an inhibitor is suspected, dilution of the sample (i.e. using less DNA) may result in successful amplification. If degradation is suspected, quantitation by UV absorbance may not change, but the performance of another assay in which a larger fragment is successfully amplified helps to rule out degradation. When extracting DNA from paraffin blocks, microtome blades and gloves should be changed after each sample to avoid contamination with wild-type DNA (i.e. from another sample or from desquamated skin cells of the technician, which might still have better quality DNA that is more easily amplified than the fixed DNA). No matter what the source of tissue or DNA, specimens should be prepared and stored at sites physically separated from locations where PCR amplification is performed or PCR products (i.e. running gels) are otherwise used, so as to avoid contaminating the sample with amplified PCR products. Nonetheless, to confirm that contamination has not occurred, a negative control (i.e. PCR of a PCR reaction mixture, set up during the time that samples are to be analysed, but without the addition of template DNA) must be included with every set of samples (we use one per row of gel - 20 samples) to monitor and identify sample-to-sample contamination. These controls must be carried through all phases of sample processing and amplification. Positive controls carrying a known sequence are also useful but should be included only as the final sample to reduce cross-contamination.

After the extraction of DNA, some laboratories place small aliquots of DNA in several tubes so as to avoid repeated freezing and thawing of samples. Furthermore, it may be advantageous to put aliquots of DNA into tubes or on plates used for PCR at the time of extraction, and then to store the DNA at -20ºC. In this way, when an assay is performed the samples are already in aliquots and the chances of contamination are reduced. Other methods of standardization may include making enough buffer, NTP mixes, primers, etc., for an

entire study, so that consistency is achieved in the reagents. However, these too should be divided into aliquots.

The validation of an assay requires more than identifying the predicted base-pair length: a pseudogene might be identical in length. Validation can be accomplished through direct sequencing of the PCR product for homozygous individuals and comparison with published sequences. However, if the PCR product contains another polymorphic site that causes a shift in the sequence (i.e. a nucleotide deletion), the sequencing methods cannot be used unless the PCR fragment alleles are cloned first. An alternative approach would be to perform the assay for members of families and prove Mendelian inheritance. Large families are needed, with multiple generations, and these are available commercially (Coriell Institute, Camden, NJ). This has the advantage of allowing the investigator to practise on a large number of samples and learn to interpret the gels before valuable field samples are used.

Positive controls are important. A known standard for each informative genotype should be included in each experiment to verify that the assay is working properly. Further, possible inhibitors in the sample itself or highly degraded sample DNA may lead to false negative results, which would be suggested if a positive control amplifies but the samples do not.

Problems for the PCR include false priming, which results in the amplification of a non-specific product. One cause is a low annealing temperature, so that the primers anneal to genes with similar homology. Hot-start methods or raising the annealing temperature helps to exclude this problem. The simplest approach for hot starts is the addition of the polymerase after template denaturation. This method is not recommended, however, for large numbers of samples, because the chance of cross-contamination is increased by handling hot tubes (condensation at the walls and cap). Another approach for hot starts, which is time-consuming, is that of separating the polymerase and reaction mixture by a wax barrier, which liquefies after template denaturation and allows the reagents to mix (Sparkman, 1992). Alternativly, it is possible to use a Taq™ polymerase bound to an antibody so as to release the active enzyme after completion of template denaturation.

PCR mistakes can be based on polymerase errors. Further, inter- and intramolecular homology of primers can result in a primer-dimer product of similar size. Primer-dimers are template-independent, duplex PCR products (50-60 bp) composed of the extension added to one primer using the second primer as template. Once initiated, primer-dimer products are amplified very efficiently and limit the amplification of the target DNA. The complementarity between the two 3' ends of the primer set has been shown to enhance primer-dimer formation products. On the other hand, the presence or absence of primer-dimers can be used as indicator of Taq™ polymerase function and whether the source DNA contains inhibitory substances.

Independently of the above sources of misclassification, another problem can arise when attempts are made to amplify sequences that are members of a related gene family or for which one or more pseudogenes are present in the genome. The latter is often the case in studies on metabolic polymorphisms. It is possible for such artefacts to be generated when primers are not unique. Statistically, primers need to have at least 17 bases to be unique in the human genome (Thein & Wallace, 1986) but they must also be designed to anneal with regions that are unique among the related sequences. If such primers cannot be found, specific amplification can often be achieved by using primers that have at least three unique bases at their 3' end. Furthermore, products of similar genes or pseudogenes can frequently be distinguished by means of restriction enzyme digests. The specificity of different primer pairs can therefore be easily controlled by digestion of the products with restriction enzymes. An alternative approach to excluding the amplification of homologous genes is to predigest the template DNA before the PCR and thus eliminate amplification from the allele retaining the restriction site.

The correct choice of gel for the detection of amplified or enzymatically digested fragments is important for increasing the accuracy of the assay. The matrix must be adequate to achieve sufficient resolution of PCR products. We have found that polyacrylamide gels are among the best for resolution but the most cumbersome with which to work. NuSieve (FMC Products, Rockland, ME) or Metaphor (FMC Products, Rockland, ME) gels are useful for the detection of small fragments and fragments that need to be resolved and have similar base-pair lengths (i.e. a VNTR of 4-16 bases).

The interpretation of assay results and the reading of gels requires experience. Typically, amplified fragments have different intensities after ethidium bromide staining, and shorter fragments are less intense than longer ones because less dye is taken up. Also, heterozygote bands are half as intense as homozygote bands. Thus, each sample needs to be interpreted in the context of the other samples on the gel and the positive controls. For example, we do not report results for a sample where there is an upper band and no lower band if there is not another sample on the same row which has a less intense upper band and a lower band. When reading gels, our laboratory uses two independent blind reviewers. The first reads the results and enters the data in a database. The second then reads the gels, and the first cross-checks the database. Repeats are done for discrepant results, and if there are not two results that are clearly interpretable and agree the sample is eliminated from the analysis. We do repeats on either 20% or 100% of the samples, depending on the difficulty of the assay or the quality of the DNA; 100% is used for the more difficult assays.

References

Anker, P., Stroun, M. & Maurice, P.A. (1975) Spontaneous release of DNA by human blood lymphoctyes as shown in an *in vitro* system. *Cancer Res.*, 35, 2375-2382

Barnes, W.M. (1994) PCR amplification of up to 35-kb DNA with high fidelity and high yield from lambda bacteriophage templates. *Proc. Natl. Acad.. Sci. USA*, 91, 2216-2220

Bertilsson, L., Alm, C., De Las Carreras, C., Widen, J., Edman, G. & Schalling, D. (1989) Debrisoquine hydroxylation polymorphism and personality. *Lancet*, 1, 555

Botstein, D., White, R.L., Skolnick, M. & Davis, R.W. (1980) Construction of a genetic linkage map in man using restriction fragment length polymorphisms. *Am. J. Hum. Genet.*, 32, 314-331

Broly, F., Marez, D., Sabbagh, N., Legrand, M., Millecamps, S., Lo Guidice, J.M., Boone, P. & Meyer, U.A. (1995) An efficient strategy for detection of known and new mutations of the CYP2D6 gene using single strand conformation polymorphism analysis. *Pharmacogenetics*, 5, 373-384

Budowle, B. & Baechtel, F.S. (1990) Modifications to improve the effectiveness of restriction fragment length polymorphism typing. *Appl. Theor. Electrophor.*, 1, 181-187

Chan, C.Y., Lee, S.D., Hwang, S.J., Lu, R.H., Lu, C.L. & Lo, K.J. (1995) Quantitative branched DNA assay and genotyping for hepatitis C virus RNA in Chinese patients with acute and chronic hepatitis. *Chin. J. Infect. Dis.*, 171, 443-446

Chehab, F.F., Doherty, M., Cai, S.P., Kan, Y.W., Cooper, S. & Rubin, E.M. (1987) Detection of sickle cell anaemia and thalassaemias. *Nature*, 329, 293-294 [erratum in *Nature*, 329, 678]

Chehab, F.F. & Kan, Y.W. (1989) Detection of specific DNA sequences by fluorescence amplification: a colour complementation assay. *Proc. Natl. Acad. Sci. USA*, 86, 9178-9182

Cheng, S., Chang, S.Y., Gravitt, P. & Respess, R. (1994a) Long PCR. *Nature*, 369, 684-685

Cheng, S., Fockler, C., Barnes, W.M. & Higuchi, R. (1994b) Effective amplification of long targets from cloned inserts and human genomic DNA. *Proc. Natl. Acad. Sci. USA*, 91, 5695-5699

Conner, B.J., Reyes, A.A., Morin, C., Itakura, K., Teplitz, R.L & Wallace, R.B. (1983) Detection of sickle cell beta S-globin allele by hybridization with synthetic oligonucleotides. *Proc. Natl. Acad. Sci. USA*, 80, 278-282

Cosma, G., Crofts, F., Currie, D., Wirgin, I., Toniolo, P. & Garte, S.J. (1993) Racial differences in restriction fragment length polymorphisms and messenger RNA inducibility of the human CYP1A1 gene. *Cancer Epidemiol. Biomarkers Prev.*, 2, 53-57

Day, I.N. & Humphries, S.E. (1994) Electrophoresis for genotyping: microtiter array diagonal gel electrophoresis on horizontal polyacrylamide gels, hydrolink, or agarose. *Anal. Biochem.*, 222 (2), 389-395

De Lamballerie, X., Zandotti, C., Vignoli, C., Bollet, C. & de Micco, P. (1992) A one-step microbial DNA extraction method using "Chelex 100" suitable for gene amplification. *Res. Microbiol.*, 143, 785-790

Donis-Keller, H., Green, P., Helms, C., Cartinhour, S., Weiffenbach, B., Stephens, K., Keith, T.P., Bowden, D.W., Smith, D.R., Lander, E.S., Botstein, D., Akots, G., Rediker, K.S., Gravius, T., Brown, V.A., Rising, M.B., Parker, C., Powers, J.A., Watt, D.E., Kauffman, E.R., Bricker, A., Phipps, P., Muller-Kahle, H., Fulton, T.R., Ng, S., Schumm, J.W., Braman, J.C., Knowlton, R.G., Barker, D.F., Crooks, S.M., Lincoln, S.E., Daly, M.J. & Abrahamson, J. (1987) A genetic linkage map of the human genome. *Cell*, 51, 319-337

Erlich, H.A., Gelfand, D. & Sninsky, J.J. (1991) Recent advances in the polymerase chain reaction. *Science*, 252, 1643-1651

Fearon, E.R. & Vogelstein, B. (1990) A genetic model for colorectal tumorigenesis. *Cell*, 61, 759-767

Fey, M.F., Pilkington, S.P., Summers, C. & Wainscoat, J.S. (1987) Molecular diagnosis of haematological disorders using DNA from stored bone marrow slides. *Br. J. Haematol.*, 67, 489-492

Forsthoefel, K.F., Papp, A.C., Snyder, P.J. & Prior, T.W. (1992) Optimization of DNA extraction from formalin-fixed tissue and its clinical application in Duchenne muscular dystrophy. *Am. J. Clin. Pathol.*, 98, 98-104

Garcia-Pacheco, J.M., Mantilla, P., Garcia-Olivares, E. & Manzano-Fernandez, M.N. (1995) Routine HLA DRB/DQB oligonucleotide typing by a non-radioactive dot-blot micromethod. *J. Immunol. Methods*, 180, 35-43

Gasparini, P., Savoia, A., Pignatti, P.F., Dallapiccola, B. & Novelli, G. (1989) Amplification of DNA from epithelial cells in urine. *N. Engl. J. Med.*, 320, 809

Goelz, S.E., Hamilton, S.R. & Vogelstein, B. (1985) Purification of DNA from formaldehyde-fixed and paraffin-embedded human tissue. *Biochem. Biophys. Res. Commun.*, 130, 118-126

Goodfellow, P.N. (1992) Human genome project. Variation is now the theme. *Nature*, 359, 777-778

Goodman, M.F., Creighton, S., Bloom, L.B. & Petruska, J. (1993) Biochemical basis of DNA replication fidelity. *Crit. Rev. Biochem. Mol. Biol.*, 28, 83-126

Greer, C.E., Wheeler, C.M. & Manos, M.M. (1994) Sample preparation and PCR amplification from paraffin-embedded tissues. *PCR Methods Appl.*, 3, S113-122

Gustincich, S., Manfioletti, G., Del Sal, G., Schneider, C. & Carninci, P. (1991) A fast method for high-quality genomic DNA extraction from whole human blood. *Biotechniques.*, 11, 298-300, 302

Han, C.Y., Lin, B.K & Lin, H.J. (1992) Methanol for preparing hair bulbs for PCR. *Nucleic Acids Res.*, 20, 6419-6420

Hayashi, K., Orita, M., Suzuki, Y. & Sekiya, T. (1989) Use of labelled primers in polymerase chain reaction (LP-PCR) for a rapid detection of the product. *Nucleic Acids Res.*, 17, 3605

Hayashi, K. (1991) PCR-SSCP: a simple and sensitive method for detection of mutations in the genomic DNA. *PCR. Methods Appl.*, 1, 34-38

Heller, M.J., Robinson, R.A., Burgart, L.J., TenEyck, C.J. & Wilke, W.W. (1992) DNA extraction by sonication: a comparison of fresh, frozen, and paraffin-embedded tissues extracted for use in polymerase chain reaction assays. *Mod. Pathol.*, 5, 203-206

Higuchi, R., Bowman, B., Freiberger, M., Ryder, O.A. & Wilson, A.C. (1984) DNA sequences from the quagga, an extinct member of the horse family. *Nature*, 312, 282-284

Higuchi, R., von Beroldingen, C.H., Sensabaugh, G.F. & Erlich, H.A. (1988) DNA typing from single hairs. *Nature*, 332, 543-546

Hillier, L. & Green, P. (1991) OSP: a computer program for choosing PCR and DNA sequencing primers. *PCR. Methods Appl.*, 1, 124-128

Hochmeister, M.N., Budowle, B., Jung, J., Borer, U.V., Comey, C.T. & Dirnhofer, R. (1991) PCR-based typing of DNA extracted from cigarette butts. *Int. J. Legal Med.*, 104, 229-233

Jackson, D.P., Lewis, F.A., Taylor, G.R., Boylston, A.W. & Quirke, P. (1990) Tissue extraction of DNA and RNA and analysis by the polymerase chain reaction. *J. Clin. Pathol.*, 43, 499-504

Jeanpierre, M. (1987) A rapid method for the purification of DNA from blood. *Nucleic Acids Res.*, 15, 9611

Jinks, D.C., Minter, M., Tarver, D.A., Vanderford, M., Hejtmancik, J.F. & McCabe, E.R. (1989) Molecular genetic diagnosis of sickle cell disease using dried blood specimens on blotters used for newborn screening. *Hum.Genet.*, 81, 363-366

Kallio, P., Syrjanen, S., Tervahauta, A. & Syrjanen, K. (1991) A simple method for isolation of DNA from formalin-fixed paraffin-embedded samples for PCR. *J. Virol. Methods*, 35, 39-47

Kato, N., Yokosuka, O., Omata, M., Hosoda, K. & Ohto, M. (1990) Detection of hepatitis C virus ribonucleic acid in the serum by amplification with polymerase chain reaction. *J. Clin. Invest.*, 86, 1764-1767

Kato, S., Shields, P.G., Caporaso, N.E., Sugimura, H., Trivers, G.E., Tucker, M.A., Trump, B.F., Weston, A. & Harris, C.C. (1994) Analysis of cytochrome P450 2E1 genetic polymorphisms in relation to human lung cancer. *Cancer Epidemiol. Biomarkers Prev.*, 3, 515-518

Keen, J., Lester, D., Inglehearn, C., Curtis, A. & Bhattacharya, S. (1991) Rapid detection of single base mismatches as heteroduplexes on hydrolink gels. *Trends Genet.*, 7, 5

Kerem, B., Rommens, J.M., Buchanan, J.A., Markiewicz, D., Cox, T.K., Chakravarti, A., Buchwald, M. & Tsui, L.C. (1989) Identification of the cystic fibrosis gene: genetic analysis. *Science*, 245, 1073-1080

Kuppuswamy, M.N., Hoffmann, J.W., Kasper, C.K., Spitzer, S.G., Groce, S.L & Bajaj, S.P. (1991) Single nucleotide primer extension to detect genetic diseases: Experimental application to haemophilia B (factor IX) and cystic fibrosis genes. *Proc. Natl. Acad. Sci. USA*, 88, 1143-1147

Kwok, S., Mack, D.H., Sninsky, G.D., Ehrlich, B.J., Poiesz, B.J., Dock, N.L., Alter, H.J., Mildvan, D. & Grieco, M.H. (1989) Diagnosis of human immunodeficiency virus in seropositive individuals: enzymatic amplification of HIV viral sequences in peripheral blood mononuclear cells. In: *HIV Detection by Genetic Engineering Methods*. New York, Marcel Dekker, Inc

Lagarde, J.P., Benlian, P., Zekraoui, L. & Raisonnier, A. (1995) [Genotyping of apolipoprotein E (alleles epsilon 2, epsilon 3 and epsilon 4) from capillary blood]. *Ann. Biol. Clin. (Paris)*, 53, 15-20

Landegren, U., Kaiser, R., Sanders, J. & Hood, L. (1988) A ligase-mediated gene detection technique. *Science*, 241, 1077-1080

Lander, E.S. (1989) DNA fingerprinting on trial. *Nature*, 339, 501-505

Lau, J.Y., Mizokami, M., Kolberg, J.A., Davis, G.L., Prescott, L.E., Ohno, T., Perrillo, R.P., Lindsay, K.L., Gish, R.G., Qian, K.P., Kohara, M., Simmonds, P. & Urdea, M.S. (1995) Application of six hepatitis C virus genotyping systems to sera from chronic hepatitis C patients in the United States. *J. Infect. Dis.*, 171, 281-289

Leon, S.A., Shapiro, B., Sklaroff, D.M. & Yaros, M.J. (1977) Free DNA in the serum of cancer patients and the effect of therapy. *Cancer Res*, 37, 646-650

Lew, A.M. & Kelly, J. (1991) Capture of chromosomal DNA by anti-histone antibodies for PCR. *Nucleic Acids Res.*, 19, 3459

Lin, H.J., Han, C.Y., Bernstein, D.A., Hsiao, W., Lin, B.K. & Hardy, S. (1994) Ethnic distribution of the glutathione transferase Mu 1-1 (GSTM1) null genotype in 1473 individuals and application to bladder cancer susceptibility. *Carcinogenesis*, 15, 1077-1081

Maekawa, B., Cole, T.G., Seip, R.L. & Bylund, D. (1995) Apolipoprotein E genotyping methods for the clinical laboratory. *J. Clin. Lab. Anal.*, 9, 63-69

Martin, M., Carrington, M. & Mann, D. (1992) A method for using serum or plasma as a source of DNA for HLA typing. *Hum Immunol.*, 33, 108-113

Myers, R.M., Maniatis, T. & Lerman, L.S. (1987) Detection and localization of single base changes by denaturing gradient gel electrophoresis. *Methods Enzymol.*, 155, 501-527

Nakamura, Y., Leppert, M., O'Connell, P., Wolff, R., Holm, T., Culver, M., Martin, C., Fujimoto, E., Hoff, M., Kumlin, E. & White, R. (1987) Variable number of tandem repeat (VNTR) markers for human gene mapping. *Science*, 235, 1616-1622

Newton, C.R., Graham, A., Heptinstall, L.E., Powell, S.J., Summers, C., Kalsheker, N., Smith, J.C. & Markham, A.F. (1989) Analysis of any point mutation in DNA. The amplification refractory mutation system (ARMS). *Nucleic Acids Res.*, 17, 2503-2516

Nickerson, D.A., Kaiser, R., Lappin, S., Stewart, J., Hood, L. & Landegren, U. (1990) Automated DNA diagnostics using an ELISA-based oligonucleotide ligation assay. *Proc. Natl. Acad. Sci. USA*, 87, 8923-8927

Nikiforov, T.T., Rendle, R.B., Goelet, P., Rogers, Y.H., Kotewicz, M.L., Anderson, S., Trainor, G.L. & Knapp, M.R. (1994) Genetic bit analysis: a solid phase method for typing single nucleotide polymorphisms. *Nucleic Acids Res.*, 22, 4167-4175

Orita, M., Suzuki, Y., Sekiya, T. & Hayashi, K. (1989) Rapid and sensitive detection of point mutations and DNA polymorphisms using the polymerase chain reaction. *Genomics*, 5, 874-879

145

Paabo, S. (1985) Molecular cloning of Ancient Egyptian mummy DNA. *Nature*, 314, 644-645

Paabo, S. (1989) Ancient DNA: extraction, characterization, molecular cloning, and enzymatic amplification. *Proc. Natl. Acad. Sci. USA*, 86, 1939-1943

Panaccio, M., Georgesz, M. & Lew, A.M. (1993) FoLT PCR: a simple PCR protocol for amplifying DNA directly from whole blood. *Biotechniques*, 14, 238-243

Panaccio, M. & Lew, A. (1991) PCR based diagnosis in the presence of 8% (v/v) blood. *Nucleic Acids Res*, 19, 1151

Peinado, M.A., Fernandez-Renart, M., Capella, G., Wilson, L. & Perucho, M. (1993) Mutations in the p53 suppressor gene do not correlate with c-K-ras oncogene mutations in colorectal cancer. *Int. J. Oncol.*, 2, 123-134

Petersen, M.B., Economou, E.P., Slaugenhaupt, S.A., Chakravarti, A. & Antonarakis, S.E. (1990) Linkage analysis of the human HMG14 gene on chromosome 21 using a GT dinucleotide repeat as polymorphic marker. *Genomics*, 7, 136-138

Ramos, M.D., Lalueza, C., Girbau, E., Perez-Perez, A., Quevedo, S., Turbon, D. & Estivill, X. (1995) Amplifying dinucleotide microsatellite loci from bone and tooth samples of up to 5000 years of age: more inconsistency than usefulness. *Hum. Genet.*, 96, 205-212

Rebrov, L.B., Kozel'tsev, V.L., Shishkin, S.S. & Debov, S.S. (1983) [Various enzymatic aspects of postmortem autolysis]. *Vestn. Akad. Med. Nauk. SSSR*, 10, 82-89

Saiki, R.K., Bugawan, T.L., Horn, G.T., Mullis, K.B. & Erlich, H.A. (1986) Analysis of enzymatically amplified beta-globin and HLA-DQ alpha DNA with allele-specific oligonucleotide probes. *Nature*, 324, 163-166

Saiki, R.K., Walsh, P.S., Levenson, C.H. & Erlich, H.A. (1989) Genetic analysis of amplified DNA with immobilized sequence-specific oligonucleotide probes. *Proc. Natl. Acad.. Sci. USA*, 86, 6230-6234

Sajantila, A., Budowle, B., Strom, M., Johnsson, V., Lukka, M., Peltonen, L. & Ehnholm, C. (1992) PCR amplification of alleles at the DIS80 locus: comparison of a Finnish and a North American Caucasian population sample, and forensic casework evaluation. *Am. J. Hum. Genet.*, 50, 816-825

Sambrook, J., Fritsch, E.F. & Maniatis, T. (1989) *Molecular Cloning, a Laboratory Manual. Vol. I.* New York, Cold Spring Harbor Press

Secchiero, P., Carrigan, D.R., Asano, Y., Benedetti, L., Crowley, R.W., Komaroff, A.L., Gallo, R.C. & Lusso, P. (1995) Detection of human herpesvirus 6 in plasma of children with primary infection and immunosuppressed patients by polymerase chain reaction. *J. Infect. Dis.*, 171, 273-280

Shapiro, B., Chakrabarty, M., Cohn, E.M. & Leon, S.A. (1983) Determination of circulating DNA levels in patients with benign or malignant gastrointestinal disease. *Cancer*, 51, 2116-2120

Shibata, D. (1992) The polymerase chain reaction and the molecular genetic analysis of tissue biopsies. In: Herrington, C.S. & McGee, J.O., eds, *Diagnostic Molecular Pathology: a Practical Approach.* Oxford, IRL Press, p. 85

Smith, L.J., Braylan, R.C., Nutkis, J.E., Edmundson, K.B., Downing, J.R. & Wakeland, E.K. (1987) Extraction of cellular DNA from human cells and tissues fixed in ethanol. *Anal. Biochem.*, 160, 135-138

Smits, H.L., Tieben, L.M., Tjong-A-Hung, S.P., Jebbink, M.F., Minnaar, R.P., Jansen, C.L. & ter Schegget, J. (1992) Detection and typing of human papillomaviruses present in fixed and stained archival cervical smears by a consensus polymerase chain reaction and direct sequence analysis allow the identification of a broad spectrum of human papillomavirus types. *J. Gen. Virol.*, 73, 3263-3268

Sorenson, G.D., Pribish, D.M., Valone, F.H., Memoli, V.A., Bzik, D.J. & Yao, S.L. (1994) Soluble normal and mutated DNA sequences from single-copy genes in human blood. *Cancer Epidemiol. Biomarkers Prev.*, 3, 67-71

Southern, E.M. (1975) Detection of specific sequences among DNA fragments separated by gel electrophoresis. *J. Mol. Biol.*, 98, 503-517

Sparkman, D.R. (1992) Paraffin wax as a vapour barrier for the PCR. *PCR. Methods Appl.*, 2, 180-181

Steen, V.M., Andreassen, O.A., Daly, A.K., Tefre, T., Borresen, A.L., Idle, J.R. & Gulbrandsen, A.K. (1995) Detection of the poor metabolizer-associated CYP2D6(D) gene deletion allele by long-PCR technology. *Pharmacogenetics*, 5, 215-223

Stein, E.L., Santoso, S., Behrens, G., Mueller-Eckhardt, C. & Bux, J. (1995) Genotyping of the granulocyte-specific NA antigens from small quantities of blood or serum. *Tissue Antigens*, 45, 69-72

Sugimura, H., Caporaso, N.E., Shaw, G.L., Modali, R.V., Gonzalez, F.J., Hoover, R.N., Resau, J.H., Trump, B.F., Weston, A. & Harris, C.C. (1990) Human debrisoquine hydroxylase gene polymorphisms in cancer patients and controls. *Carcinogenesis*, 11, 1527-1530

Syvanen, A.C., Aalto-Setala, K., Harju, L., Kontula, K. & Soderlund, H. (1990) A primer-guided nucleotide incorporation assay in the genotyping of apolipoprotein E. *Genomics*, 8, 684-692

Syvanen, A.C., Sajantila, A. & Lukka, M. (1993) Identification of individuals by analysis of biallelic DNA markers, using PCR and solid-phase minisequencing. *Am. J. Hum. Genet.*, 52, 46-59

Thein, S.L. & Wallace, R.B. (1986) The use of synthetic oligonucleotides as specific hybridization probes in the diagnosis of genetic disorders. In: Davies, K.E., ed, *Human Genetic Diseases*. Oxford, IRL Press, p. 33

Vasioukhin, V., Anker, P., Maurice, P., Lyautey, J., Lederrey, C. & Stroun, M. (1994) Point mutations of the N-ras gene in the blood plasma DNA of patients with myelodysplastic syndrome or acute myelogenous leukaemia. *Br. J. Haematol.*, 86, 774-779

Walsh, P.S., Metzger, D.A. & Higuchi, R. (1991) Chelex 100 as a medium for simple extraction of DNA for PCR-based typing from forensic material. *Biotechniques*, 10, 506-513

Westwood, S.A. & Werrett, D.J. (1990) An evaluation of the polymerase chain reaction method for forensic applications. *Forensic. Sci. Int.*, 45, 201-215

Wu, D.Y., Ugozzoli, L., Pal, B.K. & Wallace, R.B. (1989) Allele-specific enzymatic amplification of beta-globin genomic DNA for diagnosis of sickle cell anemia. *Proc. Natl. Acad. Sci. USA*, 86, 2757-2760

Corresponding author
Peter G. Shields
Molecular Epidemiology Section,
Laboratory of Human Carcinogenesis,
National Cancer Institute,
Building 37, Room 2C16,
37 Convent Drive MSC 4255,
Bethesda, MD 20892-4255, USA

Metabolic Polymorphisms and Susceptibility to Cancer
W. Ryder
IARC Scientific Publications No. 148
International Agency for Research on Cancer, Lyon, 1999

Chapter 14. Ah receptor gene polymorphisms and human cancer susceptibility

Seymour Garte and Kazuhiro Sogawa

The Ah receptor (Ahr) gene occupies a central role in the metabolic pathways involved in the detoxification of important environmental carcinogens. The structures of the rodent and human genes have been elucidated, and the molecular details of the receptor function, including its interaction with other proteins such as Arnt and hsp90, have been thoroughly investigated. The Ahr gene is polymorphic in mice and in humans. In mice, good correlations have been found between structural polymorphisms in the gene and functional variants in various genetic strains. In humans, work on polymorphisms and their possible role in gene function as well as cancer susceptibility is just beginning.

The Ah receptor (Ahr) gene is potentially one of the most important metabolic genes involved in determining individual susceptibility to xenobiotics, including several classes of chemical carcinogens. More than two decades ago the existence of this receptor was postulated to be a critical feature of the Ah (aromatic hydrocarbon) locus, responsible for the induction of enzymatic activities involved in the detoxification of polycyclic aromatic hydrocarbons (PAH) and related compounds such as dioxin or TCDD. Mouse strain differences were demonstrated in the induction of aryl hydrocarbon hydroxylase (AHH) enzymatic activity in response to PAH (Poland *et al.*, 1974; Nebert & Jones, 1989; Greenlee and Poland, 1979; Niwa *et al.*, 1975). This difference was attributed to a gene or genes that followed Mendelian inheritance. The genes that encode this enzymatic activity are members of the phase I cytochrome P450 family, including CYP1A1, CYP1A2 and CYP1B1, which are thoroughly discussed elsewhere in this volume. It has been established that all of the pleiotypic responses of animals to exposure to TCDD, including induction of the CYP1A1 gene, result from agonist binding to a specific cytosolic receptor (Poland & Bradfield, 1992), the Ah receptor, which is coded for by the Ahr gene (Bock, 1994; Okey *et al.*, 1994; Nebert *et al.*, 1993; Hankinson, 1995). Because of technical difficulties in the purification of the Ah

receptor protein (Poland & Bradfield, 1992)), the Ahr gene was not cloned from mice until 1992 (Burbach *et al.*,1992; Ema *et al.*, 1992); the human cDNA was described the following year (Dolwick *et al.*, 1993; Eguchi *et al.*, 1994).

Ahr gene function

Activation of the Ahr gene is responsible for a variety of tissue and species-specific toxic responses in animals and humans. These include immunosuppression, a wasting syndrome (in mice), teratogenicity, chloracne (in humans), as well as carcinogenicity and/or tumour promotion. The specific mechanisms responsible for these diverse toxic responses are unknown, although there is good evidence that the initial steps, binding of ligand to receptor, transfer to the nucleus, formation of a ternary complex with another transcription factor called Arnt (see below), followed by binding to response elements upstream of the relevant target gene, occur for each of these complex multifactorial diseases. The identification of the target genes involved in each case will provide the crucial information necessary to elucidate the precise mechanisms involved.

An important issue in this field is the role of Ahr as a mediator of carcinogenesis induced by its ligands, especially TCDD. While the mechanisms and dose response characteristics of human carcinogenesis by TCDD are still under intense investigation, it appears quite likely that the initial steps of the process must involve the Ahr gene and its gene product, which must bind to the agonist before further cellular events can ocurr. The implications of such a receptor-based mechanism for dose-response modelling are of great interest but cannot be dealt with further here.

Although much of the research related to the Ah locus has concentrated on the metabolism of model inducers such as TCDD and aromatic hydrocarbons via the CYP1A1 gene, it is vitally important to remember that this gene is only one of many whose transcriptional control is affected by binding of the Ah receptor-ligand complex. Other genes known or postulated to be under the control of Ahr include CYP1A2, glutathione-S-transferaseYa, aldehyde-3-dehydrogenase, NAD(P)H quinone oxidoreductase, plasminogen activator inhibitor PAI-2 and IL-1 beta (Bock, 1994; Safe & Krishnan, 1995). This list includes other phase 1 and phase 2 detoxification genes, as well as other genes important in growth and homeostasis regulation.

In addition to its role as a mediator of agonist-induced gene expression, the Ahr locus can act to inhibit expression of certain genes (Whitelaw et al., 1994). Most of these genes are induced by estrogen, and the mechanism of inhibition by Ahr agonists probably resides in interference with the normal binding and/or function of the estrogen receptor system. The genes thus affected include epidermal growth factor, c-fos, progesterone receptor, estrogen receptor and cathepsin D. Safe and Krishnan (1995) have shown that the Ah receptor complex binds to an imperfect recognition sequence in an enhancer region of these genes, which results in the inhibition of estrogen-induced gene expression. Therefore the Ah receptor complex may act as a negative transcription factor via a mechanism similar to its action in the induction of gene expression.

The pleiotropic activity of Ahr is one reason that it is such an important candidate for studies on differential susceptibility to carcinogens as well as other toxicants. A single loss or decrement of function polymorphism in this gene can have a wide array of consequences for a number of downstream processes that depend on the various target genes or processes described above.

Ahr gene structure

The Ahr has long been postulated to be a member of the steroid/thyroid/retinoic acid receptor superfamily, because the molecular mechanism of activation of the Ahr apparently resembles that of steroid hormone receptors such as the glucocorticoid hormone receptor (Sugawa & Fujii-Kuriyama, 1993). The steroid receptors are generally members of the ErbA family of zinc finger proteins. However, structural analysis of the Ahr cDNA revealed that it does not exhibit similarity to steroid hormone receptors, but is instead characterized by two domains, the basic helix-loop-helix (bHLH) domain and the PAS domain, localized in the N-terminal half of the molecule (Burbach et al., 1992; Ema et al., 1992). The HLH family of proteins is often found in transcription factors critical for cell growth and differentiation, such as the c-myc group and the Myo D group. The PAS domain was designated as a common region found in the Drosophila circadian rhythm protein Per (period), human Arnt, and the Drosophila neurogenic protein Sim (single minded) (Nambu et al., 1991). The PAS domain comprises approximately 250 to 300 amino acids, and contains two 50 amino acid repeats. Proteins containing bHLH domains are generally involved in protein-protein interaction, without the participation of small ligands. Ahr thus represents a new class of ligand-binding receptors.

The molecular biology of Ahr

The heterodimeric partner protein of the Ahr, designated Ah receptor nuclear translocator (Arnt), also contains HLH and PAS domains (Hankinson, 1995; Hoffman et al., 1991; Sogawa et al., 1995a). The amino acid homology of HLH and PAS domains between Ahr and Arnt was 25% and 18%, respectively. The Ahr and Arnt proteins form heterodimers through the HLH and PAS domains, and bind to response elements in enhancer regions of target genes such as CYP1A1 (Denison et al.,1988) through the adjacent basic region. These response elements, called xenobiotic response elements (XRE) (Fujisawa-Sehara et al., 1987), or dioxin response elements (DRE), have the consensus sequence CACGCNA/T. Arnt is able to homodimerize and heterodimerize with Ahr and other factors containing HLH and PAS domains (Sogawa *et al.*, 1995a). In the C-terminal half of the PAS domain of the Ahr, a ligand binding region and a region necessary for association with the 90 kD heat shock protein (Hsp 90) are overlapped (Burbach *et al.*, 1992; Antonsson *et al.*,1995). Transcriptional activation domains are localized in the C-terminal half of Ahr and Arnt, (Whitelaw *et al.*, 1994; Sogawa *et al.*, 1995b; Li *et al.*, 1994).

The primary structures of the human (Dolwick *et al.*, 1993; Eguchi *et al.*, 1994; Ema *et al.*, 1994a), mouse (Burbach *et al.*, 1992; Ema *et al.*, 1992), and rat (Carver *et al.*, 1994) Ahr, consisting of 848, 805 and 853 amino acids respectively, were deduced from their cDNAs. The mouse Ahr gene is 37.5 kb long and is separated into 11 exons (Schmidt *et al.*, 1993; Mimura *et al.*, 1994). It is a TATA-less gene, but has several GC boxes in the promoter region. The presence of other cis-acting elements such as an AP-1 binding site, E box, and CRE are also reported (Schmidt *et al.*, 1993; Mimura *et al.*, 1994). Deletion analysis of the upstream region of the Ahr gene suggests that various combinations of these cis-acting elements function in a cell-type specific manner in the transcription of the gene (FitzGerald *et al.*, 1996).

The calculated size of the mouse protein is 90 kD, and that of the human protein is 96 kD (Dolwick *et al.*, 1993). These sizes differ from the observed molecular weights (see below), probably because of post-translational modification. There is strong sequence homology (98-100%) between the mouse and human genes in the N terminal region, comprising the basic and helix loop helix portions of the genes. However, the homology is quite poor in the glutamine rich (Q-rich) carboxy terminal domain which may be called a hyper-variable domain (Dolwick *et al.*, 1993). Both Ahr and Arnt exhibit a number of stop codons at the 3' end of the gene, and polymorphisms at these sites are responsible for the variable sizes of the various forms of Ahr protein. The major human transcript is a 6.6 kb message which is easily detected in human tissues although to varying degrees (Dolwick *et al.*, 1993).

Chromosomal localization of human AhR was assigned to 7p21 (Le Beau *et al.*, 1994; Ema *et al.*, 1994). The mouse AhR gene has been localized on chromosome 12 (Schmidt *et al.*, 1993). This is logical, since mouse chromosome 12 carries a region homologous to a part of human chromosome 7.

The human Arnt gene was mapped to chromosome1q21 (Johnson *et al.*, 1993), a different chromosome from that of the AhR gene.

Even before the cloning of the Ah receptor gene, many of the molecular details of the function of the Ah locus were discovered. The Ahr is stably associated with hsp90 in the latent, ligand-free form in the cytosol (Perdew, 1988; Wilhelmsson *et al.*, 1990). The role of hsp90 is believed to be to maintain a ligand-binding conformation of the Ahr, and to repress the DNA-binding activity of the Ahr. It is not known whether the dissociation of Ahr from hsp90 occurs in the cytosol or in the nucleus. No evidence has been reported that Arnt interacts with hsp90. After entering cells, the xenobiotic ligand (such as TCDD or benzo(a)pyrene) binds to a heteroduplex comprised of the Ah receptor protein and Hsp90 in the cytosol (Denis *et al.*, 1988).

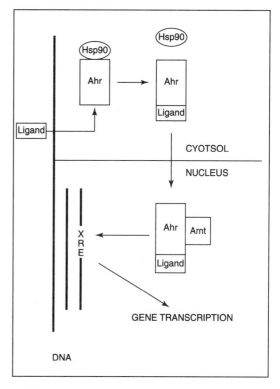

Figure 1. Schematic model showing the interactions between an inducing xenobiotic ligand, the Ah receptor, heat shock protein and Arnt.   XRE = xenobiotic response element, sometimes called the dioxin response element (DRE), in the promoter regions of numerous genes.

Following binding of the ligand and release of the Hsp90, the ligand receptor complex moves into the nucleus, where it binds to Arnt (Hankinson, 1995; Hoffman *et al.*, 1991; Sogawa *et al.*, 1995). This ternary complex then binds to the response elements of a variety of genes, which results in a strong induction of gene transcription. (Pollenz *et al.*, 1993; Hord & Perdew, 1994). Fig. 1 illustrates this model on the basis of work done in several laboratories.

Examination of the DNA-binding mode of the Ahr-Arnt complex revealed that the basic sequence of Arnt recognizes the CAC half site of the XRE core sequence, and that of the Ahr recognizes the other half site (Sogawa *et al.*, 1995; Bacsi *et al.*, 1995). The enhancer activity of the XRE is synergistically activated by a GC box localized in the vicinity of the TATA box of the CYP1A1 gene and other TCDD-inducible drug metabolizing genes. In accordance with this observation, the HLH and PAS domains of the Ahr and Arnt directly interact with zinc finger domains of Sp1, a factor which binds to the GC box sequences (Kobayashi *et al.*, 1996).

In vitro dephosphorylation experiments demonstrated that DNA binding of the complex is dependent on phosphorylation. Protein kinase C has been implicated in regulation of the Ahr function (Carrier *et al.*, 1992; Berghard *et al.*, 1993). Down regulation of protein kinase C by prolonged exposure to phorbol esters results in a loss of DNA binding of the Ahr in human keratinocytes (Carrier *et al.*, 1992). In addition, long-term treatment of mice *in vivo* with the phorbol ester blocks the TCDD-elicited Ahr activation to the DNA-binding form (Okino *et al.*, 1992). Using specific kinase inhibitors it has been found that tyrosine phosphorylation of the receptor is also necessary for its DNA-binding in keratinocytes (Gradin *et al.*, 1994). Recently, two phosphorylated regions in the C-terminal half of the Ahr were estimated using the ^{32}P-labelled Ahr by the chemical cleavage methods (Mahon & Gasiewicz, 1995).

Ahr gene expression

Hayashi *et al.* (1994) isolated genomic clones of human Ahr and Arnt, and developed a quantitative RT-PCR assay for the expression of these genes in human tissues. They found that the mRNAs for both genes were widely expressed in human tissues and that a high level occurred in lung. Inter-individual differences in the level of expression of both genes were seen in liver, lung and blood. The authors observed a correlation between the levels of expression of the Ahr and Arnt genes and that of CYP1A1, and also found an association with cigarette smoking. The phenotypic differences between individual humans were not examined with respect to any genotypic differences in polymorphic forms of the gene. Dolwick *et al.* (1993) also reported differential tissue-specific levels of Ahr gene expression in humans, the highest being in lung and placenta.

Ahr polymorphism in mice

The Ahr genes are highly polymorphic in mice and humans (Fujii-Kuriyama *et al.*, 1995). A number of mouse gene polymorphisms have been identified and some of these correspond to the interstrain functional polymorphisms produced in response to induction by TCDD, which were delineated years ago. A number of different inbred strains of mice were compared for sensitivity to the CYP1A1-inducing activity of TCDD. The C57BL mouse strain is far more sensitive to induction of the Ah locus, including all the toxic and biochemical consequences of this induction, than the DBA strain. The Ahr allele from the C57BL strain is termed the Ahr^{b-1} allele, while the allele from DBA mice is called Ahr^d. The Ahr^{b-1} allele encodes a 95 kD receptor protein, while the Ahr^d allele codes for a 104 kD gene product (Chang *et al.*, 1993). The ligand-binding affinity of the Ahr^{b-1} allele is 15-20 times higher than that of the Ahr^d allele. A third allele, the Ahr^{b-2}, found in BALB/c and other strains of mice, has similar affinity to the Ahr^{b-1} allele, but the encoded protein is 104 kD as is the case for the Ahr^d allele (Schmidt *et al.*, 1993). There are ten nucleotide differences between the Ahr^{b-1} and Ahr^d alleles, five of which are silent. One of the sequence polymorphisms changes a termination codon in Ahr^{b-1} to Arg in Ahr^d, which extends the length of the protein by 43 amino acids and accounts for the size difference between the two alleles. Another sequence polymorphism in the Ahr^d allele replaces a leucine with a proline. This polymorphism may be responsible for the differences in agonist-binding affinity between the Ah receptors of these two strains of mice (Chang *et al.*, 1993). Another laboratory has reported on an alanine to valine mutation at position 375 (Ema *et al.*, 1994b) between the

Ahr[b-1] and Ahr[d] alleles. These authors found that an analogous mutation to aspartate in the human Ahr gene at position 381 completely abolished ligand binding of the human Ahr gene. The Ahr[b-1] and Ahr[b-2] alleles are nearly homologous, with only a few sequence differences between them (Schmidt *et al.*, 1993). However, one of these differences occurs in a termination codon, leading to the increased observed transcript and protein sizes, analogous to the situation with the Ahr[d] allele.

Ahr polymorphism in humans

The situation with respect to sequence polymorphisms in the human Ahr gene is currently complex and fluid. In addition to the mutation discussed above, several other laboratories have reported on polymorphic forms of the human Ahr gene and receptor protein. Kawajiri *et al.* (1995) detected an arginine to lysine polymorphism at codon 554 by SSCP screening. These workers studied the population frequency and possible involvement of this polymorphism in cancer susceptibility (see below). Another group has reported on an Msp1 restriction-length polymorphism (RFLP) that results in the presence or absence of a restriction fragment at 2.7 kb when the human gene is digested with Msp1 (Jones *et al.*, 1994). No information was given as to the site or functional significance of this polymorphism but the frequency of the null allele is at least 37%. A more rare Msp1 RFLP was detected in 7 % of the sample of 27 individuals. In four different human cell lines two Ahr proteins were found with sizes of 104 and 106 kD, but only the 106 kD protein was photoaffinity-labelled by the TCDD agonist, implying a difference in binding affinities similar to that seen in mice (Perdew & Hollenback, 1995). Considering the size of the gene, the modest level of interspecies homology (especially at the 3' region), the existence of multiple polymorphic alleles in the mouse gene, and the known differences in phenotype between individuals, it would not be surprising if several more sequence polymorphisms of the human Ahr gene were discovered in the near future and if some of them proved to be important factors in interindividual differences in susceptibility to xenobiotic exposure (Nebert *et al.*, 1993). At least one polymorphism, an Msp1 RFLP, has been discovered in the human Arnt gene (Johnson *et al.*, 1992).

Ahr polymorphism and cancer susceptibility

Only one study has been published which has explored a possible association between Ahr sequence polymorphisms and human susceptibility to carcinogenesis. Kawajiri *et al.* (1995), who have already made important contributions in this field with respect to the CYP1A1 gene (see Chapter 15), examined 25 Japanese individuals for the presence of polymorphisms in the Ahr gene using single-strand conformational polymorphism analysis (SSCP). This method is faster and simpler than complete sequencing and is often used as a screen to detect mutations in a panel of samples. Two polymorphic regions were found in coding regions of the gene. One of these, in exon 2, proved to be silent, whereas the other, in exon 10, results in the replacement of an arginine by a lysine. In a population sample of 277 Japanese the Arg allele had a population frequency of 0.57 while the Lys allele had one of 0.43. The authors discovered no difference in the inducibility of AHH enzyme activity as a function of this genotype. On the basis of a chi-square analysis of genotype distributions in a case-control study of lung cancer the authors reported no effect of the polymorphism on risk of any lung cancer type. However, if one calculates the odds ratios for the heterozygous and homozygous polymorphisms from their data a small but statistically significant effect of the heterozygous polymorphism in all lung cancers and in Kreyberg type 1 is seen. The latter is the lung cancer histological type most associated with tobacco smoking. Although the effects are small and limited to the heterozygous group, further study is required to be certain of the role of the Arg/Lys polymorphism in cancer susceptibility in this population. No linkage was observed between this Ahr polymorphism and the CYP1A1 Msp polymorphism (Kawajiri *et al.*, 1995) among the cases.

Conclusion

Work on Ahr polymorphisms as potential genetic susceptibility factors is only just beginning. In the light of the many efforts made to elucidate the role of such polymorphisms in genes like CYP1A1 and CYP2E1 and the GST genes (see Chapters 15, 19 and 21), much more research on Ahr polymorphisms is clearly required before any definitive conclusion can be drawn. It is critical, for example, to assess the association of these polymorphisms (and perhaps others not yet discovered) with several types of cancer for different ethnic populations, since both the genotypic distribution (Cosma *et al.*, 1993; Stephens *et al.*, 1994) and the effect of genetic variants (Hirvonen *et al.*, 1992; Kawajiri *et al.*, 1990; Taioli *et al.*, 1995) have been shown to depend strongly on ethnicity. It will also be important to examine the role of carcinogen dose (for example, in the case of smoking), since several groups have demonstrated an important difference in the magnitude of alteration in sensitivity to environmental exposures based on dose in other susceptibility genes such as CYP1A1 and NAT (Nakachi *et al.*, 1991; Vineis *et al.*, 1994; Nakachi *et al.*, 1993). In fact this work has shown that a form of gene-environment interaction occurs such that in individuals with low exposure levels the increased risk due to the presence of the genetic polymorphism risk factor is greater than in highly exposed individuals. Finally, considering the complexity of the possible gene-gene interactions between the Ahr gene and its downstream target genes, future studies should attempt to present a global view of all the interrelated genotypes in individuals rather than focusing solely on single polymorphisms in one gene at a time (Nakachi *et al.*, 1993; Ichiba *et al.*, 1994). The issue of linkage between polymorphisms in different genes should also be addressed.

After years of intensive effort all the important genes in the human Ah locus have been cloned or characterized. Once the situation with respect to human Ahr gene polymorphisms has been clarified it will become possible to perform case-control studies of the Ahr polymorphisms as potential carcinogenesis susceptibility markers. In the next few years we should be able to understand clearly how an individual composite genotype of this locus (as well as other related genes discussed elsewhere in this volume) relates to risk of cancer from exposure to a large and important class of environmental chemical carcinogens.

References

Antonsson, C., Whitelaw, M.L., McGuire, J., Gustafsson, J.-A. & Poellinger, L. (1995) Distinct roles of the molecular chaperone hsp90 inmodu-lating dioxin receptor function via the basic helix-loop-helix and PAS domains. *Mol. Cell. Biol.*, 15, 756-765

Bacsi, S.G., Reisz-Porszasz, S. & Hankinson, O. (1995) Orientation of the heterodimeric aryl hydrocarbon (dioxin) receptor complex on its asymmetric DNA recognition sequence. *Mol. Pharmacol.*, 47, 432-438

Berghard, A., Gradin, K., Pongratz, I., Whitelaw, M. L. & Poellinger, L. (1993) Cross-coupling of signal transduction pathway: the dioxin receptor mediates induction of cytochrome P-450IA1 expression via a protein kinase C-dependent mechanism. *Mol. Cell. Biol.*, 13, 677-689

Bock, K.W. (1994) Aryl hydrocarbon or dioxin receptor: biologic and toxic responses. *Rev. Physiol. Biochem. Pharmacol.*,125,1-42

Burbach, K.M., Poland, A. & Bradfield C.A. (1992) Cloning of the Ah-receptor cDNA reveals a distinctive ligand-activated transcription factor. *Proc. Natl. Acad. Sci. USA*, 89, 8185-8189

Carrier, F., Owens, R. A., Nebert, D. W. & Puga, A. (1992) Dioxin-dependent activation of murine cyp1a-1 gene transcription requires protein kinase C-dependent phosphorylation. *Mol. Cell. Biol.*, 12, 1856-1863

Carver, L. A., Hogenesch, J. B. & Bradfield, C. (1994) Tissue-specific expression of the rat Ah-receptor and ARNT mRNAs. *Nucleic Acids Res.*, 22, 3038-3044

Chang, C., Smith, D.R., Prasad, V.S., Sidman, C.L., Nebert, D.W. & Puga, A. (1993) Ten nucleotide differences, five of which cause amino acid changes, are associated with the Ah receptor locus polymorphism of C57BL/6 and DBA/2 mice. *Pharmacogenetics*, 3(6),312-321

Cosma, G., Crofts, F., Currie, D., Wirgin, I., Toniolo, P. & Garte, S.J. (1993) Racial differences in restriction fragment length polymorphisms and messenger RNA inducibility of the human CYP1A1 gene. *Cancer Epidemiol. Biomarkers Prev.*, 2, 53-57

Denis, M., Cuthill, S., Wikstrom, A.C., Poellinger, L. & Gustafsson, J.A. (1988) Association of the dioxin receptor with 90,000 heat shock protein: a structural kinship with the glucocorticoid receptor. *Biochem. Biophys. Res. Commun.*, 155, 801-807

Denison, M.S., Fisher, J.M. & Whitlock J.P. (1988) The DNA recognition site for the dioxin-Ah receptor complex. *J. Biol. Chem.*, 263, 17221-17224

Dolwick, C.M., Schmidt, J.V., Carver, L.A., Swanson H.I. & Bradfield, C.A. (1993) Cloning and expression of a human Ah receptor cDNA. *Mol. Pharmacol.*, 44, 911-917

Eguchi, H., Hayashi, S., Watanabe, J., Gotoh, O. & Kawajiri K. (1994) Molecular cloning of the human AH receptor gene promoter. *Biochem. Biophys. Res. Commun.*, 203(1), 615-622

Ema, M., Matsushita, N., Sogawa, K., Ariyama, T., Inazawa, J., Nemoto,T., Ota, M., Oshimura, M. & Fujii-Kuriyama, Y. (1994a) Human aryl hydrocarbon receptor: functional expression and chromosomal assignment to 7p21. *J. Biochem.*, 116, 845-851

Ema, M., Ohe, N., Suzuki, M., Mimura, J., Sogawa, K., Ikawa, S. & Fujii-Kuriyama, Y. (1994b) Dioxin-binding activities of polymorphic forms of mouse and human arylhydrocarbon receptors. *J. Biol. Chem.*, 269(44), 27337-27343

Ema, M., Sogawa, K., Watanabe, N., Chujoh, Y., Matsushita, N., Gotoh,O., Funae, Y. & Fujii-Kuriyama, Y. (1992) cDNA cloning and structure of mouse putative Ah receptor. *Biochem. Biophys. Res. Commun.*, 184, 246-253

FitzGerald, C. T., Fernandez-Salguero, P., Gonzalez, F. J., Nebert, D.W. & Puga, A. (1996) Differential regulation of mouse Ah receptor gene expression in cell lines of different tissue origins. *Arch. Biochem. Biophys.*, 333, 170-178

Fujii-Kuriyama, Y., Ema, M., Mimura, J., Matsushita, N. & Sogawa, K. (1995) Polymorphic forms of the Ah receptor and induction of the CYP1A1 gene. *Pharmacogenetics*, 5, S149-153

Fujisawa-Sehara, A., Sogawa, K., Yamane, M. & Fujii-Kuriyama, Y. (1987) Characterization of xenobiotic responsive elements upstream from the drug-metabolizing cytochrome P-450c gene: a similarity to glucocorticoid regulatory elements. *Nucleic Acids Res.*, 15, 4179-4191

Gradin, K., Whitelaw, M. L., Toftgard, R., Poellinger, L. & Berghard, A. (1994) A tyrosine kinase-dependent pathway regulates ligand-dependent activation of the dioxin receptor in human keratinocytes. *J. Biol. Chem.*, 269, 23800-23807

Greenlee, W.F. & Poland, A. (1979) Nuclear uptake of 2,3,7,8-tetrachlorodibenzo-p-dioxin in C57BL/6J and DBA/2J mice. Role of the hepatic cytosol receptor protein. *J. Biol. Chem.*, 254, 9814-9821

Hankinson, O. (1995) The aryl hydrocarbon receptor complex. *Annu. Rev. Pharmacol. Toxicol.*, 35, 307-340

Hayashi, S., Watanabe, J., Nakachi, K., Eguchi, H., Gotoh, O. & Kawajiri, K. (1994) Interindividual difference in expression of human Ah receptor and related P450 genes. *Carcinogenesis*, 15(5), 801-806

Hirvonen, A., Pursiainen, K.H., Karjalainen, A., Anttila, S. & Vainio, H. (1992) Point mutational Msp1 and Ile-Val polymorphism closely linked in the CYP1A1 gene: lack of association with susceptibility to lung cancer in a Finnish study population. *Cancer Epidemiol. Biomarkers Prev.*, 1, 485-489

Hoffman, E.C., Reyes, H., Chu, F.F., Sander, F., Conley, L.H., Brooks, B.A. & Hankinson, O. (1991) Cloning of a factor required for activity of the Ah (dioxin) receptor. *Science*, 252, 954-958

Hord, N.G. & Perdew, G.H. (1994) Physicochemical and immunochemical analysis of the aryl hydrocarbon receptor nuclear translocator: characterizartion of two monoclonal antibodies to the aryl hydrocarbon receptor nuclear translocator. *Mol. Pharmacol.*, 46, 618-626

Ichiba, M., Hagmar, L., Rannug, A., Hogstedt, B., Alexandrie, A.K., Carstensen, U. & Hemminki, K. (1994) Aromatic DNA adducts, micronuclei and genetic polymorphism for CYP1A1 and GST1 in chimney sweeps. *Carcinogenesis*, 15(7), 1347-1352

Johnson, B.S., Brooks, B.A., Reyes, H., Hoffman, E.C. & Hankinson, O. (1992) An MspI RFLP in the human ARNT gene, encoding a subunit of the nuclear form of the Ah (dioxin) receptor. *Hum. Mol. Genet.*, 1(5), 351

Jones, J.E., Huckaby, C.S., Stafford, M.D. & Linnoila, R.I. (1994) An MspI RFLP of the human AHR gene. *Hum. Mol. Genet.*, 3(11), 2083

Kawajiri, K., Nakachi, K., Imai, K., Yoshii, A., Shinoda, N. & Watanabe, J. (1990) Identification of genetically high-risk individuals to lung cancer by DNA polymorphisms of the cytochrome p4501A1 gene. *FEBS Lett.*, 263 (1) 131-133

Kawajiri, K., Watanabe, J., Eguchi, H., Nakachi, K., Kiyohara, C. & Hayashi, S. (1995) Polymorphisms of human Ah receptor gene are not involved in lung cancer. *Pharmacogenetics*, 5(3),151-158

Kobayashi, A., Sogawa, K. & Fujii-Kuriyama, Y. (1996) Cooperative interaction between AhR/Arnt and Sp1 for the drug-inducible expression of CYP1A1 Gene. *J. Biol. Chem.*, 271, 12310-12316

Le Beau, M.M., Carver, L.A., Espinosa, R., 3rd, Schmidt, J.V. & Bradfield, C.A. (1994) Chromosomal localization of the human AHR locus encoding the structural gene for the Ah receptor to 7p21—>p15. *Cytogenet. Cell Genet.*, 66(3), 172-176

Li, H., Dong, L. & Whitlock, J.P. Jr. (1994) Transcriptional activation function of the mouse Ah receptor nuclear translocator. *J. Biol. Chem.*, 269, 28098-28105

Mahon, M.J. & Gasiewicz, T.A. (1995) Ah receptor phosphorylation: location of phosphorylation sites to the C-terminal half of the protein. *Arch. Biochem. Biophys.*, 318, 166-174

Mimura, J., Ema, M., Sogawa, K., Ikawa, S. & Fujii-Kuriyama, Y. (1994) A complete structure of the mouse Ah receptor gene. *Pharmacogenetics*, 4, 349-354

Nakachi, K., Imai, K., Hayashi, S. & Kawajiri, K. (1993) Polymorphisms of the CYP1A1 and glutathione S-transferase genes associated with susceptibility to lung cancer in relation to cigarette dose in a Japanese population. *Cancer Res.*, 53, 2994-2999

Nakachi, K., Imai, K., Hayashi, S., Watanabe, J. & Kawajiri, K. (1991) Genetic susceptibility to squamous cell carcinoma of the lung in relation to cigarette smoking dose. *Cancer Res.*, 51, 5177-5181

Nambu, J.R., Lewis, J.O., Wharton, Jr., K.A. & Crews, S. T. (1991) The *Drosophila* single-minded gene encodes a helix-loop-helix protein that acts as a master regulator of CNS midline development. *Cell*, 67, 1157-1167

Nebert, D.W. & Jones, J.E. (1989) Regulation of the mammalian cytochrome P1-450 (CYP1A1) gene. *Int. J. Biochem.*, 21, 243-52

Nebert, D.W., Puga, A. & Vasiliou, V. (1993) Role of the Ah receptor and the dioxin-inducible [Ah] gene battery in toxicity, cancer, and signal transduction. *Ann. NY Acad. Sci.*, 685: 624-640

Niwa, A., Kumaki, K., Nebert, D.W. & Poland A.P. (1975) Genetic expression of aryl hydrocarbon hydroxylase activity in the mouse. Distinction between the "responsive" homozygote and heterozygote at the Ah locus. *Arch. Biochem. Biophys.*, 166, 559-564

Okey, A.B., Riddick, D.S. & Harper, P.A. (1994) Molecular biology of the aromatic hydrocarbon (dioxin) receptor. *Trends Pharmacol. Sci.*, 15: 226-232

Okino, S.T., Pendurthi, U.R. & Tukey, R.H. (1992) Phorbol esters inhibit the dioxin receptor-mediated transcriptional activation of the mouse Cyp1a-1 and Cyp1a-2 genes by 2,3,7,8-tetra-chlorodibenzo-p-dioxin. *J. Biol. Chem.*, 267, 6991-6998

Perdew, G. H. (1988) Association of the Ah receptor with the 90 kD heat shock protein. *J. Biol. Chem*, 263, 13802-13805

Perdew, G.H. & Hollenback, C.E. (1995) Evidence for two functionally distinct forms of the human Ah receptor. *J. Biochem. Toxicol.*, 10(2): 95-102

Poland, A. & Bradfield, C. (1992) A brief review of the Ah locus. *Tohoku J. Exp. Med.*,168, 83-87

Poland, A.P. , Glover, E., Robinson, J.R. & Nebert D.W. (1974) Genetic expression of aryl hydrocarbon hydroxylase activity. Induction of monooxygenase activities and cytochrome P1-450 formation by 2,3,7,8-tetrachlorodibenzo-p-dioxin in mice genetically "nonresponsive" to other aromatic hydrocarbons. *J. Biol. Chem.*, 249, 5599-5606

Pollenz, R. S., Sattler, C. A. & Poland, A. (1993) The aryl hydrocarbon receptor and aryl hydrocarbon receptor nuclear translocator protein show distinct subcellular localizations in Hepa 1c1c7 cells by immunofluorescence microscopy. *Mol. Pharmacol.*, 45, 428-438

Safe, S. & Krishnan, V. (1995) Cellular and molecular biology of aryl hydrocarbon (Ah) receptor-mediated gene expression. *Arch. Toxicol.*, 17, 99-115

Schmidt, J.V., Carver, L.A. & Bradfield, C.A. (1993) Molecular characterization of the murine Ahr gene. Organization, promoter analysis, and chromosomal assignment. *J. Biol. Chem.*, 268(29), 22203-22209

Sogawa, K. & Fujii-Kuriyama, Y. (1993) Regulation of cytochrome P450 expression. In: Schenkman, J.B. & Greim, H., eds, *Handbook of Experimental Pharmacology, Vol.105, Cytochrome P450.* Berlin, Heidelberg; Springer-Verlag; pp. 493-501

Sogawa, K., Nakano, R., Kobayashi, A., Kikuchi, Y., Ohe, N., Matsushita, N. & Fujii-Kuriyama, Y. (1995a) Possible function of Ah receptor nuclear translocator (Arnt) homodimer in transcriptional regulation. *Proc. Natl. Acad. Sci. USA*, 92(6), 1936-1940

Sogawa, K., Iwabuchi, K., Abe, H. & Fujii-Kuriyama, Y. (1995b) Transcriptional activation domains of the Ah receptor and Ah receptor nuclear translocator. *J. Cancer Res. Clin. Oncol.*,121(9-10), 612-620

Stephens, E.A, Taylor, J.A, Kaplan, N., Yang, C.H., Hsieh, L.L., Lucier, G.W. & Bell, D.A. (1994) Ethnic variation in the CYP2E1 gene: polymorphism analysis of 695 African-Americans, European-Americans and Taiwanese. *Pharmacogenetics*, 4(4), 185-192

Taioli, E., Trachman, J. ,Chen, X.,Toniolo, P. & Garte, S.J. (1995) CYP1A1 RFLP is associated with breast cancer in African American women. *Cancer Res.*, 55, 3757-3758

Vineis, P., Bartsch, H., Caporaso, N., Harrington, A., Kadlubar, F.F., Landi, M.T., Malaveille, C., Shields, P.G., Skipper, P., Talaska, G. & Tannenbaum, S.R. (1994) Genetically based N-acetyltransferase metabolic polymorphism and low-level environmental exposure to carcinogens. *Nature*, 369, 154-156

Whitelaw, M.L., Gustafsson, J.A. & Poellinger, L. (1994) Identification of transactivation and repression functions of the dioxin receptor and its basic helix-loop-helix/PAS partner factor Arnt: inducible versus constitutive modes of regulation. *Mol. Cell. Biol.*, 14(12), 8343-8355

Wilhelmsson, A., Cuthill, S., Denis, M., Wikstrom, A.-C.,Gustafsson, J.-A. & Poellinger, L. (1990) The specific DNA binding activity of the dioxin receptor is modulated by the 90 kd heat shock protein. *EMBO J.*, 9, 69-76

Corresponding author

Seymour Garte
Environmental and Occupational Health Sciences Institute, UMDNJ,
170 Frelinghuysen Road,
Piscataway, NJ, USA

and

Sci. Dir.
Genetics Research Institute
Milan, Italy

Metabolic Polymorphisms and Susceptibility to Cancer
W. Ryder
IARC Scientific Publications No. 148
International Agency for Research on Cancer, Lyon, 1999

Chapter 15. CYP1A1

Kaname Kawajiri

CYP1A1 plays an important role in the metabolism of polycyclic hydrocarbons that occur in the environment and several studies suggest that the genetic polymorphism of the gene may play a role in the predisposition to cancer. In order to evaluate the function of CYP1A1 *in vivo* as a host factor determinant of enviromentally-caused cancers in humans, additional investigations are needed involving not only molecular epidemiological approaches in different ethnic populations but also more direct approaches such as the use of gene-targeted mice as a model system.

The *CYP1A1* gene is of critical importance for the metabolism of polycyclic aromatic hydrocarbons (Omura *et al.*, 1993; Guengerich & Shimada, 1991; Kawajiri & Fujii-Kuriyama, 1991). The gene product, aromatic hydrocarbon hydroxylase (AHH), catalyses the first step in the conversion of many environmental carcinogens, such as benzo(a)pyrene in cigarette smoke, to their ultimate DNA-binding, carcinogenic form. Human CYP1A1 protein is composed of 512 amino acid residues, which is smaller by 12 amino acids than its rodent equivalent. In experimental animals, 1A1 is induced in both the liver and extrahepatic tissues by exogenous polycyclic aromatic hydrocarbons, such as benzo(a)pyrene, 3-methylcholan-threne and TCDD. In contrast, 1A1 in humans is considered to function primarily as an extrahepatic enzyme, because considerable amounts of both mRNA and protein can be detected in lung, lymphocytes, and placenta, in contrast to undetectable levels in most human livers examined.

In animal model systems, genetically regulated levels of AHH activity are associated with susceptibility to chemically developed skin or lung carcinomas (Kouri & Nebert, 1977). Marked differences in the metabolism of polycyclic aromatic hydrocarbons and susceptibility to chemically induced cancer among strains of mice can be designated from a genetic polymorphism of Ah receptor (Ema *et al.*, 1994), a regulatory transcription factor of the 1A1 protein. In humans, reports from numerous laboratories have suggested a relationship between higher levels of AHH inducibility in certain tissues, such as peripheral blood lymphocytes, and the incidence of lung, larynx, renal and ureter cancers (Kellermann *et al.*, 1973b; Emery *et al.*, 1978; Gahmberg *et al.*, 1979; Korsgaad *et al.*, 1984; Kouri

et al., 1982). The rationale for such an association was that individuals with high AHH inducibility could readily and efficiently activate polycyclic aromatic hydrocarbons in our environment. However, there are reports from other laboratories suggesting a lack of any relationship between high AHH inducibility in human-derived tissues and susceptibility to cancers (Paigen *et al.*, 1977, 1979; Ward *et al.*, 1978; Karki *et al.*, 1987). At present there is no consensus concerning the role of AHH inducibility in the etiology of cancer susceptibility associated with cigarette smoke. (Caporaso *et al.*, 1991; Nebert *et al.*, 1991).

The *CYP1A1* gene has been localized to chromosome 15 near the MPI locus at 15q22-24 (Hildebrand *et al.*, 1985), and several *CYP1A1* RFLP patterns have been reported (Spurr *et al.*, 1987; Bale *et al.*, 1987; Haugen *et al.*, 1990). Clearly, it might be helpful in predicting the individual risk of cancer if some of the genetic polymorphisms were correlated with cancer susceptibility. Three polymorphisms of the *CYP1A1* gene have been studied extensively in relation to cancer susceptibility (Fig. 1); two genetically-linked polymorphisms, one producing an *Msp* I recognition site in the 3' non-coding region and the other a one-base substitution of adenine to guanine in the haem-binding region of exon 7 (*Ile-Val* polymorphism), have been associated with an increased risk of smoking-induced lung cancer in Asians but not in Caucasians (Kawajiri *et al.*, 1993). A novel *Msp* I RFLP in the 3' non-coding region of the *CYP1A1* gene found only in an African-American population (Crofts *et al.*, 1993) has also been studied. The present chapter briefly reviews the current status of the relationship between metabolic polymorphisms of CYP1A1 and cancer susceptibility in human (Tables 1-3).

Table 1. Distribution of CYP1A1 genotypes (Msp I) in cancer patients and healthy controls

Populations		CYP1A1 genotypes			
		A(m1/m1)	B(m1/m2)	C(m2/m2)	Total
Kawajiri 1998, Kawajiri *et al.* 1993	Control	166 (44.3)	169 (45.1)	40 (10.6)	375
(Japan)	Lung	130 (39.9)	144 (44.1)	52 (16.0)	326
	Sq	38 (36.1)	43 (41.0)	24 (22.9)	105
	Ad	69 (46.1)	66 (44.0)	15 (10.0)	150
Okada *et al.* 1994 (Japan)	Lung	98 (36.7)	124 (46.4)	45 (16.9)	267
	Sq	33 (38.4)	35 (40.7)	18 (20.9)	86
Kihara *et al.* 1995 (Japan)	Control	81 (43.8)	71 (38.4)	33 (17.8)	185
	Lung	36 (37.1)	45 (46.4)	16 (16.5)	97
Tefre *et al.* 1991 (Norway)	Control	167 (78.8)	43 (20.3)	2 (0.9)	212
	Lung	172 (77.8)	47 (21.3)	2 (0.9)	221
	Sq	59 (73.8)	20 (25.0)	1 (1.2)	80
Hirvonen *et al.* 1992 (Finland)	Control	95 (78.5)	24 (19.8)	2 (1.7)	121
	Lung	65 (74.5)	22 (25.5)	0 (0)	87
	Sq	30 (68.2)	14 (31.8)	0 (0)	44
Drakoulis *et al.* 1994 (Germany)	Control	146 (85.4)	25 (14.6)	0 (0)	171
	Lung	119 (83.8)	22 (15.5)	1 (0.7)	296
	Sq	87 (81.3)	8 (16.8)	2 (1.9)	107
Sugimura *et al.* 1994 (Brazil)	Nonblacks				
	Control	56 (62.2)	27 (30.0)	7 (7.8)	90
	Lung	7 (64.8)	25 (28.4)	6 (6.8)	88
	Blacks				
	Control	14 (63.7)	6 (27.2)	2 (9.1)	22
	Lung	12 (54.5)	7 (31.8)	3 (13.7)	22
Shields *et al.* 1993 (USA)	Control	43 (76.8)	11 (19.6)	2 (3.6)	56
	Lung	33 (68.8)	12 (25.0)	3 (6.3)	48
Kawajiri 1998, Kawajiri *et al.* 1993	Control	166 (44.3)	169 (45.1)	40 (10.6)	375
(Japan)	Stomach	45 (45.3)	50 (48.0)	9 (8.7)	104
	Colorectal	37 (47.5)	32 (41.0)	9 (11.5)	78
	Breast	15 (48.4)	13 (41.9)	3 (9.7)	31
Okada *et al.* 1994 (Japan)	Pancreas	29 (53.7)	21 (38.9)	4 (7.4)	54
Taioli *et al.* 1995b (USA)	African-Americans				
	Control	51 (60.0)	31 (36.5)	3 (3.5)	85
	Breast	7 (33.4)	10 (47.6)	4 (19.0)	21
	Caucasians				
	Control	146 (79.8)	32 (17.5)	5 (2.7)	183
	Breast	22 (77.3)	8 (26.7)	0 (0)	30
Sivaraman *et al.* 1994 (USA)	Control	23 (49.0)	22 (47.0)	2 (4.0)	47
	Colorectal	23 (53.0)	10 (23.0)	10 (23.0)	43

Sq. = squamous cell carcinoma of the lung; Ad. = adenocarcinoma of the lung

Table 2. Distribution of CYP1A1 genotypes (Ile-Val) in cancer patients and healthy controls

Populations		CYP1A1 genotypes			
		Ile/Ile	Ile/Val	Val/Val	Total
Kawajiri 1998, Kawajiri *et al.* 1993	Control	233 (65.1)	108 (30.2)	17 (4.7)	358
(Japan)	Lung	188 (57.5)	103 (31.5)	36 (11.0)	327
	Sq	61 (58.7)	30 (28.8)	13 (12.5)	104
	Ad	89 (59.0)	48 (31.8)	14 (9.2)	151
Kihara *et al.* 1995 (Japan)	Control	101 (55.5)	70 (38.5)	11 (6.0)	182
	Lung	59 (61.1)	31 (32.6)	5 (5.3)	95
Drakoulis *et al.* 1994 (Germany)	Control	160 (93.6)	11 (6.4)	0 (0)	171
	Lung	125 (88.0)	15 (10.6)	2 (1.4)	142
Hamada *et al.* 1995 (Brazil)	Control	91 (84.3)	15 (13.9)	2 (1.8)	108
	Lung	70 (70.7)	27 (27.3)	2 (2.0)	99
Alexandrie *et al.* 1994 (Sweden)	Control	306 (93.0)	23 (7.0)	0 (0)	329
	Lung	280 (94.6)	16 (5.4)	0 (0)	296
	Sq	98 (91.6)	9 (8.4)	0 (0)	107
Kawajiri 1998, Kawajiri *et al.* 1993	Control	233 (65.1)	108 (30.2)	17 (4.7)	358
(Japan)	Stomach	54 (56.8)	37 (39.0)	4 (4.2)	95
	Colorectal	59 (69.4)	21 (24.7)	5 (5.9)	85
	Breast	65 (66.5)	29 (29.6)	4 (4.1)	98
Katoh *et al.* 1995 (Japan)	Control	57 (56.4)	39 (38.6)	5 (5.0)	101
	Urothelial	50 (60.2)	30 (36.2)	3 (3.6)	83
Taioli *et al.* 1995b (USA)	African-Americans				
	Control	78 (94.0)	5 (6.0)	0 (0)	83
	Breast	20 (100)	0 (0)	0 (0)	20
	Caucasians				
	Control	145 (82.9)	28 (16.0)	2 (1.1)	175
	Breast	24 (82.8)	5 (17.2)	0 (0)	29
Ambrosone *et al.* 1995 (USA)	Control	195 (85.5)	31 (13.6)	2 (0.9)	228
	Breast	140 (79.5)	32 (18.2)	4 (2.3)	176
Sivaraman *et al.* 1994 (USA)	Control	33 (70.2)	14 (29.8)	0 (0)	47
	Colorectal:	32 (74.4)	9 (20.9)	2 (4.7)	43

Sq. = squamous cell carcinoma of the lung; Ad. = adenocarcinoma of the lung

CYP1A1 phenotype

Measurement

The CYP1A1-dependent phenotype has been determined through assay of the AHH metabolism of benzo(a)pyrene in human-derived tissues, usually peripheral blood lymphocytes (Nebert, 1978). Basal AHH activity in lymphocytes is so weak that a mitogen, such as phytohaemagglutinin or poke-weed, must be introduced into the medium. Further induction with 3-methylcholanthrene, dibenzanthracene or TCDD may be required. AHH activity is measured using benzo(a)pyrene as a substrate by the fluorometric method, and one unit of AHH activity is defined as the amount of enzyme that catalyses the substrate with the formation of fluorescence equivalent to 1 pmol 3-hydroxy-

Table 3. Distribution of CYP1A1 genotypes (AA) in cancer patients and healthy controls

Populations		CYP1A1 genotypes			
		AA	Aa	aa	Total
Taioli et al. 1995a (USA)	Control	103 (83.7)	20 (16.3)	0 (0)	123
	Lung	63 (82.9)	12 (14.0)	1 (1.1)	86
	Sq	24 (92.3)	2 (7.7)	0 (0)	26
	Ad	20 (66.7)	9 (30.0)	1 (3.3)	30
Kelsey et al. 1994 (USA)	Control	74 (76.3)	21 (21.6)	2 (2.1)	97
	Lung	60 (83.3)	11 (15.3)	1 (1.4)	72
Taioli et al. 1995b (USA)	African-Americans				
	Control	72 (83.7)	14 (16.2)	0 (0)	86
	Breast	17 (81.0)	4 (19.0)	0 (0)	21
	Caucasian				
	Control	183 (100)	0 (0)	0 (0)	183
	Breast	30 (100)	0 (0)	0 (0)	30

Sq. = squamous cell carcinoma of the lung; Ad. = adenocarcinoma of the lung

benzo(a)pyrene in 45 min. In lymphocytes, AHH inducibility has been expressed as the ratio of AHH activity in induced cultures to that in uninduced mitogen-stimulated cultures. The viability of lymphocytes can be determined by the assay of NADH-cytochrome c reductase.

Experimental studies of the role of CYP1A1 phenotype in carcinogenesis

The Ah receptor (Ahr) is a ligand-dependent transcription factor that positively regulates inducible expression of AHH activity (CYP1A1 phenotype). In mice the single Ah locus has been found to govern the genetic differences in the inducibility of AHH for metabolic activation of aromatic hydrocarbons among various inbred strains and, therefore, to be related to the susceptibility of the experimental animals to chemical carcinogenesis (Nebert, 1978). It was reported that responder mice, such as C57BL/6, were at high risk of carcinogenesis induced by these carcinogens, while non-responder mice, such as DBA/2J, were relatively resistant. The Ah receptor exhibits considerable functional and structural variability among inbred strains of mice, and this polymorphism is known to arise from multiple genetic alleles at the Ah locus. Non-responsive strain DBA/2J mice possessed Ahr with an affinity for agonist that was 15-20 times lower than that of the receptor in the responsive C57BL/6 strain. Ema et al. (1994) showed that two polymorphisms were involved in different ligand affinity between the two strains of mice; 43 extra amino acids at the C-terminal originated by a codon change from Opal (C57BL) to Arg (DBA) and one amino acid replacement at 375 from Ala (C57BL) to Val (DBA) led to low ligand affinity of the Ahr protein in the DBA (K^d = 1.66 nM for TCDD) compared with that of C57BL mice (K^d = 0.27 nM for TCDD).

Epidemiological evidence of the role of CYP1A1 phenotype in carcinogenesis

Kellermann et al. (1973a) reported that inducibility of AHH showed a trimodal distribution in cultured, mitogen-stimulated lymphocytes, thereby suggesting a genetic basis for this variation. This was supported by family pedigree analysis, which revealed that the different AHH activities were under genet-

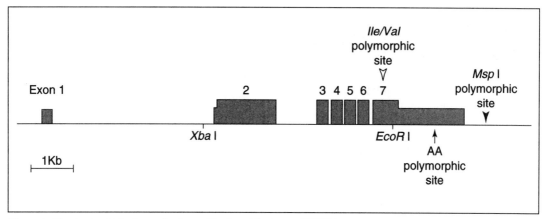

Figure 1. Structural organization and polymorphic sites of the human CYP1A1 gene.

ic control. Reproducibility and trimodal distribution of AHH inducibility in lymphocytes among humans were reconfirmed recently by a strictly developed analysis (Kouri *et al.*, 1982; Trell *et al.*, 1985). On the basis of these results a model was proposed in which the groups with low and high AHH inducibilities are homozygous for two different alleles, and the group with intermediate AHH activity is heterozygous for two alleles. These population studies provided a basis for the hypothesis that susceptibility to smoking-induced cancer may be associated with genetically determined metabolic polymorphism of AHH inducibility.

Kellermann *et al.* (1973a) measured AHH inducibility in mitogen-stimulated lymphocytes from 121 patients with bronchogenic carcinoma and 230 healthy control individuals. The majority of patients were found to be in groups with genetically increased AHH activity (30.6%, 37/121), and only a small proportion had a genetically low AHH activity (5.0%, 6/121). In contrast, high and low AHH groups comprised 10.9% (25/230) and 42.2% (97/230) of the healthy control individuals respectively. In patients with cancer of the larynx the distribution of AHH activity was similar to that of lung cancer patients. It was concluded that individuals with a genetically high AHH activity were at greater risk for developing smoking-associated cancers if they were heavy smokers than were individuals with low AHH activity. Emery *et al.* (1978) showed that the proportion of high AHH inducibility (induced to uninduced AHH activity greater than 4.0) was significantly greater among patients with squamous cell carcinoma (69.4%,

43/62) of the lung than among healthy controls (33.9%, 21/62) matched for age, sex and smoking habits. Gahmberg *et al.* (1979) reported that high induced AHH activity (induced to uninduced AHH activity greater than 1.5) was found in 39% of patients with lung cancer, but in only 15% (61/404) of normal subjects. However, only 17% of the patients with other malignancies had high AHH activity. Korsgaad *et al.* (1984) studied the relationship between AHH inducibility and smoking-associated cancers. In 34 patients with carcinomas of the oral cavity, 41 with larynx cancer and 22 with pulmonary carcinomas there was a highly significant overrepresentation of high AHH inducibility, whereas 30 patients with carcinomas of the renal pelvis and ureter and 46 with urinary bladder carcinomas did not differ significantly in this respect from a control population comprising 92 subjects.

However, an absence of association between AHH inducibility and cancer susceptibility has also been reported. Paigen *et al.* (1977, 1979) conducted two similar studies, using lung (n = 17) and bladder (n = 16) cancer patients. They found that the inducibility of AHH activity in the progeny of bladder cancer patients (n = 53) did not differ from that of their parents and of matched healthy controls (n = 53), whereas half of the lung cancer patients showed a lower AHH inducibility than their progeny (n = 57) and healthy controls (n = 57). Ward *et al.* (1978) reported a hospital-based case-control study of 32 lung cancer patients, 27 larynx cancer patients and 58 controls. The mean AHH inducibility was 3.2 ± 0.02

in patients who had lung cancer, 2.96 ± 0.18 in patients with larynx cancer and 3.29 ± 0.04 for the controls. These values and the distribution of AHH inducibility in pecentiles do not suggest differences between cases and controls. Karki *et al.* (1987) conducted a hospital-based case-control study on AHH inducibility using lymphocytes from 34 patients with pulmonary carcinoma and from 43 non-smoking and 37 smoking controls. The mean inducibility ratio was very similar in all three groups, ranging from 4.5 to 5.5.

A more likely explanation for these contradictory results may relate to the myriad technical difficulties involved in achieving reproducible mitogen activation and subsequent AHH induction in human peripheral blood lymphocytes. Using cryopreserved lymphocytes to improve the assay system, Kouri *et al.* (1982) carried out a case-control study on 51 individuals, 21 of them with lung cancer and 30 with non-malignant pulmonary diseases. All the 14 highest AHH/NADH-cytochrome c reductase levels were in patients with lung cancer. Mean AHH/cytochrome c reductase was 0.89 for lung cancer patients and 0.47 for non-cancer patients. However, whether or not the higher AHH inducibility levels are the cause or the result of primary lung cancer remains to be determined. Although the genetic difference in the susceptibility of mice to chemically induced carcinogenesis is governed by polymorphism of the Ahr, as previously mentioned, no germ line polymorphism of the human Ahr showed a significant association with AHH inducibility or with lung cancer incidence (Kawajiri *et al.*, 1995; Micka *et al.*, 1997).

CYP1A1 genotype
Measurement

(a) Msp I polymorphism in the human CYP1A1 gene
Southern blot analysis

Human lymphocyte DNA (8 µg) is digested with restriction nuclease *Msp* I for 2 hours at 37°C and the products are subjected to electrophoresis in 0.8% agarose for Southern blot analysis (Kawajiri *et al.*, 1990). The DNA fragments are transferred to a nitrocellulose or nylon membrane filter. The filter is hybridized to the ^{32}P-labelled *Xba* I-*Eco* RI fragment of the cloned *CYP1A1* gene in a hybridiza-

tion solution at 65°C overnight and washed twice with 0.1x SSC containing 0.1% SDS at 65°C for 30 min followed by autoradiography against a Kodak XAR-5 film at -80°C with an intensifying screen. An individual with genotype *A(m1/m1)* is a predominant homozygote, where the *Msp* I site (264th downstream from the poly(A) additional signal) is absent. An individual homozygous for the rare allele is genotype *C (m2/m2)*, derived from a one-base substitution of thymine with cytosine to form the *Msp* I, as confirmed by PCR-direct sequencing. An individual with genotype *B(m1/m2)* is heterozygous for the alleles.

PCR-restriction nuclease digestion analysis

Two synthetic oligonucleotide primers of 21 bases (C47: 5'-CAGTGAAGAGGTGTAGCCGCT-3' and C44: 5'-TAGGAGTCTTGTCTCATGCCT-3' from the 130th to the 150th and from the 449th to the 469th bases respectively, counting from the poly (A) additional signal) are prepared (Hayashi *et al.*, 1991). PCR is carried out with 25 cycles under the following conditions: 1 minute at 95°C for denaturation, 1 minute at 68° C and 1 minute at 72°C for primer annealing and primer extension. The amplified fragments, including the *Msp* I site, are digested with *Msp* I for 2 hours at 37°C and the products subjected to electrophoresis in a 1.8% agarose gel. Genotype *A* is characterized by a 0.34 kb fragment; genotype *B* by 0.14, 0.20 and 0.34 kb; and genotype *C* by 0.14 and 0.20 kb. The genotypes of the *CYP1A1* gene ascribed to the *Msp* I site are identified as restriction fragment length polymorphisms (RFLPs) by the PCR and are in complete agreement with the results of Southern blot analysis.

(b) Ile-Val polymorphism in the human CYP1A1 gene

Difference in one base at position 4889 in the 7th exon of the *CYP1A1* gene was found by PCR direct sequencing (Hayashi *et al.*, 1991). This novel point mutation resulted in the replacement of Ile by Val at residue 462 in the HR2 region, which was well conserved among the P450 families (Gotoh *et al.*, 1983). The RFLP method cannot be used to detect this polymorphism because there is no suitable restriction site. For screening purposes, therefore, allele-specific PCR amplification (Hayashi *et al.*, 1991) and SSCP (Kawajiri *et al.*, 1996b) analyses have been adopted.

Allele-specific PCR amplification method

Two oligonucleotides of 20-mer (1A1A; 5'-GAAGTGTATCGGTGAGACCA-3' and 1A1G; 5'-GAAGTGTATCGGTGAGACCG-3'), both of which contain the polymorphic site at the 3' end, are synthesized and each is used as a primer for allele-specific PCR amplification together with another strand of 21-mer primer (C53; 5'-GTAGACA-GAGTCTAGGCCTCA-3') located about 190 bp downstream of a polymorphic site detected by sequencing (Hayashi *et al.*, 1991). PCR is performed with 30 cycles under the following conditions: 1 minute at 95°C for denaturation, annealing at 65°C for 1 minute, and extension at 72°C for 1 minute. The PCR products are then subjected to electrophoresis in a 1.8% agarose gel.

Single-strand conformational polymorphism (SSCP)

A pair of primers (5'-GAACTGCCACTTCAGCT-GTCT-3' and 5'-GTAGACAGAGTCTAGGCCTCA-3') are used for screening the *Ile-Val* polymorphism by SSCP analysis (Kawajiri *et al.*, 1996). Genomic DNA (50 ng) is used in a 5-µl PCR reaction mixture containing 10 mM Tris-HCl (pH 8.3), 1.5 mM MgCl$_2$, 50 mM KCl, 0.01% gelatin (w/v), 1.25 mM each of four deoxynucleotide triphosphates except for dCTP, which has a concentration of 0.125 mM, 1µM of each primer, and 0.2 µl of [α-^{32}P]dCTP (3000Ci mmole^{-1}) and Taq DNA polymerase. The PCR is programmed as follows: initial denaturation, 1 minute at 95°C; amplification for 20 seconds at 95°C, 2 minutes at 60°C for 30 cycles; elongation for 1 minute at 72°C. After completion of the PCR the product is diluted 1:100 in loading buffer (95% formamide, 20 mM EDTA, 0.05% bromphenol blue and 0.05% xylene cyanol). The DNA fragments are subjected to electrophoresis at 35 W for approximately 3 hours in 5% non-denaturing polyacrylamide gel with 5% glycerol at room temperature. Upon complete migration the gels are dried and subjected to autoradiography against a Kodak XAR-5 film at -80°C with an intensifying screen. The results given by these two methods are fully consistent with those obtained by direct sequencing.

(c) Race-specific AA RFLP in the CYP1A1 gene

A new *Msp* I RFLP in the *CYP1A1* gene has been found in African-Americans but not in Caucasians or Asians (Crofts *et al.*, 1993). The polymorphism results from a single A-T to G-C transition in the 3' non-coding region about 300 bp upstream from the polyadenylation site. For analysis of the AA RFLP the following two 20-mer primers are used: 5'-GGCTGAGCAATCTGACCC-TA-3' and 5'-ATACCCCCCCCTCACTCC-3'. PCR is performed using initial denaturation at 95°C for 4 minutes followed by 40 cycles of 94°C for 20 seconds, 60°C for 20 seconds and 70°C for 20 seconds, with a final extension at 72°C for 10 minutes. This generates a 221-bp fragment, which is then subjected to digestion with *Msp* I. The digested product is visualized on a 2.5% agarose gel; variant alleles are digested into separate fragments of 125 bp and 96 bp. Genotypes AA, Aa and aa represent the predominant homozygous, heterozygous and rare homozygote respectively (London *et al.*, 1995).

Epidemiological evidence of the association between the CYP1A1 genotypes and cancer susceptibility

(a) Relationship between the Msp I or Ile-Val polymorphisms and cancer

Lung cancer

The genetic association between the *Msp* I and *Ile-Val* polymorphisms of the human *CYP1A1* gene was investigated in Japanese (Hayashi *et al.*, 1991), German (Drakoulis *et al.*, 1994) and Finnish (Hirvonen *et al.*, 1992) general populations revealing that these two loci were very closely associated. A recent population study on the *CYP1A1* genotypes was conducted mainly by PCR-nuclease digestion (*Msp* I polymorphism) or allele-specific PCR amplification (*Ile-Val* polymorphism) analyses.

Since first investigating an association of the *Msp* I polymorphism of the *CYP1A1* gene with predisposition to lung cancer (Kawajiri *et al.*, 1990), especially to smoking-associated squamous cell carcinoma, using Southern blot analysis, we have greatly increased the numbers of cases and healthy controls. In our study, lymphocyte DNAs of 2500 Japanese were isolated from a cohort of a general population and used as controls (Nakachi *et al.*, 1991). The genotypes of 375 randomly selected subjects were determined. Genotypes *A*, *B* and *C* were found in 166 (44%), 169 (45%) and 40 (11%) individuals respectively among the healthy controls. This result showed a good fit with Hardy-Weinberg equilibrium, in which the relative frequencies p^2, $2pq$, and q^2 of genotypes estimated from the gene frequencies p and q must be equal to the observed, with a gene frequency of 0.67 for $m1$ and 0.33 for $m2$ (Kawajiri et al., 1993). However, when 105 patients with squamous cell carcinoma of the lung were analysed the C genotype was found in 24 patients (23%), about twice the frequency among the controls. We also looked at the distribution of three genotypes of the Ile-Val polymorphism in cancer patients and healthy controls. The genotypes of Ile/Ile, Ile/Val and Val/Val were found in 233 (65%), 108 (30%) and 17 (5%) individuals respectively among 358 controls (Kawajiri et al., 1993). In 104 patients with squamous cell carcinoma of the lung, genotype Val/Val was found in 13 patients (13%). In a population of 86 patients with squamous cell carcinoma of the lung, Okada et al. (1994) reported that genotype C appeared in 21% (18/86), which was twice as high as in the control subjects.

In contrast, the association of adenocarcinoma of the lung with cigarette smoking is less clear than that of squamous cell carcinoma, and the frequencies of genotype C and Val/Val have not been significantly distinguished from those in healthy populations (Kawajiri et al., 1993). This may be partly ascribed to the heterogeneity of adenocarcinoma of the lung on the basis of the clinical and histopathological characteristics, and the etiologies may be complicated and different among the adenocarcinomas (Suzuki et al., 1990). From this point of view we classified adenocarcinoma of the lung by differentiation grades and examined the involvement of CYP1A1 polymorphisms (Nakachi et al., 1995). The highest proportion of current or ex-smokers and their cigarette consumption was among the poorly differentiated cases. The two polymorphisms of CYP1A1 were examined among current or ex-smokers with three differentiated grades, revealing that poorly differentiated adenocarcinoma included significantly elevated frequencies of genotype C (26%; 12/46) and Val/Val (11%; 5/46), which have been found to be 'susceptible' in squamous cell carcinoma of the lung.

In a study on 221 lung cancer patients and 212 healthy controls in a Norwegian population, Tefre et al. (1991) demonstrated the absence of a correlation between the Msp I polymorphism and an increased risk of lung cancer. They also found an absence of associations with particular histological types of lung cancer, cigarette smoking history or occupational exposure to asbestos. Hirvonen et al. (1992) reported a lack of an association between Msp I RFLP and lung cancer risk using 87 lung cancer patients and 121 healthy controls in a Finnish population. A similar lack of association between Msp I RFLP and lung cancer incidence was reported by Shields et al. (1993), who studied the DNA of 78 subjects who were African-Americans and Caucasians. Drakoulis et al. (1994) conducted a case-control study on association between the Msp I or Ile-Val polymorphism and lung cancer risk in an ethnically homogeneous German population. Although no statistically significant difference was found in the distribution of Msp I RFLP between all cell types of lung cancer (n = 142) and controls (n = 171), a trend to overrepresentation of the m2 allele of the Msp I RFLP was observed among 52 squamous cell carcinoma patients. In contrast, the frequency of Val-coded allele in lung cancer patients was 2-fold higher than in the control group (OR = 2.16; 95% CI; 0.96-5.11, P = 0.033). They also found that there was a close genetic linkage of the two polymorphisms of the CYP1A1 gene in the controls, but no linkage was observed among lung cancer patients. In a Brazilian population the Msp I polymorphism was not associated with lung cancer susceptibility (110 cases; 112 controls) (Sugimura et al., 1994), while the Ile-Val polymorphism was found to be associated with lung cancer (99 cases; 108 controls; OR = 2.26; 95% CI, 1.14-4.47) (Hamada et al., 1995). These results indicate that the site responsible for cancer susceptibility is the Ile-Val polymorphism in the catalytic site of CYP1A1.

Other cancer sites

In Japanese people the frequency distributions of the Msp I or Ile-Val genotypes in patients with other cancer sites, such as stomach (n = 95), colon (n = 85) and breast (n = 98) were the same as in healthy controls (Kawajiri et al., 1993). No association was found with pancreatic cancer (n = 54) (Okada et al., 1994). Taioli et al. (1995b) reported an association of the Msp I polymorphism with an increased risk of breast cancer in African-Americans (21 cases; 85 controls; OR = 9.7; 95% CI, 2.0-47.9), but no association in Caucasians (30 cases; 183 controls). Sivaraman *et al.* (1995) reported a positive correlation between the *Msp* I polymorphism and colorectal cancer in Japanese (P = 0.008) and Hawaiian/part-Hawaiian subjects (P<0.001), although the study lacked the capacity to detect a similar association in Caucasians.

(b) Relationship between race-specific AA RFLP and cancer

Lung cancer

In a study on 76 lung cancer patients and 123 healthy controls in an African-American population, Taioli *et al.* (1995a) demonstrated the absence of a correlation between race-specific AA RFLP and an increased risk of all cell types of lung cancer. However, analysis by histological type showed an association between adenocarcinoma (n = 30) of the lung and the AA RFLP genotypes Aa+aa with an odds ratio of 2.6 (95% CI, 1.1-6.3). The mean numbers of packs of cigarettes-year in adenocarcinoma patients with and without at least one variant allele were 5.0 ± 2.5 and 37.2 ± 6.5 (P<0.05) respectively. A lower dose of cigarette smoking is sufficient to exert a carcinogenic effect on the incidence of adenocarcinoma patients carrying the susceptible allele. The absence of an association between AA RFLP and all cell types of lung cancer was also reported by Kelsey *et al.* (1995) (72 cases; 97 controls) and London *et al.* (1995) (144 cases; 230 controls) in an African-American population. Furthermore, London *et al.* did not confirm (in 51 cases) that AA RFLP may be an important risk factor for adenocarcinoma of the lung in the African-American population reported by Taioli *et al.* (1995a).

Other cancer sites

Taioli *et al.* (1995) also examined the role of AA RFLP in susceptibility to breast cancer in African-Americans (21 cases; 86 controls) and Caucasians (30 cases; 86 controls) and found no association in either group.

Discussion

Most P450 metabolism results in the detoxification of a wide variety of xenobiotics, although certain chemicals are activated in this process to electrophilic forms that can damage DNA and sometimes produce carcinogenic transformation of the cells (Omura *et al.*, 1993; Guengerich & Shimada, 1991; Kawajiri & Fujii-Kuriyama, 1991). Since this P450-mediated bioactivation is an initial and obligatory step in chemical carcinogenesis, interindividual variation in the metabolic activity of P450s may influence subsequent steps, including detoxification by Phase II enzymes, the formation of DNA-carcinogen adducts and ultimate cancer consequence.

The genetic difference in phenotypic expression and/or structure of P450 genes is worthy of study in order to explain the interindividual or interracial difference in cancer susceptibility (Kawajiri & Fujii-Kuriyama, 1991; Gonzalez, 1995). Most studies in this area compare the frequency of metabolic phenotypes or genotypes of a P450 enzyme between cancer patients and controls. In metabolic phenotype comparison studies it may be necessary to pay more attention to the development of methods of determining phenotypes, and also to the examination of the possible influences of medication on both patients and controls (especially hospital controls), since some P450s can be induced by chemicals (Omura *et al.*, 1993). Even a simple case-control comparison of phenotype or genotype frequency should examine the selection bias of controls, who must be representative of the general population from which patients are drawn. In this sense, hospital controls are, in general, not desirable because they are a more or less biased population. A large DNA library from a general population may be appropriate as a control pool, and a follow-up study using the DNA library can confirm the results of case-control studies.

A close association of smoking-associated lung cancer incidence with the *Msp* I or *Ile-Val* polymorphisms of the human *CYP1A1* gene was found in Japanese people but not in Caucasians. A major reason for this discrepancy was an ethnic difference in the allelic frequency of these polymorphisms. In *Msp* I polymorphism the frequency of the susceptible allele of *m2* was 0.332 in 375 healthy Japanese people (Kawajiri *et al.*, 1993), while frequencies of *m2* in Norwegian (Telfre *et al.*, 1991), Finnish (Hirvonen *et al.*, 1992) and German (Drakoulis *et al.*, 1994) subjects were 0.115, 0.12 and 0.073 respectively. On the basis of the Hardy-Weinberg equation these data suggest that the frequency of genotype C (m2/m2) is 110/1000 among Japanese people and about 6-14/1000 among Caucasians, i.e. almost 8 to 18 times more frequent among Japanese subjects than in Caucasians. Clearly, studies involving a large number of subjects will be required to disclose associations of the Msp I and Ile-Val polymorphisms with lung cancer in different ethnic populations. It is of interest that there is a moderate risk elevation of heterozygous genotype B in Finnish (OR = 1.85; P = 0.125) (Hirvonen et al., 1992) or Norwegian (OR = 1.24) (Telfre et al., 1991) study populations. The possibility exists that in Caucasians the heterozygous genotype B and Ile/Val contribute substantially to the attributable risk of lung cancer.

As for the relationship between CYP1A1 genotypes and phenotypic expressions, Petersen et al. (1991), using family pedigree analysis, demonstrated that a high CYP1A1 inducible phenotype segregated concordantly with the m2 allele having the Msp I site. We constructed and expressed the cDNA for Ile- and Val-coded CYP1A1 in yeast cells and compared the catalytic activities (Kawajiri et al., 1993). Both AHH activity and mutagenic activity towards benzo(a)pyrene were studied and we found that the Val-type of CYP1A1 showed a higher AHH activity and mutagenicity than the Ile-type, although the enzyme activities were expressed at low levels. Recently, Zhang et al. (1996) reported that benzo(a)pyrene-7,8- and 9,10-dihydrodiol formation were comparable when purified CYP1A1-Ile[462] catalysed the reconstituted reaction compared with catalysis by CYP1A1-Val[462]. Kiyohara et al. (1996) reported that AHH inducibility was correlated with the Msp I polymorphism (P<0.0001) but no association was found for the Ile-Val polymorphism (P = 0.509). Age-adjusted AHH inducibility in lymphocytes with genotype A (n = 38), B (n = 37) and C (n = 7) was 4.89 ± 0.36, 4.82 ± 0.29 and 13.61 ± 1.44 respectively. They also found that basal AHH activity in lymphocytes with a homozygous mutant Val/Val genotype was significantly higher than that of the Ile-homozygote (P<0.05).

Frequency comparison should be followed by a well-designed case-control study. The relative risk is then estimated for phenotypes or genotypes and levels of exposure to carcinogens. The risk estimate of environmental exposures in different phenotypes or genotypes is important not only in the identification of susceptible individuals but also to clarify whether the observed genetic risk elevation results from an interaction of a susceptible genotype with environmental carcinogens or is determined prior to gene-enviroment interaction. Dose-response relationships between phenotypes or genotypes can provide decisive information on this matter. We investigated the difference in susceptibility to squamous cell carcinoma of the lung in terms of CYP1A1 genotypes, taking the amount of cigarettes consumed into account (Nakachi et al., 1991, 1993, 1995). Patients with a susceptible homozygous genotype of the Msp I or Ile-Val polymorphisms contracted the carcinoma after smoking fewer cigarettes than those with other genotypes. A case-control study revealed that individuals with the susceptible Msp I or Ile-Val genotype were at remarkably high risk, with an odds ratio of 6.55 or 8.46 respectively (95% CI, 2.49-17.24 or 2.48-28.85 respectively), at a low dose level of cigarette smoking. On the other hand this relative susceptibility of genotype C or Val/Val compared to genotype A or Ile/Ile decreased about 1.5-fold at the higher cigarette dose level. Although the risk of all genotypes increases at higher dose levels the genetic difference in cancer risk tends to reduce at high dose levels where the environmental influence outweighs genetic predispositions. It has also been reported that a lower cigarette dose is sufficient to exert carcinogenic effects on adenocarcinoma carrying the AA polymorphism (Taioli et al., 1995a).

However, the mechanisms of genetic predisposition to lung cancer remain largely obscure. Lung carcinogenesis seems to start from a clonal expansion of the cells that gained a selective growth advantage through early genetic change in the cells. Thus, genetic predisposing factors to smoking-associated lung cancer, such as CYP1A1 polymorphisms, may affect the mutational frequencies of target genes in early genetic alterations. In this respect, we examined p53 mutations in relation to CYP1A1 polymorphisms, using surgical specimens of 148 non-small-cell lung cancer (NSCLC) patients who were smokers (Kawajiri et al., 1996a). The frequency of p53 mutations among heavy smokers was higher than in patients who had never smoked (P<0.01; OR = 3.74; 95% CI, 1.46-9.56). Smokers with susceptible rare homozygous alleles, such as either the *Msp* I or *Ile-Val* polymorphism of the *CYP1A1* gene, exhibit a 4.5-fold (P<0.005; OR, 4.48; 95% CI, 1.64-12.26) or 5.5-fold (P<0.01: OR, 5.52; 95% CI, 1.55-19.64) higher risk of having a mutation of the *p53* gene than those with non-susceptible predominant homozygous alleles of the gene. A recent report showed that susceptibility to hepatocellular carcinoma induced by aflatoxin B_1 was associated with low activity of the detoxification enzyme epoxide hydrolase and *GSTM1* genotypes, resulting in increased *p53* mutation (McGlynn *et al.*, 1995). It has been reported that *p53* mutations in patients with NSCLC were associated not only with the genesis and progression of lung cancer but also with shortened survival as predictors of poor prognosis (Mitsudomi *et al.*, 1993; Horio *et al.*, 1993). We have recently shown that a germ line *Msp* I polymorphism of the *CYP1A1* gene is associated with various clinical parameters responsible for the poorer prognosis in patients with NSCLC; it is also an independent factor indicative of prognostic significance at the non-resectable advanced stage of the disease (Goto *et al.*, 1996).

References

Alexandrie, A.-K., Sundberg, M.I., Seidegard, J., Tornling, G. & Rannug, A. (1994) Genetic susceptibility to lung cancer with special emphasis on CYP1A1 and GSTM1: a study on host factors in relation to age at onset, gender and histological cancer types. *Carcinogenesis*, 15, 1785-1790

Ambrosone, C.B., Freudenheim, J.L., Graham, S., Marshall, J.R., Vena, J.E., Brasure, J.R., Laughlin, R., Nemoto, T., Michalek, A.M., Harrington, A., Ford, T.D. & Shields, P. Cytochrome (1995) P4501A1 and glutathione S-transferase (M1) genetic polymorphisms and postmenopausal breast cancer risk. *Cancer Res.*, 55, 3483-3485

Bale, A.E., Nebert, D.W. & McBride, O.W. (1987) Subchromosomal localization of the dioxin-inducible P_1-450 locus (CYP1) and description of two RFLPs detected with a 3' P_1-450 cDNA probe. *Cytogenet. Cell. Genet.*, 46, 574-575

Caporaso, N., Landi, M.T. & Vineis, P. (1991) Relevance of metabolic polymorphisms to human carcinogenesis: evaluation of epidemiological evidence. *Pharmacogenetics*, 1, 4-19

Crofts, F., Cosma, G.N., Currie, D., Taioli, E., Toniolo, P. & Garte, S. (1993) A novel *CYP1A1* gene polymorphism in African-Americans. *Carcinogenesis*, 14, 1729-1731

Drakoulis, N.D., Cascorbi, I., Brockmöller, C.R. & Roots, G.I. (1994) Polymorphisms in the human *CYP1A1* gene as susceptibility factors for lung cancer: exon-7 mutation (4889 A to G), and a T to C mutation in the 3'-flanking region. *Clin. Investig.*, 72, 240-248

Ema, M., Ohe, N., Suzuki, M., Mimura, J., Sogawa, K., Ikawa, S. & Fujii-Kuriyama, Y. (1994) Dioxin-binding activities of polymorphic forms of mouse and human Ah receptors. *J. Biol. Chem.*, 269, 27337-27343

Emery, A.E.H., Anand, R., Danford, N., Duncan, W. & Paton, L. (1978) Aryl-hydrocarbon-hydroxylase inducibility in patients with cancer. *Lancet*, 1, 470-472

Gahmberg, C.G., Sekki, A., Kosunen, T.U., Holsti, L.R. & Makela, O. (1979) Induction of aryl hydrocarbon hydroxylase activity and pulmonary carcinoma. *Int. J. Cancer*, 23, 302-305

Gonzalez, F.J. (1995) Genetic polymorphism and cancer susceptibility: Fourteenth Sapporo Cancer Seminar. *Cancer Res.*, 55, 710-715

Goto, I., Yoneda, S., Yamamoto, M. & Kawajiri, K. (1996) Prognostic significance of germ line polymorphisms of the *CYP1A1* and glutathione *S*-transferase genes in patients with non-small-cell lung cancer. *Cancer Res.*, 56, 3725-3730

Gotoh, O., Tagashira, Y., Iizuka, T. & Fujii-Kuriyama, Y. (1983) Structural characteristics of cytochrome P-450. Possible location of the haeme-binding cysteine in determined amino-acid sequence. *J. Biochem.*, 93, 807-817

Guengerich, F.P. & Shimada, T. (1991) Oxidation of toxic and carcinogenic chemicals by human cytochrome P-450 enzymes. *Chem. Res. Toxicol.*, 4, 391-407

Hamada, G.S., Sugimura, H., Suzuki, I., Nagura, K., Kiyohara, E., Iwase, T., Tanaka, M., Takahashi, T., Watanabe, S., Kino, I. & Tsugane, S. (1995) The heme-binding region polymorphism of cytochrome P450 IA1 (*CypIA1*), rather than the *Rsa* I polymorphism of IIE1(*CypIIE1*), is associated with lung cancer in Rio de Janeiro. *Cancer Epidemiol. Biomarkers Prev.*, 4, 63-67

Haugen, A., Willey, J., Borresen, A.L. & Tefre, T. (1990) *Pst* I polymorphism at the human P_1-450 gene on chromosome 15. *Nucleic Acids Res.*, 18, 3114

Hayashi, S.-I., Watanabe, J., Nakachi, K. & Kawajiri, K. (1991) Genetic linkage of lung cancer-associated *Msp* I polymorphism with amino acid replacement in the haeme binding region of the cytochrome P450 IA1 gene. *J. Biochem.*, 110, 407-411

Hildebrand, C.E., Gonzalez, F.J., McBride, O.W. & Nebert, D.W. (1985) Assignment of the human 2,4,7,8-tetrachlorodibenzo-*p*-dioxin-inducible cytochrome P_1-450 gene to chromosome 15. *Nucleic Acids Res.*, 13, 2009-2016

Hirvonen, A., Husgafvel-Pursianinen, K., Karjalainen, A., Anttila, S. & Vainio, H. (1992) Point-mutational *Msp* I and *Ile-Val* polymorphisms closely linked in the *CYP1A1* gene: Lack of association with susceptibility to lung cancer in a Finnish study population. *Cancer Epidemiol. Biomarkers Prev.*, 1, 485-489

Horio, Y.,Takahashi, T., Kuroishi, T., Hibi, K., Suyama, M., Niimi, T., Shimokata, K., Yamakawa, K., Ueda, R. & Takahashi, T. (1993) Prognostic significance of *p53* mutations and 3p deletions in primary resected non-small cell lung cancer. *Cancer Res.*, 53 1-4

Karki, N., Pokela, R., Nuutinen, L. & Pelkonen, O. (1987) Aryl hydrocarbon hydroxylase in lymphocytes and lung tissue from lung cancer patients and controls. *Int. J. Cancer*, 39, 565-570

Katoh, T., Inatomi, H., Nagaoka, A. & Sugita, A. (1995) Cytochrome P4501A1 gene polymorphism and homozygous deletion of the glutathione S-transferase M1 gene in urothelial cancer patients. *Carcinogenesis*, 16, 655-657

Kawajiri, K. (1998) Molecular epidemiology of lung cancer. In: Puga, A. & Wallace, K., eds, *Molecular Biology in Toxicology.* Washington DC, Taylor and Francis

Kawajiri, K., Eguchi, H., Nakachi, K., Sekiya, T. & Yamamoto, M. (1996a) Association of *CYP1A1* germ line polymorphisms with mutations of the *p53* gene in lung cancer. *Cancer Res.*, 56, 72-76

Kawajiri, K. & Fujii-Kuriyama, Y. (1991) P450 and human cancer. *Jpn. J. Cancer Res.*, 82, 1325-1335

Kawajiri, K., Nakachi, K., Imai, K., Watanabe, J. & Hayashi, S.-I. (1993) The *CYP1A1* gene and cancer susceptibility. *Crit. Rev. Oncol. Hematol.*, 14, 77-87

Kawajiri, K., Nakachi, K., Imai, K., Yoshii, A., Shinoda, N. & Watanabe, J. (1990) Identification of genetically high-risk individuals to lung cancer by DNA polymorphisms of the cytochrome P450 IA1 gene. *FEBS Lett.*, 263, 131-133

Kawajiri, K., Watanabe, J., Eguchi, H., Nakachi, K., Kiyohara, C. & Hayashi, S.-I. (1995) Polymorphisms of human Ah receptor gene are not involved in lung cancer. *Pharmacogenetics*, 5, 151-158

Kawajiri, K., Watanabe, J. & Hayashi, S.-I. (1996b) Identification of allelic variants of human *CYP1A1* gene. *Methods Enzymol.*, 272, 226-232

Kellermann, G., Luyten-Kellermann, M. & Shaw, C.R. (1973a) Genetic variation of aryl hydrocarbon hydroxylase in human lymphocytes. *Am. J. Hum. Genet.*, 25, 327-331

Kellermann, G., Shaw, C.R. & Luyten-Kellermann, M. (1973b) Aryl hydrocarbon hydroxylase inducibility and bronchogenic carcinoma. *N. Engl. J. Med.*, 289, 934-937

Kelsey, K.T., Wiencke, J.K. & Spitz, M.R. (1994) A race-specific polymorphism in the *CYP1A1* gene is not associated with lung cancer in African-Americans. *Carcinogenesis*, 15, 1121-1124

Kihara, M., Kihara, M. & Noda, K. (1995) Risk of smoking for squamous and small cell carcinomas of the lung modulated by combinations of CYP1A1 and GSTM1 gene polymorphisms in a Japanese population. *Carcinogenesis*, 16, 2331-2336

Kiyohara, C., Hirohata, T. & Inutsuka, S. (1996) The relationship between aryl hydrocarbon hydroxylase and polymorphisms in the *CYP1A1* gene. *Jpn. J. Cancer Res.*, 87, 18-24

Korsgaad, R., Trell, E., Simonsson, B.G., Stiksa, G., Janzon, L., Hood, B. & Oldbring, J. (1984) Aryl hydrocarbon hydroxylase induction levels in patients with malignant tumours associated with smoking. *J. Cancer Res. Clin. Oncol.*, 108, 286-289

Kouri, R.E., McKinney, C.E., Slomiany, D.J., Snodgrass, D.R., Wray, N.P. & McLemore, T.L. (1982) Positive correlation between high aryl hydrocarbon hydroxylase activity and primary lung cancer as analysed in cryopreserved lymphocytes. *Cancer Res.*, 42, 5030-5037

Kouri, R.E. & Nebert, D.W. (1977) Genetic regulation of susceptibility to polycyclic-hydrocarbon-induced tumours in the mouse. In: *Origins of Human Cancer*. Cold Spring Harbor, Cold Spring Harbor Laboratory Press, pp. 811-835

London, S.J., Daly, A.K., Fairbrother, K.S., Holmes, C., Carpenter, C.L., Navidi, W.C. & Idle, J.R. (1995) Lung cancer risk in African-Americans in relation to a race-specific *CYP1A1* polymorphism. *Cancer Res.*, 55, 6035-6037

McGlynn, K.A., Rosvold, E.A., Lustbader, E.D., Hu, Y., Clapper, M.L., Zhou, T., Wild, C.P., Xia, X.-L., Baffoe-Bonnie, A., Ofori-Adjei, D., Chen, G-C., London, W.T., Shen, F.-M. & Buetow, K.H. (1995) Susceptibility to hepatocellular carcinoma is associated with genetic variation in the enzymatic detoxification of aflatoxin B_1. *Proc. Natl. Acad. Sci. USA*, 92, 2384-2387

Micka, J., Milatovich,, A., Menon, A., Grabowski, G.A., Puga, A. & Nebert, D. (1997) Human Ah receptor (AHR) gene: localization to 7p15 and suggestive correlation of polymorphism with CYP1A1 inducibility. *Pharmacogenetics*, 7, 95-101

Mitsudomi,T., Oyama, T., Kusano, T., Osaki, T., Nakanishi, R. & Shirakusa, T. (1993) Mutations of the *p53* gene as a predictor of poor prognosis in patients with non-small-cell lung cancer. *J. Natl. Cancer Inst.*, 85, 2018-2023

Nakachi, K., Hayashi, S.-I., Kawajiri, K. & Imai, K. (1995) Association of cigarette smoking and *CYP1A1* polymorphisms with adenocarcinoma of the lung by grades of differentiation. *Carcinogenesis*, 16, 2209-2213

Nakachi, K., Imai, K., Hayashi, S.-I. & Kawajiri, K. (1993) Polymorphisms of the *CYP1A1* and glutathione S-transferase genes associated with susceptibility to lung cancer in relation to cigarette dose in a Japanese population. *Cancer Res.*, 53, 2994-2999

Nakachi, K., Imai, K., Hayashi, S.-I., Watanabe, J. & Kawajiri, K. (1991) Genetic susceptibility to squamous cell carcinoma of the lung in relation to cigarette smoking dose. *Cancer Res.*, 51, 5177-5180

Nebert, D.W. (1978) Genetic differences in microsomal electron transport: the Ah locus. *Methods Enzymol.*, LII, 226-240

Nebert, D.W., Petersen, D.D. & Puga, A. (1991) Human AH locus polymorphism and cancer: inducibility of *CYP1A1* and other genes by combustion products and dioxin. *Pharmacogenetics*, 1, 68-78

Okada, T., Kawashima, K., Fukushi, S., Minakuchi, T. & Nishimura, S. (1994) Association between a cytochrome CYP IA1 genotype and incidence of lung cancer. *Pharmacogenetics*, 4, 333-340

Omura, T., Ishimura, Y. & Fujii-Kuriyama, Y. (1993) *Cytochrome P-450*. Second edition. Tokyo, Kodansha

Paigen, B., Gurtoo, H.L., Minowada, J., Houten, L., Vincent, R., Paigen, K., Parker, N.B., Ward, E. & Hayner, N.T. (1977) Questionable relation of aryl hydrocarbon hydroxylase to lung cancer risk. *N. Engl. J. Med.*, 297, 346-350

Paigen, B., Ward, E., Steenland, K., Havens, M. & Sartori, P. (1979) Aryl hydrocarbon hydroxylase inducibility is not altered in bladder cancer patients or their progeny. *Int. J. Cancer*, 23, 312-315

Petersen, D.D., McKinney, C.E., Ikeya, K., Smith, H.H., Bale, A.E., McBride, O.W. & Nebert, D.W. (1991) Human *CYP1A1* gene: Cosegregation of the enzyme inducibility phenotype and an RFLP. *Am. J. Hum. Genet.*, 48, 720-725

Shields, P.G., Caporaso, N.E., Falk, R.T., Sugimura, H., Trivers, G.E., Trump, B.F., Hoover, R.N., Weston, A. & Harris, C.C. (1993) Lung cancer, race, and a *CYP1A1* genetic polymorphism. *Cancer Epidemiol. Biomarkers Prev.*, 2, 481-485

Sivaraman, L., Leatham, M.P., Yee, J., Wilkens, L.R., Lau, A.F. & Marchand, L.L. (1994) *CYP1A1* genetic polymorphisms and *in situ* colorectal cancer. *Cancer Res.*, 54, 3692-3695

Spurr, N.K., Gough, A.C., Stevenson, K. & Wolf, C.R. (1987) *Msp* I polymorphism detected with a cDNA probe for the P-450 I family on chromosome 15. *Nucleic Acids Res.*, 15, 5901

Sugimura, H., Suzuki, I., Hamada, S.G., Iwase, H., Takahashi, T., Nagura, K., Iwata, H., Watanabe, S., Kino, I. & Tsugane, S. (1994) Cytochrome P-450 IA1 genotype in lung cancer patients and controls in Rio de Janeiro, Brazil. *Cancer Epidemiol. Biomarkers Prev.*, 3, 145-148

Suzuki, T., Sobue, T., Fujimoto, I., Doi, O. & Tateishi, R. Association of adenocarcinoma of the lung with cigarette smoking by grade of differentiation and subtype. *Cancer Res.*, 50, 444-447

Taioli, E., Crofts, F., Trachman, J., Demopoulos, R., Toniolo, P. & Garte, S.J. (1995a) A specific African-American *CYP1A1* polymorphism is associated with adenocarcinoma of the lung. *Cancer Res.*, 55, 472-473

Taioli, E., Trachman, J., Chen, X., Toniolo, P. & Garte, S. (1995b) A *CYP1A1* restriction fragment polymorphism is associated with breast cancer in African-American women. *Cancer Res.*, 55, 3757-3758

Tefre, T., Ryberg, D., Haugen, A., Nebert, D.W., Skaug, V., Brogger, A. & Borresen, A.-L. (1991) Human *CYP1A1*(cytochrome P_1-450) gene: lack of association between the *Msp* I restriction fragment length polymorphism and incidence of lung cancer in a Norwegian population. *Pharmacogenetics*, 1, 20-25

Trell, L., Korsgaad, R., Janzon, L. & Trell, E. (1985) Distribution and reproducibility of aryl hydrocarbon hydroxylase inducibility in a prospective population study of middle-aged male smokers and nonsmokers. *Cancer*, 56, 1988-1994

Ward, E., Paigen, B., Steenland, K., Vincent, R., Minowada, J., Gurtoo, H., Sartori, P. & Havens, M.B. (1978) Aryl hydrocarbon hydroxylase in persons with lung or laryngeal cancer. *Int. J. Cancer*, 22, 384-389

Zhang, Z.-F., Fasco, M.J., Huang, L., Guengerich, F.P. & Kaminsky, S. (1996) Characterization of purified human recombinant cytochrome P4501A1-IIe[462] and -Val[462]: assessment of a role for the rare allele in carcinogenesis. *Cancer Res.*, 56, 3926-3933

Kaname Kawajiri
Department of Biochemistry,
Saitama Cancer Center Research Institute,
818 Komuro, Ina, Saitama 362, Japan

Metabolic Polymorphisms and Susceptibility to Cancer
W. Ryder
IARC Scientific Publications No. 148
International Agency for Research on Cancer, Lyon, 1999

Chapter 16. Human cytochrome P4501A2

M. T. Landi, R. Sinha, N. P. Lang and F. F. Kadlubar

CYP1A2, a member of the cytochrome P450 superfamily (CYPs), is involved in the metabolic activation of several carcinogens, among them aromatic and heterocyclic amines, nitroaromatic compounds, mycotoxins and estrogens. Several drugs are also metabolized by CYP1A2. Individual differences in CYP1A2 activity may thus influence individual susceptibility to cancer risk and the therapeutic efficacy of some drugs.

In humans, CYP1A2 has been detected only in the liver, where it seems to be regulated by at least two mechanisms, one controlling constitutive levels of expression and another regulating inducibility.

Wide interindividual differences in CYP1A2 activity have been described. They may be due to factors such as gender, race, genetic polymorphisms, and exposure to inducers. Higher activity has been shown in men than in women.

Wide variation across racial/ethnic groups has been reported. Overall, slow and intermediate CYP1A2 metabolizers represent about 50% of Caucasians, while their frequency in Japanese subjects seems to be much lower. No nucleotide differences that could explain the phenotypic variability of the CYP1A2 gene have been found in any exons, exon-intron junctions, or 5'-flanking regions of the gene. However, two genetic variants have been identified which seem to be associated with CYP1A2 inducibility only. Induction of CYP1A2 activity has been reported as a consequence of cigarette smoking, dietary factors, several drugs, chronic hepatitis, and exposure to polybrominated biphenyls and 2,3,7,8-tetrachlorodibenzo-p-dioxin.

Several epidemiological studies have been conducted into the relationship between CYP1A2 activity, alone or in combination with other CYPs, and cancer risk. In the absence of a genotypic assay, only the CYP1A2 phenotype can be assessed at present. Many compounds have been tested as in vitro probes to assess CYP1A2 activity in humans. Currently, caffeine has the best potential for use in epidemiological studies: metabolites of caffeine after coffee consumption are measured as an index of CYP1A2 activity. Variable results have been obtained with caffeine-based methods, the use of some caffeine metabolite ratios having given bimodal or trimodal distributions while others have suggested normal or unimodal distributions.

Although the epidemiological studies are limited because only phenotyping data are available, there is a suggestion of increased risk of colon cancer and bladder cancer in subjects with rapid CYP1A2 activity. A higher level of 4-aminobiphenyl-haemoglobin adducts has also been found in moderate smokers with rapid CYP1A2 phenotype than in subjects with slow activity.

Molecular biology and biochemistry of cytochrome P4501A2

Cytochrome P4501A2 (CYP1A2) belongs to a superfamily of about 30 cytochrome P450s (CYPs) that are known to be expressed in human tissues (Nelson et al., 1996). There are two other closely related CYPs, CYP1A1 and CYP1B1, which bear 72% and 40% amino acid sequence similarity to CYP1A2 (Sutter et al., 1994) and together represent the products of the CYP1 gene family. The CYP1A2 and CYP1A1 genes each consist of 7 exons and are located in tandem on chromosome 15 (15q22-qter), while CYP1B1 is located on chromosome 2 and consists of 3 exons. The CYP1A2 and CYP1A1 genes undoubtedly arose as a consequence of gene duplication during speciation in mammals, while the divergence of CYP1B1 from CYP1As occurred much earlier. A unique feature of the human *CYP1* genes is the presence of a non-coding first exon. In addition, CYP1A2, CYP1A1 and CYP1B1 each show tissue-specific constitutive expression as well as tissue-specific inducibility. Interestingly, while CYP1A2 and CYP1A1 exhibit distinct but broad substrate specificity, CYP1B1 has a narrower spectrum of substrates yet has overlapping specificity with CYP1A2 and CYP1A1. The *CYP1A2* gene is well conserved across mammalian species (>70%) and retains remarkably similar substrate specificity, although tissue-specific expression and inducibility are species- and strain-dependent. In humans, there is also wide interindividual variation in CYP1A2 enzyme activity, depending on ethnic origin, gender and interaction between host and environment/diet.

Substrates and mechanisms of oxidation

A variety of therapeutic drugs, environmental and dietary carcinogens, and endogenous estrogens are known substrates for human CYP1A2 (Table 1). These comprise several chemical classes and involve oxidation of both nitrogen and carbon atoms to form *N*-hydroxy arylamines, phenols, epoxides, and carbinols, the latter often being unstable and leading to dealkylated products (Kadlubar & Hammons, 1987; Lemoine *et al.*, 1993; Bertilsson *et al.*, 1994; Eaton *et al.*, 1995; Shimada *et al.*, 1996; Carlson *et al.*, 1995; Spaldin *et al.*, 1995; Sharer & Wrighton, 1996).

While the catalytic mechanism for CYPs is generally thought to involve formation of radical intermediates prior to oxygen rebound (Guengerich & MacDonald, 1984), there is evidence that CYP1A2 differs by forming an enzyme-substrate complex that consists of a 2-electron oxidized intermediate-hydroxyl ion transition state that collapses to form the metabolic product (Hammons *et al.*, 1985). Such a mechanistic difference could account for the regioselectivity of CYP1A2 vs. other CYPs (e.g. *N*-oxidation vs. *ring*-oxidation of arylamines, which are often catalysed preferentially by CYP1A2 and CYP1A1 respectively).

Table 1. Classes of substrates for CYP1A2

CHEMICAL CLASS	SUBSTRATES[a]	REACTION TYPE
Drugs	Caffeine, theophylline, phenacetin, acetaminophen, nicotine, tacrine, imipramine, antipyrine, aminopyrine, clozapine	Dealkylation, *ring*-oxidation
Aromatic amines	4-aminobiphenyl, 2-naphthylamine, 2-aminofluorene, aminoanthracene, 2-acetylaminofluorene	*N*-oxidation, *ring*-oxidation
Heterocyclic amines	PhIP, IQ, MeIQx, AaC, Trp-P2, Glu-P1, MeIQ, DiMeIQx	*N*-oxidation, *ring*-oxidation
Nitrosamines	4-(methylnitrosamino)-1-(3-pyridyl)-1-butanone	Dealkylation
Mycotoxins	Aflatoxin B₁, ipomeanol, sterigmatocystin	Epoxidation, *ring*-oxidation
Nitroaromatics	6-nitrochrysene	Epoxidation
Estrogens	17β-estradiol	*ring*-oxidation

[a] The substrates listed are those in which CYP1A2 has been shown to be the major CYP involved in the catalysis. PhIP, 2-amino-6-phenylimidazo[4,5-*b*]pyridine; IQ, 2-amino-3-methylimidazo[4,5-*f*]quinoline; MeIQx, 2-amino-3,8-dimethylimidazo[4,5-*f*] quinoxaline; AC, 2-amino-α-carboline; Trp-P2, 3-amino-1-methyl-5*H*-pyrido[4,3-*b*]indole; Glu-P1, 2-amino-6-methyldipyrido [1,2-α: 3,2'-*d*]-imidazole; MeIQ, 2-amino-3,5-dimethylimidazo[4,5-*f*]quinoline; DiMeIQx, 2-amino-3,4,8-trimethylimidazo[4,5-*f*]quinoxaline.

Tissue distribution

In humans, CYP1A2 has been detected only in the liver. Using immunochemical and/or enzymatic assays, no significant levels (<0.1% of the liver) have been found in peripheral lung (Shimada *et al.*, 1992), larynx (Degawa *et al.*, 1994), small intestinal or colon mucosa, kidney, urinary bladder epithelium, prostate, breast, placenta or lymphocytes (Kadlubar & Guengerich, unpublished data). In contrast, CYP1A1 is expressed in lung, larynx, kidney, placenta, lymphocytes and fetal liver (Guengerich & Shimada, 1991; Degawa *et al.*, 1994; Pasanen & Pelkonen, 1994; Hakkola *et al.*, 1994); while CYP1B1 has been measured in breast, ovary, prostate, and uterine myometrium (Liehr *et al.*, 1995; Shimada *et al.*, 1996).

Constitutive expression and induction

Phenotyping studies (see below) have suggested that CYP1A2 is regulated by at least two mechanisms: one that controls constitutive levels of expression and another that regulates inducibility (Butler *et al.*, 1992; Sinha *et al.*, 1994; Lang *et al.*, 1994; Kadlubar, 1994). Induction of CYP1A2 activity has been reported as a consequence of cigarette smoking, consumption of charbroiled or high-temperature cooked meats, dosing with indole-3-carbinol (and ingestion of large amounts of cruciferous vegetables, which also contain indole-3-carbinol), omeprazole (an anti-ulcer drug), phenytoin (an anti-epileptic drug), rifampin (a tuberculostatic drug), environmental exposure to polybrominated biphenyls, and chronic pancreatitis (Guengerich & Shimada, 1991; Eaton *et al.*, 1995;

Wietholtz *et al.*, 1989, 1995; Chaloner *et al.*, 1990). Consequently, a polymorphic distribution of CYP1A2 activity is often observed and is generally bimodal or trimodal. Comparisons of smokers vs. non-smokers and of persons consuming high-temperature vs. low-temperature cooked meat indicate that the polymorphic distribution exists in both induced and uninduced populations and that there are individuals with both high and low levels of CYP1A2 activity who are either inducible or non-inducible.

Examination of the 5'-flanking region of the *CYP1A2* gene using cultured human cell lines, *CYP1A2* sequence-reporter gene constructs, and gel mobility shift analyses with nuclear lysates has revealed several putative regulatory elements (Eaton *et al.*, 1995; Chung & Bresnick, 1995; Muntané-Relat *et al.*, 1995). These include: 1) "xenobiotic-responsive element-like" sequences that may be bound by an aromatic hydrocarbon receptor (AhR) complex; 2) potential binding sites for transcription factors including NF-1/CCAAT, SP-1, HNF-1 and AP-1; and 3) "antioxidant-responsive" and "interleukin-6-responsive" elements. However, none of these putative regulatory regions has yet been associated with individual differences in hepatic CYP1A2 phenotype. Furthermore, sequencing of the *CYP1A2* gene, including the 5'-flanking region (up to -3 kb from exon 1), all 7 exons, and the intron-exon junctions, from persons with both high and low activity, has not yet shown any genetic basis for a CYP1A2 polymorphism (Nakajima *et al.*, 1994). Moreover, the mechanism of CYP1A2 induction can involve both AhR-dependent and AhR-inde-

Table 2. Tissue distribution and induction of the human CYP1 family

CYP1	TISSUE	ENZYME INDUCERS
CYP1A1	Lung, placenta, lymphocytes, larynx, kidney, fetal liver	Tobacco smoke, polychlorinated biphenyls, 2,3,7,8-tetrachlorodibenzo-*p*-dioxin
CYP1A2	Liver	Charbroiled or high-temperature cooked meat, tobacco smoke, omeprazole, phenytoin, rifampin, polybrominated biphenyls, chronic pancreatitis, 2,3,7,8-tetrachlorodibenzo-*p*-dioxin
CYP1B1	Kidney, breast, ovary, prostate, uterine myometrium	2,3,7,8-tetrachlorodibenzo-*p*-dioxin

pendent pathways (Daujat *et al.*, 1992). Accordingly, whatever mechanisms are eventually found to be operative for polymorphic CYP1A2 expression and inducibility will need to account for: 1) tissue-specific inducibility and expression of CYP1A2 in the liver; and 2) refractoriness for CYP1A1 and CYP1B1 inducibility/expression in liver but not in extrahepatic tissues.

It should also be noted that there is a lack of correlation between CYP1 mRNA levels and protein levels in various tissues (Hakkola *et al.*, 1996a, 1996b). For example, CYP1A2 protein levels do not correlate well with CYP1A2 mRNA levels in the liver; moreover, there is abundant CYP1A1 mRNA in many human livers but no detectable CYP1A1 protein levels (Schweikl *et al.*, 1993; Hakkola *et al.*, 1994; Kamataki *et al.*, unpublished data). In contrast, human CYP1A1 protein is expressed in fetal liver, in primary hepatocyte cultures, and even in precision-cut liver slices (Donato *et al.*, 1995; Lake *et al.*, 1996). Thus, there must also exist tissue-specific mRNA translational controls for CYP1 protein expression (Table 2).

In vivo *inhibitors of CYP1A2*
Although a number of chemical inhibitors of CYP1A2 activity have been identified *in vitro* (e.g. α-naphthoflavone, which also inhibits CYP1A1 and CYP1B1, but not other known CYPs), relatively few compounds appear to inhibit CYP1A2 activity *in vivo*. Among those that do are several drugs, including fluvoxamine, enoxacin, ciprofloxacin, furafylline (Eaton *et al.*, 1995), cimetidine (Loi *et al.*, 1993), idrocilamide (Brazier *et al.*, 1980), mexiletene (Joeres & Richter, 1987), verapamil (Fuhr *et al.*, 1992b), 5-methoxypsoralen (Bendriss *et al.*, 1996) and caffeine (Iqbal *et al.*, 1995). Of these, furafylline is a specific mechanism-based inactivator of CYP1A2 (Kunz & Trager, 1993). In addition, grapefruit juice and its major constituent, naringenin, has been reported to inhibit CYP1A2 activity in humans (Fuhr & Kummert, 1995). Evidence for decreased levels of CYP1A2, based on caffeine or theophylline clearance data, has also been obtained in subjects with chronic liver disease (Rodopoulos *et al.*, 1995), in individuals consuming low-protein diets (Kappas *et al.*, 1965), and in women during pregnancy (Brazier *et al.*, 1983) or taking oral contraceptives (Abernethy & Todd, 1985).

Interspecies comparisons
In rodents and humans, CYP1A2, CYP1A1 and CYP1B1 show high amino acid sequence homologies across species (72%-90%; Sutter *et al.*, 1994) and remarkably similar substrate specificity (Shimada *et al.*, 1989; Butler *et al.*, 1989a, 1989b; Guengerich & Shimada, 1991, Shimada *et al.*, 1996) for aromatic and heterocyclic amines and polycyclic aromatic hydrocarbons, but not for 17-estradiol (Dannan *et al.*, 1986). Humans also differ in the specificity of CYP1A induction. In all other mammalian species examined, treatment with enzyme inducers results in co-induction of both CYP1A1 and CYP1A2 *in vivo* in the liver (Bullock *et al.*, 1995); in humans, only CYP1A2 is induced or constitutively expressed in liver (see above).

CYP1A2 phenotyping
Role of CYP1A2 in metabolic activation pathways
CYP1A2 is involved in the metabolism of several chemical carcinogens, such as aromatic and heterocyclic amines, nitroaromatic compounds, mycotoxins, and estrogens (see above).

The carcinogenicity of aromatic amines has been well established in both humans and experimental animals, particularly for the urinary bladder (Garner *et al.*, 1984). Aromatic amines, such as 4-aminobiphenyl (ABP), 2-naphthylamine (2-NA) and *o*-toluidine, are found in cigarette smoke (IARC Monograph, 1986), as well as in coal- and shale-derived oils and in agricultural chemicals (Kadlubar & Hammons, 1987). The *N*-oxidation of ABP and other aromatic amines is preferentially catalysed by CYP1A2 and can produce an *N*-hydroxy intermediate that can enter the circulation, undergo renal filtration, enter the urinary bladder lumen, and be reabsorbed across the epithelium where arylamine-DNA adduct formation can occur (Kadlubar *et al.*, 1991; Badawi *et al.*, 1995).

Heterocyclic aromatic amines (HAAs) are produced during the cooking of meats and fish when juices pyrolyse (Sugimura *et al.*, 1988; Hatch *et al.*, 1992) and their amounts increase with longer cooking times and higher temperatures (Knize *et al.*, 1994). Pan-fried meat diets containing high levels of HAAs and minimal levels of PAHs are able to induce CYP1A2 activity (Sinha *et al.*, 1994). An association between consumption of "well done" (Schiffman et al., 1990; Lang et al., 1994) , "barbecued" (Peters et al., 1989), "browned" (Gerhardsson et al., 1991), and "red meat" (Giovannucci et al., 1994) with colorectal cancer has been shown; and this risk may be due to the quantity of HAAs produced during cooking procedures. HAAs also need to be metabolically activated in order to act as carcinogens and, like the aromatic amines, the first step is generally CYP1A2-dependent (Kato, 1986). In vitro studies have clearly shown that the metabolic activation of compounds such as 2-amino-1-methyl-6-phenylimidazo[4,5-b]pyridine (PhIP), 2-amino-3-methylimidazo[4,5-f]quinoline (IQ), 2-amino-3,8-dimethylimidazo[4,5-f]quinoxaline (MeIQx), 2-amino-α-carboline (AC), 3-amino-1-methyl-5H-pyrido[4,3-b]indole (Trp-P2), 2-amino-6-methyldipyrido[1,2-a:3,2'-d]imidazole (Glu-P1), 2-amino-3,5-dimethylimidazo[4,5-f]quinoline (MeIQ), 2-amino-3,4,8- trimethylimidazo[4,5-f]quinoxaline (DiMeIQx), and 2-amino-3,8-dimethylimidazo[4,5-f]quinoxaline (MeIQx) proceeds almost entirely through CYP1A2-dependent N-oxidation (Turesky et al., 1991; Lynch et al., 1995; Raza et al., 1996). Once oxidized, the N-hydroxy HAA metabolites are then O-acetylated in the liver or in another appropriate organ, predominantly by the polymorphic N-acetyltransferase (NAT2), and may form arylamine-DNA adducts (Kaderlik et al., 1994).

Some nitrosamines are also metabolized by CYP1A2. 4-methyl-nitrosamino-1-(3-pyridyl)-1-butanone (NNK) is one of the most potent carcinogens contained in tobacco smoke, mostly derived from nicotine during tobacco curing (Hecht & Hoffmann, 1988). In cell lines expressing human P450, NNK is activated by CYP1A2 to mutagenic metabolites (Crespi et al., 1991). A recent study showed that subjects who smoke blond (flue-cured) tobacco, which contains less aromatic amines but higher tobacco-specific nitrosamines than black (air-cured) tobacco, have higher CYP1A2 activity (Landi et al., 1996).

6-nitrochrysene, a potent liver and lung carcinogen in mice (Busby et al., 1985; Wislocki et al., 1986), derived mostly from diesel exhaust (Pasche et al., 1992), is metabolized by CYP1A2 to the proximate carcinogen trans-1,2-dihydroxy-6-nitrochrysene in human microsomes (Chae et al., 1993).

Aflatoxin B_1 (AFB$_1$) is the most potent of the difuranocoumarin mycotoxins that have been associated with liver cancer in developing countries, mostly in combination with endemic viral hepatitis (Qian et al., 1994; Hall & Wild, 1994). AFB$_1$ requires oxidation at the 8,9 vinyl bond to produce a reactive intermediate, AFB$_1$-exo-8,9-epoxide (AFBO), which forms a DNA adduct at the N7-guanyl position (Raney et al., 1993). Human cell lines selectively expressing CYP1A2 can activate AFB$_1$ to mutagenic metabolites at low substrate concentrations (Crespi et al., 1991). In human liver microsomes, CYP1A2 seems to be a high-affinity P450 enzyme (CYP3A4 exhibits a lower affinity) and is active at low AFB$_1$ substrate concentrations approaching those of dietary exposure (Gallagher et al., 1994). CYP1A2 is also involved in the detoxification of AFB1 to AFM1, while CYP3A4 also catalyses the detoxification of AFB1 to AFQ1.

Many steroid hormones are oxidized by P450 enzymes. In extracts of HepG2 cells, CYP1A2 was the most efficient enzyme for the 2-hydroxylation of estradiol and therefore may be the principal P450 involved in estradiol metabolism at this position (Aoyama et al., 1990). A role for CYP1A2 in androstenedione 6-hydroxylation ($r = 0.48$) was also sugggested by another study using human liver microsomes (Waxman et al., 1988).

Laboratory methods

Several compounds have been tested as in vitro and in vivo probes to assess CYP1A2 activity in humans. The analgesic drug phenacetin was widely used to measure the CYP1A2-dependent phenacetin O-deethylation in vitro and in vivo (Distlerath et al., 1985; Sesardic et al., 1988; Conney et al., 1976) until it was recognized as a potential human carcinogen (Bengtsson et al., 1978). Theophylline (1,3-dimethylxanthine; 13X) has also been used as a CYP1A2 probe in vitro and in vivo (Guengerich & Turvey, 1991; Murray et al., 1993; Miller et al., 1985), and its use is supported by the demonstration that the generation of 3-methylxanthine (3X) and 1,3-dimethyluric acid (13U) from theophylline is selectively catalysed by CYP1A2 (Sarkar & Jackson, 1994; Zhang & Kaminsky, 1995). However, only a proportion of total theophylline metabolism generates 3X and 13U (Gu et al.,

1992), and this may constitute a limit in the use of theophylline for measuring CYP1A2 activity. Currently, caffeine (1,3,7-trimethylxanthine; 137X), a widely used, relatively innocuous drug, has the best potential for use as a probe in epidemiological studies. Caffeine is almost completely metabolized in the body with the initial formation of paraxanthine (1,7-dimethylxanthine; 17X) as the major metabolite through 3-demethylation (Alvarez *et al.*, 1979; Berthou *et al.*, 1992). The 3-demethylation of caffeine is catalysed by CYP1A2 (Butler *et al.*, 1989b) and, at a lower rate, by CYP1A1; but since CYP1A1 is not constitutively expressed in the liver (Murray *et al.*, 1993), caffeine metabolism reflects hepatic CYP1A2 activity. CYP2E1 may also contribute to primary caffeine metabolism, but only to a minor extent at high substrate concentrations (Tassaneeyakul *et al.*, 1994).

Caffeine-based procedures (Table 3) for assessing CYP1A2 activity *in vivo* utilize caffeine concentrations in plasma or saliva (caffeine clearance), urinary or plasma caffeine metabolite ratios, and ^{14}C- or ^{13}C-[N-3-methyl]-caffeine breath tests (Butler *et al.*, 1992; Tanaka *et al.*, 1992; Kalow & Tang, 1993; Lang *et al.*, 1994; Lambert *et al.*, 1986; McQuilkin *et al.*, 1994) and have also been proposed or used in a variety of cancer epidemiology studies (Table 3).

These methods are based on secondary or tertiary metabolites, which do not arise exclusively from CYP1A2 metabolism, and may vary with urinary flow rates, interethnic differences in CYP activity and renal function, various induction conditions, and the use of different sampling procedures (Kalow & Tang, 1993; Fuhr & Rost, 1995; Kadlubar *et al.*, 1996). These factors may account for the variability in results obtained by different studies. In fact, the use of some caffeine metabolite ratios has resulted in bimodal or trimodal distributions, consistent with family studies and *in vitro* metabolism data (see below), while others have suggested normal or unimodal distributions (see Table 3). Efforts to clarify the reasons for het-

Table 3. Caffeine phenotyping methods for CYP1A2

METHODS	ASSAY PROCEDURE	FREQUENCY DISTRIBUTION
Caffeine breath test	^{13}C-caffeine dosing, $^{13}CO_2/^{12}CO_2$ at 1 hr, isotope dilution MS	Unimodal, trimodal[a,b]
Caffeine metabolites	Caffeine tablets or coffee extraction & HPLC analysis	
17X/137X in urine (3-6 hr)		Trimodal/bimodal[c,d]
17X/137X in plasma (5-7 hr)		Bimodal[e]
17X/137X in saliva (5-7 hr)		Bimodal[e]
(17X + 17U)/137X in urine (4-5 hr)		Trimodal/bimodal[f,g]
(AFMU + 1X + 1U)/17U in urine (2-24 hr)		Unimodal[h]
(AAMU + 1X + 1U)/17U in urine (2-24 hr)		Unimodal[i]

[a] Lambert *et al.*, 1990; [b]Kadlubar *et al.*, in preparation; [c]Kadlubar *et al.*, 1990; [d]McQuilkin *et al.*, 1995; [e]Fuhr & Rost, 1994; [f]Butler *et al.*, 1992; [g]Nakajima *et al.*, 1994; [h]Campbell *et al.*, 1987; [i]Kalow & Tang, 1991. The abbreviations used are: MS, mass spectrometry; HPLC, high performance liquid chromatography; 17X, 1,7-dimethylxanthine (paraxanthine); 137X, 1,3,7-trimethylxanthine (caffeine); 17U, 1,7-dimethyluric acid; AFMU, 5-acetyl-6-formylamino-3-methyluracil; 1X, 1-methylxanthine; 1U, 1-methyluric acid; AAMU, 5-acetyl-6-amino-3-methyluracil.

erogeneity of results have been made. One of the major criticisms (Tang & Kalow, 1996) made of the (17X+17U)/137X ratio (Butler *et al.*, 1992) derives from work by Tang *et al.* (1994), who reported that caffeine (137X) excretion depends on urine flow; the bimodal distribution observed by the (17X+17U)/137X ratio thus only reflects a polymorphism in renal clearance of caffeine. Others (Lang *et al.*, 1994) have reported that, under controlled experimental conditions and methods of analysis, urinary caffeine concentrations are not dependent on urine flow, as previously shown by Birkett & Miners (1991). A recent study (Kadlubar et al., 1996; Kadlubar *et al.*, in preparation) has shown a urinary constituent that often co-migrates with caffeine on a variety of HPLC columns to be highly dependent on urine flow rate. This unknown constituent, probably of dietary origin, is present in 20%-50% of urine samples and has required the use of computerized photodiode-array detection systems to assure peak purities by comparison with spectral libraries of authentic standards. These authors think that the differences in results may also be due to a lack, in many studies, of diode array UV detection and spectral matching to assure analytical separation of this constituent from caffeine. In addition, the ratio (AAMU+1X+1U)/17U may also reflect CYP2E1 activity (Fuhr *et al.*, 1996) and confound study results. An extensive pharmacokinetic modelling study by Rostami-Hodjegan *et al.* (1996), utilizing the data of Tang *et al.* (1994) and concluding that the (17X+17U)137X ratio is invalid, may likewise be unfounded because of this analytical problem.

Another important point of discussion is related to the variable urine collection times (Table 3). The ratio (AAMU+1X+1U)/17U is measured in 24-hr urines (Kalow & Tang, 1991) or in spot urines (Denaro *et al.*, 1996), and appears to be more suitable for large studies, partly because measurements can be taken in subjects while they consume single or multiple doses of caffeine. In contrast, the (17X+17U)/137X ratio is measured in urine collected over the four to five hours after the consumption of a standardized cup of coffee, and subjects are instructed to avoid coffee consumption the day before the study (Butler *et al.*, 1992). This procedure is felt to be more accurate because the smallest peak on the HPLC elution profile is always caffeine and at four to five hours

the urine sample usually contains the highest concentration of caffeine, since at this time the blood caffeine concentrations are highest (Bonati *et al.*, 1982).

Many studies regard caffeine clearance, both in plasma and in saliva (caffeine half-life or paraxanthine/caffeine ratio in a spot sample), as the best possible reflection of CYP1A2 in liver (Tang *et al.*, 1994; Notarianni *et al.*, 1995; Denaro *et al.*, 1996; Rostami-Hodjegan *et al.*, 1996; Miners & Birkett, 1996), but the health and dietary conditions of the host may strongly influence the results. Furthermore, no strong experimental support has been shown for this assumption. Others (Kadlubar *et al.*, in preparation; Kadlubar *et al.*, 1996) consider the pulmonary excretion of $^{13}CO_2$ from a labelled caffeine dose in the caffeine breath test (Lambert *et al.*, 1983; Lambert *et al.*, 1990) as the most direct measure of CYP1A2-catalysed caffeine 3-demethylation in the liver, although the results may be influenced by the respiratory quotient and thus by physical activity, health conditions and diet (Fuhr & Rost, 1994).

These controversies underline the large variability found in CYP1A2 data. Earlier evidence for interindividual variability and polymorphisms are found in metabolic studies on CYP1A2 substrates, including phenacetin (Shahidi, 1968; Alvares *et al.*, 1979; Devonshire *et al.*, 1983), aromatic amines (Hammons *et al.*, 1985; Minchin *et al.*, 1985; Butler *et al.*, 1989a, 1989b) and heterocyclic amines (Yamazoe *et al.*, 1988).

At the molecular level, fifteenfold to sixtyfold CYP1A2 mRNA or protein levels have been found in liver samples (Sesardic *et al.*, 1988; Ikeya *et al.*, 1989; Butler *et al.*, 1989b; Schweickl *et al.*, 1993).

Intraindividual variability

CYP1A2 activity in humans appears to be a consequence of both heritable and environmental components. Nakajima *et al.* (1994) investigated the urinary (17U+17X)/137X ratio in 12 subjects (eight non-smokers and four smokers) on two occasions 11 months apart. The correlation between the first determination and second determination was 0.87. The coefficient of variation ranged from 0.7% to 84.5%. The difference between the two times may be due to either measurement error or various environmental factors such as diet, which was not controlled.

To study intraindividual variation in the caffeine metabolic ratio, Carillo & Benitez (1994) repeated six monthly determinations in ten subjects. They found no significant differences within each subject and the coefficients of variation for N-1-, N-3- and N-7-demethylations of caffeine were 5.2%, 13.7% and 14.1% respectively.

In the study reported by Sinha et al. (1994), 66 subjects were phenotyped by urinary caffeine metabolite on three occasions: at the start of the study when the subjects were on their normal diets; after one week on a diet containing minimal levels of known inducers; and after one week when the subjects were consuming high heterocyclic amine in meat cooked at high temperature. Apart from the method used to cook the meat, the diets for weeks one and two were identical. The investigators found that the CYP1A2 levels were induced in a majority of the subjects but there was a underlying "fixed" component to the CYP1A2 phenotype (correlation between CYP1A2 at the end of week one and at the end of week 2 was $r = 0.54$).

Interindividual variability

Interindividual differences in CYP1A2 phenotype may be due to different factors such as gender, race and environmental exposure to inducers. Some phenotyping studies show that age and gender differences do not account for large interindividual variation in CYP1A2 activity; while others have shown a higher CYP1A2 index among men than among women (Relling et al., 1992; Nakajima et al., 1994; Horn et al., 1995; Ross et al., 1996). Horn et al. (1995) showed a statistically significant difference between nulliparous and parous women. Parous women had CYP1A2 activity values (measured by the caffeine breath test) similar to those in men, whereas the results for women who had never given birth were lower. Decrease in caffeine clearance in pregnant women has been also reported (Knutti et al., 1981). The implication of these studies is that female hormones may have a role in the gender difference, and this is supported by evidence of impairment of caffeine clearance in females using low-dose estrogens (Abernethy & Todd, 1985) and by the finding that there is lower CYP1A2 activity in females using oral contraceptives than in females not using them (Catteau et al., 1995).

Caffeine toxicity in females, but not males, has also been associated with lower CYP1A2 activity (Carrillo & Benitez, 1996), suggesting the occurrence of drug-drug interactions.

In contrast to the hypothesis that hormonal factors are responsible for decreased CYP1A2 levels in women, Ross et al. (1996) have reported that females have significantly lower CYP1A2 activity than males when consuming their normal diet. However, when both groups were consuming a controlled diet in a metabolic study (Sinha et al., 1994) the difference in CYP1A2 activity between the genders was no longer present after one week. This implies that there is some component in the diet that can influence CYP1A2 activity which is consumed in different amounts by males and females.

A wide variation across racial/ethnic groups is one factor that may influence the results on the phenotypic distribution of slow, intermediate and rapid metabolizers of CYP1A2, as well as on the inducibility of this gene. Overall, slow CYP1A2 metabolizers represent about 10% in Caucasians, while their frequency in Japanese people seems to be much lower (Nakajima et al., 1994). Interestingly, the induction of CYP1A2 by cigarette smoking has recently been confirmed in Caucasians but not in Chinese or in African-Americans (Lang et al., 1994; Kadlubar, 1994). African-American subjects had lower CYP1A2 ratios than the Caucasians (Relling et al., 1992), while rural Shona children in Zimbabwe had lower CYP1A2 activity than urban children in this country as well as children and adults from Canada (Masimirenbwa et al., 1995).

The composition of study groups also varies widely. CYP1A2 is known to be induced by several drugs and environmental and dietary compounds (see above). All of the studies reporting a polymodal distribution analysed smokers and non-smokers separately, whereas the studies showing a log normal distribution did not. Not only the number of cigarettes smoked seems to be an important modifier but also the type of tobacco (Butler et al., 1992; Landi et al., 1996). Studies should have taken this factor into account, although even among non-smokers the levels of CYP1A2 are subject to large interindividual variation (Vistisen et al., 1992; Schweikl et al., 1993).

Dietary constituents that are known to induce CYP1A2, such as charcoal-broiled beef (Conney et al., 1976; Kappas et al., 1978; Kall & Clausen, 1995), pan-fried meat (Sinha et al., 1994), cruciferous vegetables (Pantuck et al., 1979; Vistisen et al., 1991; McDanell et al., 1992; Kall et al., 1996) may also differ widely between groups, along with alcohol (Horn et al., 1995) and drug consumption (Abernethy & Todd, 1985). Since a number of genetic determinants and environmental exposures are likely to influence CYP1A2 phenotype there is a need for further information on CYP1A2 expression or inducibility, particularly at the gene level.

Application to epidemiological studies
As discussed, CYP1A2 has an important role in the activation of several environmental and dietary carcinogens. Individual differences in constitutive and/or inducible expression of CYP1A2 may thus influence individual susceptibility to environmentally-related cancer risk. Several epidemiological studies have been conducted to investigate the relationship between CYP1A2 activity, alone or in combination with other CYPs, and cancer risk (see below). Other end points have been examined which may be related to cancer risk, e.g. the levels of ABP-haemoglobin adduct in relation to CYP1A2 phenotype in both smokers and nonsmokers (Landi et al., 1996). However, since the genetic polymorphism or polymorphisms responsible for CYP1A2 interindividual variability in humans have not yet been determined, all of these studies suffer limitations because only phenotyping data are available. Phenotype can be extremely useful in at-risk categories (Rothman et al., 1993) because of the large variability within this group and the importance of identifying subgroups at increased risk (Le Marchand et al., 1996). However, phenotype may exhibit continuous and overlapping variability due to numerous genetic and environmental factors, and separating the influence of the genetic background from environmental induction may be extremely difficult. For example, the study of the frequency of CYP1A2-dependent rapid metabolizers among smokers as a possible determinant of cancer risk can be confounded by the smoking-dependent induction of CYP1A2 activity. Conversely, it is improbable

that one would be able to select a group of pure genetically-determined rapid CYP1A2 individuals to investigate the effect of environmental exposures on cancer risk in those subjects. Moreover, in order to control for environmental inducers it would be necessary to have large sample sizes, and feasibility limitations could arise.

An effort has been made to detect genetic variations in CYP1A2 metabolism, and graphical methods, such as histograms and probit plots have been widely used. However, these methods can be subject to misinterpretation. Inflections of probit plots may arise from environmental factors acting differentially on subjects who are genetically identical at the determining loci. Conversely, an apparently normal distribution may conceal genetic heterogeneity (Vesell & Gaylor, 1995). It has been suggested that, if probit plots show apparent inflections, goodness of fit tests should be applied for comparing the measurements (in this case, the CYP1A2 activity level) of individuals to a specified type of statistical distribution (Jackson et al., 1989). However, these tests lack the power to detect subtle effects. Other graphical methods have been proposed, such as the normal test variable (Endrenyi & Patel, 1991) and diagnostic mixture detection plots (Roeder, 1994), but they may have similar limitations. Genetic analyses, possibly at molecular level (Vesell & Gaylor, 1995), in combination with phenotype procedures, therefore seem imperative.

CYP1A2 genotyping
CYP1A2 gene regulation
The human CYP1A2 gene (7.8 kilobases long and comprising seven exons and six introns), 3255 base pairs of the 5'-flanking region, and about 1500 base pairs of the 3'-non-coding region have been sequenced (Quattrochi & Tukey, 1989; Ikeya et al., 1989; as modified in GeneBank) and mapped to chromosome 15 (Jaiswal et al., 1987). The mRNA is 3119 bases in length, including the first non-coding exon (55 bases), and encodes a 515 amino acid sequence resulting in a protein with molecular weight of 58 294 daltons. The initiation codon starts with nucleotide 10 of exon 2. There is 79-83% similarity among human, mouse and rabbit CYP1A2 in exons 2 to 6 (Ikeya et al., 1989) and 80-91% similarity between exons 2, 4, 5 and 6 of human CYP1A1 and CYP1A2. The

high level of conserved nucleotides in these exons suggests that the encoded protein domain of such an exon is important in the catalytic function of both CYP1A1 and CYP1A2 enzymes. However, in general, there is more similarity in the human and mouse CYP1A2 than between human CYP1A1 and CYP1A2.

Three possible transcription regulatory sequences were found immediately upstream of the transcriptional start site (Eaton *et al.*, 1995). The three sequences are a TATA box at -27, two SP1 recognition sites (5'-GGGCGG-3'or 5'-CCGC-CC-3') at -37 and -907, and eight CCAAT elements spanning 3 kb of the 5'-flanking region, including one at -50 which is nearest to the transcription initiation site. In addition, three canonical 5-base pair boxes (CACGC), found upstream of all mammalian *CYP1A1* genes that are believed to interact with the aromatic hydrocarbon receptor complex, are present in the *CYP1A2* 5'-flanking region of human *CYP1A2* (Quattrochi & Tukey, 1989; Ikeya *et al.*, 1989; as modified in *GeneBank*). Interestingly, conserved regions were found in intron 1 of the human, mouse and rat *CYP1A2* gene, similar to the highly conserved regions found on alignment of the sequences in the upstream 5'-flanking region, in exon 1, and in intron 1 of *CYP1A1* genes in humans, mouse and rat. This suggests that the regulatory elements controlling the *CYP1A2* gene may have similarities to those controlling the *CYP1A1* gene.

The molecular mechanism of induction of CYP1A2 by various compounds was initially studied by Quattrochi *et al.* (1989, 1994). They subcloned the *CYP1A2* gene promoter sequence, a 3700 base pair fragment from the 5'-flanking region of *CYP1A2*, to the procaryotic chloramphenicol acetyltransferase (*CAT*) reporter gene and then transfected this construct into a transformed human hepatoma cell line (HepG2). These cells generated a twofold to threefold increase in CYP1A2-directed CAT activity when treated with 3-methylcholanthrene (3-MC). The DNA fragment located between -3202 to -1595 base pairs exhibited the strongest CAT response when induced by 3-MC. But when this CYP1A2-responsive element was transfected into human breast carcinoma (MCF7) cell lines, no induction by 3-MC was observed. This result implies that the induction of CYP1A2 by this responsive element may be regulated in a tissue-specific manner (Quattrochi & Tukey, 1989). Further detailed dissection of the 5'-flanking portion of the *CYP1A2* gene resulted in the identification of two regions that contributed the overall induction of CAT by 3-MC. The two xenobiotic-responsive element-like sequences were designated X1 (located between -2532 to -2423) and X2 (-2259 to -1987) respectively.

The induction of the *CYP1A2* gene is controlled by a number of different regulatory factors. The binding of X1 to the AhR complex is important for the overall expression of the CYP1A2 gene, but removal of the X1 region of the DNA does not completely eliminate the induction response (Quattrochi *et al.*, 1994; Eaton *et al.*, 1995). This suggests that additional regulatory elements support PAH-induced transcriptional activation of the human *CYP1A2* gene. Quattrochi *et al.* (1994) also found several potential AP1 binding sites and a conserved TATA sequence in the DNA fragment -2259 to -1970. An antioxidant-responsive element is present at -1555 to -1545 of the *CYP1A2* gene (Eaton *et al.*, 1995), but it is not thought to be involved in the 3-MC-initiated induction of the gene (Quattrochi *et al.*, 1994). Furthermore, Chung & Bresnick (1995) have identified two functional important cis elements in the 5'-flanking region which regulate the constitutive expression of human CYP1A2, one at the proximal 42-base pair DNA sequence from -72 to -31 and the other a distal 259-base pair DNA from -2352 to -2094. These results suggest that the 259-base pair DNA fragment contains positive regulator binding sites (activator protein-1, nuclear factor-E1.7, and one-half hepatic nuclear factor-1 binding consensus sequence) and that hepatic nuclear factor-1 could contribute to the liver-specific expression of human *CYP1A2*. There is also evidence that CYP1A2 activity or expression can be downregulated in rat and human hepatocytes in primary cultures by inflammatory mediators (Baker *et al.*, 1992, Abdel-Razzak *et al.*, 1994), transforming growth factors (Abdel-Razzak *et al.* 1994), and oxidative stress (Barker *et al.* 1994). Barker *et al.* (1992) found that interleukin-1 rapidly suppressed the transcription rate of both *CYP1A1* and *CYP1A2* in isolated rat hepatocytes induced by TCDD. As many of the actions of the inflammatory mediators are mimicked by oxidative stress,

Baker et al. (1994) treated rodent hepatocyte primary cultures with hydrogen peroxide to determine the effect on expression of these genes. They concluded that CYP1A1 and CYP1A2 gene transcription was responsive to oxidative stress and that the majority of this responsiveness could be modified by cellular redox potential. Abdel-Razzak et al. (1994), using primary human hepatocyte culture, found that tumour necrosis factor 1 produced nearly 100% inhibition of 3-MC and benzo[a]pyrene-induced CYP1A1 and CYP1A2 mRNA and EROD activity. Furthermore, they found that protein synthesis was required for the suppressive effect of the cytokine. Other cytokines also had a suppressive effect but to a lower extent than that seen for tumour necrosis factor 1.

The genetic basis for the phenotypic differences in CYP1A2 was investigated by Nakajima et al. (1994). The differences in nucleotide sequence between poor metabolizers and extensive metabolizers were determined; however, no nucleotide differences in exon, exon-intron junctions, and 5'-flanking regions (up to -2.6 kilobases) were found. Recently, however, two genetic variants of the intron 1 sequence of CYP1A2 were identified; they appear to be associated with CYP1A2 inducibility, but not constitutive expression (Yokoi et al., in preparation).

As TCDD and PAHs induce at least six genes (coding for CYP1A1, CYP1A2, NADPH:quinone oxidoreductase, aldehyde dehydrogenase, UDP-glucuronosyltransferases and the a-class GSTs) via a functional AhR, there may be functional relationships between these genes. Some preliminary data from a smoking cessation study (MacLeod et al., 1996) and the work of Sinha et al. (1994) indicate that CYP1A1, CYP1A2 and GSTM1 gene-gene interactions could be important. CYP1A2 activity was higher in individuals who possessed the GSTM1 null allele than in those expressing the GSTM1*A,B allele. CYP1A1 genotype in individuals with the Ile/Ile variant had greater mean CYP1A2 activity than in those with the heterozygous Ile/Val allelic variant. On exposure to the inducer, cigarette smoke or high temperature cooked meat, individuals possessing the heterozygous form of CYP1A1 gene had increased CYP1A2 activity compared to the more common Ile/Ile CYP1A1 genotype. Vaury et al. (1995) demonstrated an association between two of the genes that belong to the AhR complex, CYP1A1 and GSTs. There was high inducibility of CYP1A1 gene transcription by TCDD only in the presence of GSTM1 null genotype, while there were low levels of mRNA induction when there was at least one GSTM1 allele present. Furthermore, CYP1A1 expression was associated with the AhR as well as AhR nuclear translocator expression in various tissues of 20 subjects (Hayashi et al., 1994). Vickers et al. (1989) also found that estrogen receptor status of breast cancer cells was associated with distinct patterns of expression of both phase I (aryl hydrocarbon hydroxylase and CYP1A1) and phase II (GST) drug-metabolizing enzymes.

CYP1A2 family studies

Interindividual variation in the elimination of theophylline and antipyrine was studied in unrelated adults and families (Penno & Vesell, 1983; Miller et al., 1985). Both the drugs used are metabolized by different isoforms of hepatic CYPs. In the study carried out by Penno & Vesell (1983), 83 unrelated adults and 61 members of 13 families were administered antipyrine; urines were collected at regular intervals for 72 hours; and various antipyrine metabolites were measured. A trimodal distribution was obtained when antipyrine rate constants were plotted for the unrelated subjects. For each family, pedigree analysis was used to identify the mode of transmission of these three phenotypes, and the investigators concluded that the phenotypes were under monogenic control. Miller et al. (1985) used theophylline elimination to determine whether or not interindividual variation was under genetic control. Theophylline was administered to 79 unrelated adults, six sets of monozygotic twins, six sets of dizygotic twins, and six two-generation families. Urines were collected at regular intervals for 48 hr, and three principal metabolites were measured. The twin study revealed that the elimination of this drug was predominantly under genetic control. As with the antipyrine study, each of the theophylline metabolites appeared to be trimodally distributed in the unrelated adults. In the six families, the pedigree analysis of the three phenotypes was consistent with control by two alleles at a single gene locus and with autosomal codominant transmission. Furthermore, in respect of the three families in which both antipyrine and theophylline were studied, it was found that the correlation was 0.7 for the overall elimination rate constant, the implication being that there was a common regulatory element for both the antipyrine and theophylline polymorphisms. However, there is a suggestion that there is more than a single genetic polymorphism, as different gene frequencies for the antipyrine and theophylline polymorphisms have been demonstrated (Miller *et al.*, 1985).

Segregation analyses were performed on 68 families (Catteau *et al.*, 1995). A generational effect was observed where children had a greater mean value for a CYP1A2 activity index than parents. There was no significant familial resemblance and no major gene was detected. The authors concluded that there was no underlying genetic model to explain the variability of the phenotype. An alternative explanation, which may also apply to the previously described family studies, is that the power was not sufficient to differentiate the models. Multiple environmental mechanisms may be involved in the induced CYP1A2 phenotype. However, there may be influence of yet unknown inducers and inhibitors in the diet and the environment which could obscure the detection of genetic polymorphisms by adding to the 'noise'.

CYP1A2 population studies
Kadlubar (1994) compared the distribution of CYP1A2 phenotypes in subjects from Australia, China, Italy, and Japan and from Arkansas and Georgia in the USA. He found a trimodal distribution of CYP1A2 phenotypes in all the populations except the Japanese, who appeared to have a bimodal distribution. The results indicated a wide variation in metabolic proficiency for CYP1A2 across racial/ethnic groups.

Epidemiological and clinical studies
The wide range of expression seen in humans and the ability of CYP1A2 to activate environmental chemicals to proximate carcinogens suggests the need for epidemiological studies in order to assess the impact of CYP1A2 activity on cancer risks. Concern also exists because of the known interactions of CYP1A2 with commonly administered

pharmaceuticals used in humans, either as important routes of metabolism or as inhibitors of CYP1A2 activity and consequently of the metabolism of concurrently administered drugs. Studies published to date have focused on CYP1A2 activity level alone or combined with other metabolic polymorphisms.

Colorectal cancer
On the basis of *in vitro* studies of heterocyclic aromatic amine activation by CYP1A2 (see above) a case-control study of colon cancer and colon polyps was performed (Lang *et al.*, 1994) with a view to identifying the relationship between phenotype, environmental exposure and risk of colon neoplasia. The investigators found that a combination of rapid CYP1A2 phenotype with rapid NAT2 phenotype showed the greatest risk. Moreover, this disease risk was further increased by apparent exposure to heterocyclic aromatic amines as measured by the subjects' preference for cooked meat that was "well done". Confirmation of these findings must await the results of larger case-control studies now in progress.

Urinary bladder cancer
CYP1A2 has been reported as a risk factor for bladder cancer in a case-control study conducted in an Asian population with no history of occupational exposure (Lee *et al.*, 1994). In 100 bladder cancer patients and 84 controls, CYP1A2, CYP2D6 and NAT2 phenotypes were measured using theophylline, metoprolol and isoniazid urinary metabolites respectively. Variables such as age, gender and smoking were controlled for in the analysis. No differences were noted between cases and controls for CYP2D6 and NAT2 phenotypes. However, the 1-methyluric acid recovery ratio from theophylline was significantly higher in cases than in controls ($p < 0.05$).

Other cancers
Kellermann *et al.* (1980) reported increased antipyrine clearance to be a risk factor for lung cancer on the basis of findings in a study of lung cancer patients who had stopped smoking and of non-smoking controls. While the authors interpreted this activity as being due to aryl hydrocarbon hydroxylase, current understanding ascribes

this function to CYP1A2 in the light of reports of high correlations between clearance of antipyrine and theophylline (Schellens et al., 1989) and the identification of CYP1A1 and CYP2C9 as major contributors to aryl hydrocarbon hydroxylase activity in hepatic and extrahepatic tissues respectively (Shimada et al., 1992). Several studies of the role of CYP1A2 in colon polyps, breast cancer, prostate cancer and endometrial cancer are currently being conducted.

Cardiovascular disease
The hypothesis that CYP1A2 and/or NAT2 may be involved in the pathogenesis of peripheral arterial disease was investigated in a case-control study (Ilett et al., 1993). CYP1A2 and NAT2 phenotypes were determined from urinary metabolite patterns after an oral dose of caffeine. The NAT2 phenotype was similar in both atherosclerotic patients (43.3% rapid) and control subjects (42.0% rapid). Similarly, CYP1A2 metabolism values in atherosclerotic and control non-smokers and smokers did not show major differences. The authors concluded that the metabolism of environmental agents via the acetylation (NAT2) or N-oxidation (CYP1A2) pathways was unlikely to play a role in determining the risk of developing cardiovascular disease.

Clinical implications
Several important drugs are metabolized by CYP1A2, including warfarin (Rettie et al., 1992), antipyrine (Engel et al., 1992; Dahlqvist et al., 1984), caffeine (Butler et al., 1989b), theophylline (Schellens et al., 1989) acetaminophen (Patten et al., 1993), imipramine (Lemoine et al., 1993), tacrine (Spaldin et al., 1995) and estrogens (see above). Several pharmaceuticals are capable of CYP1A2 inhibition to varying degrees and can lead to acute toxicity. These agents include fluvoxamine (Brosen et al., 1993), enoxacin (Davis et al., 1995), ciprofloxacin (Batty et al., 1995), cimetidine (Loi et al., 1993), mexiletene (Joeres et al., 1987) and verapamil (Koleva et al., 1995).

Two important groups of drugs that influence CYP1A2 are the serotonin re-uptake inhibitors and the quinolone antibacterials. Fluvoxamine is a serotonin re-uptake inhibitor with a very potent inhibitory effect against O-deethylation of phenacetin (catalysed by CYP1A2). Other serotonin re-uptake inhibitors (citalopram, N-desmethycitalopram, fluoxetine, norfluoxetine, paroxetine, sertraline and litoxetin) either did not inhibit or weakly inhibited O-deethylation of phenacetin (Brosen et al., 1993).

The quinolones more commonly inhibit CYP1A2, as measured by the inhibition of 3-demethylation of caffeine in human liver microsomes. Reduction in CYP1A2 activity after administration of quinolones has been reported as follows: enoxacin acid - 66.6%; pipemidic acid - 59.3%; norfloxacin - 55.7%; lomefloxacin - 23.4%; pefloxacin - 22.0%; amifloxacin - 21.4%; difloxacin 21.3%; ofloxacin - 11.8%; temafloxacin - 10.0%; fleroxacin - no effect (Fuhr et al., 1992b).

The clinical effects of these agents are determined by the degree of inhibition, the therapeutic range of the agent whose metabolism is being inhibited and the impact of drug levels outside the therapeutic range. Prolongation of caffeine or theophylline half-life, due to smoking cessation or administration of a quinolone antibiotic, can result in acute toxic effects, particularly when subjects are being treated with other agents concurrently (Batty et al., 1995).

Acknowledgements
Support for this work was provided in part by USA NCI grants RO1-CA55751, RO1-CA74982, and USA EPA grant R825280.

References
Abdel-Razzak, Z., Corcos, L., Fautrel,. A., Campion, J.-P. & Guillouzo, A. (1994) Transforming growth factor-1 down-regulates basal and polycyclic aromatic hydrocarbon-induced cytochromes P-450 1A1 and 1A2 in adult human hepatocytes in primary culture. Mol. Pharmacol., 46, 1100-1110

Abernethy, D.R. & Todd, E.L. (1985) Impairment of caffeine clearance by chronic use of low-dose estrogen-containing oral contraceptives. Eur. J. Clin. Pharmacol., 28, 425-428.

Alvares, A.P., Kappas, A., Eiseman, J.L., Anderson, K.E., Pantuck, C.B., Pantuck, E.J., Hsiao, K.C., Garland, W.A. & Conney, A.H. (1979) Interindividual variation in drug metabolism. Clin. Pharmacol. Ther., 26, 407-419

Aoyama, T., Korzekwa, K., Nagata, K., Gillette, J., Gelboin, H.V. & Gonzales, F.J. (1990) Estradiol metabolism by complementary deoxyribonucleic acid expressed human cytochrome P450s. *Endocrinology*, 126, 3101-3106

Badawi, A.F., Hirvonen, A., Bell, D.A. & Kadlubar, F.F. (1995) Role of aromatic amine acetyltransferases, NAT1 and NAT2, in carcinogen-DNA adduct formation in the human urinary bladder. *Cancer Res.*, 55, 5230-5237

Barker, C.W., Fagan, J.B. & Pasco, D.S. (1992) Interleukin-1 beta suppresses the induction of P4501A1 and P4501A2 mRNAs in isolated hepatocytes. *J. Biol. Chem.*, 267, 8050-8055

Barker, C.W., Fagan, J.B. & Pasco, D.S. (1994) Down-regulation of P450IA1 and P4501A2 mRNA expression in isolated hepatocytes by oxidative stress. *J. Biol. Chem.*, 269, 3985-3990

Batty, K.T., Davis, T.M., Ilett, K.F., Dusci, L.J. & Langton, S.R. (1995) The effect of ciprofloxacin on theophylline pharmacokinetics in healthy subjects. *Br. J. Clin. Pharmacol.*, 39, 305-311

Bendriss, E.K., Bechtel, Y., Bendriss, A., Humbert, P., Paintaud, G., Magnette, J., Agache, P. & Bechtel, P.R. (1996) Inhibition of caffeine metabolism by 5-methoxypsoralen in patients with psoriasis. *Br. J. Clin. Pharmacol.*, 41, 421-424

Bengtsson, U., Johansson, S. & Angervall, L. (1978) Malignancies of the urinary tract and their relation to analgesic abuse. *Kidney Int.*, 13, 107-113

Berthou, F., Guillois, B., Riche, C., Dreano, Y., Jacqz-Aigrain, A.E. & Beaune, P.H. (1992) Interspecies variations in caffeine metabolism related to cytochrome P4501A enzymes. *Xenobiotica*, 22, 671-680

Bertilsson, L., Carrilo, J.A., Dahl, M.-L., Llerena, A., Alm, C., Bondesson, U., Lindstrom, L., Rodriguez de la Rubia, I., Ramos, S. & Benitez, J. (1994) Clozapine disposition covaries with CYP1A2 activity determined by a caffeine test. *Br. J. Clin. Pharm.*, 39, 471-473

Birkett, D.J. & Miners, J.O. (1991) Caffeine renal clearance and urine caffeine concentrations during steady state dosing. Implications for monitoring caffeine intake during sports events. *Br. J. Clin. Pharmacol.*, 31, 405-408

Bonati, M., Latini, R., Galletti, F., Young, J.F., Tognoni, G. & Garattini, S. (1982) Caffeine disposition after oral doses. *Clin. Pharmacol. Ther.*, 32, 98-106

Brazier, J.L., Descotes, J., Lery, N., Ollagnier, M. & Evreux, J.-C. (1980) Inhibition by idrocilamide of the disposition of caffeine. *Eur. J. Clin. Pharmacol.*, 17, 37-43

Brazier, J.L., Ritter, J., Berland, M., Khenfer, D. & Faucon, G. (1983) Pharmacokinetics of caffeine during and after pregnancy. *Dev. Pharmacol. Ther.*, 6, 315-322

Brosen, K., Skjelbo, E., Rasmussen, B.B., Poulsen, H.E. & Loft, S. (1993) Fluvoxamine is a potent inhibitor of cytochrome P4501A2. *Biochem. Pharmacol.*, 45, 1211-4

Bullock, P., Pearce, R., Draper, A., Podval, J., Bracken, W., Veltman, J., Thomas, P. & Parkinson, A. (1995) Induction of liver microsomal cytochrome P450 in cynomolgus monkeys. *Drug Metab. Dispos.*, 23, 736-748

Busby, W.F., Garner, R.C., Chow, F.L., Martin, C.N., Stevens, E.K., Newberne, P.M.. & Wogan, G.N. (1985) 6-nitrochrysene is a potent tumorigen in newborn mice. *Carcinogenesis*, 6, 801-803

Butler, M.A., Guengerich, F.P. & Kadlubar, F.F. (1989a) Metabolic oxidation of the carcinogens 4-aminobiphenyl and 4,4'-methylene*bis*(2-chloroaniline) by human hepatic microsomes and by purified rat hepatic cytochrome P-450 monooxygenases. *Cancer Res.*, 49, 25-31

Butler, M.A., Iwasaki, M., Guengerich, F.P. & Kadlubar, F.F. (1989b) Human cytochrome P-450$_{PA}$(P-4501A2), the phenacetin *O*-deethylase, is primarily responsible for the hepatic 3-demethylation of caffeine and *N*-oxidation of carcinogenic arylamines. *Proc. Natl. Acad. Sci. USA*, 86, 7696-7700

Butler, M.A., Lang, N.P., Young, J.F., Caporaso, N.E., Vineis, P., Hayes, R.B., Teitel, C.H., Massengill, J.P., Lawsen, M.F. & Kadlubar, F.F. (1992) Determination of CYP1A2 and NAT2 phenotypes in human populations by analysis of caffeine urinary metabolites. *Pharmacogenetics*, 2, 116-127

Carrillo, J.A. & Benitez, J. (1994) Caffeine metabolism in a healthy Spanish population: *N*-acetylator phenotype and oxidation pathways. *Clin. Pharmacol. Ther.*, 55, 293-304

Carrillo J.A. & Benitez, J. (1996) CYP1A2 activity, gender and smoking, as variables influencing the toxicity of caffeine. *Br. J. Clin. Pharmacol.*, 41, 605-608

Catteau, A., Bechtel,Y.C., Poisson, N., Bechtel, P.R. & Bonaiti-Pellie, C. (1995) A population and family study of CYP1A2 using caffeine urinary metabolites. *Eur. J. Clin. Pharmacol.*, 47, 423-430

Campbell, M.E., Spielberg, S.P. & Kalow, W. (1987) A urinary metabolite ratio that reflects systemic caffeine clearance. *Clin. Pharmacol. Ther.*, 42, 157-165

Carlson, T.J., Jones, J.P., Peterson, L., Castagnoli, N., Iyer, K.R. & Trager, W.F. (1995) Stereoselectivity and isotope effects associated with cytochrome P450-catalysed oxidation of (S)-nicotine. *Drug Metab. Dispos.*, 23, 749-756

Chae, Y.-H., Yun, C.H., Guengerich, F.P., Kadlubar, F.F. & El-Bayoumy, K. (1993) Roles of human hepatic and pulmonary cytochrome P450 enzymes in the metabolism of the environmental carcinogen 6-nitrochrysene. *Cancer Res.*, 53, 2028-2034

Chaloner, C., Sandle, L.N., Mohan, V., Snehalatha, C., Viswanathan, M. & Braganza, J.M. (1990) Evidence for induction of cytochrome P-450I in patients with tropical chronic pancreatitis. *Int. J. Clin. Pharm. Ther. Toxicol.*, 28, 235-240

Chung, I. & Bresnick, E. (1995) Regulation of the constitutive expression of the human CYP1A2 gene: cis elements and their interactions with proteins. *Mol. Pharm.*, 47, 677-685

Conney, A.H., Pantuck, E.J., Hsiao, K.-C., Garland, W.A., Anderson, K.E., Alvarez, A.P. & Kappas, A. (1976) Enhanced phenacetin metabolism in human subjects fed charcoal-broiled beef. *Clin. Pharmacol. Ther.*, 20, 633-642

Crespi, C.L., Penman, B.W., Gelboin, H.V. & Gonzales, F.J. (1991) A tobacco-smoke derived nitrosamine, 4-(methylnitrosamino)-1-(3-pyridyl)-1-butanone, is activated by multiple human cytochrome P450s including the polymorphic human cytochrome P4502D6. *Carcinogenesis*, 12, 1197-1201

Crowley, J.J., Cusack, B.J., Jue, S.G., Koup, J.R. & Vestal, R.E. (1987) Cigarette smoking and theopylline metabolism: effects of phenytoin. *Clin. Pharmacol. Ther.*, 42, 334-340

Dahlqvist, R., Bertilsson, L., Birkett, D.J., Eichelbaum, M., Säwe, J. & Sjöqvist, P. (1984) Theophylline metabolism in relation to antipyrine, debrisoquine, and sparteine metabolism. *Clin. Pharmacol. Ther.*, 35, 815-821

Dannan, G.A., Porubek, D.J., Nelson, S.D., Waxman, D.J. & Guengerich, F.P. (1986) 17β-estradiol 2- and 4-hydroxylation catalysed by rat hepatic cytochrome P-450: roles of individual forms, inductive effects, developmental patterns, and alterations by gonadectomy and hormone replacement. *Endocrinology*, 118, 1952-1960

Daujat, M., Peryt, B., Lesca, P., Fourtanier, G., Domergue, J. & Maurel, P. (1992) Omeprazole, an inducer of human CYP1A1 and 1A2, is not a ligand for the Ah receptor. *Biochem. Biophys. Res. Commun.*, 188, 820-825

Davis, J.D., Aarons, L. & Houston, J.B. (1995) Metabolism of theophylline and its inhibition by fluoroquinolones in rat hepatic microsomes. *Xenobiotica*, 25, 563-573

Degawa, M., Stern, S.J., Martin, M.V., Guengerich, F.P., Fu, P.P., Ilett, K.F., Kaderlik, R.K. & Kadlubar, F.F. (1994) Metabolic activation and carcinogen-DNA adduct detection in human larynx. *Cancer Res.*, 54, 4915-4919

Denaro, C.P., Wilson, M., Jacob, P. 3rd & Benowitz N.L. (1996) Validation of urine caffeine metabolite ratios with the use of stable isotope-labelled caffeine clearance. *Clin. Pharmacol. Ther.*, 59, 284-296

Devonshire, H.W., Kong, I., Cooper, M., Sloan, T.P., Idle, J.R. & Smith, R.L. (1983) The contribution of genetically determined oxidation status to interindividual variation in phenacetin disposition. *Br. J. Clin. Pharmacol.*, 16, 157-166

Distlerath, L.M., Reilly, P.E.B., Martin, M.V., Davis, G.G., Wilkinson, G.R. & Guengerich, F.P. (1985) Purification and characterization of the human liver cytochromes P-450 involved in debrisoquine 4-hydroxylation and phenacetin O-deethylation, two prototypes for genetic polymorphism in oxidative drug metabolism. *J. Biol. Chem.*, 260, 9057-9067

Donato, M.T., Castell, J.V. & Gomez-Lechon, M.J. (1995) Effect of model inducers on cytochrome P450 activities of human hepatocytes in primary culture. *Drug Metab. Dispos.*, 23 553-558

Eaton, D.L., Gallagher, E.P., Bammler, T.K. & Kunze, K.L. (1995) Role of cytochrome P4501A2 in chemical carcinogenesis: implications for human variability in expression and enzyme activity. *Pharmacogenetics*, 5, 259-274

Endrenyi, L. & Patel, M. (1991) A new, sensitive graphical method for detecting deviations from the normal distribution of drug responses: the NTV plot. *Br. J. Clin. Pharmacol.*, 32, 159-166

Engel, G., Knebel, N.G., Hofman, U. & Eichelbaum, M. (1992) *In vitro* characterization of human P450-enzymes involved in antipyrine metabolism. In: Abstracts of 23rd European Workshop on Drug Metabolism

Fuhr, U., Anders, E.M., Mahr, G., Sorgel, F. & Staib, A.H. (1992a) Inhibitory potency of quinolone antibacterial agents against cytochrome P450IA2 activity *in vivo* and *in vitro*. *Antimicrob. Agents Chemother.*, 36, 942-948

Fuhr, U., Woodcock, B.G. & Siewert, M. (1992b) Verapamil and drug metabolism by the cytochrome P450 isoform CYP1A2. *Eur. J. Clin. Pharmacol.*, 42, 463-464

Fuhr, U. & Kummert, A.L. (1995) The fate of naringin in humans: a key to grapefruit juice-drug interactions. *Clin. Pharmacol. Ther.*, 58, 365-373

Fuhr, U. & Rost K.L. (1994) Simple and reliable CYP1A2 phenotyping by the paraxanthine/caffeine ratio in plasma and saliva. *Pharmacogenetics*, 4, 109-116

Fuhr, U., Rost, K.L., Engelhardt, R., Sachs, M., Liermann, D., Belloc, C., Beaune, P., Janezic, S., Grant, D., Meyer, U.A. & Staib, A.H. (1996) Evaluation of caffeine as a test drug for CYP1A2, NAT2 and CYP2E1 phenotyping in man by *in vivo* versus *in vitro* correlations. *Pharmacogenetics*, 6, 159-176

Gallagher, E.P., Wienkers, L.C., Stapleton, P.L., Kunze, K.L. & Eaton, D.L. (1994) Role of human microsomal and human complementary DNA-expressed cytochromes P4501A2 and P4503A4 in the bioactivation of aflatoxin B_1. *Cancer Res.*, 54,101-108

Garner, R.C., Martin, C.N. & Clayson, D.B. (1984) Carcinogenic aromatic amines and related compounds. In: Searle, C.E., ed, *Chemical Carcinogens*. Washington, American Chemical Society, Monograph No.182, 2nd Edition, Vol.1, pp. 175-276

Gerhardsson de Verdier, M., Hagman, U., Peters, R.K., Steineck, G. & Övervik, E. (1991) Meat, cooking methods and colorectal cancer: a case-referent study in Stockholm. *Int. J. Cancer*, 49, 520-525

Giovannucci, E., Rimm, E.B., Stamfer, M.J., Colditz, G.A., Ascherio, A. & Willett, W.C. (1994). Intake of fat, meat, and fibre in relation to risk of colon cancer in men. *Cancer Res.*, 54,2390-2397

Gu, L., Gonzales, F.J., Kalow, W. & Tang, B.K. (1992) Biotransportation of caffeine, paraxanthine, theobromine and theophylline by cDNA-expressed human CYP1A2 and CYP2E1. *Pharmacogenetics*, 2, 73-77

Guengerich, F.P. & MacDonald, T.L. (1984) Chemical mechanisms of catalysis by cytochromes P-450: a unified view. *Acc. Chem. Res.*, 17, 9-16

Guengerich, F.P. & Shimada, T. (1991) Oxidation of toxic and carcinogenic chemicals by human cytochrome P-450 enzymes. *Chem. Res. Toxicol.*, 4, 319-407

Guengerich, F.P. & Turvy, C.G. (1991) Comparison of levels of several human microsomal P-450 enzymes and epoxide hydrolase in normal and disease states using immunochemical analysis of surgical liver samples. *J. Pharmacol. Exp. Ther.*, 256, 1189-1194

Hakkola, H., Pasanen, M., Purkunen, R., Saarikoski, S., Pelkonen, O., Maenpaa, J., Rane, A. & Raunio, H. (1994) Expression of xenobiotic-metabolizing cytochrome P-450 forms in human adult and fetal liver. *Biochem. Pharmacol.*, 48, 59-64

Hakkola, H., Raunio, H., Purkunen, R., Pelkonen, O., Saarikoski, S., Cresteil, T. & Pasanen, M. (1996a) Detection of cytochrome P450 gene expression in human placenta in first trimester of pregancy. *Biochem. Pharmacol.*, 52, 379-383

Hakkola, H., Pasanen, M., Hukkanen, J., Pelkonen, O., Maenpaa, J., Edwards, R.J., Boobis, A.R. & Raunio H. (1996b) Expression of xenobiotic-metabolizing cytochrome P450 forms in human full-term placenta. *Biochem. Pharmacol.*, 51, 403-411

Hall, A.J. & Wild, C.P. (1994) Epidemiology of aflatoxin-related disease. In: Eaton, D.L. & Groopman, J.D., eds, *The Toxicology of Aflatoxins: Human Health, Veterinary and Agricultural Significance*. New York, Academic Press, pp. 233-258

Hammons, G.J., Guengerich, F.P., Weis, C.C., Beland, F.A. & Kadlubar, F.F. (1985) Metabolic activation of carcinogenic arylamines by rat, dog, and human hepatic microsomes and by purified flavin-containing and cytochrome P-450 monooxygenases. *Cancer Res.*, 45, 3578-3585

Hatch, F.T., Knize, M.G., Moore, D.H. & Felton, J.S. (1992) Quantitative correlation of mutagenic and carcinogenic potencies for heterocyclic amines from cooked foods and additional aromatic amines. *Mutat. Res.*, 271, 269-287

Hayashi, S., Watanabe, J., Nakachi, K., Eguchi, H., Gotoh, O. & Kawajiri, K. (1994) Interindividual difference in expression of human Ah receptor and related P450 genes. *Carcinogenesis*, 15, 801-806

Hecht, S.S. & Hoffman, D. (1988) Tobacco-specific nitrosamines, an important group of carcinogens in tobacco smoke. *Carcinogenesis*, 9, 875-884

Horn, E.P., Tucker, M.A., Lambert, G., Silverman, D., Zametkin, D., Sinha, R., Hartge, T., Landi, M.T. & Caporaso, N.E. (1995) A study of gender-based cytochrome P4501A2 variability: a possible mechanism for the male excess of bladder cancer. *Cancer Epidemiol. Biomarkers Prev.*, 4, 529-533

IARC Monographs on the Evaluation of the Carcinogenic risk of Chemicals to Humans. Vol. 38. Tobacco Smoking. (1986) Lyon, IARC, pp. 83-126

Ikeya, K., Jaiswal, A.K., Owens, R.A., Jones, J.E., Nebert, D.W. & Kimura, S. (1989) Human CYP1A2: sequence, gene structure, comparison with the mouse and rat orthologous gene, and differences in liver 1A2 mRNA expression. *Mol. Endocrinol.*, 3, 1399-1408

Ilett, K.F., Castleden, W.M., Vandongen, Y.K., Stacey, M.C., Butler, M.A. & Kadlubar, F.F. (1993) Acetylation phenotype and cytochrome P450IA2 phenotype are unlikely to be associated with peripheral arterial disease. *Clin. Pharmacol. Therap.*, 54, 317-322

Iqbal, N., Ahmad, B., Janbaz, K.H., Gilani, A.-U.H. & Niazi, S.K. (1995) The effect of caffeine on the pharmacokinetics of acetaminophen in man. *Biopharm. Drug Dispos.*, 16, 481-487

Jackson, P.R., Tucker, G.T. & Woods, H.F. (1989) Testing for bimodality in frequency distributions of data suggesting polymorphisms of drug metabolism - histograms and probit plots. *Br. J. Clin. Pharmacol.*, 28, 647-653

Jaiswal, A.K., Nebert, D.W., McBride, O.W. & Gonzalez, F.J. (1987) Human P3450: cDNA and complete protein sequence, repetitive *alu* sequences in the 3' nontranslated region, and localization of gene to chrome 15. *J. Exp. Pathol.*, 3, 1-17

Joeres, R. & Richter, E. (1987) Mexiletine and caffeine elimination. *N. Engl. J. Med.*, 317, 117

Kaderlik, K.R., Minchin, R.F., Mulder, G.J., Ilett, K.F., Daugaard-Jenson, M., Teitel, C.H. & Kadlubar, F.F. (1994) Metabolic activation pathway for the formation of DNA adducts of the carcinogen 2-amino-1-methyl-6-phenylimidazo[4,5-b]pyridine (PhIP) in rat extrahepatic tissues. *Carcinogenesis*, 15, 1703-1709

Kadlubar, F.F. (1994) Biochemical individuality and its implications for drug and carcinogen metabolism. Recent insights from acetyltransferase and cytochrome P4501A2 phenotyping and genotyping in humans. *Drug Metab. Dispos.*, 26, 37-46

Kadlubar, F.F., Dooley, K.L., Teitel, C.H., Roberts, D.W., Benson, R.W., Butler, M.A., Bailey, J.R., Young, J.F., Skipper, P.W. & Tannenbaum, S.R. (1991) Frequency of urination and its effects on metabolism, pharmacokinetics, blood haemoglobin adduct formation, and liver and urinary DNA bladder adduct levels in beagle dogs given the bladder carcinogen 4-aminobiphenyl. *Cancer Res.*, 51, 4371-4377

Kadlubar F.F. & Hammons, G.J. (1987) The role of cytochrome P-450 in the metabolism of chemical carcinogens. In: Guengerich, F.P., ed, *Mammalian Cytochromes P-450, Vol II*. Boca Raton, Florida; CRC Press, Inc.; pp. 81-130

Kadlubar, F.F., Talaska, G., Butler, M.A., Teitel, C.H., Massengill, J.P. & Lang, N.P. (1990) Determination of carcinogenic arylamine N-oxidation phenotype in humans by analysis of caffeine urinary metabolites. In: Mendelsohn, M.L. & Albertini, R.J., eds, *Mutation and the Environment. Part B: Metabolism, Testing Methods, and Chromosomes*. New York, John Wiley and Sons, pp. 107-114

Kadlubar, F.F., Young, J.F., Lang, N.P., Caporaso, N.E., Sinha, R. & Landi, M.T. (1996) Correspondence re: letter to the editor by B.K. Tang and W. Kalow on CYP1A2 phenotyping using caffeine. *Cancer Epidemiol. Biomarkers Prev.*, 5, 757-758

Kall, M.A. & Clausen J. (1995) Dietary effect on mixed function P450 1A2 activity assayed by estimation of caffeine metabolism in man. *Human & Exp. Toxicol.*, 14, 801-807

Kall, M.A., Vang, O. & Clausen, J. (1996) Effects of dietary broccoli on human *in vivo* drug metabolizing enzymes: evaluation of caffeine, oestrone and chlorzoxazone metabolism. *Carcinogenesis*, 17, 791-799

Kalow, W. & Tang, B.K. (1991) Use of caffeine metabolites ratios to explore CYP1A2 and xanthine oxidase activities. *Clin. Pharmacol. Ther.*, 50, 508-519

Kalow, W. & Tang, B.K. (1993) The use of caffeine for enzyme assays: a critical appraisal. *Clin. Pharmacol. Ther.*, 53, 503-514

Kappas, A., Alvares, A.P., Anderson, K.E., Pantuck, E.J., Pantuck, C.B., Chang, R.& Conney, A.H. (1978) Effect of charcoal-broiled beef on antipyrine and theophylline metabolism. *Clin. Pharmacol. Ther.*, 23, 445-450

Kappas, A., Anderson, K.E., Conney, A.H. & Alvares, A.P. (1965) Influence of dietary protein and carbohydrate on antipyrine and theophylline metabolism in man. *Clin. Pharmacol. Ther.*, 20 643-653

Kato, R. (1986). Metabolic activation of mutagenic heterocyclic amines from protein pyrolysates. *CRC Crit. Rev. Toxicol.*, 16, 307-348

Kellermann, G., Jett, J.R., Luyten-Kellermann, M., Moses, H.L. & Fontana R.S. (1980) Variation of microsomal mixed function oxidase(s) and human lung cancer. *Cancer*, 45, 1438-1442

Knize, M.G., Dolbeare, F.A., Carroll, K.L., Moore, D.H. 2nd & Felton, J.S. (1994) Effects of cooking time and temperature on the heterocyclic amine content of fried-beef patties. *Food. Chem. Toxicol.*, 32, 595-603

Knutti, R., Rothweiler, H. & Schlatter, C. (1981) Effect of pregnancy on the pharmacokinetics of caffeine. *Eur. J. Clin. Pharmacol.*, 21, 121-126

Koleva, M.R. & Stoychev, T.S. (1995) Effect of nifedipine, verapamil and diltiazem on the enzyme-inducing activity of phenobarbital and beta-naphthoflavone. *Gen. Pharmacol.*, 26, 225-228

Kunze, K.L. & Trager, W.F. (1993) Isoform-selective mechanism-based inhibition of human cytochrome P450 1A2 by furafylline. *Chem. Res. Toxicol.*, 6, 649-656

Lake, B.G., Charzat, C., Tredger, J.M., Renwick, A.B., Beamand, J.A. & Price, R.J. (1996) Induction of cytochrome P450 isoenzymes in cultured precision-cut rat and human liver slices. *Xenobiotica*, 26, 297-306

Lambert, G.H., Schoeller, D.A., Humphrey, H.E.B., Kotake, A.N., Lietz, H., Campbell, M., Kalow, W., Spielberg, S.P. & Budd, M. (1990) The caffeine breath test and caffeine urinary metabolite ratios in the Michigan cohort exposed to polybrominated biphenyls: a preliminary study. *Environ. Health Perspect.*, 89, 175-181

Lambert, G.H., Schoeller, D.A., Kotake, A.N., Flores, C. & Hay, E. (1986) The effect of age, gender, and sexual maturation on the caffeine breath test. *Dev. Pharmacol. Ther.*, 9, 375-388

Landi, M.T., Zocchetti, C., Bernucci, I., Kadlubar, F.F., Tannenbaum, S., Skipper, P., Bartsch, H., Malaveille, C., Shields, P., Caporaso, N.E. & Vineis P. (1996) Cytochrome P4501A2: enzyme induction and genetic control in determining 4-aminobiphenyl-hemoglobin adduct levels. *Cancer Epidemiol. Biomarkers Prev.*, 5, 693-698

Lang, N.P., Butler, M.A., Massengill, J., Lawson, M., Stotts, R.C., Hauer-Jansen, M.. & Kadlubar, F.F. (1994) Rapid metabolic phenotypes for acetyltransferase and cytochrome P4501A2 and putative exposure to food-borne heterocyclic amines

increase the risk for colorectal cancer of polyps. *Cancer Epidemiol. Biomarkers Prev.*, 3, 675-682

Lee, S.W., Jang, I.J., Shin, S.G., Lee, K.H., Yim, D.S., Kim, S.W., Oh, S.J. & Lee, S.H. (1994) CYP1A2 activity as a risk factor for bladder cancer. *J. Korean Med. Sci.*, 9, 482-489

Le Marchand, L., Sivaraman, L., Franke, A.A., Custer, L.J., Wilkens, R.L., Lau, A.F. & Cooney, R.V. (1996) Predictors of N-acetyltransferase activity: Should caffeine phenotyping and *NAT2* genotyping be used interchangeably in epidemiological studies? *Cancer Epidemiol. Biomarkers Prev.*, 5, 449-455

Lemoine, L., Gautier, J.C., Azoulay, D., Kiffel, L., Belloc, C., Guengerich, F.P., Maurel, P., Beaune, P. & Leroux, J.P. (1993) Major pathway of imipramine metabolism is catalysed by cytochromes P-450 1A2 and P-450 3A4 in human liver. *Mol. Pharmacol.*, 43, 827-832

Liehr, J.G., Ricci, M.J., Jefcoate, C.R., Hannigan, E.V., Hokanson, J.A. & Zhu, B.T. (1995) 4-hydroxylation of estradiol by human uterine myometrium and myoma microsomes: implications for the mechanism of uterine tumorigenesis. *Proc. Natl. Acad. Sci. USA*, 92, 9220-9224

Loi, C.-M., Parker, B.M., Cusack, B.J. & Vestal, R.E. (1993) Individual and combined effects of cimetidine and ciprofloxacin on the theophylline metabolism in male nonsmokers. *Br. J. Clin. Pharmacol.*, 36, 195-200

Lynch, A.M., Murray, S., Gooderham, N.J. & Boobis, A.R. (1995) Exposure to and activation of dietary heterocyclic amines in humans. *Crit. Rev. Oncol. Hematol.*, 21, 19-31

MacLeod, S., Sinha, R., Kadlubar, F.F. & Lang, N.P. (1997) Polymorphisms of CYP1A1 and GSTM1 influence the *in vivo* function of CYP1A2. *Mutat. Res.*, 376, 135-142

Masimirembwa, C.M., Beke, M., Hasler, J.A., Tang, B.K. & Kalow, W. (1995) Low CYP1A2 activity in rural Shona children of Zimbabwe. *Clin. Pharmacol. Ther.*, 57, 25-31

McDanell, R.E., Henderson, L.A., Russell, K. & McLean, A.E.M. (1992) The effect of *Brassica* vegetable consumption on caffeine metabolism in humans. *Hum. Exp. Toxicol.*, 11, 167-172

McQuilkin, S.H., Nierenberg, D.W. & Bresnick, E. (1995) Analysis of within-subject variation of caffeine metabolism when used to determine cytochrome P4501A2. *Cancer Epidemiol. Biomarkers Prev.*, 4, 139-146

Miller, C.A., Slusher, L.B. & Vesell, E.S. (1985) Polymorphism of theophylline metabolism in man. *J. Clin. Invest.*, 75, 1415-1425

Minchin, R.F., McManus, M.E., Boobis, A.R., Davies, D.S. & Thorgeirsson, S.S. (1985) Polymorphic metabolism of the carcinogen 2-acetylaminofluorene in human liver microsomes. *Carcinogenesis*, 6, 1721-1724

Miners, J.O. & Birkett, D.J. (1996) The use of caffeine as a metabolic probe for human drug metabolizing enzymes. *Gen. Pharmacol.*, 27, 245-249

Muntané-Relat, J., Ourlin, J-C., Domergue, J. & Maurel, P. (1995) Differential effects of cytokines on the inducible expression of CYP1A1, CYP1A2, and CYP3A4 in human hepatocytes in primary culture. *Hepatology*, 22, 1143-1153

Murray, B.P., Edwards, R.J., Murray, S., Singleton, A.M., Davies, D.S. & Boobis, A.R. (1993) Human hepatic CYP1A1 and CYP1A2 content, determined with specific anti-peptide antibodies, correlates with the mutagenic activation of PhIP. *Carcinogenesis*, 14, 585-592

Nakajima, M., Yokoi, T., Mitzutani, M., Shin, S., Kadlubar, F.F. & Kamataki, T. (1994) Phenotyping of CYP1A2 in Japanese population by analysis of caffeine urinary metabolites: absence of mutation prescribing the phenotype in the *CYP1A2* gene. *Cancer Epidemiol. Biomarkers Prev.*, 3, 413-421

Nelson, D.R., Koymans, L., Kamataki, T., Stegeman, J.J., Feyereisen, R., Waxman, D.J., Waterman, M.R., Gotoh, O., Coon, M.J., Estabrook, R.W., Gunsalus, I.C. & Nebert, D.W.

(1996) P450 superfamily: update on new sequences, gene mapping, accession numbers and nomenclature. *Pharmacogenetics*, 6, 1-42

Notarianni, L.J., Oliver, S.E., Dobrocky, P., Bennet, P.N. & Silverman, B.W. (1995) Caffeine as a metabolic probe: comparison of the metabolic ratios used to assess CYP1A2 activity. *Br. J. Clin. Pharmacol.*, 39, 65-69

Pantuck, E.J., Pantuck, C.B., Garland, W.A., Min, B.H., Wattenberg, L.W., Anderson, K.E., Kappas, A. & Conney, A.H. (1979) Stimulatory effect of Brussels sprouts and cabbage on human drug metabolism. *Clin. Pharmacol. Ther.*, 25, 88-95

Pasanen, M. & Pelkonen, O. (1994) The expression and environmental regulation of P450 enzymes in human placenta. *Crit. Rev. Toxicol.*, 24, 211-229

Pasche, T., Hathorfne, S.B., Miller, D.J. & Wenclaviack, B. (1992) Supercritical fluid extraction of nitrated polycyclic aromatic hydrocarbons and polycyclic aromatic hydrocarbons from diesel exhaust particulate matter. *J. Chromatogr.*, 609, 333-340

Patten, C.J., Thomas, P.E., Guy, R.L., Lee, M., Gonzalez, F.J., Guengerich, F.P. & Yang, C.S. (1993) Cytochrome P450 enzymes involved in acetaminophen activation by rat and human liver microsomes and their kinetics. *Chem. Res. Toxicol.*, 6, 511-518

Penno, M.B. & Vesell, E.S. (1983) Monogenic control of variations in antipyrine metabolite formation. *J. Clin Invest.*, 71, 1968-1709

Peters, R.K., Garabrant, D.H., Yu, M.C. & Mack, T.M. (1989) A case-control study of occupational and dietary factors in colorectal cancer in young men by subsite. *Cancer Res.*, 49, 5459-5468

Qian, G.-S., Ross, R.K., Yu, M.C., Yuan, J.-M., Gao, Y.-T., Henderson, B.E., Wogan, G.N. & Groopman, J.D. (1994) A follow-up study of urinary markers of aflatoxin exposure and liver cancer risk in Shanghai, People's Republic of China. *Cancer Epidemiol. Biomarkers Prev.*, 3, 3-10

Quattrochi, L.C. & Tukey, R.H. (1989) The human cytochrome *CYP1A2* gene contains regulatory elements responsive to 3-methylcholanthrene. *Mol. Pharmacol.*, 36, 66-71

Quattrochi, L.C., Vu, T. & Tukey, R.H. (1994) The human *CYP1A2* gene and induction by 3-methylcholanthrene. *J. Biol. Chem.*, 269 (9), 6949-6954

Raney, V.M., Harris, T.M. & Stone, M.P. (1993) DNA conformation mediates aflatoxin B_1-DNA binding and the formation of guanine N7 adducts by aflatoxin B_1 8,9-exo-epoxide. *Chem. Res. Toxicol.*, 6, 64-68

Raza, H., King, R.S., Squires, R.B., Guengerich, F.P., Miller, D.W., Freeman, J.P. & Kadlubar, F.F. (1996) Metabolism of 2-amino-α-carboline, a food-borne heterocyclic amine mutagen and carcinogen, by human and rodent liver microsomes and by human cytochrome P4501A2. *Drug Metab. Dispos.*, 24: 395-400

Relling, M.V., Lin, J.S., Ayers, G.D. & Evans, W.E. (1992) Pharmacoepidemiology and drug utilization. Racial and gender differences in *N*-acetyltransferase, xanthine oxidase, and CYP1A2 activities. *Clin. Pharmacol. Ther.*, 52, 643-658

Rettie, A.E., Korzekwa, K.R., Kunze, K.L., Lawrence, R.F., Eddy, A.C., Aoyama, T., Gelboin, H.V., Gonzalez, F.J. & Trager, W.F. (1992) Hydroxylation of warfarin by human cDNA-expressed cytochrome P-450: a role for P-4502C9 in the etiology of *(S)*-warfarin drug interactions. *Chem. Res. Toxicol.*, 5, 54-59

Rodopoulos, N., Wisen, W. & Norman, A. (1995) Caffeine metabolism in patients with chronic liver disease. *Scand. J. Clin. Lab. Invest.*, 55, 229-242

Roeder, K. (1994) A graphical technique for determining the number of components in a mixture of normals. *J. Am. Stat. Assoc.*, 89, 487-495

Ross, S., Sinha, R., Patterson, B., Rothman, N., Lang, N.P. & Kadlubar, F.F. (1996) Gender differences in cytochrome P4501A2 (CYP1A2) activity before and after a controlled diet. *Proc. Am. Assoc. Cancer Res.*, 37,1754

Rostami-Hodjegan, A., Nurminen, S., Jackson, P.R. & Tucker, G.T. (1996) Caffeine urinary metabolite ratios as markers of enzyme activity: a theoretical assessment. *Pharmacogenetics*, 6, 121-149

Rothman, N., Hayes, R.B., Bi, W., Caporaso, N., Broly, F., Woosley, R.L., Yin, S., Feng, P., You, X. & Meyer, U.A. (1993) Correlation between *N*-acetyltransferase activity and *NAT2* genotype in Chinese males. *Pharmacogenetics*, 3, 250-255

Sarkar, M.A. & Jackson, B.J. (1994) Theophylline *N*-demethylation as probes for P4501A1 and P4501A2. *Drug. Metab. Dispos.*, 22, 827-834

Schellens, J.H., Janssens, A.R., van der Wart, J.H., van der Velde, E.A. & Breimer D.D. (1989) Relationship between the metabolism of antipyrine, hexobarbital and theophylline in patients with liver disease as assessed by a 'cocktail' approach. *Eur. J. Clin. Invest.*, 19, 472-479

Schiffman, M.H. & Felton, J.S. (1990) Fried foods and the risk of colon cancer. *Am. J. Epidemiol.*, 131, 376-378

Schweikl, H., Taylor, J.A., Kitareewan, S., Linko, P., Nagorney, D. & Goldstein, J.A. (1993) Expression of *CYP1A1* and *CYP1A2* genes in human liver. *Pharmacogenetics*, 3, 239-249

Sesardic, D., Boobis, A.R., Edwards, R.J. & Davies, D.S. (1988) A form of cytochrome P450 in man, orthologous to form d in the rat, catalyses the *O*-deethylation of phenacetin and is inducible by cigarette smoking. *Br. J. Clin. Pharmacol.*, 26, 363-372

Shahidi, N.T. (1968) Acetophenetidin-induced methemoglobinemia. *Ann. NY Acad. Sci.*, 151, 822-832

Sharer, J.E. & Wrighton, S.A. (1996) Identification of the human hepatic cytochromes P450 involved in the *in vitro* oxidation of antipyrine. *Drug Metab. Dispos.*, 24, 487-494

Shimada, T., Hayes, C.L., Yamazaki, H., Amin, S., Hecht, S.S., Guengerich, F.P. & Sutter, T.R. (1996) Activation of chemically diverse procarcinogens by human cytochrome P-450 1B1. *Cancer Res.*, 56, 2979-2984

Shimada, T., Iwasaki, M., Martin, M.V. & Guengerich, F.P. (1989) Human liver activation microsomal cytochrome P-450 enzymes involved in the bioactivation of procarcinogens detected by *umu* gene response in *Salmonella typhimurium* TA 1535/pSK1002. *Cancer Res.*, 49, 3218-3228

Shimada, T., Yun, C.-H., Yamazaki, H., Gautier, J.-C., Beaune, P.H. & Guengerich, F.P. (1992) Characterization of human lung microsomal cytochrome P-450 1A1 and its role in the oxidation of chemical carcinogens. *Mol. Pharmacol.*, 41, 856-864

Sinha, R., Rothman, N., Brown, E.D., Mark, S.D., Hoover, R.N., Caporaso, N.E., Levander, O.A., Knize, M.G., Lang, N.P. & Kadlubar, F.F. (1994) Pan-fried meat containing high levels of heterocyclic aromatic amines but low levels of polycyclic aromatic hydrocarbons induces cytochrome P4501A2 activity in humans. *Cancer Res.*, 54, 6154-6159

Spaldin, V., Madden, S., Adams, D.A., Edwards, R.J., Davies, D.S. & Park, B.K. (1995) Determination of human hepatic cytochrome P4501A2 activity *in vitro* use of tacrine as an isoenzyme-specific probe. *Drug Metab. Dispos.*, 23, 929-934

Sugimura, T., Sato, S. & Wakabayashi, K. (1988) Mutagens/carcinogens in pyrolysate of amino acids and proteins and in cooked foods: heterocyclic aromatic amine. In: Woo, Y.T., Lai, D.Y., Arcos, J.C. & Argus, M..F., eds, *Chemical Induction of Cancer, Structural Bases and Biological Mechanisms*. New York; Academic Press, Inc.; pp. 681-710

Sutter, T.R., Tang, Y.M., Hayes, C.L., Wo, Y.-Y., Jabs, E.W., Li, X., Yin, H., Cody, C.W. & Greenlee, W.F. (1994) Complete cDNA sequence of a human dioxin-inducible mRNA identifies a new gene subfamily of cytochrome P450 that maps to chromosome 2. *J. Biol. Chem.*, 269, 13092-13099

Tanaka, E., Ishikawa, A., Yamamoto, Y., Osada, A., Tsuji, K., Fukao, K., Misawa, S. & Iwasaki, Y. (1992) A simple useful method for the determination of hepatic function in patients with liver cirrhosis using caffeine and its three major dimethylmetabolites. *Int. J. Clin. Pharmacol. Ther. Toxicol.*, 30, 336-341

Tang, B.K. & Kalow, W. (1996) CYP1A2 phenotyping using caffeine. *Cancer Epidemiol. Biomarkers Prev.*, 5, 231

Tang, B.K., Zhou, Y., Kadar, D. & Kalow, W. (1994) Caffeine as a probe for CYP1A2 activity: potential influence of renal factors on urinary phenotypic trait measurements. *Pharmacogenetics*, 4, 117-124

Tassaneeyakul, W., Birkett, D.J., McManus, M.E., Tassaneeyakul, W., Veronese, T., Andersson, T., Tukey, R.H. & Miners, J.O. (1994) Caffeine metabolism by human hepatic cytochromes P450: contributions of 1A2, 2E1 and 3A isoforms. *Biochem. Pharmacol.*, 47, 1767-1776

Turesky, R.J., Lang, N.P., Butler, M.A., Teitel, C.H. & Kadlubar, F.F. (1991) Metabolic activation of carcinogenic heterocyclic aromatic amines by human liver and colon. *Carcinogenesis*, 12, 1839-1845

Vaury, C., Laine, R., Noguiez, P., de Coppett, P., Jaulin, C., Praz, F., Pompon, D. & Amor-Gueret, A. (1995) Human glutathione S-transferase *M1* null genotype is associated with a high inducibility by cytochrome *P450 1A1* gene transcription. *Cancer Res.*, 55, 5520-5523

Vesell, E.S. & Gaylor, D.W. (1995) Limitations of probit plots in pharmacogenetics: requirement of genetic analyses to test hypotheses based on graphical methods. *Pharmacogenetics*, 5, 18-23

Vickers, P.J., Dufresne, M.J. & Cowan, K.H. (1989) Relation between cytochrome P450IA1 expression and extrogen receptor content of human breast cancer cells. *Mol. Endocrinol.*, 3, 157-164

Vistisen, K., Loft, S. & Poulsen, H.E. (1991) Cytochrome P450 1A2 activity in man measured by caffeine metabolism: effect of smoking, broccoli and exercise. *Adv. Exp. Med. Biol.*, 283. 407-411

Vistisen, K., Poulsen, H.E. & Loft, S. (1992) Foreign compound metabolism capacity in man measured from metabolites of dietary caffeine. *Carcinogenesis*, 13, 1561-1568

Waxman, D.J., Attisano, C., Guengerich, F.P. & Lapenson, D.P. (1988) Human liver microsomal steroid metabolism: identification of the major microsomal steroid hormone 6 beta-hydroxylase cytochrome P450 enzyme. *Arch. Biochem. Biophys.*, 263, 424-436

Wietholtz, H., Zysset, T., Kreiten, K., Kohl, D., Buschel, R. & Matern, S. (1989) Effects of phenytoin, carbamazepine, and valproic acid on caffeine metabolism. *Eur. J. Clin. Pharmacol.*, 36, 401-406

Wietholtz, H., Zysset, T., Marschall, H.-U., Generet, K. & Matern, S. (1995) The influence of rifampin treatment on caffeine clearance in healthy man. *J. Hepatol.*, 22, 78-81

Wislocki, P.G., Bagan, E.S., Lu, A.Y.H., Dooley, K.L., Fu, P.P., Han-Hsu, H., Beland, F.A. & Kadlubar, F.F. (1986) Tumorigenicity of nitrated derivatives of pyrene, benz[a]anthracene, chrysene and benzo[a]pyrene in the newborn mouse assay. *Carcinogenesis*, 7, 1317-1322

Yamazoe, Y., Abu-Zeid, M., Yamauchi, K. & Kato, R. (1988) Metabolic activation of pyrolysate arylamines by human liver microsomes: possible involvement of a P-448-H type cytochrome P450. *Jpn. J. Cancer Res.*, 79, 1159-1167

Zhang, Z.-Y. & Kaminsky, L.S. (1995) Characterization of human cytochromes P450 involved in theophylline 8-hydroxylation. *Biochem. Pharmacol.*, 50, 205-211

Corresponding author
Maria Teresa Landi
Genetic Epidemiology Branch,
EPN 400 - 6130 Executive Boulevard,
Bethesda, MD 20892, USA

Metabolic Polymorphisms and Susceptibility to Cancer
W. Ryder
IARC Scientific Publications No. 148
International Agency for Research on Cancer, Lyon, 1999

Chapter 17. The CYP2A subfamily: function, expression and genetic polymorphism

Hannu Raunio, Arja Rautio and Olavi Pelkonen

The CYP2A6 gene is one of the three members of the human CYP2A gene subfamily, the others being CYP2A7 and CYP2A13. The CYP2A6 enzyme catalyses the oxidation of several compounds that have clinical or toxicological interest, including pharmaceuticals, procarcinogens, and tobacco smoke constituents. CYP2A6 is expressed mainly in liver, and only trace amounts are found in extrahepatic tissues. Coumarin is a high-affinity substrate for CYP2A6, and a phenotyping test based on coumarin 7-hydroxylation has been developed. Two mutant alleles of the CYP2A6 gene have been found, i.e. CYP2A6*2 and CYP2A6*3. Homozygosity for both mutated alleles appears to confer a poor metabolizer (PM) phenotype, detectable by slow or non-existent 7-hydroxylation of coumarin. Very little is known about the inducibility and regulation of CYP2A6, but studies on the mouse orthologue, CYP2A5, have revealed novel pathways for induction. Since CYP2A6 polymorphism was found fairly recently, nothing is known presently about associations between variant CYP2A6 alleles and diseases or other adverse outcomes of exposure to toxins. Such studies, however, are clearly warranted, given the wide range of procarcinogens and other toxins metabolized by the CYP2A6 enzyme.

Cytochrome P450 (CYP) enzymes mediate the oxidative metabolism of numerous exogenous and endogenous compounds (Nelson *et al.*, 1996). Individual CYP forms have been shown to catalyse the metabolic activation and inactivation of numerous procarcinogens and promutagens (Gonzalez, 1992; Guengerich, 1993), and genetic polymorphisms of CYP genes affect the risk of acquiring xenobiotic-induced cancer (Wolf *et al.*, 1994; Raunio *et al.*, 1995). CYP2A is one of the seven CYP2 subfamilies known to be present in humans (Fernandez-Salguero & Gonzalez, 1995). The purpose of this Chapter is to review the existing knowledge of the function and expression of members in the CYP2A subfamily. The newly discovered polymorphism of CYP2A6 and its possible significance are also discussed.

Function of CYP2A forms

CYP2A6 is the best-characterized enzyme in this subfamily (Pelkonen *et al.*, 1993). It is a high-affinity coumarin 7-hydroxylating enzyme, and it also catalyses the O-deethylation of 7-ethoxycoumarin (Pelkonen & Raunio, 1995; Chang & Waxman,

1996). CYP2A6 has also been shown to catalyse the metabolism of several pharmaceuticals as well as compounds that are of toxicological significance, such as nitrosamines and aflatoxin B_1. Currently known CYP2A6 substrates are listed in Table 1. It should be noted that the furanocoumarin derivatives commonly used as anticoagulants, such as warfarin, are not metabolized by CYP2A6 but rather by members of the CYP2C subfamily (Honkakoski *et al.*, 1992).

Many of the procarcinogenic compounds listed in Table 1 have been tested only in bioassays, and the kinetic parameters such as affinities towards CYP2A6 enzyme have not been thoroughly characterized in most cases. Nicotine, because of its widespread use, is an especially interesting substrate. The inactivation of nicotine via C-oxidation to cotinine may be mediated by CYP2A6 (Cashman *et al.*, 1992; Nakajima *et al.*, 1996b), and the 3'-hydroxylation of cotinine is mediated by CYP2A6. Thus, any interindividual variations in CYP2A6 levels may affect nicotine inactivation rates and smoking patterns. Many other agents of toxicological interest are also substrates for the CYP2A6 enzyme (Table 1).

Table 1. CYP2A6 substrates

Compound	Assay/end point	Reference
Pharmaceuticals		
Coumarin	7-hydroxylation	(Yamano *et al.*, 1990)
(7-ethoxycoumarin)	O-deethylation	(Miles *et al.*, 1990)
		(Yun *et al.*, 1991)
		(Salonpää *et al.*, 1993)
Methoxyflurane	Dehalogenation	(Kharasch *et al.*, 1995)
Halothane	Reduction	(Spracklin *et al.*, 1996)
SM-12502	S-oxidation	(Nunoya *et al.*, 1996)
Losigamone	Oxidation	(Torchin *et al.*, 1996)
Toxic agents		
Nicotine	*N*-1'-oxidation	(Cashman *et al.*, 1992)
		(Nakajima *et al.*, 1996b)
Cotinine	3'-hydroxylation	(Nakajima *et al.*, 1996a)
NNK	Inhibition studies	(Yamazaki *et al.*, 1992
	Cell transformation	(Tiano *et al.*, 1993)
NDEA	Mutagenicity	(Crespi *et al.*, 1990)
	Inhibition studies	(Yamazaki *et al.*, 1992)
	Inhibition studies	(Camus *et al.*, 1993)
AFB$_1$	Ames test	(Aoyama *et al.*, 1990)
	Mutagenicity	(Crespi *et al.*, 1990
	Umu gene expression	(Yun *et al.*, 1991)
MOCA	*N*-oxidation	(Yun *et al.*, 1992)
1,3-butadiene	Monoxide formation	(Duescher & Elfarra, 1994)
Quinoline	1-oxidation	(Reigh *et al.*, 1996)
3-methylindole	Methylene imine formation	(Thornton-Manning *et al.*, 1996)
DCBN	Protein adduct formation	(Ding *et al.*, 1996)

SM-12502, 3,5-dimethyl-2-(3-pyridyl)thiazolidin-4-one hydrochloride; NNK, 4-methylnitrosamino-1-(3-pyridyl)-1-butanone; NDEA, *N*-nitrosodiethylamine; AFB$_1$, aflatoxin B$_1$; MOCA, 4,4'-methylene-bis(2-chloroaniline); DCBN, 2,6-dichlorobenzonitrile.

Expression of CYP2A genes

Measurements of liver coumarin 7-hydroxylation activities have revealed substantial interindividual differences in small-scale population studies. Large interindividual differences also exist at the CYP2A6 apoprotein and mRNA levels (Pelkonen *et al.*, 1993; Pelkonen & Raunio, 1995). In immunoblotting experiments using purified human CYP forms as standards, CYP2A6 protein constitutes 1-10% of the total liver CYP content (Yun *et al.*, 1991; Shimada *et al.*, 1994; Imaoka *et al.*, 1996).

The organization and structure of the entire human *CYP2A* gene cluster was recently characterized (Fernandez-Salguero *et al.*, 1995; Hoffman et al., 1995). The cluster consists of three genes (*CYP2A6*, *CYP2A7* and *CYP2A13*) and two *CYP2A7* pseudogenes localized within a 350-kb region in the long arm of chromosome 19 (Hoffman *et al.*, 1995). *CYP2A7* encodes a non-functional protein (Yamano *et al.*, 1990), and no full-length *CYP2A13* cDNA has yet been found. The elucidation of the *CYP2A* gene structures made it possible to assess their level of expression in human tissues. Using gene-specific RT-PCR, we recently screened several tissues for the presence or absence of CYP2A transcripts. Transcripts for all three genes (CYP2A6, CYP2A7 and CYP2A13) were found in liver. CYP2A6 was the most abundant form, followed by CYP2A7, and very little CYP2A13 mRNA was present. In comparison with liver, nasal mucosa contained a low amount of CYP2A6 and a relatively high level of CYP2A13 transcripts. Kidney, duodenum, lung, alveolar macrophages, peripheral lymphocytes, placenta and uterine endometrium were negative for all transcripts (Koskela *et al.*, unpublished).

Regulation of expression of CYP2A genes

While only scant information is available on the regulation of the human *CYP2A6* gene, the CYP2A6 orthologue in mice, CYP2A5, has been thoroughly studied. CYP2A5 is inducible by phenobarbital, the archetypal inducer, but in contrast to almost all other CYP forms, CYP2A5 is elevated by several hepatotoxic compounds (Pellinen *et al.*, 1993; Pellinen *et al.*, 1994; Camus-Randon *et al.*, 1996), heavy metals (Legrum *et al.*, 1979; Hahnemann *et al.*, 1992), and agents that interfere with cellular haeme metabolism (Salonpää *et al.*, 1995). Biological insults, such as integration of hepatitis B-virus (HBV) in hepatocyte DNA (Kirby *et al.*, 1994a) and infestation with the liver fluke *Opisthorchiasis viverrini* (Kirby *et al.*, 1994b) also result in an elevation of hepatic CYP2A5. Second messenger pathways are involved in the induction process, since cAMP-elevating agents induce CYP2A5 in mouse hepatocytes (Salonpää *et al.*, 1994). The increases in CYP2A5 are regulated both at the pretranscriptional and posttranscriptional levels (Aida & Negishi, 1991; Geneste *et al.*, 1996). These findings indicate that murine CYP2A5 is regulated in a very complex manner, possibly involving several independent cellular pathways.

Studies with primary human hepatocytes showed that at least phenobarbital and rifampicin are capable of inducing CYP2A6 (Dalet-Beluche *et al.*, 1992). Epileptic patients receiving drug therapy (carbamazepine, clonazepam, phenobarbital and phenytoin) exhibit an increased capacity to form 7-hydroxycoumarin *in vivo* (Sotaniemi *et al.*, 1995). Also in humans, fibrosis and infestation of the liver with *Opisthorchiasis viverrini* enhance coumarin 7-hydroxylation *in vivo* (Satarug *et al.*, 1996). The observation that overexpression of the HBV core protein leads to focal elevation of CYP2A5 in mouse liver (Kirby *et al.*, 1994a) suggested that similar events could occur in humans with chronic HBV infection, and a recent study (Kirby *et al.*, 1996) indicates that this is indeed the case. In sections of human liver infected with HBV, an elevated level of CYP2A6 protein was found by immunostaining in hepatocytes expressing the HBV core antigen (Kirby *et al.*, 1996). This provides a possible explanation for the observed synergistic effect on the development of hepatocellular carcinoma between HBV carrier status and aflatoxin exposure (IARC, 1993). An increase in liver CYP2A6 content by HBV integration could alter liver metabolism towards more effective activation of aflatoxins and nitrosamines, leading to an increase in the amount of initiated hepatocytes. This scenario is theoretical and has not yet been tested.

CYP2A6 polymorphism

Phenotyping studies

Coumarin can be used as a probe drug to assess CYP2A6 status *in vivo*. This phenotyping test involves administration of 5 mg of coumarin perorally, collection of the urine for up to 24 hours and measurement of the urine 7-hydroxycoumarin content (Rautio *et al.*, 1992). Since coumarin is rapidly absorbed and metabolized, the 2-hour 7-hydroxycoumarin excretion rate has proved to be a reliable index of CYP2A6 function. The coumarin test for CYP2A6 is one of the most specific CYP phenotyping tests available at the moment, since no other human CYP form has the capacity to catalyse coumarin 7-hydroxylation to a significant degree (Waxman *et al.*, 1991).

Using the coumarin test, some potentially modifying factors of coumarin 7-hydroxylation *in vivo* have been investigated. In a study with 20 young healthy volunteers (Rautio *et al.*, 1994), the excretion rate of 7-hydroxycoumarin did not change after acute alcohol ingestion or after treatment with rifampicin or cimetidine, suggesting that some known inhibitors and inducers of CYP enzymes do not affect CYP2A6 function *in vivo*. On the other hand, 7-hydroxycoumarin excretion was slightly lower in both female and male smokers compared to non-smokers (Iscan *et al.*, 1994). Methoxsalen (8-methoxypsoralen), an anti-psoriatic agent, has been shown to inhibit the *in vivo* formation of 7-hydroxycoumarin in humans (Mäenpää *et al.*, 1994) and Merkel *et al.*

(1994) have shown that grapefruit juice flavonoids inhibit 7-hydroxycoumarin formation in healthy volunteers. Wheat germ juice also inhibits 7-hydroxycoumarin formation, while vegan diet has no significant effect (Rauma *et al.*, 1996). Epileptic patients treated with enzyme-inducing antiepileptic drugs have increased 7-hydroxycoumarin excretion velocities (Sotaniemi *et al.*, 1995).

Initial population phenotyping studies, each involving less than 110 individuals, revealed a rather wide distribution of coumarin 7-hydroxylation activity in British (Cholerton *et al.*, 1992), Finnish (Rautio *et al.*, 1992), Turkish (Iscan *et al.*, 1994) and Chinese (Rautio et al, unpublished) populations. Fig. 1 summarizes the coumarin 7-

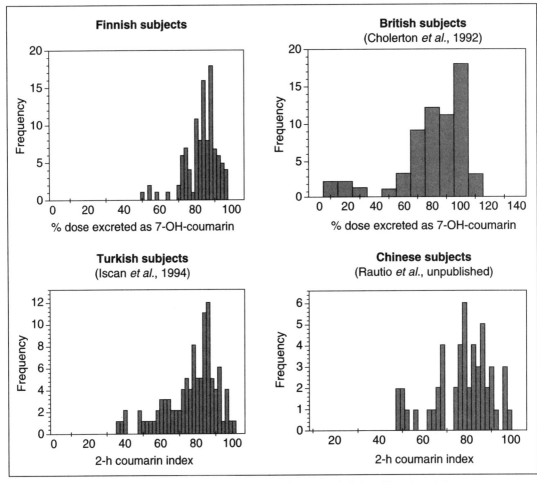

Figure 1.. Frequency distribution histograms of coumarin 7-hydroxylation capacity in four different populations.

hydroxylation distribution frequencies in these population studies. In all these studies there were outliers from the main clusters, but statistical analysis indicated the distribution to be uni-modal or non-polymorphic in each case. However, subsequent phenotyping studies have revealed that there are individuals in both Caucasian and Oriental populations who com-pletely lack coumarin 7-hydroxylating capacity, as discussed in detail below.

Genotyping studies

Three alleles of the *CYP2A6* gene have been found, initially designated wild-type, *CYP2A6v1* and *CYP2A6v2* (Fernandez-Salguero et al., 1995). The new designations for these alleles are *CYP2A6*1, *CYP2A6*2* and *CYP2A6*3*, respective-ly (Daly et al., 1996). *CYP2A6*2* has a point mutation in codon 160 leading to a Leu-His amino acid change. The resulting enzyme appears to produce a defective enzyme not capa-ble of coumarin 7-hydroxylation (Yamano et al., 1990). *CYP2A6*3* differs from the wild-type allele in regions within exons 3, 6, and 8, which bear sequence relatedness with the corresponding exons of the *CYP2A7* gene. A PCR-based method for determining CYP2A6 alleles from genomic DNA was developed (Fernandez-Salguero et al., 1995). Initial population studies have shown that there are considerable interethnic variations in the frequencies of the variant alleles (Table 2). The number of individuals so far studied has been rather low in most populations, and the

allele frequencies listed in Table 2 can be expect-ed to change once a greater number of DNA sam-ples has been assayed in each population. The apparently higher number of variant alleles in the Japanese population is consistent with the recent observation that a higher percentage of Japanese people lack hepatic coumarin 7-hydrox-ylation compared with Caucasians (Shimada et al., 1996).

After completion of the population studies which, presumably due to the limited number of individuals studied, revealed no clear phenotyp-ic polymorphism of CYP2A6 (Cholerton et al., 1992; Rautio et al., 1992; Iscan et al., 1994), sev-eral individuals were found in the Caucasian population who did not produce 7-hydroxy-coumarin in the coumarin test. These individuals were either *CYP2A6*2/CYP2A6*2* or *CYP2A6*3/CYP2A6*3* homozygotes. All the *CYP2A6 *3/*3* individuals who have been found up to the present lack coumarin 7-hydroxylating capacity, but some *CYP2A6 *2/*2* individuals with an intermediate capacity for coumarin 7-hydroxylation have been identified (Gullsten et al., unpublished). Homozygosity for *CYP2A6*2* and *CYP2A6*3* thus confers a poor metabolizer (PM) phenotype, whereas wild-type (*CYP2A6*1*) homozygotes and heterozygotes are extensive metabolizers (EM). However, this genotype-phe-notype correlation is not unequivocal, and fur-ther studies are needed to establish the exact relationship between the different *CYP2A6* hap-lotypes and the phenotype.

Table 2. Allelic frequencies of CYP2A6 gene in different populations				
Population	CYP2A6*1	CYP2A6*2	CYP2A6*3	Number of alleles analysed
Caucasian				
English	76	17	7	58
Finnish	89	9	2	88
Spanish	88	4	9	820
Asian				
Japanese	52	20	28	40
Taiwanese	83	11	6	178
African-American	98	0	2	40

Data from Fernandez-Salguero et al., 1995; Gullstén et al., 1997.

Consequences of CYP2A6 polymorphism

In theory, CYP2A6 polymorphism could have the following consequences:

- Clinically used drugs that are metabolized by CYP2A6 could accumulate and possibly cause toxic side-effects in persons lacking CYP2A6 activity.
- CYP2A6 status, by mediating the metabolism of nicotine to cotinine, could affect smoking patterns.
- Extensive metabolizers could be at an increased risk of cancer or other toxic outcomes caused by procarcinogens and promutagens that are activated by CYP2A6.

As yet, none of these possibilities has been rigorously tested. CYP2A6 is not a rate-limiting enzyme for the metabolism of any commonly used clinical drug, but since the systematic exploration of form-specific metabolism of drugs has just begun (Pelkonen *et al.*, 1995) we can expect that several drug substrates for CYP2A6 will emerge in the near future. The platelet-activating factor antagonist SM-12502 and the anticonvulsant losigamone are examples of novel CYP2A6 drug substrates (Nunoya *et al.*, 1996; Torchin *et al.*, 1996).

Nicotine maintains tobacco addiction and has therapeutic value in aiding smoking cessation and possibly in treating other conditions (Benowitz, 1996). Besides being involved in the formation of cotinine from nicotine (Cashman *et al.*, 1992), CYP2A6 appears to mediate the 3'-hydroxylation of cotine (Nakajima *et al.*, 1996a). This raises the possibility that variations in CYP2A6, through determining levels of nicotine metabolites, affect smoking patterns or the disposition to begin smoking. This is clearly worth testing, especially as attempts to link CYP2D6 polymorphism with smoking habits have yielded negative results (Benowitz *et al.*, 1996; Cholerton *et al.*, 1996).

A plausible consequence of CYP2A6 polymorphism is that PM and EM individuals have a different level of risk of acquiring cancer caused by exogenous procarcinogens, especially aflatoxins and nitrosamines. Since these agents are activated by CYP2A6, individuals with a PM phenotype could be protected from cancer initiation. This hypothesis was tested in a Spanish population exposed to low levels of mycotoxins. In this study

(Gullstén *et al.*, 1997), 90 patients with liver cancer, 83 with liver cirrhosis, and 237 healthy controls were genotyped for *CYP2A6* status. There was no significant difference in the distribution of different CYP2A6 genotypes between liver cancer and control groups, whereas there was a clear tendency towards underrepresentation of PM genotypes in the cirrhosis group (Gullstén *et al.*, 1997). This result suggests that in a population exposed to low levels of mycotoxins, *CYP2A6* status does not affect liver cancer risk. CYP2A6 poor metabolizers could, however, be protected from developing liver cirrhosis. This is an intriguing finding that needs to be verified in larger populations, since the frequency of PM genotypes is low in Caucasians.

The procarcinogenic compounds identified as CYP2A6 substrates appear to differ greatly in their affinities to the enzyme. The exact kinetics of activation of most procarcinogenic substrates by the CYP2A6 enzyme are largely unknown, and the contribution of CYP2A6 to the overall metabolism of these procarcinogens deserves further attention. For example, the nitrosamine NDEA is a high-affinity substrate for CYP2A6 but is also metabolized by CYP2E1 (Crespi *et al.*, 1990; Yamazaki *et al.*, 1992; Camus *et al.*, 1993). The *N*-oxidation of MOCA (4,4'-methylene-bis(2-chloroaniline)) is catalysed by expressed CYP2A6 enzyme, but in human liver microsomes the reaction is mainly catalysed by CYP3A4 with virtually no contribution by CYP2A6 (Yun *et al.*, 1991; Yun *et al.*, 1992).

In conclusion, CYP2A6 polymorphism has been established both at gene and phenotype levels. In analogy with variant *CYP2D6*, *N-acetyltransferase 1/2*, and *glutathione S-transferase M1/T1* genes, no apparent adverse health effects are attributable to dysfunction of the CYP2A6 gene. These deviant genetic traits become manifest only if an individual is exposed to relevant substrates, e.g. clinical drugs that produce side-effects at high serum concentrations, or procarcinogens activated by the corresponding enzymes. In addition to the currently recognized CYP2A6 substrates, a number of new compounds are expected to be found which are metabolized by this CYP form. Associations of CYP2A6 variant genotypes with various diseases and smoking habits will undoubtedly be explored in detail in the near future.

Acknowledgements

Work in the authors' laboratory has been supported by the Finnish Academy of Sciences (contracts 1051029 and 29456) and the European Commission Biomed1 and Biomed2 Programmes.

References

Aida, K. & Negishi, M. (1991) Post-transcriptional regulation of coumarin 7-hydroxylase (P450Coh) induction by xenobiotics in mouse liver: mRNA stabilization by pyrazole. *Biochemistry*, 30, 8041-8045

Aoyama, T., Yamano, S., Guzelian, P.S., Gelboin, H.V. & Gonzalez, F.J. (1990) Five of 12 forms of vaccinia virus-expressed human hepatic cytochrome P450 metabolically activate aflatoxin B_1. *Proc. Natl. Acad. Sci. USA*, 87, 4790-4793

Benowitz, N.L. (1996) Pharmacology of nicotine: addiction and therapeutics. *Annu Rev. Pharmacol. Toxicol.*, 36, 597-613

Benowitz, N.L., Jacob, P. & Perez-Stable, E. (1996) CYP2D6 phenotype and the metabolism of nicotine and cotinine. *Pharmacogenetics*, 6, 239-242

Camus, A.-M., Geneste, O., Honkakoski, P., Bereziat, J.-C., Henderson, C.J., Wolf, C.R., Bartsch, H. & Lang, M.A. (1993) High variability of nitrosamine metabolism among individuals: role of cytochromes P450 2A6 and 2E1 in the dealkylation of N-nitrosodimethylamine and N-nitrosodiethylamine in mice and humans. *Mol. Carcinog.*, 7, 268-275

Camus-Randon, A.-M., Raffalli, F., Bereziat, J.-C., McGregor, D., Konstandi, M. & Lang, M.A. (1996) Liver injury and expression of cytochrome P450: evidence that regulation of CYP2A5 is different from that of other major xenobiotic metabolizing CYP enzymes. *Toxicol. Appl. Pharmacol.*, 138, 140-148

Cashman, J.R., Park, S.B., Yang, Z.-C., Wrighton, S.A., Jacob, P. & Benowitz, N.L. (1992) Metabolism of nicotine by human liver microsomes: steroselective formation of *trans*-nicotine N'-oxide. *Chem. Res. Toxicol.*, 5, 639-646

Chang, T.K.H. & Waxman, D.J. (1996). The CYP2A subfamily. In: Ioannides, C., ed, *Cytochromes P450. Metabolic and Toxicological Aspects*. Boca Raton: CRC Press, pp. 99-134

Cholerton, S., Boustead, C., Taber, H., Arpanahi, A. & Idle, J.R. (1996) *CYP2D6* genotypes in cigarette smokers and non-tobacco users. *Pharmacogenetics*, 6, 261-263

Cholerton, S., Idle, M.E., Vas, A., Gonzalez, F.J. & Idle, J.R. (1992) Comparison of a novel thin-layer chromatographic-fluorescence detection method with a spectrofluorometric method for the determination of 7-hydroxycoumarin in human urine. *J. Chromatogr.*, 575, 325-330

Crespi, C.L., Penman, B.W., Leakey, J.A.E., Arlotto, M.P., Stark, A., Parkinson, A., Turner, T., Steimel, D.T., Rudo, K., Davies, R.L. & Langenbach, R. (1990) Human cytochrome P450IIA3: cDNA sequence, role of the enzyme in the metabolic activation of promutagens, comparison to nitrosamine activation by human cytochrome P450IIE1. *Carcinogenesis*, 11, 1293-1300

Dalet-Beluche, I., Boulenc, X., Fabre, G., Maurel, P. & Bonfils, C. (1992) Purification of two cytochrome P450 isozymes related to CYP2A and CYP3A gene families from monkey (baboon, Papio papio) liver microsomes. Cross reactivity with human forms. *Eur. J. Biochem.*, 204, 641-648

Daly, A.K., Brockmöller, J., Broly, F., Eichelbaum, M., Evans, W.E., Gonzalez, F.J., Huang, J.-D., Idle, J.R., Ingelman-Sundberg, M., Ishizaki, T., Jacqz-Aigrain, E., Meyer, U.A., Nebert, D.W., Steen, V.M., Wolf, C.R. & Zanger, U.M. (1996) Nomenclature for human *CYP2D6* alleles. *Pharmacogenetics*, 6, 193-201

Ding, X., Spink, D.C., Bhama, J.K., Sheng, J.J., Vaz, A.D.N. & Coon, M.J. (1996) Metabolic activation of 2,6-dichlorobenzonitrile, an olfactory-specific toxicant, by rat, rabbit and human cytochromes P450. *Mol. Pharmacol.*, 49, 1113-1121

Duescher, R.J. & Elfarra, A.A. (1994) Human liver microsomes are efficient catalysts of 1,3-butadiene oxidation: evidence for major roles by cytochromes P450 2A6 and 2E1. *Arch. Biochem. Biophys.*, 311, 342-349

Fernandez-Salguero, P., Hoffman, S.M.G., Cholerton, S., Mohrenweiser, H., Raunio, H., Rautio, A., Pelkonen, O., Huang, J., Evans, W.E., Idle, J.R. & Gonzalez, F.J. (1995) A genetic polymorphism in coumarin 7-hydroxylation: sequence of the human CYP2A genes and identification of variant CYP2A6 alleles. *Am. J. Hum. Genet.*, 57, 651-660

Fernandez-Salguero, P. & Gonzalez, F.J. (1995) The CYP2A gene subfamily: species differences, regulation, catalytic activities and role in chemical carcinogenesis. *Pharmacogenetics*, 5, S123-S128

Geneste, O., Raffalli, F. & Lang, M.A. (1996) Identification and characterization of a 44 kDa protein that binds specifically to the 3' untranslated region of CYP2a5 mRNA: inducibility, subcellular distribution and possible role in mRNA stabilization. *Biochem. J.*, 313, 1029-1037

Gonzalez, F.J. (1992) Human cytochromes P450: problems and prospects. *Trends Pharmacol. Sci.*, 13, 346-352

Guengerich, F.P. (1993) Bioactivation and detoxication of toxic and carcinogenic chemicals. *Drug Metab. Dispos.*, 21, 1-6

Gullstén, H., Agundez, J.A.G., Benitez, J., Läärä, E., Ladero, J.M., Diaz-Rubio, M., Fernandez-Salguero, P., Gonzalez, F., Rautio, A., Pelkonen, O. & Raunio, H. (1997) CYP2A6 gene polymorphism and risk of liver cancer and cirrhosis. *Pharmacogenetics*, 7, 247-250

Hahnemann, B., Salonpää, P., Pasanen, M., Mäenpää, J., Honkakoski, P., Juvonen, R., Lang, M.A., Pelkonen, O. & Raunio, H. (1992) Effect of pyrazole, cobalt and phenobarbital on mouse liver cytochrome P-450 2a-4/5 (Cyp2a-4/5) expression. *Biochem. J.*, 286, 289-294

Hoffman, S.M.G., Fernandez-Salguero, P., Gonzalez, F.J. & Mohrenweiser, H.W. (1995) Organization and evolution of the cytochrome P450 CYP2A-2B-2F subfamily gene cluster on human chromosome 19. *J. Molec. Evolut.*, 41, 894-900

Honkakoski, P., Arvela, P., Juvonen, R., Lang, M.A., Kairaluoma, M. & Pelkonen, O. (1992) Human and mouse liver coumarin 7-hydroxylases do not metabolize warfarin in vitro. *Br. J. Clin. Pharmacol.*, 33, 313-317

IARC (1993). *IARC Monographs on the Evaluation of Carcinogenic Risks to Humans. Volume 56. Some Naturally Occurring Substances: Food Items and Constituents, Heterocyclic Aromatic Amines and Mycotoxins.* IARC, Lyon, France.

Imaoka, S., Yamada, T., Hiroi, T., Hayashi, K., Sakaki, T., Yabusaki, Y. & Funae, Y. (1996) Multiple forms of human P450 expressed in *Saccharomyces cerevisiae*, systematic characterization and comparison with those of the rat. *Biochem. Pharmacol.*, 51, 1041-1050

Iscan, M., Rostami, H., Guray, T., Pelkonen, O. & Rautio, A. (1994) A study on the interindividual variability of coumarin 7-hydroxylation in a Turkish population. *Eur. J. Clin. Pharmacol.*, 47, 315-318

Kharasch, E.D., Hankins, D.C. & Thummel, K.E. (1995) Human kidney methoxyflurane and sevoflurane metabolism. Intrarenal fluoride production as a possible mechanism of methoxyflurane nephrotoxicity. *Anesthesiology*, 82, 689-699

Kirby, G.M., Batist, G., Alpert, L., Lamoureux, E., Cameron, R.G. & Alaoui-Jamali, M.A. (1996) Overexpression of cytochrome P-450 isoforms involved in aflatoxin B1 bioactivation in human liver with cirrhosis and hepatitis. *Toxicol. Pathol.*, 24, 458-467

Kirby, G.M., Chemin, I., Montesano, R., Chisari, F.V., Lang, M.A. & Wild, C.P. (1994a) Induction of specific cytochrome P450s involved in aflatoxin B1 metabolism in hepatitis B virus transgenic mice. *Mol. Carcinog.*, 11, 74-80

Kirby, G.M., Pelkonen, P., Vatanasapt, V., Camus, A.-M., Wild, C.P. & Lang, M.A. (1994b) Association of liver fluke (Opisthorchis viverrini) infestation with increased expression of cytochrome P450 and carcinogen metabolism in male hamster liver. *Mol. Carcinog.*, 11, 81-89

Legrum, W., Stuehmeier, G. & Netter, K.J. (1979) Cobalt as a modifier of microsomal monooxygenase in mice. *Toxicol. Appl. Pharmacol.*, 48, 195-204

Mäenpää, J., Juvonen, R., Raunio, H., Rautio, A. & Pelkonen, O. (1994) Methoxsalen and coumarin interactions in man and mouse. *Biochem. Pharmacol.*, 48, 1363-1369

Merkel, U., Sigusch, H. & Hoffmann, A. (1994) Grapefruit juice inhibits 7-hydroxylation of coumarin in healthy volunteers. *Eur. J. Clin. Pharmacol.*, 46, 175-177

Miles, J.S., McLaren, A.W., Forrester, L.M., Glancey, M.J., Lang, M.A. & Wolf, C.R. (1990) Identification of the human liver cytochrome P-450 responsible for coumarin 7-hydroxylase activity. *Biochem. J.*, 267, 365-371

Nakajima, M., Yamamoto, T., Nunoya, K.-I., Yokoi, T., Nagashima, K., Inoue, K., Funae, Y., Shimada, N., Kamataki, T. & Kuroiwa, Y. (1996a) Characterization of CYP2A6 involved in 3'-hydroxylation of cotinine in human liver microsomes. *J. Pharmacol. Exp. Ther.*, 277, 1010-1015

Nakajima, M., Yamamoto, T., Nunoya, K.-I., Yokoi, T., Nagashima, K., Inoue, K., Funae, Y., Shimada, N. & Kuroiwa, Y. (1996b) Role of human cytochrome P4502A6 in C-oxidation of nicotine. *Drug Metab. Dispos.*, 24, 1212-1217

Nelson, D.R., Koymans, L., Kamataki, T., Stegeman, J.J., Feyereisen, R., Waxman, D.J., Waterman, M.R., Gotoh, O., Coon, M.J., Estabrook, R.W., Gunsalus, I.C. & Nebert, D.W. (1996) P450 superfamily: update on new sequences, gene mapping, accession numbers and nomenclature. *Pharmacogenetics*, 6, 1-42

Nunoya, K.-I., Yokoi, T., Kimura, K., Kodama, T., Funayama, M., Inoue, K., Nagashima, K., Funae, Y., Shimada, N., Green, C. & Kamataki, T. (1996) (+)-Cis-3,5-dimethyl-2-(3-pyridyl) thiazolidin-4-one hydrochloride (SM-12502) as a novel substrate for cytochrome P450 2A6 in human liver microsomes. *J. Pharmacol. Exp. Ther.*, 277, 768-774

Pelkonen, O. & Raunio, H. (1995) Individual expression of carcinogen-metabolizing enzymes: cytochrome P4502A. *J. Occup. Environ. Med.*, 37, 19-24

Pelkonen, O., Raunio, H., Rautio, A., Mäenpää, J. & Lang, M.A. (1993) Coumarin 7-hydroxylase: characteristics and regulation in mouse and man. *J. Irish Coll. Phys. Surg.*, 22, 24-28

Pelkonen, O., Rautio, A. & Raunio, H. (1995). Specificity and applicability of probes for drug metabolizing enzymes. In: Alvan, G., Balant, L.P., Bechtel, P.R., Boobis, A.R., Gram, L.F., Paintaud, G. & Pithan, K., eds, *European Cooperation in the Field of Scientific and Technical Research - COST B1 Conference on the Variability and Specificity in Drug Metabolism*. Luxembourg, European Commission, pp. 147-158

Pellinen, P., Stenbäck, F., Raunio, H., Pelkonen, O. & Pasanen, M. (1994) Modification of hepatic cytochrome P450 profile by cocaine-induced hepatotoxicity in DBA/2 mouse. *Eur. J. Pharmacol. Environ. Toxicol. Pharmacol.*, 292, 57-65

Pellinen, P., Stenbäck, F., Rautio, A., Pelkonen, O., Lang, M.A. & Pasanen, M. (1993) Response of mouse liver coumarin 7-hydroxylase activity to hepatotoxins: dependence on strain and agent and comparison to other monooxygenases. *Naunyn-Schmiedeberg Arch. Pharmacol.*, 348, 435-443

Rauma, A.-L., Rautio, A., Pasanen, M., Pelkonen, O., Törrönen, R. & Mykkänen, H. (1996) Coumarin 7-hydroxylation in long-term adherents of a strict uncooked vegan diet. *Eur. J. Clin. Pharmacol.*, 50, 133-137

Raunio, H., Husgafvel-Pursiainen, K., Anttila, S., Hietanen, E., Hirvonen, A. & Pelkonen, O. (1995) Diagnosis of polymorphisms in carcinogen-activating and inactivating enzymes and cancer susceptibility-review. *Gene*, 159, 113-121

Rautio, A., Kraul, H., Kojo, A., Salmela, E. & Pelkonen, O. (1992) Interindividual variability of coumarin 7-hydroxylation in healthy individuals. *Pharmacogenetics*, 2, 227-233

Rautio, A., Salmela, E., Arvela, P., Pelkonen, O. & Sotaniemi, E.A. (1994). Assessment of CYP2A6 and CYP3A4 activities *in vivo* in different diseases in man. In: Lechner, M.C., ed, *Cytochrome P450. Biochemistry, Biophysics and Molecular Biology.* Paris, John Libbey Eurotext, pp. 519-521

Reigh, G., McMahon, H., Ishizaki, M., Ohara, T., Shimane, K., Esumi, Y., Green, C., Tyson, C. & Ninomiya, S. (1996) Cytochrome P450 species involved in the metabolism of quinoline. *Carcinogenesis,* 17, 1989-1996

Salonpää, P., Hakkola, J., Pasanen, M., Pelkonen, O., Vähäkangas, K., Battula, N., Nouso, K. & Raunio, H. (1993) Retrovirus-mediated stable expression of human CYP2A6 in mammalian cells. *Eur. J. Pharmacol. Environ. Toxicol. Pharmacol.,* 248, 95-102

Salonpää, P., Krause, K., Pelkonen, O. & Raunio, H. (1995) Up-regulation of CYP2A5 expression by porphyrinogenic agents in mouse liver. *Naunyn-Schmiedeberg Arch. Pharmacol.,* 351, 446-452

Salonpää, P., Pelkonen, O., Kojo, A., Pasanen, M., Negishi, M. & Raunio, H. (1994) CYP2A5 expression and inducibility by phenobarbital is modulated by cAMP in mouse primary hepatocytes. *Biochem. Biophys. Res. Commun.,* 205, 631-637

Satarug, S., Lang, M.A., Yongvanit, P., Sithithaworn, P., Mairiang, E., Mairiang, P., Pelkonen, P., Bartsch, H. & Haswell-Elkins, M.R. (1996) Induction of cytochrome P450 2A6 expression in humans by the carcinogenic parasite infection, *Opisthorchiasis viverrini. Cancer Epidemiol. Biomarkers. Prev.,* 5, 795-800

Shimada, T., Yamazaki, H. & Guengerich, F.P. (1996) Ethnic-related differences in coumarin 7-hydroxylation activity catalysed by cytochrome P2402A6 in liver microsomes of Japanese and Caucasians populations. *Xenobiotica,* 26, 395-403

Shimada, T., Yamazaki, H., Mimura, M., Inui, Y. & Guengerich, F.P. (1994) Interindividual variations in human liver cytochrome P-450 enzymes involved in the oxidation of drugs, carcinogens and toxic chemicals: studies with liver microsomes of 30 Japanese and 30 Caucasians. *J. Pharmacol. Exp. Ther.,* 270, 414-423

Sotaniemi, E.A., Rautio, A., Bäckström, M., Arvela, P. & Pelkonen, O. (1995) Hepatic cytochrome P450 isozyme (CYP2A6 and CYP3A4) activities and fibrotic process in liver. *Br. J. Clin. Pharmacol.,* 39, 71-76

Spracklin, D.K., Thummel, K.E. & Kharasch, E.D. (1996) Human reductive halothane metabolism *in vitro* is catalysed by cytochrome P450 2A6 and 3A4. *Drug Metab. Dispos.,* 24, 976-983

Thornton-Manning, J., Appleton, M.L., Gonzalez, F.J. & Yost, G.S. (1996) Metabolism of 3-methylindole by vaccinia-expressed P450 enzymes: correlation of 3-methyleneindolenine formation and protein-binding. *J. Pharmacol. Exp. Ther.,* 276, 21-29

Tiano, H.F., Hosokawa, M., Clulada, P.C., Smith, P.B., Wang, R., Gonzalez, F.J., Crespi, C.L. & Langenbach, R. (1993) Retroviral mediated expression of human cytochrome P450 2A6 in C3H/10T1/2 cells confers transformability by 4-(methylnitrosamino) -1 - (3- pyridyl) 1 -butanone (NNK). *Carcinogenesis,* 14, 1421-1427

Torchin, C.D., McNeilly, P.J., Kapetanovic, I.M., Strong, J.M. & Kupferberg, H.J. (1996) Stereoselective metabolism of a new anticonvulsant drug candidate, losigamone, by human liver microsomes. *Drug Metab. Dispos.,* 24, 1002-1008

Waxman, D.J., Lapenson, D.P., Aoyama, T., Gelboin, H.V., Gonzalez, F.J. & Korzekwa, K. (1991) Steroid hormone hydroxylase specificities of eleven cDNA-expressed human cytochrome P450s. *Arch. Biochem. Biophys.,* 290, 160-166

Wolf, C.R., Smith, C.A.D. & Forman, D. (1994) Metabolic polymorphisms in carcinogen metabolizing enzymes and cancer susceptibility. *Brit. Med. Bulletin,* 50, 718-731

Yamano, S., Tatsuno, J. & Gonzalez, F.J. (1990) The CYP2A3 gene product catalyses coumarin 7-hydroxylation in human liver microsomes. *Biochemistry,* 29, 1322-1329

Yamazaki, H., Inui, Y., Yun, C.-H., Guengerich, F.P. & Shimada, T. (1992) Cytochrome P450 2E1 and 2A6 enzymes as major catalysts for metabolic activation of N-nitrosodialkylamines and tobacco-related nitrosamines in human liver microsomes. *Carcinogenesis,* 13, 1789-1794

Yun, C.-H., Shimada, T. & Guengerich, F.P. (1991) Purification and characterization of human liver microsomal cytochrome P-450 2A6. *Mol. Pharmacol.,* 40, 679-685

Yun, C.-H., Shimada, T. & Guengerich, F.P. (1992) Contributions of human liver cytochrome P450 enzymes to the N-oxidation of 4,4'-methylene-bis(2-chloroaniline). *Carcinogenesis,* 13, 217-222

Corresponding author
H. Raunio
Department of Pharmacology and Toxicology, University of Oulu, Oulu, FIN 90220, Finland

Metabolic Polymorphisms and Susceptibility to Cancer
W. Ryder
IARC Scientific Publications No. 148
International Agency for Research on Cancer, Lyon, 1999

Chapter 18. Cytochrome P450 CYP2D6

C. Roland Wolf and Gillian Smith

Altered expression of CYP2D6 (debrisoquine hydroxylase), resulting from genetic polymorphism at the CYP2D6 gene locus, is responsible for pronounced interindividual variation in the metabolism of many clinically important drugs. Although CYP2D6 substrates are structurally diverse, most are small molecules that interact with the protein via an electrostatic interaction between a basic nitrogen which is common to the majority of CYP2D6 substrates and an aspartic acid residue in the active site of the protein. As CYP2D6 substrates have a wide range of pharmacological functions, any variation in CYP2D6 expression can have profound clinical consequences.

CYP2D6 activity can be determined both by phenotyping methods with a variety of probe drugs and by genotyping methods where PCR-based techniques are used to investigate the inheritance of individual CYP2D6 alleles. Allele frequencies have been shown to vary widely between populations of different racial origin. For example, the PM genotype is particularly rare in Orientals. The inheritance of certain CYP2D6 allelic variants has been associated with altered susceptibility to Parkinson's disease and several types of cancer.

Functions and substrates for CYP2D6

Cytochrome P450 CYP2D6 (debrisoquine hydroxylase) was first purified from human liver (Distlerath *et al.*, 1985) in an attempt to rationalize interindividual variation in oxidative drug metabolism. The now well-defined genetic polymorphism at the CYP2D6 gene locus was the first defect in drug metabolism to be specifically associated with altered expression of a P450 enzyme (Gonzalez *et al.*, 1988). This defect has been shown to be responsible for pronounced interindividual variation in the metabolism of many clinically important drugs, including the marker substrates debrisoquine and sparteine. Approximately 6% of the Caucasian population inherit one or more gene-inactivating CYP2D6 mutations (Mahgoub *et al.*, 1977; Sachse *et al.*, 1997). These individuals do not express functional CYP2D6 protein and are therefore unable to metabolize compounds that are CYP2D6 substrates.

CYP2D6 substrates are structurally diverse and, as a consequence, can perform many different pharmacological functions. Indeed, recent estimates suggest that CYP2D6 may be responsible for the metabolism of up to 25 % of all prescribed drugs (Benet *et al.*, 1996), examples of which are given in Table 1. The majority of substrates for CYP2D6 are small molecules containing a basic nitrogen atom. Although structurally diverse, the majority of CYP2D6 substrates are thought to interact with the protein through an electrostatic interaction between the substrate basic nitrogen and a negatively charged aspartate residue in the active site of the protein. Using homology modelling to predict the active site structure of CYP2D6, we have identified a specific aspartic acid residue (Asp 301) that lies within the active site of the protein and mediates interaction between protein and substrate (Ellis *et al.*, 1995; Modi *et al.*, 1996). Analysis of a series of mutant CYP2D6 proteins, where residue 301 was altered by site-directed mutagenesis, has confirmed that the retention of a negative charge at position 301 in CYP2D6 is an important determinant of the catalytic activity of the enzyme (Ellis *et al.*, 1995).

The ability to predict *a priori* whether a substrate can be accommodated in an energetically favourable conformation within the active site of CYP2D6 is an important goal, both in the *ab initio* identification of drugs that may be CYP2D6 substrates and therefore subject to polymorphic metabolism, and in the rationalization of experi-

Table 1. CYP2D6 substrates

β-blockers:

alprenolol, metoprolol, timolol, bufuralol, propranolol, guanoxan, indoramine, bupranolol

Antiarrythmics:

sparteine, N-propylajmaline, propafenone, mexiletine, flecainide, encainide, procainamide

Tricyclic antidepressants:

nortriptyline, desipramine, clomipramine, imipramine, amitryptiline, minaprine, fluvoxamine

Antipsychotics:

perphenazine, thioridazine, zuclopenthixol, haloperidol, tomoxetine, paroxetine, amiflavine,

methoxyphenamine, fluoxetine, levomepromazine, olanzapine

Analgesics:

codeine, ethylmorphine

Antihistamines:

loratadine, promethazine

Others:

debrisoquine (antihypertensive), 4-hydroxy amphetamine (central nervous system stimulant), phenformin, perhexiline, MDMA (Ecstasy), dextromethorphan (antitussive), ritonavir (HIV 1 protease inhibitor), dolasetron (antiemetic), ondansetron, tropisetron (5-HT$_3$ receptor antagonists), nicergoline (vasodilator), mexilitine (diabetes), dexfenfluramine (appetite suppressant), MPTP (1-methyl-4-phenyl-1,2,3,6-tetrahydropyridine, neurotoxin)

mentally obtained metabolites. For example, we and others have recently demonstrated that the Parkinsonism-inducing neurotoxin MPTP (1-methyl-4-phenyl-1,2,3,6-tetrahydropyridine) is a substrate for CYP2D6 (Coleman et al., 1996; Gilham et al., 1997). In experiments involving the use of recombinant enzyme we have shown that two products are formed following the reaction of MPTP with CYP2D6, only one of which is dependent on the presence of a negative charge at position 301 (Gilham et al., 1997; Modi et al., 1997). Modelling MPTP in the active site of CYP2D6 has allowed us to rationalize these experimental obser-

vations, and has revealed that the CYP2D6 active site can accommodate MPTP in two distinct conformations, only one of which involves binding of MPTP to Asp 301 (Modi et al., 1997). The ability of CYP2D6 to metabolize MPTP is of particular interest because the inheritance of the CYP2D6 PM genotype has been associated with increased incidence of Parkinson's disease (see below).

Interindividual variation in drug metabolism as a result of aberrant CYP2D6 expression can influence both drug pharmacokinetics and pharmacodynamics, thereby producing a variety of pharmacological consequences. Certain reactions catalysed by CYP2D6 result in the conversion of a prodrug that is inactive, or has only minimal activity, to its active form. For example, the analgesic codeine is 0-demethylated to morphine by CYP2D6 (Chen *et al.*, 1988). Poor metabolizing (PM) individuals are unable to perform this metabolic conversion and therefore do not obtain the desired therapeutic effect when codeine is used as an analgesic. In contrast, many CYP2D6 drug substrates including β-blockers, tricyclic antidepressants and antiarrythmics fail to be efficiently eliminated from the body by PM, and this results in higher plasma concentrations of active drugs. Unless interindividual differences in the metabolism of these compounds is taken into account at the time of prescription, exposure to many of these can lead to the development of unpleasant or even life-threatening side-effects in PM individuals (Tucker, 1994).

The extent to which lack of CYP2D6 expression is of clinical significance is largely determined by the width of the therapeutic window of the drug in question, i.e. the range of concentrations between the minimum dose required to achieve the desired therapeutic effect and that at which toxicity occurs. For example, the therapeutic window is relatively wide for beta-blockers such as metoprolol and timolol but is much narrower for the antiarrhythmics flecainide and propafenone.

The clinical relevance of polymorphism at the CYP2D6 gene locus is also determined by the extent to which CYP2D6 is the major route of metabolism of the compound of interest. For example, perhexiline is almost uniquely metabolized by CYP2D6 and, as a consequence, the therapeutic usefulness of the drug in CYP2D6 poor metabolizers is severely compromised by associated side-effects (Shah *et al.*, 1982). In contrast, propranolol can be metabolized by other P450 enzymes and is also excreted at relatively high concentrations as unchanged drug; variation in CYP2D6 expression is therefore relatively unimportant (Walle *et al.*, 1985).

Certain drugs, such as cimetidine, ranitidine and quinidine, are inhibitors of CYP2D6. Exposure to these agents can lead to "phenocopying", the development of a PM phenotype in an individual who is genetically an extensive metabolizer. Several drugs that are substrates for CYP2D6 can also be metabolized by other P450 isozymes, often leading to the generation of alternative metabolites. These secondary routes of metabolism may become increasingly important in CYP2D6 PMs and may necessitate alteration of the prescribed dose and/or monitoring for the formation of novel or undesirable metabolites.

The mechanisms by which the expression of CYP2D6 is regulated are not clearly understood and few endogenous substrates have been proposed for the enzyme. However, Martinez *et al.* (1997) identified tryptamine as a CYP2D6 substrate and demonstrated that CYP2D6 can catalyse the metabolic conversion of tryptamine to tryptophol, a final metabolite in a secondary catabolic pathway of L-tryptophan.

Unlike the majority of Family 2 P450 proteins, CYP2D6 expression does not seem to be inducible following xenobiotic challenge. Phenotyping studies with both metoprolol and dextromethorphan, however, indicate that CYP2D6 activity is increased during pregnancy (Högstedt *et al.*, 1983; Wadelius *et al.*, 1997). CYP2D6 expression also varies during the menstrual cycle, where the metabolic ratio for debrisoquine is significantly lower in the luteal phase than in the ovulatory phase (Llerena *et al.*, 1996). These findings imply that CYP2D6 expression may be influenced by steroid hormones. In support of this we have demonstrated that only a very minor change to the active site structure of CYP2D6 is required to allow the enzyme to accommodate and metabolize the steroid nucleus. The alteration of a single amino acid (Phe to Ile) in the substrate-binding site of CYP2D6 leads to the creation of an enzyme that has acquired the ability to metabolize testosterone to a unique stereospecific and regiospecific product (Smith *et al.*, 1997).

CYP2D6 catalyses the biotransformation of codeine to the analgesic morphine (Chen *et al.*, 1988). There is some evidence, however, that morphine can also be formed endogenously in the central nervous system in addition to its administration as a prescribed drug. CYP2D6 is thought to be present in a functional form in human brain (Niznik *et al.*, 1990; Kalow & Tyndale, 1992; Gilham *et al.*, 1997), raising the possibility that it may catalyse reactions in the central nervous system (CNS). Supporting this hypothesis is the fact that PM individuals are less tolerant to tonic pain (Sindrup *et al.*, 1993), a finding rationalized on

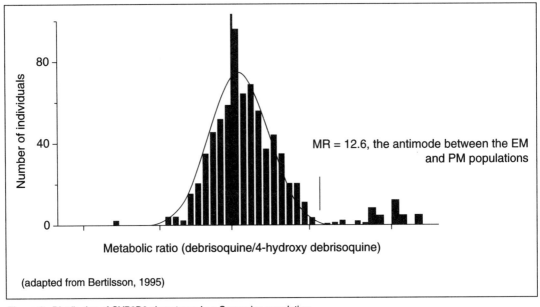

(adapted from Bertilsson, 1995)

Figure 1. Distribution of CYP2D6 phenotypes in a Caucasian population.
Frequency distribution of CYP2D6 metabolic ratios (MRs) in a Caucasian population (n = 1011). Individuals with MR < 12.6 are designated extensive metabolizers (EMs) while those with MR > 12.6 are designated poor metabolizers (PMs). MR is defined as the ratio of debrisoquine to 4-hydroxy debrisoquine excreted in urine.

the basis of an inherited deficiency in the ability to metabolically convert codeine to morphine. On the premise that CYP2D6 may indeed play a fundamental role in central nervous system metabolism, attempts have been made to correlate the CYP2D6 phenotype with personality (Bertilsson *et al.*, 1989; Llerena *et al.*, 1993). Similar studies in Sweden (Bertilsson *et al.*, 1989) and Spain (Llerena *et al.*, 1993) suggest that CYP2D6 PM are more anxiety prone and have less well developed social skills than extensive metabolizers. Whether these observations are linked to the newly proposed function of CYP2D6 in tryptamine metabolism (Martinez *et al.*, 1997) and the possible involvement of the enzyme in dopaminergic/serotoninergic neurotransmission remains to be determined. Accurate quantification of such data is not easily achieved and the results of these studies remain speculative.

Molecular and biochemical characterization of the CYP2D6 polymorphism

Characterization of the polymorphism at the CYP2D6 gene locus arose from early observations that 5-10% of the Caucasian population were

inefficient metabolizers of either debrisoquine, an adrenergic antihypertensive agent (Mahgoub *et al.*, 1977), or sparteine, an alkaloid used in the treatment of arrhythmia (Eichelbaum *et al.*, 1979). As a consequence, certain patients showed an exaggerated clinical response following prescription of these drugs.

Phenotyping studies in affected individuals, in which the metabolism of a subclinical dose of either debrisoquine or sparteine was monitored by measuring the relative amount of parent compound and metabolite excreted in the urine (the metabolic ratio), revealed that this defect in oxidative metabolism was under monogenic control and was inherited as an autosomal recessive trait (Mahgoub *et al.*, 1977). Analysis of metabolic ratios for debrisoquine and sparteine in large study populations demonstrated a bimodal distribution pattern for drug clearance, dividing the population into extensive (EM) metabolizers with normal drug pharmacokinetics and PM with compromised metabolism (Fig. 1).

A combination of linkage mapping, *in situ* hybridization and analysis of somatic cell hybrids has made it possible to localize the CYP2D6 gene

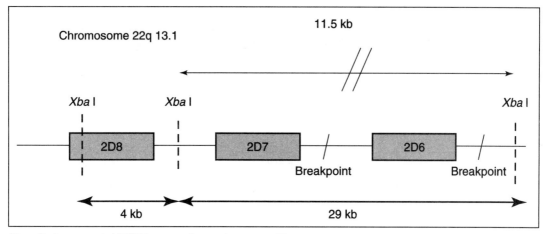

Figure 2. Arrangement of CYP2D genes on human chromosome 22.
The relative position of each of the CYP2D genes on chromosome 22 is illustrated. Restriction fragment sizes following RFLP analysis with Xba 1 are shown. Approximate positions of the breakpoint regions in the CYP2D6*5 (gene deletion allele) are marked.

to human chromosome 22q 13. 1 (Gough *et al.*, 1992), where it occurs in a cluster with the highly homologous but inactive pseudogenes CYP2D7 and CYP2D8 (Heim & Meyer, 1992; Fig. 2). While CYP2D8 is a true pseudogene, containing many frame-disrupting mutations, CYP2D7 has only a single T insertion at position 226 in the first exon, leading to a disrupted reading frame (Kimura *et al.*, 1989). The presence and sequence of the CYP2D pseudogenes appears to be conserved between individuals and also in different ethnic groups. On current evidence, polymorphism at the CYP2D gene locus seems to be confined to CYP2D6. CYP2D6 is localized in close proximity to the immunoglobulin gene locus on chromosome 22, a region of high genetic instability, and this may provide a mechanistic rationale for the high level of polymorphism in CYP2D6.

Multiple allelic variants at the CYP2D6 gene locus have been described (Table 2). Eight of these include one or more gene-inactivating mutations that have arisen as a consequence of single nucleotide substitutions or deletions, splice-junction alterations, or, uniquely in the case of the CYP2D6*5 allele, deletion of the entire CYP2D6 gene. In addition, a minority of individuals have increased catalytic activity towards CYP2D6 substrates as a consequence of an aberrant gene duplication event resulting in the inheritance of multiple copies of CYP2D6 (alleles CYP2D6*2x2, CYP2D6*2x3, CYP2D6*2x4, CYP2D6*2x5 and CYP2D6*2x13) arranged in tandem (Johansson *et al.*, 1993). Such individuals, termed ultra-rapid metabolizers, are extremely efficient at metabolizing compounds that are CYP2D6 substrates. They therefore require increased doses of these drugs in order to achieve an appreciable pharmacological effect (Bertilsson *et al.*, 1993).

Initial characterization of the CYP2D6 polymorphism at the molecular level was achieved by RFLP analysis with the restriction enzyme *Xba 1*. This revealed the presence of restriction fragments of 44kb, 29kb and 11.5kb, which co-segregate with the PM phenotype (Skoda *et al.*, 1988; Kagiomoto *et al.*, 1990). The most common gene-inactivating allelic variants of CYP2D6 both give 29 kb fragments following *Xba I* digestion - CYP2D6*3 (29A, CYP2D6A), which has a single nucleotide deletion in Exon 5 resulting in a frameshift and CYP2D6*4 (29B, CYP2D6B), which contains several silent single nucleotide substitutions and a point mutation in the consensus sequence for the splice site at the intron 3/exon 4 splice junction. Together with CYP2D6*5 (the gene deletion), which gives a characteristic 11.5 kb band on *Xba I* RFLP analysis, these alleles account for >95% of all CYP2D6 PM alleles in the Caucasian population.

The remaining CYP2D6 alleles are relatively rare in Caucasians and, with the exception of the CYP2D6*2A (gene amplification) alleles, the phenotypic consequences of inheriting many of

Table 2. CYP2D6 alleles		
Allele[1]	Trivial name[2]	Enzyme activity[3]
CYP2D6*1A	WILD-TYPE	normal
CYP2D6*1B		normal
CYP2D6*1C		normal
CYP2D6*2	CYP2D6L1	decreased
CYP2D6*2x2	CYP2D6L2	increased
CYP2D6*2x3		increased
CYP2D6*2x4	CYP2D6L2x2	increased
CYP2D6*2x5		increased
CYP2D6*2x13	CYP2D6L2x12	increased
CYP2D6*2B		normal
CYP2D6*3	CYP2D6A	inactive
CYP2D6*4A	CYP2D6B	inactive
CYP2D6*4B		inactive
CYP2D6*4C	K29-1	inactive
CYP2D6*4D		inactive
CYP2D6*4E		inactive
CYP2D6*5	CYP2D6D	inactive
CYP2D6*6A	CYP2D6T	inactive
CYP2D6*6B		inactive
CYP2D6*7	CYP2D6E	inactive
CYP2D6*8	CYP2D6G	inactive
CYP2D6*9	CYP2D6C	reduced
CYP2D6*10A	CYP2D6J	reduced
CYP2136*10B	CYP2D6Ch1	reduced
CYP2D6* 10C	CMD6Ch2	reduced
CYP2D6* 11	CYP2D6F	inactive
CYP2D6* 12		inactive

Table 2 (Contd). CYP2D6 alleles		
Allele[1]	Trivial name[2]	Enzyme activity[3]
CYP2D6* 13		inactive
CYP2D6* 14		inactive
CYP2D6* 15		inactive
CYP2D6* 16	CYP2D6D2	inactive
CYP2D6* 17	CYP2D6Z	reduced

[1]Allele nomenclature according to Daly et al., 1996.

[2] Two further CYP2D6 alleles have been reported since the publication of the1996 nomenclature paper: (a) G → T transversion at position 1846 of CYP2D6, leading to a frameshift and the creation of a premature stop codon (Broly et al., 1995); and (b) a 9-base pair insertion in exon 9 of CYP2D6, leading to an increase in catalytic activity of the enzyme (Yokoi et al., 1996).

[3]Activities of each allele are given relative to CYP2D6* 1, the wild-type enzyme; in general, activities have been determined towards a single substrate only.

these rarer forms of CYP2D6 are not fully understood. Several alleles, particularly those within the CYP2D6*9 and CYP2D6*10 subgroups, have retained the ability to bind haem and produce functional protein, although the catalytic activities and substrate specificities of these CYP2D6 forms have not been fully characterized. Alleles CYP2D6*13 and CYP2D6*16 are thought to have arisen from gene conversion events, where regions of the inactive pseudogene CYP2D7 are incorporated into CYP2D6 (Panserat et al., 1995; Daly et al., 1996).

A unified nomenclature system for CYP2D6 alleles has recently been published (Daly et al., 1996) in which the molecular structure of each of the allelic variants is described. Subsequently, however, further CYP2D6 alleles have been identified (Table 2; Broly et al., 1995; Yokoi et al., 1996; Sachse et al., 1997). Several of these contain gene-inactivating mutations, although the frequency of each within the Caucasian population is extremely low. A further candidate CYP2D6 allelic variant has been described (Crespi et al., 1995; Ellis et al., 1996) which differs by a single amino acid substitution (methionine to valine) at position 374. The CYP2D6 cDNA sequence, CYP2D6-Met, first published by Gonzalez et al. (1998) contained methionine at position 374, but a valine residue was present at the same position in the corresponding genomic sequence, CYP2D6-Val (Kimura et al., 1989). Experiments where both forms of the protein were expressed in mammalian cells (Crespi et al., 1995) and in yeast (Ellis et al., 1996) revealed minor differences in catalytic activity between the two forms of the protein towards a range of CYP2D6 substrates. PCR-based assays have been used to investigate whether the two sequences do indeed exist as true allelic variants but have failed to detect the presence of the CYP2D6-Met allele in either of the Caucasian populations studied.

Phenotype and genotype tests - accuracy, reproducibility and feasibility

A number of probe drugs have been used in CYP2D6 phenotyping studies, including debrisoquine, sparteine and the current drug of choice, dextromethorphan. Although phenotyping analysis can give an accurate overall assessment of an individual's drug-metabolizing capacity, there is not always a direct correlation with CYP2D6 genotype. A variety of factors, including other interfering medications, particularly other drugs that are CYP2D6 substrates or inhibitors, can interfere with an experimentally determined phenotype. Environmental influences (food,

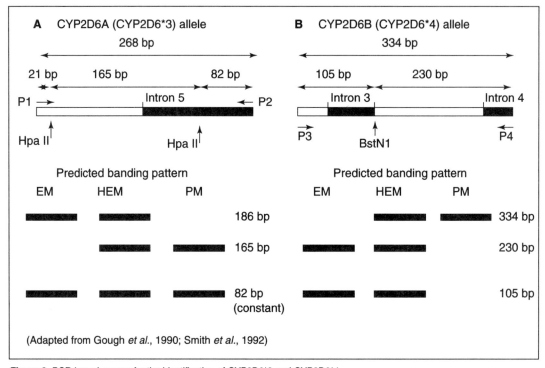

A CYP2D6A (CYP2D6*3) allele

268 bp

21 bp   165 bp   82 bp

P1 →   Intron 5   ← P2

Hpa II   Hpa II

Predicted banding pattern

EM   HEM   PM

186 bp

165 bp

82 bp
(constant)

B CYP2D6B (CYP2D6*4) allele

334 bp

105 bp   230 bp

Intron 3   Intron 4

P3   BstN1   P4

Predicted banding pattern

EM   HEM   PM

334 bp

230 bp

105 bp

(Adapted from Gough *et al.*, 1990; Smith *et al.*, 1992)

Figure 3. PCR-based assays for the identification of CYP2D6*3 and CYP2D6*4.
PCR-based strategies to identify the CYP2D6*3 and CYP2D6*4 alleles are shown, along with predicted banding patterns following digestion with the restriction enzymes Hpa II and Bst NI.

smoking, alcohol), physiological status (age, hormones) and pathological conditions including impaired liver or kidney function are also important modulators of drug metabolism. For many drugs the dose-response curves are significantly altered with age, and therefore individual phenotypes do not necessarily remain constant with time.

The CYP2D6 phenotype can be determined quickly and accurately, usually by HPLC-based methods that analyse the relative concentrations of parent drug and metabolites in urine. The values obtained, however, are not always reproducible, and these methods can be inconvenient for the patient; for instance, urine collection is often required over an extended period. The possibility that unwanted or even dangerous side-effects, e.g. the development of hypotension in PM individuals during phenotypic assessment of CYP2D6 activity, is also an important consideration. The major advantage of phenotypic assessment of CYP2D6 activity, however, is that it is a

measure of true individual metabolizing capacity at the time of study. Genotyping analysis, in contrast, gives an unequivocal genetically-based prediction of individual drug metabolism, but does not allow for the effects of liver function, exposure to environmental chemicals, alcohol consumption or a range of other factors that may influence enzyme activity.

Genotyping analysis for CYP2D6, where metabolic capacity can be predicted on the basis of the exact allelic inheritance of each individual, is now routinely performed, using a variety of complementary PCR-based techniques. The most commonly used of these use PCR amplification of the regions of CYP2D6 of interest, coupled with restriction enzyme analysis to detect the presence of the most frequently inherited inactive CYP2D6 alleles - CYP2D6*3 and CYP2D6*4 (Gough *et al.*, 1990; Heim & Meyer, 1990; Smith *et al.*, 1992; Fig. 3). As CYP2D6*3 and CYP2D6*4 together account for the majority of PM alleles, routine analysis is often restricted to analysing for the presence of these alleles alone. Several studies have compared the predictive power of this limited analysis of CYP2D6 genotype and have found the results to be accurately predictive of phenotype in more than 95% of individuals (Evans & Relling, 1991; Graf et al., 1992).

Further PCR or SSCP assays have been described which can be used to detect the presence of the rarer allelic variants (see Daly et al., 1996 and references therein). PCR-based methods have also been described for confirming the presence of the CYP2D6*5 allele, in which the entire CYP2D6 gene is deleted (Johansson et al., 1996; Steen et al., 1995), and the multi-copy CYP2D6*2 alleles (Johansson et al., 1996). These methods are less precise, however, and do not permit the identification of individuals heterozygous for CYP2D6*5 and another CYP2D6 allele. The identification of such individuals may be particularly important when the second allele is not gene-inactivating. Accurate assessment of individual drug-metabolizing ability in these cases could be considered to be a limitation in the genetic assessment of CYP2D6 activity. The assessment of CYP2D6 activity is equally complicated in other, relatively rare, cases. For example an individual may inherit one copy of the CYP2D6*2A allele with two copies of the gene arranged in tandem and a second allele which is gene-inactivating. Such individuals, termed intermediate metabolizers, have metabolic ratios within the tails of the EM or PM population distributions (Fig. 1). In such cases, assessment of individual CYP2D6 activity can only be made with any degree of accuracy by phenotyping analysis. In general, however, genetically based assessment of individual CYP2D6 activities is more accurate and less invasive than corresponding phenotyping procedures.

For genotyping analysis to be a truly accurate predictor of individual drug-metabolizing ability, it is necessary to identify all the variant alleles within the population to be studied and to understand the phenotypic consequences of inheriting each of them. Otherwise certain allelic variants may be erroneously classified as wild-type, making it more difficult to rationalize idiosyncratic responses to drug treatment. For CYP2D6 the alleles so far reported account for a very high percentage of PM individuals, identified by phenotyping analysis. Genetic analysis of a highly poly-

morphic gene locus such as CYP2D6 is not trivial. Multiplex PCR assays have been reported (Stuven et al., 1996; Sachse et al., 1997) in which the presence of multiple allelic variants of CYP2D6 can be determined simultaneously, but these methods are not yet fully optimized and do not, for example, permit the identification of CYP2D6*5 heterozygotes. Technologies are being developed in which oligonucleotides, representing the sequences of all possible CYP2D6 allelic variants, are deposited on a chip. This is then probed with genomic DNA from each individual of interest. Hybridization between the test DNA and the chip-bound oligos occurs only at exact sequence matches. Computer imaging of the resultant fluorescence quenching permits accurate assessment of genotype.

Distribution of CYP2D6 genotype and phenotype in different populations

There are marked differences in both CYP2D6 genotype and phenotype in populations of different racial origin (Kalow, 1982; reviewed by Bertilsson, 1995). Direct comparison of allele frequencies in different populations is not always straightforward, however, due to differences in individual methods used to assign genotype and/or phenotype. This is exemplified by two studies designed to investigate CYP2D6 PM frequency in the Nigerian population, one of which reported a PM frequency of 8.1 % (Mbafeno et al., 1980) while the other, analysing a comparable population, failed to detect any PMs (Iyun et al., 1986). This may be partly explained by the almost exclusive use of debrisoquine as a probe drug in early phenotyping studies. In recent years, dextromethorphan has been more commonly used to assign CYP2D6 phenotype.

With the advent of molecular genetic techniques that can unequivocally assign CYP2D6 genotype, genotyping has largely overtaken phenotyping as the method of choice for predicting individual CYP2D6 activity. Many population studies, however, have been based on phenotypic assessment of CYP2D6 activity. Therefore, direct comparison of the results of these studies with genetically based assessments of CYP2D6 allele frequencies in different populations should perhaps be approached with some caution. With this caveat in mind, CYP2D6 PM frequencies reported for different racial groups are summarized in Table 3.

Table 3. CYP2D6 PM frequencies in different populations

Population	PM frequency	Genotyping/ Phenotyping (G/P)	n	Reference
British	4.3	G	720	Wolfe et al., 1992
	10.4	P	234	Ayesh et al., 1984
	8.7	P	104	Law et al., 1989
German	7.0	G/P	589	Sasche et al., 1997
	10.4	P	402	Roots et al., 1988
	9.5	G	137	Kerb et al., 1992
French	7.9	P	254	Duche et al., 1991
Belgian	7.2	P	167	Horsmans et al., 1991
Finnish	5.7	G	122	Hirvonen et al., 1993
Swedish	6.3	P	1011	Bertilsson et al., 1992
	5.9	G	68	Rannug et al., 1995
Norwegian	5.4	G	220	Tefre et al., 1992
Spanish	5.0	G	258	Agundez et al., 1994
	7.0	P	143	Benitez et al., 1991
Jordanian	2.9	P	241	Irshaid et al., 1993
Ghanaian	6.0	P	100	Woolhouse et al., 1979
Nigerian	8.1	P	123	Mbanefo et al., 1980
	0.0	P	137	Iyun et al., 1986
Ethiopian	1.8	G	122	Aklillu et al., 1996
Egyptian	1.4	P	84	Mahgoub et al., 1979
Saudi Arabian	0.1	P	92	Islam et al., 1980
South African	18.8	P	46	Sommers et al., 1988
Black American	1.9	G	127	Evans et al., 1993
USA	6.1	P	49	Caporaso et al., 1990
Chinese	0.7	P	269	Lou et al., 1987
	1.01	P	695	Bertilsson et al., 1992
Japanese	0.0	P	100	Nakamura et al., 1985
	2.0	P	84	Ishizaki et al., 1987
Singaporean	0.0	P	76	Lee et al., 1988
Thai	1.1	P	93	Wanwimolruk et al., 1990
New Zealand Maori	5.0	P	101	Wanwimolruk et al., 1990

PM, poor metabolizer

The most striking difference in PM frequency is seen between Caucasian and Oriental populations. On average, the PM frequency in the Caucasian population is 7%. This was validated by Sachse *et al.* (1997), who conducted a detailed study of CYP2D6 genotype and phenotype in 589 German individuals, using a series of multiplex PCR reactions to detect the presence of all known CYP2D6 alleles. All PM individuals were represented by only five loss-of-function alleles (CYP2D6*3, CYP2D6*4, CYP2D6*5, CYP2D6*6 and CYP2D6*15). The remaining functionally inactive alleles (CYP2D6*8, CYP2D6*11, CYP2D6*12, CYP2D6*13 and CYP2D6*14), which had previously been described in Caucasian populations, were not detected. The value of screening such a relatively large population for mutations in CYP2D6 was demonstrated by the discovery of three new CYP2D6 allelic variants.

It has been recognized for some time that although the PM frequency is significantly lower, mean CYP2D6 activity is also lower in Orientals than in Caucasians. Many Orientals consequently have a reduced ability to metabolize antidepressant and neuroleptic drugs that are substrates for CYP2D6 (Lou *et al.*, 1990; Lin & Finder, 1983). Indeed, many antidepressants are prescribed at lower doses in Oriental populations because of the higher mean metabolic ratio for CYP2D6 substrates and the lower associated plasma clearance time. The molecular basis of this difference has been attributed to the relatively low frequency (< 0.5%) of the CYP2D6*3 and CYP2D6*4 alleles, which are the most abundant gene-inactivating allelic variants in Caucasians, in Oriental populations (Johansson *et al.*, 1991). In contrast, the most abundant CYP2D6 allele in Orientals, comprising 51% of Chinese alleles, is CYP2D6*10B (CYP2D6Chl), which contains a Pro → Ser change at codon 34, a substitution thought to influence protein stability and to result in a form of CYP2D6 with reduced catalytic activity (Johansson *et al.*, 1994). CYP2D6*10B, which is not present in the Caucasian population, is thought to be derived from CYP2D6*4A, the most common gene-inactivating allele in Caucasians. Oriental populations also have a relatively high frequency of CYP2D6*10C (CYP2D6Ch2), which contains a 49bp substitution in exon 9 originating from the pseudogene CYP2D7 (Johansson *et al.*, 1994). A further allele, CYP2D6*10A (CYP2D6J) has been described in the Japanese population, which is closely related to the most common Chinese allele, CYP2D6*1OB (CYP2D6Ch 1) (Yokota *et al.*, 1993).

Unlike CYP2D6*3 and CYP2D6*4, CYP2D6*5, the gene deletion, is present at approximately equivalent frequencies (~5% of all PM alleles) in all the populations studied, suggesting that the gene deletion preceded both the divergence of the races and the development of further mutations in CYP2D6. The gene amplification alleles have also been detected outside the Caucasian population. In Chinese people resident in Sweden, for example, the CYP2D6*2x2 allele occurred at a frequency of 0.9% (Johansson *et al.*, 1994). In contrast, almost 30% of the Ethiopian population have duplicated CYP2D6 alleles (Akillu *et al.*, 1996). This finding, combined with the relatively low (1.8%) PM frequency, highlights the considerable racial heterogeneity in CYP2D6 structure and activity in different racial groups.

There is relatively little information about CYP2D6 allele frequencies and the molecular basis of the PM phenotype in other populations. It is interesting to note that PM frequencies remain relatively constant in all the Caucasian (European and Scandinavian) populations studied. Similarly, the Chinese, Japanese, Singaporean and Thai populations show comparable CYP2D6 allele frequencies. Somewhat surprisingly in view of their geographical localization, the New Zealand Maoris have a PM frequency much closer to the Caucasian average than to the Oriental average (Wamwimolruk *et al.*, 1990).

The role of CYP2D6 in carcinogenesis in humans: potential bias and confounders

Up to 80% of all human cancers are thought to arise from exposure to environmental agents (Doll & Peto, 1981) It therefore seems reasonable to propose that interindividual variation in the expression of xenobiotic metabolizing enzymes, including CYP2D6, may determine individual cancer risk. The development of rapid DNA-based methods for investigating CYP2D6 genotype has allowed numerous studies on the evaluation of the inheritance of the CYP2D6 PM genotype in various cancer types. Logically, interindividual variation in CYP2D6 expression may influence cancer susceptibility in several ways. If CYP2D6 catalyses the detoxification of a particular toxin or carcinogen, PM individuals will be at an increased risk of disease. In contrast, if the metabolic activation of a particular carcinogenic substrate is catalysed by CYP2D6, PM individuals will be protected. In addition, the possibility that this enzyme may be involved in hormone homeostasis or other metabolic processes cannot be excluded. However, making predictions about the inci-

dence of specific cancer types on the basis of the functions of CYP2D6 has been difficult, largely due to the paucity of candidate carcinogens recognized as CYP2D6 substrates. The situation is further complicated by differences between the findings of different studies.

This difficulty is particularly well illustrated by the results of studies investigating the frequency of CYP2D6 PMs in lung cancer (Table 4). The CYP2D6 PM phenotype was first reported to be protective in lung cancer (Ayesh et al., 1984;

Table 4. CYP2D6 PM frequencies in lung cancer patients and controls

Country	PM frequency (cancers)	n	PM frequency (controls)	n	Genotyping/ Phenotyping (G/P)	Reference
1. UK	1.9	106	8.9	258	P	Hetzel et al., 1980
2. UK	1.6	245	10.4	234	P	Ayesh et al., 1984
3. UK	1.9	104	8.7	104	P	Law et al., 1989
4. UK	1.1	89	13.0	92	P	Caporaso 1990
5. Germany	7.0	270	11.1	270	P	Roots et al., 1988
6. UK	9.8	82	7.4	94	P	Speirs et al., 1990
7. Italy	0.86	116	5.3	854	P	Puchetti et al., 1994
8. France	6.5	153	8.5	264	P	Duche et al., 1991
9. France	7.8	128	12	145	P	Bouchardy, et al., 1996
10. Belgium	5.5	91	7.2	167	P	Horsmans et al., 1991
11. Spain	4.8	84	7.0	143	P	Benitez et al., 1991
12. USA	8.7	335	7.2	373	P	Shaw et al., 1995
13. Finland	0.9	106	5.7	122	G	Hirvonen et al., 1993
14. UK	3.6	361	5.0	720	G	Wolf et al., 1992
15. Germany	4.7	170	7.6	198	G	Roots et al., 1993
16. Norway	9.8	204	5.1	117	G	Tefre et al., 1994
17. France	6.8	249	5.5	271	G	Stucker et al., 1995
18. Spain	0.0	89	7.0	98	G	Agundez et al., 1994
19. Slovenia	2.5	200	6.5	107	G	Dolzan et al., 1995
20. USA	4.4	343	4.9	710	G	London et al., 1997

PM, poor metabolizer

Caporaso *et al.*, 1990; Law *et al.*, 1989; Puchetti *et al.*, 1994). However, further studies identified inheritance of the CYP2D6 PM genotype as a statistically significant risk factor (Roots *et al.*, 1988; Benitez *et al.*, 1991; Duche *et al.*, 1991; Shaw *et al.*, 1995; Horsmans *et al.*, 1991; Speirs *et al.*, 1990), while others (Wolf *et al.*, 1992; Stucker *et al.* 1995) reported only a very weak association. These data were subsequently confirmed by meta-analysis of data from all published studies (Wolf *et al.*, 1994; d'Errico *et al.*, 1995; Christensen *et al.*, 1997) and a recent population-based case control study which co-analysed a number of variables including smoking history and occupational exposure to environmental pollutants (London *et al.*, 1997). Bouchardy *et al.* (1996) analysed CYP2D6 phenotype in French lung cancer patients and controls for whom detailed information on smoking history was available. A statistically significant association was found between inheritance of the CYP2D6 extensive metabolizer phenotype, i.e. CYP2D6 PM protective, and susceptibility to lung cancer, but this was only evident for heavy smokers. The variation in PM frequencies in control populations and in lung cancer patients in the different study populations is summarized in Table 4.

Such marked variation in the PM frequencies in both cases and controls in the different studies makes the significance of the data difficult to determine. The variation could be attributable to a range of factors, including the methods used to assign CYP2D6 phenotype and genotype. Selection of the control population may also be an important issue, where the absence of age and sex matching in control populations in some of the published studies could be a confounding factor. There is no evidence, however, that this is an important variable in the case of CYP2D6, although the possibility of some controls developing disease at a later date cannot be ruled out, particularly if the control and disease populations are not age matched. While the majority of authors analysed PM frequencies in healthy controls, in certain studies the controls were hospital inpatients. Although these individuals had no history of malignancy they were not, by definition, disease-free. It is difficult to estimate what effect individual diseases have on CYP2D6 phenotype.

Although smoking is the primary cause of lung cancer, not all smokers develop the disease. Other factors that determine individual disease susceptibility include the number of cigarettes smoked, the type of tobacco used, and exposure to other synergistic risk factors, such as alcohol. These factors can vary widely in populations of different ethnic origin and may therefore influence the relative importance of polymorphism in CYP2D6. Many CYP2D6 alleles are present at different frequencies in different populations and it is therefore important to know the ethnic origin of all participants in studies. This is particularly true when the results of several studies are combined, e.g. in meta-analysis.

The largest differences in PM frequencies between cases and controls were found when PM status was determined by phenotyping analysis. The average PM frequency in the different control groups was also significantly higher in the populations studied by phenotyping. More recent studies have predominantly used genotyping methods to determine CYP2D6 activity. Direct comparison of the results obtained from these studies with those of earlier phenotyping analysis must therefore be approached with caution.

Lung cancer is unique among the cancer types that have been studied, in that a specific substrate, NNK (4-(methylnitrosamine)-1-(3-pyridyl)-1-butanone), which is a nitrosamine known to be metabolically activated by CYP2D6, has been identified in tobacco smoke (Crespi *et al.*, 1991). Nitrosamine-DNA adducts are reduced in CYP2D6 PMs (Kato *et al.*, 1995), suggesting that the PM phenotype may be protective against the effects of these mutagenic chemicals. NNK can also be metabolized by several further P450 isozymes, however, making the relative contribution of CYP2D6 to the overall metabolism and toxicity of the chemical difficult to estimate. Nicotine is also known to be a substrate for CYP2D6 (McCracken *et al.*, 1992; Cholerton *et al.*, 1994). CYP2D6 is one of the enzymes that catalyses the metabolism of nicotine to cotinine and therefore plays a significant role in determining individual nicotine levels. CYP2D6 PMs have significantly higher plasma concentrations of nicotine than EMs with similar smoking habits (Cholerton *et al.*, 1994). By extrapolation, therefore, it follows that PM individuals may receive the same nicotine "high" at a lower dose, i.e. lower cigarette consumption. If this were true it would be expected that average cigarette consumption would be lower in PMs and that they would have a concomitant reduction in lung cancer risk. However, analysis of the combined results of lung cancer studies in which smoking history has been addressed as an independent risk factor suggests that this is not the case, although inheritance of the CYP2D6 PM genotype may have a slight protective effect in light smokers (London *et al.*, 1997).

CYP2D6 PM frequencies have also been investigated in a variety of other cancer types, including breast cancer, bladder cancer, melanoma and leukaemia (Wolf *et al.*, 1992; Cartwright *et al.*, 1984; Ladero *et al.*, 1991; Jennings *et al.*, 1996). In comparison to the lung cancer data, however, relatively few studies have reported any statistically significant associations between CYP2D6 activity and susceptibility to disease. For the majority of these malignancies, no candidate carcinogen has been proposed which is a known CYP2D6 substrate. The same is true of many other human diseases whose incidences are thought to be influenced by exposure to environmental agents. Inheritance of the CYP2D6 PM phenotype has been implicated in the etiology of a wide range of diseases, e.g. rheumatoid arthritis (Beyeler *et al.*, 1994) and multiple sclerosis (Agundez *et al.*, 1995), the incidence of which is particularly high in specific geographical areas and is therefore thought to be influenced by exposure to environmental toxins. In the majority of such studies, however, no significant association with CYP2D6 genotype has been proven.

In contrast, a significant overrepresentation of CYP2D6 PMs has been reported in patients with Parkinson's disease (Smith *et al.*, 1992; Kurth & Kurth, 1993; Plante-Bordeneuve *et al.*, 1994). Although some contradictory data have also been published the current consensus is that the CYP2D6 PM genotype is twice as common in PD patients as in controls. It is therefore particularly interesting that we and others have recently been able to demonstrate that MPTP, a contaminant of synthetic meperidine narcotics, "street heroin", is a substrate for CYP2D6 (Coleman *et al.*, 1996; Gilham *et al.*, 1997; Modi *et al.*, 1997).

Interindividual variation in the expression of CYP2D6 may be one factor that determines individual disease susceptibility. It is becoming increasingly clear, however, that studying the effects of genetically controlled variation in the expression of a single enzyme in isolation, however well characterized the variation is, may not be informative. Carcinogen metabolism, both activation and detoxification, is a balance between the relative activities of all the enzymes active within the metabolic pathway of a particular compound. For example, predictions made on the basis of knowledge of interindividual variation in P450 expression can be considerably strengthened by additional information on the relative levels of expression of Phase II enzymes such as the glutathione S-transferases and N-acetyl transferases and enzymes which are involved in DNA repair. This approach was illustrated by Brockmöller *et al.* (1996), who investigated polymorphism in NAT2, GSTM1, GSTTI, microsomal epoxide hydrolase and P450 genes in a large cohort of German bladder cancer patients and controls. Such an approach permits investigation of the possibility of synergism in allelic variation at more than a single gene locus. It is also important that interindividual variations in enzyme activity are linked to carcinogen exposure, and that this is done not only in respect of agents that are easily identified as carcinogens such as tobacco and industrial pollutants but also for agents including alcohol and foodborne carcinogens which are less obviously identified as risk factors for disease.

References

Agundez, L.A., Martinez, C., Ladero, L.M., Ledesma, L.C., Ramos, L.M., Martin, R., Rodriguez, A., Jara, C. & Benitez, J. (1994) Debrisoquine oxidation genotype and susceptibility to lung cancer. *Clin. Pharmacol. Ther.*, 55, 10-14

Agundez, L.A., Arroyo, R., Ledesma, L.C., Martinez, C., Ladero, L.M., de Andreas, C., Jimenezjimenez, F.J., Molina, L.A., Alvarezcermeno, L.C., Vareladeseijas, E., Gimenezroldan, S. & Benitez, J. (1995) Frequency of CYP2D6 allelic variants in multiple sclerosis. *Acta Neurol. Scand.*, 92, 464-467

Aklillu, E., Persson, L, Bertilsson, L., Johansson, L, Rodrigues, F. & Ingelman-Sundberg, M. (1996) Frequency distribution of ultrarapid metabolizers of debrisoquine in an Ethiopian population carrying duplicated and multiduplicated functional CYP2D6 alleles. *J. Pharmacol. Exp.Ther.*, 278, 441-446

Ayesh, R., Idle, J.R., Ritchie, L.C., Crother, M.W. & Hetzel, M.R. (1984) Metabolic oxidation phenotypes as markers for susceptibility to lung cancer. *Nature*, 312, 169-170

Benet, L.Z., Kroetz, D.L. & Sheiner, L.B. (1996) Pharmacokinetics. In: Hardman, L.G., Goodman Gilman, A. & Limbird, L.E., eds, *Goodman and Gilman's Pharmacological Basis of Therapeutics*, 9th edition. New York, McGraw Hill, pp. 3-27

Benitez, L., Ladero, L.M., Jara, C., Carillo, L.A., Cobaleda, L., Llerena, A., Vargas, E. & Munro, J.J. (1991) Polymorphic oxidation of debrisoquine in lung cancer patients. *Eur.J. Cancer*, 27, 158-161

Bertilsson, L., Alm, C., de las Carreras, C., Widen, L., Edman, G. & Schalling, D. (1989) Debrisoquine hydroxylase polymorphism and personality. *Lancet*, 2, 555

Bertilsson, L., Lou, Y.Q., Du, Y.L., Liu, Y., Kuang, T.Y., Liao, X.M., Wang, K.Y., Reviriego, J., Iselins, L. & Sjoqvist, F. (1992) Pronounced differences between native Chinese and Swedish populations in the polymorphic hydroxylation of debrisoquine and S-mephenytoin. *Clin. Pharmacol. Ther.*, 51, 388-397

Bertilsson, L., Dahl, M.-L., Sjoqvist, F, Aberg-Wistedt, A., Humble, M., Johansson, I., Lundqvist, E. & Ingelman-Sundberg, M. (1993) Molecular basis for rational megaprescribing in ultrarapid hydroxylators of debrisoquine. *Lancet*, 341, 63

Bertilsson, L. (1995) Geographical/interracial differences in polymorphic drug oxidation. *Clinical Pharmacokinetics*, 29, 192-209

Beyeler, C., Daly, A.K., Armstrong, M., Astbury, C., Bird, H.A. & Idle, J.R. (1994) Phenotype/genotype relationships for the cytochrome P450 enzyme CYP2D6 in rheumatoid arthritis - influence of drug therapy and disease activity. *J. Rheumatol.*, 21, 1034-1039

Bouchardy, C., Benhamou, S. & Dayer, P. (1996) The effect of tobacco on lung cancer risk depends on CYP2D6 activity. *Cancer Res.*, 56, 251-253

Brockmöller, J., Cascorbi, L, Kerb, R. & Roots, I. (1996) Combined analysis of inherited polymorphisms in arylamine N-acetyltransferase 2, glutathione S-transferases M 1 and T 1, microsomal epoxide hydrolase and cytochrome P450 enzymes as modulators of bladder cancer risk. *Cancer Res.*, 56, 3915-3925

Broly, F., Marez, D., Lo Guidice J.-M., Sabagh, N., Legrand, M., Boone, P. & Meyer, U.A. (1995) A nonsense mutation in the cytochrome P450 CYP2D6 gene identified in a Caucasian with an enzyme deficiency. *Hum. Genet.*, 96, 601-603

Caporaso, N.E., Tucker, M.A., Hoover, R.N., Hayes, R.B., Pickle, L.W., Issaq, H.J., Muschik, G.M., Green-Gallo, L., Buivys, D., Aisner, S., Resan, J.H., Trump, B.F., Tollerud, D. Weston, A. & Harris, C.C. (1990) Lung cancer and the debrisoquine metabolic phenotype. *J. Natl. Cancer Inst.*, 82, 1264-1271

Cartwright, R.A., Philip, P.A., Rogers, H.J. & Glashan, R.W. (1984) Genetically determined debrisoquine oxidation capacity in bladder cancer. *Carcinogenesis*, 5, 1191-1192

Chen, Z.R., Somogyi, A.A. & Bochner, F. (1988) Polymorphic 0-demethylation of codeine. *Lancet*, 2, 914-915

Cholerton, S., Arpanahi, A., McCracken, N., Boustead, C., Taber, H., Johnstone, E., Leathart, L., Daly, A.K. & Idle, J.R. (1994) Poor metabolizers of nicotine and CYP2D6 polymorphism. *Lancet*, 343, 62-63

Christensen, P.M., Gotzsche, P.C. & Brosen, K. (1997) The sparteine/debrisoquine (CYP2D6) oxidation polymorphism and the risk of lung cancer: a meta-analysis. *Br. J. Clin. Pharmacol.*, 51, 389-393

Coleman, T., Ellis, S.W., Martin, L.L., Lennard, M.S. & Tucker, G.T. (1996) 1-methyl-4phenyl-1,2,3,6-tetrahy-dropyridine (MPTP) is N-demethylated by cytochromes P450 2D6, 1 A2 and 3A4 - implications for susceptibility to Parkinson's-disease. *J. Pharmacol. Exp.Ther.*, 277, 685-690

Crespi, C.L., Penman, B.W., Gelboin, H.V. & Gonzalez, F.J. (1991) A tobacco smoke-derived nitrosamine 4-(methyl l-nitrosamino)-1-(3-pyridyl) -1-butanone is activated by multiple human cytochrome P450s, including the polymorphic cytochrome P450 2D6. *Carcinogenesis*, 7, 1197-1201

Crespi, C.L., Steimel, D.T., Penman, B.W., Korzekwa, K.R., Fernandez-Salguero, P., Buters, J.T.M., Gelboin,. H.V., Gonzlez, F.J., Idle, J.R. & Daly, A.K. (1995) Comparison of substrate metabolism by wild-type CYP2D6 protein and a variant containing methionine, not valine, at position 374. *Pharmacogenetics*, 5, 234-243

Daly, A.K., Brockmöller, J., Broly, R., Eichelbaum, M., Evans, W.E., Gonzalez, F.J., Huang, J.-D., Idle, J.R., Ingelman-Sundberg, M., Ishizaki, T., Jacqz-Aigrain, E., Meyer, U.A., Nebert, D.W., Steen, V.M., Wolf, C.R. & Zanger, U.M. (1996a) Nomenclature for human CYP2D6 alleles. *Pharmacogenetics*, 6, 193-201

Daly, A.K., Fairbrother, K.S., Andreassen, O.A., London, S.L., Idle, J.R. & Steen, V.M. (1996b) Characterization and PCR-based detection of two different hybrid CYP2D7P/CYP2D6 alleles associated with the poor metabolizer phenotype. *Pharmacogenetics*, 6, 319-328

d'Errico, A., Taioli, E., Chen, X. & Vineis, P. (1996) Genetic metabolic polymorphisms and the risk of cancer: a review of the literature. *Biomarkers*, 1, 149-173

Distlerath, L.M., Reilly, P.E.B., Martin, M.V., Davis, G.G., Wilkinson, G.R. & Guengerich, F.P. (1985) Purification and characterization of the human liver cytochrome P450 involved in debrisoquine 4-hydroxylation and phenacetin O-deethylation, two prototypes for genetic polymorphism in oxidative drug metabolism. *J. Biol. Chem.*, 260, 9057-9067

Doll, R. & Peto, R. (1981) *Causes of Cancer.* Oxford, Oxford University Press

Dolzan, V., Rudolf, Z. & Breskvar, K. (1995) Human CYP2D6 gene polymorphism in Slovene cancer patients and healthy controls. *Carcinogenesis*, 16, 2675-2678

Duche, L.C., Joanne, C., Barre, L., de Cremoux, H., Dalphin, L.C., Depierre, A., Brochard, P., Tillement, J.P. & Bechtel, P. (1991) Lack of relationship between the polymorphism of debriso-quine oxidation and lung cancer. *Br. J. Clin. Pharmacol.*, 31, 533-536

Eichelbaum, M., Spannbrucker, N., Steinke, B. & Dengler, H.J. (1979) Defective N-oxidation of sparteine in man - a new pharmacogenetic defect. *Eur. J. Clin. Pharmacol.*, 16, 183-187

Ellis, S.W., Hayhurst, G.P., Smith, G., Lightfoot, T., Wong, M.S., Simula, A.P., Ackland, M.L, Sternberg, M.J.E., Lennard, M.S., Tucker, G.T. & Wolf, C.R. (1995) Evidence that aspartic acid 301 is a critical substrate-contact residue in the active site of cytochrome P450 2D6. *J. Biol. Chem.*, 270, 29055-29058

Ellis, S.W., Rowland, K., Ackland, M.L, Rekka, E., Simula, A.P., Lennard, M.S., Wolf, C.R. & Tucker, G.T. (1996) Influence of amino acid residoe 374 of cytochrome P450 2D6 (CYP2D6) on the regio- and enantioselective metabolism of metoprolol. *Biochem. J.*, 316, 647-654

Evans, W.E. & Relling, M.V. (1991) Concordance of P450 2D6 (debrisoquine hydroxylase) phenotype and genotype: inability of dextromethorphan metabolic ratio to descriminate reliably heterozygous and homozygous extensive metabolizers. *Pharmacogenetics*, 1, 143-148

Evans, W.E., Relling, M.V., Rahman, A., McLeod, H.L., Scott, E.P. & Lin, J.-S. (1993) Genetic basis for a lower prevalence of deficient CYP2D6 oxidative drug metabolism phenotypes in black Americans. *J. Clin. Invest.*, 91, 2150-2154

Gilham, D.E., Cairns, W., Paine, M.L.L., Modi, S., Poulsom, R., Roberts, G.C.K. & Wolf, C.R. (1997)

Metabolism of MPTP by cytochrome P450 2D6 and the demonstration of 2D6 messenger-RNA in human fetal and adult brain by *in situ* hybridization. *Xenobiotica*, 27, 111-125

Gonzalez, F.J., Skoda, R.C., Kimura, S., Umeno, M., Zanger, U.M., Nebert, D.W., Gelboin, H.V., Hardwick, L.P. & Meyer, U.A. (1988) Characterization of the common genetic defect in humans deficient in debrisoquine metabolism. *Nature*, 331, 442-446

Gough, A.C., Miles, L.S., Spurr, N.X, Moss, L.E., Gaedigk, A., Eichelbaum, M. & Wolf, C.R. (1990) Identification of the primary gene defect at the cytochrome P450 CYP2D locus. *Nature*, 347, 773-776

Gough, A.C., Smith, C.A.D., Howell, S.M., Wolf, C.R., Bryant, S.P. & Spurr, N.K. (1992) Localization of the CYP2D gene locus to human chromosome 22q13.1 by polymerase chain reaction, *in situ* hybridization and linkage analysis. *Genomics*, 15, 430-432

Graf, T., Broly, R, Hoffinan, R, Probst, M., Meyer, U.A. & Howald, H. (1992) Prediction of phenotype for acetylation and for debrisoquine hydroxylation by DNA-tests in healthy human volunteers. *Eur. J. Clin. Pharmacol.*, 43, 399-403

Heim, M.H. & Meyer, U.A. (1990) Genotyping of poor metabolizers of debrisoquine by allele-specific PCR amplification. *Lancet*, 336, 529-532

Heim, M. & Meyer, U. A. (1992) Evolution of a highly polymorphic human cytochrome P450 gene cluster: CYP2D6. *Genomics*, 14, 49-58

Hetzel, M.R., Law, M., Keal, E.E., Sloan, T.P., Idle, J.R. & Smith, R.L. (1980) Is there a genetic component in bronchial carcinoma in smokers? *Thorax*, 35, 709

Hirvonen, A., Husgafvel-Pursiainen, K., Antilla, S., Karjalainen, A., Pelkonen, 0. & Vainio, H. (1993) PCR-base CYP2D6 genotyping for Finnish lung cancer patients. *Pharmacogenetics*, 3, 19-27

Hogstedt, S., Lindberg, B. & Rane, A. (1983) Increased oral clearance of metoprolol in pregnancy. *Eur. J. Clin. Pharmacol.*, 24, 217-220

Horsmans, Y., Desager, L.P. & Harvengt, C. (1991) Is there a link between debrisoquine oxidation phenotype and lung cancer susceptibility? *Biomed. Pharmacother.*, 45, 359-362

Ishizaki, T., Eichelbaum, M., Horai, Y., Hashimoto, K., Chiba, K. & Dengher, H.J. (1987) Evidence for polymorphic oxidation of sparteine in Japanese subjects. *British Journal of Clin. Pharmacol.*, 23, 482-485

Islam, S.I., Idle, J.R. & Smith, R.L. (1980) The polymorphic 4-hydroxylation of debrisoquine in a Saudi Arabian population. *Xenobiotica*, 10, 819-825

Iyun, A.O., Lennard, M.S., Tucker, G.T. & Woods, H.F. (1986) Metoprolol and debrisoquine metabolism in Nigerians: lack of evidence for polymorphic oxidation. *Clin. Pharmacol. Ther.*, 40, 387-394

Jennings, M., Sweetland H., Smith, C.A.D., Wolf, C.R., Lennard, M.S., Tucker, G.T., Woods, H.F. & Rogers, K. (1996) Lack of relationships between the debrisoquine (CYP2D6) and mephenytoin (CYP2C 19) oxidation polymorphisms and susceptibility to breast cancer. *Breast*, 5, 254-258

Johansson, I., Yue, Q.Y., Dahl, M., Heim, J., Sawe, L., Bertilsson, L., Meyer, U.A., Sjoqvist, F. & Ingelman-Sundberg, M. (1991) Genetic analysis of the interethnic difference between Chinese and Caucasians in the polymorphic metabolism of debrisoquine and S-mephenytoin. *Clin. Pharmacol. Ther.*, 40, 553-556

Johansson, I., Lundqvist, E., Bertilsson, L., Dahl M.-L., Sjoqvist, F. & Ingelman-Sundberg, M. (1993) Inherited amplification of an active gene in the cytochrome P450 CYP2D locus as a cause of ultrarapid metabolism of debrisoquine. *Proc. Natl. Acad. Sci. USA*, 90, 11825-11829

Johansson, I., Oscarson, M., Yue, Q.Y., Bertilsson, L., Sjoqvist, F. & Ingelman-Sundberg, M. (1994)

Genetic analysis of the Chinese cytochrome P4502D locus: characterization of variant CYP2D6 genes present in subjects with diminished capacity for debrisoquine hydroxylation. *Mol. Pharmacol.*, 46, 452-459

Johansson, L., Lundqvist, E., Dahl M.-L. & Ingelman-Sundberg, M. (1996) PCR-based genotyping for duplicated and deleted CYP2D6 genes. *Pharmacogenetics*, 6, 351-355

Kagimoto, M., Heim, M., Kagimoto, K., Zeugin, T. & Meyer, U.A. (1990) Multiple mutations of the human cytochrome P450IID6 gene (CYP2D6) in poor metabolizers of debrisoquine. *J. Biol. Chem.*, 265, 17209-17214

Kalow, W. (1982) Ethnic differences in drug metabolism. *Clin. Pharmacokinet.*, 7, 373-400

Kalow, W. & Tyndale, R. F. (1992) Debrisoquine/sparteine monooxygenase and other P450s in brain. In: Kalow, W., ed, *Pharmacogenetics of Drug Metabolism*. Oxford, Pergamon Press, pp. 649-656

Kato, S., Bowman, E.D., Harrington, A,M., Blömeke, B. & Shields, P.G. (1995) Human lung carcinogen-DNA adduct levels mediated by genetic polymorphisms *in vivo*. *J. Natl. Cancer Inst.*, 87, 902-907

Kerb, R., Brockmöller, L., Drakoulis, N. & Roots, I. (1992) CYP2D6 and glutathione S-transferase class mu as host factors of lung cancer susceptibility. *J.Basic Clin. Physiol. Pharmacol.*, 3, 131

Kimura, S., Umeno, M., Skoda, R.C., Meyer, U.A. & Gonzalez, F.J. (1989) The human debrisoquine 4-hydroxylase (CYP2D) locus: sequence and identification of the polymorphic CYP2D6 gene, a related gene and a pseudogene. *Am. J. Hum. Genet.*, 45, 889-904

Kurth, M.C. & Kurth, J.H. (1993) Variant cytochrome P450 CYP2D6 allelic frequencies in Parkinson's disease. *Am.J. Med. Genet.*, 48, 166-168

Ladero, J.M., Benitez, L., Jara, C., Llerena, A., Valdivielso, L., Muno, J.J. & Vargas, E. (1991) Polymorphic oxidation of debrisoquine in women with breast cancer. *Oncol.*, 48, 107-110

Law, M.R., Hetzel, M.R. & Idle, J.R. (1989) Debrisoquine metabolism and genetic predisposition to lung cancer. *Br. J. Cancer*, 59, 686-687

Lee, E.J.D., Yeoh, P.N. & Gong, N.H. (1988) Oxidation phenotyping in Chinese and Malay populations. *Clin. Exp. Pharmacol. Physiol.*, 15, 889-891

Lin, K.M. & Finder, E. (1983) Neuroleptic dosage for Asians. *Am. J. Psychiatry*, 22, 451-465

Llerena, A., Edman, G., Cobaleda, L., Benitez, L., Schalling, D. & Bertilsson, L. (1993) Relationship between personality and debrisoquine hydroxylation capacity - suggestion of an endogenous neuroactive substrate or product of the cytochrome P450 2D6. *Acta Psychiatr. Scand.*, 87, 23-28

Llerena, A., Cobaleda, L., Martinez, C. & Benitez, J. (1996) Interethnic differences in drug metabolism - influence of genetic and environmental factors on debrisoquine hydroxylase phenotypes. *Eur. J. Drug Metab. Pharmacokinet.*, 21, 129-138

London, S.J., Daly, A.K., Leathart, J.B.S., Navidi, W.C., Carpenter, C.C. & Idle, J.R. (1997) Genetic polymorphism of CYP2D6 and lung cancer risk in African-Americans and Caucasians in Los Angeles county. *Carcinogenesis*, 18, 1203-1214

Lou, Y.C., Ying, L., Bertilsson, L. & Sjöqvist, F. (1987) Low frequency of slow debrisoquine hydroxylation in a native Chinese population. *Lancet*, 2, 852-853

Lou, Y.C. (1990) Differences in drug metabolism polymorphism between Orientals and Caucasians. *Drug Metab. Rev.*, 22, 451-475

Mahgoub, A., Idle, J.R., Dring, L.G., Lancaster, R. & Smith, R.L. (1977) Polymorphic hydroxylation of debrisoquine in man. *Lancet*, 2, 584-586

Mahgoub, A., Idle, J.R. & Smith, R.L. (1979) A population and familial study of the defective alicyclic hydroxylation of debrisoquine among Egyptians. *Xenobiotica*, 9, 51-56

Martinez, C., Agundez, J.A.G., Gervasini, G., Martin, R. & Benitez, J. (1997) Tryptamine: a possible endogenous substrate for CYP2D6. *Pharmacogenetics*, 7, 85-93

Mbanefo, C., Bababunmi, E.A., Mahgoub, A., Sloan, T.P., Idle, J.R. & Smith, R.L. (1980) A study of the debrisoquine hydroxylation polymorphism in a Nigerian population. *Xenobiotica*, 10, 811-818

McCracken, N.W., Cholerton, S. & Idle, J.R. (1992) Cotinine formation by cDNA expressed human cytochrome P450. *Med. Sci. Res.*, 20, 877-878

Modi, S., Paine, M.J., Sutcliffe, M.J., Lian, L.Y., Primrose, W.U., Wolf, C.R. & Roberts, G. C. K. (1996) A model for human cytochrome-p-450 2D6 based on homology modelling and nmr studies of substrate-binding. *Biochemistry*, 35, 4540-4550

Modi, S., Gilham, D.E., Sutcliffe, M.J., Lian, L.Y., Primrose, W.U., Wolf, C.R. & Roberts, G.C.K. (1997) 1-methyl-4-phenyl-1,2,3,6-tetrahydropyridine as a substrate of cytochromeP450 2D6 - allosteric effects of nadph-cytochrome P450 reductase. *Biochemistry*, 36, 4461-4470

Nakamura, K., Goto, F., Ray, W.A., McAllister, C.B., Jacqz, E., Wilkinson, G.R. & Branch, R.A. (1985) Interethnic differences in genetic polymorphism of debrisoquine and metoprolol hydroxylation between Japanese and Caucasian populations. *Clin. Pharmacol.*, 38, 402-408

Niznik, H.B., Tyndale, R.F., Sallee, F.K, Gonzalez, F.J., Hardwick, J.P., Inaba, T. & Kalow, W. (1990) The dopamine transporter and cytochrome P450I1D1 (debrisoquine 4-hydroxylase) in brain: resolution and identification of two distinct [^{3}H] GBR-12935 binding proteins. *Arch. Biochem. Biophys.*, 276, 424-432

Panserat, S., Mura, C., Gerard, N., Vincent-Viry, M., Galteau, M.M., Jacqz-Aigrain, E. & Krishnamoorthy, R. (1995) An unequal cross-over event within the CYP2D gene cluster generates a chimeric CYP2D7/CYP2D6 gene which is associated with the poor metabolizer phenotype. *Br. J. Clin. Pharmacol.*, 40, 361-367

Plante-Bordeneuve, V., Davis, M.B., Maranganore, D.M., Marsden, C.D. & Harding, A.E. (1994) Debrisoquine hydroxylase gene polymorphism in familial Parkinson's disease. *J. Neurol., Neurosurg. Psychiatry*, 57, 911-913

Puchetti, V., Faccini, G.B., Micciolo, R., Ghimenton, F., Bertrand, C. & Zatti, N. (1994) Dextromethorphan test for evaluation of congenital predisposition to lung cancer. *Chest*, 105, 449-453

Rannug, A., Alexandrie, A.X., Persson, I. & Ingelman-Sundberg, M. (1995) Genetic polymorphism of cytochromes P450 1A1, 2D6 and 2El: regulation and toxicological significance. *J. Occup. Med.*, 37, 25-36

Roots, L., Drakoulis, N., Ploch, M., Heinemeyer, G., Loddenkemper, R., Minks, T., Nitz, M., Otte, F. & Kloch, M. (1988) Debrisoquine hydroxylation phenotype, acetylation phenotype and ABO blood groups as genetic host factors of lung cancer risk. *Klin.Wochenschr.*, 66, 87-97

Roots, I., Drakoulis, N. & Brockmöller, J. (1993) Still an open question: does active CYP2D6 predispose to lung cancer? *Proceedings of the 8th International Conference on Cytochrome P450*. Lisbon

Sachse, C., Brockmöller, J., Bauer, S. & Roots, I. (1997) Cytochrome P450 2D6 variants in a Caucasian population: allele frequencies and phenotypic consequences. *Am. J. Hum. Genet.*, 60, 284-295

Shah, R.R., Oates, N.S., Idle, J.R., Smith, R.L. & Lockhart, L.D.F. (1982) Impaired oxidation of debrisoquine in patients with perhexiline neuropathy. *Br. Med. J.*, 284, 295-299

Shaw, G.L., Falk, R.T., Deslauriers, L., Frame, J.X., Nesbitt, L.C., Pass, H.I., Issaq, H.J., Hoover, R.N. & Tucker, M.A. (1995) Debrisoquine metabolism and lung cancer risk. *Cancer Epidemiol. Biomarkers Prev.*, 4, 41-48

Sindrup, S.H., Poulsen, L., Brosen, K., Arendt-Nielsen, L. & Gram, L.F. (1993) Are poor metabolizers of sparteine/debrisoquine less pain-tolerant than extensive metabolizers? *Pain*, 53, 335-349

Skoda, R.C., Gonzalez, F.J., Demierre, A. & Meyer, U.A. (1988) Two mutant alleles of the human cytochrome P-450dbl gene (P45021) associated with genetically deficient metabolism of debrisoquine and other drugs. *Proc. Natl. Acad. Sci. USA*, 85, 5240-5243

Smith, C.A.D., Gough, A.C., Leigh, P.X, Summers, B.A., Harding, A.E., Maranganore, D.M., Sturman, S.G., Schapira, A.H.V., Williams, A.C., Spurr, N.K. & Wolf, C.R. (1992) Debrisoquine hydroxylase gene polymorphism and susceptibility to Parkinson's disease. *Lancet*, 339, 1375-1377

Smith, G., Stanley, L.A., Sim, E., Strange, R.C. & Wolf, C.R. (1995) Metabolic polymorphisms and cancer susceptibility. *Cancer Surv.*, 25, 27-65

Smith, G., Modi, S., Pillai, L., Lian, L.Y., Sutcliffe, M.L, Pitchard, M.P., Friedberg, T., Roberts, G.C.K. & Wolf, C.R. (1998) Determinants of the substrate specificity of human cytochrome P450 CYP2D6: design and construction of a mutant with testosterone hydroxylase activity. *Biochem. J.*, 331, 783-792

Sommers, D.K., Moncrieff, J. & Avenant, J. (1988) Polymorphism of the 4-hydroxylation of debrisoquine in the San Bushmen of South Africa. *Southern Africa Hum. Toxicol.*, 7, 273-276

Speirs, C.L, Murray, S., Davies, D.S., Biola Modadeje, A.F. & Boobis, A.R. (1990) Debrisoquine oxidation phenotype and susceptibility to lung cancer. *Br. J. Clin. Pharmacol.*, 29, 101-109

Steen, V.M., Andreassen, O.A., Daly, A.K., Tefre, T., Borresen, A.-L., Idle, J.R. & Gulbrandsen, A.-K. (1995) Detection of the poor metabolizer-associatcd CYP2D6(D) gene deletion allele by long-PCR technology. *Pharmacogenetics*, 5, 215-223

Stucker, L., Cosme, J., Laurent, P., Cenee, S., Beaune, P., Bignon, L., Depierre, A., Milleron, B. & Hemon, D. (1995) CYP2D6 genotype and lung cancer risk according to histologic type and tobacco exposure. *Carcinogenesis*, 16, 2759-2764

Stuven, T., Griese, E.-U., Kroemer, H.K., Eichelbaum, M. & Zanger, U.M. (1996) Rapid detection of CYP2D6 null alleles by long distance and multiplex polymerase chain reaction. *Pharmacogenetics*, 6, 417-421

Tefre, T., Daly, A.K., Armstrong, M., Leathart, L.B.S., Idle, J.R., Brogger, A. & Borresen, A.L. (1994) Genotyping of the CYP2D6 gene in Norwegian lung cancer patients and controls. *Pharmacogenetics*, 4, 47-57

Tucker, G.T. (1994) Clinical implications of genetic polymorphisms in drug metabolism. *J. Pharmacol.*, 46, 417-424

Wadelius, M., Darj, E., Frenne, G. & Rane, A. (1997) Induction of CYP2D6 in pregnancy. *Clin. Pharmacol. Ther.*, 62, 400-407

Walle, T., Byington, R.P., Furberg, L.D., Mcintyre, K.M. & Vokanas, P.S. (1985) Biologic determinants of propranolol disposition: results from 1308 patients in the beta-blocker heart attack trial. *Clin. Pharmacol. Ther.*, 38, 509-518

Wanwimolruk, S., Patamusucon, P. & Lee, E.J.D. (1990) Evidence for the polymorphic oxidation of debrisoquine in New Zealand Caucasians. *Br.J. Clin. Pharmacol.*, 29, 244-247

Wanwimolruk, S., Pratt, E.L., Denton, J.R., Chalcroft, S.C.W., Barron, P.A. & Broughton, J.R. (1995) Evidence for the polymorphic oxidation of debrisoquine and proguanil in a New Zealand Maori population. *Pharmacogenetics*, 5, 193-198

Wolf, C.R., Smith, C.A.D., Gough, A.C., Moss, L.E., Vallis, K.A., Howard, G., Carey, F.L., Mills, K., McNee W., Carmichael, J. & Spurr, N. K. (1992) Relationship between the debrisoquine hydroxylase polymorphism and cancer susceptibility. *Carcinogenesis*, 13, 1035-1038

Wolf, C.R., Smith, C.A.D., Bishop, T., Forman, D., Gough, A.C. & Spurr, N.K. (1994) CYP2D6 genotyping and the association with lung cancer susceptibility. *Pharmacogenetics*, 4, 104-106

Woolhouse, N.M., Andoh, B., Mahgoub, A., Sloan, T.P., Idle, J.R. & Smith, R.L. (1979) Debrisoquine hydroxylation polymorphism among Ghanaians and Caucasians. *Clin. Pharmacol. Ther.*, 26, 584-591

Yokoi, T., Kosaka, Y, Chida, M., Chida, K, Nakamura, H., Ishizaki, T., Kinoshita, M., Sato, K., Gonzalez, F. J. & Kamataki, T. (1996) A new CYP2D6 allele with a 9bp insertion in exon 9 in a Japanese population associated with poor metabolizer phenotype. *Pharmacogenetics*, 6, 395-401

Yokota, H., Tamura, S., Furuya, H., Kimura, S., Watanabe, M., Kanazawa, L., Kondo, I. & Gonzalez, F.J. (1993) Evidence for a new variant allele CYP2D6J in a Japanese population associated with lower *in vivo* rates of sparteine metabolism. *Pharmacogenetics*, 3, 256-263

Corresponding author
C. Roland Wolf
University of Dundee Biomedical Research Centre,
ICRF Molecular Pharmacology Unit,
Ninewells Hospital and Medical School,
Dundee, DD1 9SY,
United Kingdom

Metabolic Polymorphisms and Susceptibility to Cancer
W. Ryder
IARC Scientific Publications No. 148
International Agency for Research on Cancer, Lyon, 1999

Chapter 19. The glutathione S-transferases: influence of polymorphism on cancer susceptibility

R.C. Strange and A.A. Fryer

The glutathione S-transferase supergene family is an important part of cellular enzymic defence against endogenous and exogenous chemicals, many of which have a carcinogenic potential. However, while a wide variety of chemicals can act as substrates for different members of the supergene family, the precise function of these enzymes remains unclear. The supergene family comprises several gene families that include polymorphic loci, prompting the hypothesis that allelic variants associated with less effective detoxification of potential carcinogens can confer an increased susceptibility to cancer. For example, the null genotypes at the mu class GSTM1 and theta class GSTT1 loci have attracted particular interest, and recently identified allelic variants at the mu class GSTM3 and pi class GSTP1 loci are also putative susceptibility candidates. However, while associations between GSTM1 and GSTT1 genotypes and risk have been observed in some case-control studies in lung, bladder and colon cancers, other studies have reported contrary findings, and the importance of these polymorphisms in mediating the risk of smoking-related cancers remains generally unproven. We describe the influence of glutathione S-transferase polymorphisms on the risk of several cancers, including basal cell carcinoma of skin. In the latter cancer, associations between tumour numbers, site and accrual have been observed, suggesting a role for GST enzymes in the detoxification of the products of ultraviolet radiation-induced oxidative stress. We review below current knowledge of polymorphism in GST loci, possible in vivo GST substrates, and the difficulties of determining the role of this complex gene family on the basis of available epidemiological data.

The glutathione S-transferase supergene family

The glutathione S-transferases (GSTs) comprise a supergene family of phase 2 detoxifying enzymes that catalyse a variety of reduced glutathione-dependent reactions with compounds containing an electrophilic centre (Hayes & Pulford, 1995). GST enzymes appear to be expressed in most, if not all, life forms, a finding that suggests their importance in the protection of cells from harmful chemicals. In humans, the enzymes expressed in tissue cytosols have been most intensively studied, and four major gene families have been identified: alpha on chromosome 6, mu on chromosome 1, theta on chromosome 22, and pi on chromosome 11. A further class, sigma, has been identified in non-vertebrates (Buetler & Eaton, 1992). Sequence data on enzymes of the different classes suggests the ancestral cytosolic GST gene was of the theta class with progressive divergence of the sigma class and then of the mu class GST (Hayes & Pulford, 1995). A membrane-associated GST that evolved separately to the cytosolic enzymes has been identified, although its influence on cancer susceptibility is unknown.

Polymorphism in glutathione S-transferase genes

There is evidence for allelism in GST genes in each of the alpha, mu, theta and pi gene families and it is likely that further examples of the phenomenon will be found in both the loci that have not yet been studied (e.g. GSTM5) as well as those known to exhibit polymorphism.

Alpha class gene family. Kamisaka *et al.* (1975) first reported the expression of GST enzymes now recognized as members of the alpha class family in human liver. Various isoenzymes were identified which have been shown to comprise homo- and heterodimers of the products of GSTA1 and GSTA2. Other alpha class enzymes have been described in human tissues, including a highly basic enzyme in skin (Del Boccio *et al.*, 1987) and a widely expressed acidic enzyme (Singhal *et al.*, 1994). The alpha class family, therefore, comprises two or three functional genes and at least four pseudogenes on chromosome 6p12, which appear to have evolved by gene duplication and gene conversion events (Suzuki *et al.*, 1993).Various studies have described considerable interindividual variation in the level of expression of alpha class GST enzymes in human tissues. For example, in a series of 20 brain cytosols, enzyme activity and protein were detected in only eight subjects, and within these expressers there was considerable between-individual variation (Strange *et al.*, 1992). In human liver, both A1 and A2 alpha class isoenzymes are particularly strongly expressed in hepatocytes, although occasional examples of individuals who fail to express this GST class in these cells have been reported (Board, 1981; Strange *et al.*, 1984a). However, while these data are compatible with polymorphism in GSTA1 or GSTA2, as yet there appears to be only one report of a restriction fragment length polymorphism in GSTA2 (Chen & Board,1987). The molecular basis for the observed phenotypic variation and its implications remain unknown, but studies on rats show that GSTA1 and GSTA2 subunits are readily inducible with the 5'-flanking region of GSTA2 containing cis-acting elements that respond to polycyclic aromatic hydrocarbons (PAH) or phenolic antioxidants (Rushmore *et al.*, 1993).

Mu class gene family. Five mu genes (M1-M5) situated in tandem on chromosome 1p13 have been identified (Seidegard *et al.*, 1988; Zhong *et al.*, 1993; Pearson *et al.*,1993; Ross *et al.*., 1993). Several reports have indicated the presence of mu class genes on chromosome 6 but it is unclear whether this is a functional gene, a pseudogene or a related sequence (DeJong *et al.*, 1988; DeJong *et al.*, 1991; Ross *et al.*, 1993). GSTM1 is expressed in human liver, stomach, brain and other tissues while GSTM2-GSTM5 subunits have been detected in extrahepatic tissues and cell lines (Board 1981; Strange *et al.*, 1984b; Hayes & Pulford, 1995; Mannervik & Widersten,1995).

The first polymorphism in a GST locus to be characterized was reported by Board (1981) in GSTM1. The model, based on three alleles, GSTM1*0, GSTM1*A and GSTM1*B, has been confirmed by many subsequent studies. GSTM1*0 is deleted and homozygotes (GSTM1 null genotype) express no GSTM1 protein (Seidegard *et al.*, 1988). GSTM1*A and GSTM1*B differ by only a single base in exon 7 and encode enzyme monomers that form active homo- and heterodimeric enzymes (Seidegard *et al.*, 1988; DeJong *et al.*, 1988). *In vitro* data indicate similar catalytic effectiveness of the homo- and heterodimeric enzymes resulting from these alleles.

Until recently, allelism in other mu class genes had not been reported, although variation in the level of expression of GSTM3, a gene identified by Suzuki *et al.* (1987) and subsequently cloned by Campbell *et al.* (1990), was reported in human lung and brain (Anttila *et al.*, 1995; Strange *et al.*, 1992). In 20 control and 16 astrocytoma brain samples we identified two controls and four patients with undetectable GSTM3 activity, suggesting that in some subjects, GSTM3, like GSTM1, may be deleted or may demonstrate a low activity allele (Strange *et al.*, 1992). Further evidence for variable expression of GSTM3 was reported by Nakajima *et al.* (1995), who showed that the expression of GSTM3 in human lung cytosol was significantly correlated with absence of GSTM1, suggesting GSTM1 influences expression of this and possibly other mu genes.

Inskip *et al.* (1995) tested the hypothesis that GSTM3 demonstrates a null allele by using GSTM3-specific primers to amplify across exon 6 and exon 7 (Fig. 1). In DNA samples from 244 subjects they identified amplified DNA fragments in all samples, implying that null alleles at this locus, if present, are rare. However, in 63 subjects an additional two heteroduplex bands were identified. Sequencing studies identified two alleles, GSTM3*A and GSTM3*B, that differed in intron 6 by a 3 base pair deletion in GSTM3*B. Although the difference between GSTM3*A and GSTM3*B is intronic, its importance is suggested by the presence of a recognition motif (-aagata-) for the versatile transcription factor, YY1 in GSTM3*B but

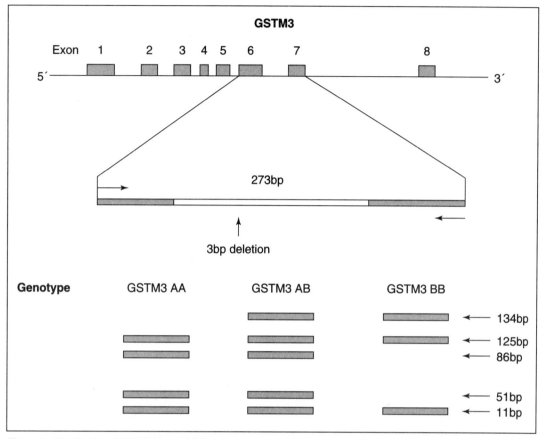

Figure 1. Identification of GSTM3*A and GSTM3*B alleles using PCR with diagnostic restriction enzyme digestion.

not in GSTM3*A. Taylor *et al.* (1991) reported the presence of conserved sequences within introns of mu class genes and suggested that this represented a selective pressure resulting from an advantageous function of these regions. Indeed, they proposed that perfect hyphenated palindromes, as seen around the site of the mutation in GSTM3, were characteristic of regulatory elements. We speculated, therefore, that expression of the GSTM3*B and GSTM3*A alleles is differently regulated through the actions of YY1 (Inskip *et al.*, 1995), and developed a PCR assay using diagnostic restriction digestion with Mnl1 to test this hypothesis (Fig. 1). Of further interest was our finding that GSTM3*B and GSTM1*A are in linkage disequilibrium (Inskip *et al.*, 1995). These data may explain the finding of variation in GSTM3 expression in the lungs of subjects with different GSTM1 genotypes (Anttila *et al.*, 1995;

Nakajima *et al.*, 1995). Thus, individuals with a GSTM1*A/GSTM3*B haplotype should express more GSTM3 than those with a GSTM1*O/GSTM3*A or GSTM1*B/GSTM3*A haplotype because GSTM3*A is not inducible by YY1. The finding of linkage dysequilibrium may also explain the discrepancy in results from case-control studies of the influence of GSTM1 genotypes on cancer susceptibility (see below).

Inskip *et al.* (1995) selected the exon 6 / exon 7 region of the gene for amplification because it presented a convenient GSTM3-specific sequence. It is possible, therefore, that other alleles exist at this locus. There are few data on allelism at other mu class genes, although Ross & Board (1993) described possible alternative splicing of GSTM4. Thus, of two GSTM4 cDNA clones isolated from a human testis library, one demonstrated excision of exon 4 and the other of exon 8.

Theta class gene family. Two theta class GSTs, GSTT1-1 and GSTT2-2, have been identified in human liver. A common null polymorphism has been identified at the GSTT1 locus (Pemble *et al.*, 1994), and this accounts for the observed phenotypic variation in GSH-related detoxification of halomethanes by human erythrocytes. Schroder *et al.* (1996) have recently reported a further theta class variant that utilizes monohalogenated methanes, ethylene oxide and dichloromethane. This variant resembles GSTT2-2 in its substrate specificity, possibly because of a common N-terminal modification that influences substrate binding.

Pi class gene family. GSTP1 is also interesting in the context of polymorphism, with the finding of alleles in the gene; one BamH1 RFLP (Kumar *et al.*, 1994) and a polymorphism in the region of pentanucleotide repeats (ATAAA) in the 5'-promoter region (Harada *et al.*, 1994). The functional significance of these polymorphisms is unknown. Recently, a further polymorphism in this GST family has been identified. Ahmad *et al.* (1990) identified two human GSTP1 isoforms that differed by one amino acid (Ile 104 or Val 104). Comparison of the enzymatic properties of the two proteins revealed differences in heat stability and affinity for 1-chloro-2,4,-dinitrobenzene (Ile-containing isoform Km = 0.8mM, Val-containing isoform Km = 3mM) (Zimniak *et al.*, 1994). The authors concluded that the residue in position 104 partly defined the geometry of the hydrophobic binding site and, consequently, specific activity for electrophilic substrates (Zimniak *et al.*, 1994). Subsequently, Ali-Osman *et al.* (1995) identified two full-length cDNAs from human glioma libraries which differed from the wild-type sequence. The first sequence differed by an A to G transition at nucleotide +313 (GSTP1b) and the second by an A to G transition at nucleotide +313 as well as a C to T transition at +341 (GSTP1c). These sequences represent allelic variants (Harries *et al.*, 1997) with the homodimeric, isoleucine-containing isoenzyme (GSTP1 AA) having greater specific activity and affinity for some (but not other) electrophilic substrates than the corresponding valine variant (GSTP1 BB) (Zimniak *et al.*, 1994; Ali-Osman *et al.*, 1995).

Substrates for glutathione S-transferase enzymes

The GSTs appear to have an absolute requirement for reduced glutathione. The sulfur atom of this thiol has a high nucleophilicity and accordingly the electrophilic centre of the other substrate can be provided by a carbon, nitrogen or sulfur atom present in arene oxides, unsaturated carbonyls, organic halides and other substances. The range of potential GST substrates is, therefore, very large, although the majority can be broadly grouped as xenobiotics or products of oxidative stress. While some substrates may be utilized by GSTs of different classes, certain GSTs appear to be effective in the detoxification of particular groups of chemicals.

The GST substrates include products of oxidative stress. Various GSTs can utilize DNA and lipid products of oxidative stress but it is not clear how these various reactions are coordinated in a cell under physiological or pathological conditions (Hayes & Strange, 1995; Smith *et al.*, 1995). Thus, a role for the alpha class enzymes in protection against oxidative stress is suggested by their high activity towards products of lipid peroxidation such as cumene hydroperoxide and 4-hydroxynonenal (Hayes & Pulford, 1995; Mannervik & Widersten, 1995). GSTT2, unlike mu and pi class enzymes, also has substantial activity towards cumene hydroperoxide. GSTT1 catalyses the detoxification of oxidized lipid and DNA (Ketterer *et al.*, 1993; Pemble *et al.*, 1994). GSTP1 appears effective in the detoxification of base propenals (e.g. thymine and uracil propenal) that arise from the oxidation of DNA (Berhane *et al.*, 1994). Other products of oxidative stress are also metabolized by other GSTs. Thus, toxic quinone metabolites of catecholamines, including aminochrome and dopachrome, are very effectively conjugated with glutathione in reactions catalysed by GSTM2-2. Adrenochrome, the oxidation product of adrenaline, is more effectively utilized by GSTM1-1 (Baez *et al.*, 1997). Other GST classes (alpha class A1-1, A2-2, A4-4; pi P1-1; theta T1-1) demonstrated negligible activities towards these substrates.

These *in vitro* studies provide support for the view that the physiological substrates for the GSTs are the various products of oxygen utilization. Thus, expression of GST is often perinuclear and mu GSTs demonstrate coordinated expression with and location in similar cell types as CuZn-superoxide dismutase and Se-glutathione peroxidase (Ketterer *et al.*, 1993; Strange, 1993). How these different antioxidant enzymes coordinate their activities is unknown, however, and for some GSTs there are only limited data on tissue patterns of expression.

The GST substrates also include environmental carcinogens. The GSTs appear to contribute to the detoxification of various potentially toxic environmental compounds encountered in food, air or medication. Of importance in the context of cancer are the PAHs found in combustion products. These chemicals generally require activation by members of the phase 1 cytochrome P450 supergene family to epoxide-containing metabolites before they become toxic. These epoxides (e.g. trans-4-phenyl-3-buten-2-one, benzo[a]-pyrene-7,8-diol-9,10-oxide) are effective substrates for mu and pi GSTs. The GSTP1 enzyme is widely expressed and can utilize a variety of potentially carcinogenic substrates, including chemicals derived from cigarette smoke, such as benzo(a)pyrene diol epoxide and acrolein, implying that allelic isoforms can confer different risks for some pathologies (Harries *et al.*, 1996). GSTT1 is also an attractive cancer susceptibility candidate as its products utilize various potential carcinogens, including chemicals used as methylating agents, pesticides and industrial solvents. Thus, substrates include monohalomethanes (e.g. methyl chloride) and ethylene oxide (Ketterer *et al.*, 1993). Furthermore, GST5-5, the rat homologue of GSTT1, has activity towards epoxides, suggesting that individuals with null genotypes at GSTM1 and GSTT1 may be at high risk of smoking-related cancers.

Data from *in vitro* studies also suggest that GSTM1 and GSTT1 enzymes protect cells from the products of phase 1 detoxification reactions (Wiencke *et al.*, 1990; Norppa *et al.*, 1995). For example, several groups have studied cytogenetic damage in host lymphocytes following exposure to a test mutagen. Thus, Wiencke *et al.* (1990) initially showed that cells from GSTM1 null individuals are more susceptible to sister chromatid exchange (SCE) following exposure to trans-stilbene oxide but not cis-stilbene oxide. These studies suggest the importance of the gene and give

an insight into specificity; cis-stilbene oxide is a poor substrate for GSTM1. Similar studies comparing the extent of SCE in subjects with GSTT1 null or expressed genotypes have been described by Hallier *et al.* (1994). GSTT1*0 homozygotes showed increased damage following exposure to methyl bromide, ethylene oxide and dichloromethane compared with GSTT1 expressers, again suggesting that this GST is important in protection against mutagen-induced damage. Norppa *et al.* (1995) extended these observations by comparing the effects of null genotypes at GSTM1 and GSTT1 on SCE frequency induced by metabolites of 1,3-butadiene, a constituent of environmental pollution. This compound is metabolized to mutagenic, mono- and di-epoxide intermediates. Exposure to the diepoxide, 1,2,3,4-diepoxybutane, resulted in increased SCE in individuals with GSTT1 null compared with GSTT1 expressers, while no differences were identified in GSTM1 null or positive subjects. Collectively, these and other studies show the importance of mu and theta GST in the protection of DNA from PAH epoxides. In particular they show the products of these genes to be influential in intact cells constitutively expressing other mutagen-metabolizing enzymes; GSTM1 influences the metabolism of monoepoxybutane, a reactive metabolite of butadiene, while GSTT1 is most effective with 1,2,3,4-diepoxybutane. Importantly, individuals who are GSTT1 expressers demonstrate lower SCE rates than subjects homozygous for GSTT1*0, suggesting that the GSTT1 enzyme is protective against background genotoxic damage (Schroder *et al.*, 1995). The same authors suggested that ethylene oxide, a substrate for GSTT1 which arises from endogenous ethylene, modulates background SCE rates. Such studies should eventually help us to understand why one gene but not another influences susceptibility to particular cancers. To date no published data are available on GSTM3 and GSTP1.

Influence of glutathione S-transferase polymorphisms on susceptibility to cancer

GST isoenzymes encoded by polymorphic members of the mu, theta and pi gene families catalyse the detoxification of a variety of reactive toxic and mutagenic compounds. It is reasonable to speculate, therefore, that homozygosity for null alleles or those encoding low activity variants are associated with a biochemical consequence. However, because of the range of potential substrates, we do not yet have a clear view of exactly which (if any) *in vivo* biochemical processes are influenced by these polymorphisms.

Identification of GST genotypes in case-control studies using the polymerase chain reaction

In spite of uncertainties regarding the true role of GSTs, the use of genotyping assays based on the polymerase chain reaction (PCR) and an increasing general interest in the role of polymorphism in determining disease susceptibility (Perera, 1996) has resulted in a considerable body of data on the influence of GST alleles on susceptibility to cancer. Robust and reliable PCR assays that identify GSTM1, GSTT1, GSTM3 and GSTP1 genotypes have been described (Comstock *et al.*, 1990; Fryer *et al.*, 1993; Pemble *et al.*, 1994; Inskip *et al.*,1995; Harries *et al.*, 1997). In the case of GSTM1, the first GST genotyping assay to be widely used, data from several laboratories show very close agreement between PCR-based identification of genotype and phenotype determined by enzyme activity measurements (Comstock *et al.*, 1990; Strange, 1993). A problem with assessing the importance of the GSTM1 polymorphism has been the inability to conveniently detect GSTM1*0, as the extent of the deletion has not been reported. Thus, while homozygotes for this allele can be identified by a failure to amplify selected regions of the gene, for instance between exon 4 and exon 5, the GSTM1*0/GSTM1*A and GSTM1*0/GSTM1*B heterozygote genotypes cannot be conveniently distinguished from the corresponding homozygous GSTM1*A and GSTM1*B genotypes. This would be possible using multiplex PCR with an internal standard, although we are not aware of studies using this approach routinely. To test the hypothesis that genotypes comprising two expressed alleles represent low-risk genotypes because they confer more effective detoxification than those heterozygous for GSTM1*0, Fryer *et al.*, (1993) devised a PCR assay using exon 7 specific primers that distinguish GSTM1*A and GSTM1*B, allowing identification of the GSTM1 null and GSTM1 A/B

(GSTM1*A/GSTM1*B) genotypes as well as the GSTM1 A (GSTM1*A/GSTM1*A and GSTM1*A-/GSTM1*0) and GSTM1 B (GSTM1*B/GSTM1*B and GSTM1*B/GSTM1*0) phenotypes. This assay has been refined by means of an approach based on an amplification refractory mutation system, and its use has allowed some conclusions to be drawn regarding the risks associated with different expressed genotypes (Heagerty *et al.*, 1994; Strange, 1996). There appears to be a gene dosage effect in at least some cancers, including basal cell carcinoma of the skin, as subjects with the GSTM1 A/B genotype are at reduced risk of multiple primary tumours.

The GSTT1 genotyping assay described by Pemble *et al.* (1994) has been widely used and shown to correlate with phenotype. Similar studies are not yet available for GSTM3 genotyping and the functional consequences of this polymorphism, if any, remain unknown.

Table 1 shows genotype frequencies for the well-characterized polymorphisms in GSTM1, GSTM3, GSTT1 and GSTP1 in control Caucasians from England and Germany, determined in our laboratory. As expected from studies on other genes there are significant differences in the frequencies of at least some of these genotypes in different ethnic groups (Zhao *et al.*, 1994; Lin *et al.*, 1994; Nelson *et al.*, 1995; Strange, 1996). For example, while the frequency of the GSTM1 null genotype is markedly lower in Nigerians (22%) than in English Caucasians (57.3%), the frequency of GSTT1 null is higher.

Influence of GST polymorphisms on susceptibility to lung cancer. The idea that GST polymorphisms might influence susceptibility to cancer was first proposed by Board (1981) following identification of the GSTM1 null genotype. Most initial studies designed to test this hypothesis concentrated on cancers associated with exposure to tobacco-derived chemicals. Thus, in a series of studies in patients with lung cancer, Seidegard *et al.*, (1988, 1990) found increased frequency of GSTM1 null in cigarette smokers with lung cancer (particularly adenocarcinoma) compared with controls. Since then there have been many studies on this cancer though conflicting data have been obtained and the influence of GSTM1 null on risk remains somewhat unclear (Zhong *et al.*,

Table 1. Glutathione S-transferase polymorphisms: genotype frequencies in control Caucasians from North Staffordshire and Berlin

GSTM1	A	B	A/B	Null	N
	26.50%	11.80%	4.30%	57.30%	211
GSTM3	AA	AB	BB		N
	73.70%	21.30%	5.00%		300
GSTT1	A	Null			N
	80.30%	19.70%			284
GSTP1*	AA	AB	BB		N
	54.30%	35.30%	10.30%		184

* Samples obtained from Berlin.

1991; Nazar-Stewart *et al.*, 1993; Nakachi *et al.*, 1993; Hirvonen *et al.*, 1993; Kerb *et al.*, 1995; Deakin *et al.*, 1996). Recent meta-analyses indicate that the null genotype confers a small increased risk of lung cancer (McWilliams *et al.*, 1995; d'Errico *et al.*, 1996). The reason for the discrepancies in GSTM1 data is unclear. One problem may be the relatively weak influence of any one genotype on susceptibility and imbalances in the distribution of confounding factors such as allelism at other relevant loci in cases and controls. Differences in exposure to carcinogens in cigarette smoke may also be important, with exaggeration of the effects of such variables in studies of small numbers of subjects. Thus, recent work suggests the effect of GSTM1 null on susceptibility to lung cancer may be more evident in patients who have smoked less than 35 pack years (Alexandrie *et al.*, 1995), although other studies have not confirmed this relationship (Deakin *et al.*, 1996). Diet may also be a confounding factor: Garcia-Closas *et al.* (1995) reported that the influence of GSTM1 null on susceptibility to squamous cell cancer of the lung was enhanced by low intake of vitamin C and other nutrients. The importance of careful selection of controls and, indeed, of what constitutes an acceptable control, has also been emphasized (Strange, 1996); while early studies on Caucasians found frequencies of GSTM1 null of about 40%, some more recent data have indicated frequencies of up to 58% in, for example, women with menorrhagia (Warwick *et al.*, 1994). In our experience the higher frequencies are typical of controls recruited among hospital inpatients and outpatients, as compared with laboratory volunteers or individuals at postmortem, although the basis for these differences is unclear. There is relatively little data on the influence of GSTT1 genotypes on susceptibility to lung cancer, but a small study by Deakin *et al.* (1996) found no differences between cases and controls. We are not aware of published data on the influence of polymorphism in GSTM3 and GSTP1 or on the importance of particular combinations of GSTM1/GSTM3 or GSTP1 genotypes.

Effects of GST genotypes on susceptibility to bladder cancer. While the concept that the consequences of GST deficiency can be expected to be most evident in smokers is attractive, because cigarette smoke contains mutagenic and carcinogenic epoxides, the data do not always support this view. Cigarette smoking is a causative factor in cervical neoplasia, cancers of the upper aerodigestive tract and bladder cancer, as well as in lung cancer. We found no significant interactions between GSTM1 or GSTT1 genotypes and smoking in women with cervical intraepithelial neoplasia and squamous cell cancer of the cervix or in patients with pharyngeal or laryngeal cancers;

thus, the combination of smoking and null genotype was not more common in cases than controls (Warwick *et al.*, 1994; Matthias *et al.*, 1996). In contrast, some but not all studies on bladder cancer demonstrate differences in genotype frequencies between cases and controls (Bell *et al.*, 1993; Zhong *et al.*, 1994; Lafuente *et al.*, 1993; Brockmöller *et al.*, 1994; Lin *et al.*, 1994), and recent meta-analysis suggests that the GSTM1 null genotype confers increased susceptibility (d'Errico *et al.*, 1996). Clearly, while these cancers share smoking as a risk factor they have very different pathogeneses. Nonetheless, the data presented show that these GST polymorphisms are not strongly associated with predisposition to smoking-related cancers, although it is possible that particular genotypes are related to certain mutational events in tumours.

Effects of GST genotypes on susceptibility to stomach and colon cancer. Allelism at GST loci might be expected to mediate the risk of gastrointestinal cancers, since various substrates, including products of inflammation and constituents of cooked meat, are implicated in the pathogeneses of these conditions. Indeed, several studies indicate that GSTM1 null confers increased risk of gastric and colon cancers (Strange *et al.*, 1991; Zhong *et al.*, 1994). Further, Zhong *et al.* (1994) found significantly higher frequencies of GSTM1 null in the proximal compared with the distal colon, although other studies have failed to reproduce this finding (Chenevix-Trench *et al.*, 1995; Szarka *et al.*, 1995; Deakin *et al.*, 1996). Two recent studies have indicated the importance of GSTT1 in mediating susceptibility to colon cancer; Chenevix-Trench *et al.* (1995) found the frequency of GSTT1 null significantly increased in patients diagnosed before 70 years of age, and Deakin *et al.* (1996) showed the frequency of this genotype was increased in cases compared with controls, although no age effect was observed.

Further support for the view that mu and theta class GST are important in the detoxification of potential toxic chemicals in the bowel comes from studies in patients with ulcerative colitis (UC) and Crohn's disease. Susceptibility to these pathologies appears to depend on genetic and environmental factors (Crotty, 1994; Sofaer, 1993). However, the identity of such putative genes is unknown. Inflammation is a prominent feature of both UC and Crohn's disease, implying that the capacity to detoxify the reactive oxygen species (ROS) and their cytotoxic products generated during inflammation may influence disease susceptibility and/or aggressiveness. The importance of detoxification is also indicated by studies showing that the risk of UC is lower in cigarette smokers and that nicotine patches have a beneficial effect on disease activity in ex-smokers. By contrast, the risk of Crohn's disease is higher in smokers. These data indicate that individual differences in the effectiveness of detoxification of electrophiles mediate susceptibility to both diseases. We found that homozygosity for GSTT1*0 is associated with increased risk of total UC. The genotype is not a general marker of susceptibility to oxidative stress in the bowel, as the association was not apparent in distal UC or Crohn's disease. The frequency distributions of GSTM1 genotypes in the Crohn's disease patients and those suffering distal UC were also found to be significantly different, and there was evidence that the products of GSTM1*B were more protective than those of GSTM1*A. Data on the possible importance of GSTM1/GSTM3 haplotypes have not yet been reported, although the finding of linkage dysequilibrium may also explain the discrepancy in results from case control studies on the influence of the GSTM1 polymorphism on susceptibility to lung and other cancers; it is thus the GSTM1/GSTM3 haplotype that determines susceptibility rather than the GSTM1 genotype alone. This hypothesis has not yet been formally tested, but case-control studies in patients with Crohn's disease, low grade cervical intraepithelial neoplasia, multiple skin tumours of different histological types and bladder cancer indicate that the GSTM1 B and GSTM1 A genotypes confer different levels of protection (Brockmöller *et al.*, 1994; Strange, 1996), although it is not yet clear if this is related to linkage dysequilibrium with GSTM3 .

Effects of GST genotypes on susceptibility to skin cancers. The view that GSTs are part of cell antioxidant defence (Ketterer *et al.*, 1993; Hayes & Strange, 1995) is supported by studies in cutaneous basal cell carcinoma (BCC). Ultraviolet (UV) radiation is a major causative factor but the

Table 2. Influence of GSTM1 and GSTM3 genotypes on number of primary BCCs

	Mean number BCCs	
	Yes	No
Male gender	2.40	1.64
Blue or green eyes	2.39	1.92
Skin type 1	2.99	2.12
GSTM1 null and skin type 1	4.57	2.00
GSTM3 AA and skin type 1	3.57	2.08

The baseline is the complement (i.e. female gender, not skin type 1, etc.).

Statistical analysis. Cross-sectional analysis. Poisson regression was used to model count data using the EGRET statistical package (SERC, Seattle, 1993). The model assumes the Poisson rate parameter (mean number BCCs) may be expressed as a function of a set of covariates; i.e. age, skin type 1, eye colour, hair colour, gender, genotypes. A rate ratio, defined as the multiplicative effect of a change of a covariate by 1, was calculated. Thus, the rate ratio for males [1] (1.43) against females [0] is mean number BCCs in males (2.40)/mean number BCCs in females (1.64), when gender alone is considered. The Poisson regression approach has the advantage that it allows study of the ratio of the mean number of BCCs corrected for other covariates, such as age and number of tumours at presentation.

relationship between exposure and risk is poorly understood. UV radiation has pleiotropic effects on skin, including the formation of reactive oxygen species (ROS), and there is evidence that these species and/or their products effect mutations in key target genes and that, via effects on cytokine expression, they influence immune modulation (Mukhtar & Elmets, 1996). Importantly, epidemiological studies have failed to link BCC with exposure to environmental pollutants (e.g. cigarette smoke). A remarkable feature of this pathology is the risk of developing further tumours (Karagas et al., 1994). This risk depends on the number of lesions already present; 27% of patients with one tumour suffer a further tumour within five years, compared with 90% of patients with ten or more lesions (Karagas et al., 1994). These data suggest that susceptibility to BCC is not merely dependent on UV radiation but also on host genetic factors. This view is supported by data showing that susceptibility to UVB-induced inhibition of contact hypersensitivity appears to be a better indicator of non-melanoma skin cancer risk than cumulative UV exposure (Schmieder et al., 1992) and that GSTM1 A/B is protective against multiple BCC (Heagerty et al., 1994).

The concept of susceptibility to BCC is complex, as genetic factors could influence both tumour numbers and accrual (Heagerty et al., 1996; Lear et al., 1996). We used an epidemiological approach to identify GSTs that influence BCC numbers and the number of lesions/year in 827 English patients. We found both GSTM1 and GSTM3 genotypes, in combination with skin type 1 (individuals who always burn but do not tan on exposure to UV) influenced the number of primary lesions (Yengi et al., 1996; Lear et al., 1996). Thus, interactions between GSTM1 null and skin type 1 or GSTM3 AA were associated with increased tumour numbers (Table 2). It is noteworthy that, individually, neither of these genotypes influenced the number of lesions, whereas in combination with skin type 1 both were associated with an increased number of lesions. In the longitudinal study, GST genotypes associated with a faster accrual were identified. Table 3 shows that male gender, number of BCCs at presentation and GSTT1 null were all associated with faster tumour accrual. The quantitative importance of each factor is given by the rate ratio. It is also noteworthy that the influence of GSTT1 null is similar to that of traditional risk factors for multiple BCC, such as male gender.

Table 3. Influence of GSTT1 genotypes and host characteristics on accrual of primary BCCs

	P value	Rate ratio	95% CI
(a) Unadjusted*			
i. Male gender	<0.001	2.260	1.793-2.848
ii. BCC number at presentation	<0.001	1.213	1.167-1.260
iii. Age at presentation	0.002	1.014	1.005-1.022
iv. GSTT1 null	<0.001	2.321	1.821-2.959
(b) Adjusted for age and number of BCCs at presentation*			
i. GSTT1 null	<0.001	2.677	2.075-3.452
ii. Male gender	<0.001	2.174	1.720-2.749
iii. Skin type 1	0.035	1.386	1.024-1.877

The baseline is the complement (i.e. female gender, not skin type 1, etc.).
* Results shown are for individual factors alone (i.e. not in the presence of other factors).

Statistical analysis. Longitudinal analysis. Poisson regression with a rate multiplier was used to adjust for the number of person-years at risk since the increase in the number of BCCs is likely to change, depending on the number of years between first presentation and August 1995. The rate multiplier therefore corrected for the different numbers of person-years at risk in different patients. Cases were omitted when appropriate data were missing for particular analyses. Only results significant at the 5% level or approaching this level of significance are described.

These studies are compatible with the view that GSTM1, GSTM3 and GSTT1 utilize products of UV-induced oxidative stress. Indeed, our finding that GSTM3 is expressed in the epidermis and basal layer of skin supports the view that this enzyme is part of local antioxidant defences (Yengi et al., 1996). Thus, the basal layer includes the stem cells believed to be the targets for UV-induced damage from which BCCs arise. Data on GSTP1 are not yet available. Further support for the importance of these genes in the protection of skin from UV comes from studies in systemic lupus erythematosus (Ollier et al., 1996): GSTM1 null is associated with increased production of anti-Ro (but not anti-La) antibodies, a phenotype associated with photosensitivity.

Overview on GST polymorphisms and cancer risk

There is now a considerable body of data supporting the view that polymorphism at different GST genes influences susceptibility to cancer. However, it remains unclear why a particular genotype is associated with an increased risk of a particular cancer but not another. Presumably different cancers have different causative substrates and this is reflected in the genes associated with susceptibility. Much work is based on studies in smoking-related cancers. In our view it remains far from clear that the GSTs play a major role in the detoxification of tobacco-derived potential carcinogens. An alternative view is that carcinogen-metabolizing enzymes such as the GSTs are involved in the metabolism of endogenous molecules and therefore exert a critical role in normal cell housekeeping activities (Nebert, 1994). We believe the data obtained in patients with BCC support this view. However, studies showing that the GSTT1 null genotype (but not GSTM1 null) is associated with increased susceptibility to astrocytoma, meningioma and myeloblastic syndromes are harder to explain (Elexpuru-Camiruaga et al., 1995; Chen et al., 1996). Thus, brain tumours are not clearly associated with exposure to environmental pollutants, although chemical carcinogens such as N-methyl-N-nitrosourea have been implicated in animal studies and the risk of glioma is linked with intake of processed meats and cheese as well as occupation. Why GSTT1 but not GSTM1 or GSTM3 influences the risk of astrocytoma is unclear (Elexpuru-Camiruaga et al., 1995; Hand et al., 1996). GSTM3 might have been expected to be a good candidate susceptibility gene for these tumours as it is usually strongly expressed in brain (Strange et al., 1992), and recent immunohisto-chemical studies show all brain cells identified in tumour and perilesional, uninfiltrated tissue demonstrate positivity for GSTM3, although expression is generally weak. However, some astrocytes at the interface between uninfiltrated and tumour tissue demonstrated strong expression. The staining of serial sections for glial fibrillary acidic protein showed the presence of many astrocytes but only a few of these demonstrated strong positivity for GSTM3 (Hand et al., 1996). Similarly, the causes of myelodysplastic syndrome are unclear, although Chen et al. (1996) interpreted their data as indicating the importance of GSTT1 in the detoxification of environmental or endogenous carcinogens. At present there appears to be no basis for predicting which cancers will be influenced by polymorphism at GST loci.

An alternative and potentially clinically important approach is the study of the influence of genotypes on the success of chemotherapy. Hall et al. (1994) studied 71 children with acute lymphoblastic leukaemia and found that GSTM1 null was associated with a better chance of remission than were other genotypes, possibly because of less effective metabolism of chemicals in the induction (vincristine, prednisolone, asparaginase) or continuing (6-mercaptopurine, methotrexate) therapies. The mechanism for this effect is unknown as these chemicals are not recognized substrates for GSTM1, although they represent an addition to the extensive literature on the role of the GSTs in determining resistance to a variety of chemotherapeutic agents (Tew, 1994; Hayes & Pulford, 1995).

Effect of GST genotypes on mutational spectrum in target tissues

Most studies on the influence of GST on risk have compared genotype frequencies in cases and controls. Since case groups may be heterogeneous in terms of the mutations leading to malignancy, studying associations between mutations in target genes and GST genotypes

may better identify the importance of these genes. Presumably, particular genotypes, alone or in combination, identify subjects who are detoxification-deficient in certain reactions and consequently more likely to suffer increased formation of carcinogen-DNA adducts (Perera, 1996) and/or particular mutations in target genes such as p53 (Perrett et al., 1995; Ryberg et al., 1994). Identifying such associations would be an important advance, both in confirming the importance of GSTs in determining individual cancer risk and in identifying the mechanism for this influence. Increasing amounts of data on this subject are becoming available. Kato et al. (1995) reported that the levels of PAH-DNA adducts in lung biopsies were related to the GSTM1 genotype, and studies in smokers with lung cancer showed that mutations in p53 and H-ras 1 were more frequent in GSTM1*0 homozygotes (Ryberg et al., 1994). Some 30% of these individuals carried GC>TC mutations within p53. Over 90% of individuals with this mutated form of p53 were also GSTM1 null. These types of mutation result from the formation of carcinogen-DNA adducts with chemicals such as benzpyrene, suggesting that GSTM1 protects p53 against mutagenesis.

We recently obtained further evidence of a protective role for GSTM1 in patients with epithelial ovarian cancer. No single causative factor has been identified but it is known that risk of this cancer increases with incessant ovulation (Goodwin et al., 1993). The cells of the ovarian surface epithelium undergo rapid cycles of cell division during repair of ovulation trauma (Goodwin et al., 1993), suggesting involvement of ROS. Various studies show genetic change in ovarian tumours with loss of heterozygosity (LOH) found on most chromosomes including 17p. This segment, on which p53 resides, shows LOH in 60% of ovarian cancers, and inappropriate expression of p53 is found in about 50% of ovarian cancers (Eccles et al., 1992; Greenblat et al., 1994). These findings show patients comprise a heterogeneous group described by different mutations, possibly because of differences in genetically-mediated ability to detoxify mutagens. Accordingly, we assessed the role of GSTM1 and GSTT1 in determining susceptibility to ovarian cancer and the relationship between allelism at these loci and expression of p53 (Sarhanis *et al.*, 1996). While we found no significant differences in genotype frequencies between the ovarian cancer cases and the controls, of 23 tumours found to be immunohistochemically positive for p53, 20 (87.0%) were GSTM1 null. The frequency distributions of GSTM1 genotypes in the p53 immunopositive and negative subjects were significantly different (exact p = 0.002) and those for GSTT1 genotypes approached significant difference (exact p = 0.057). In the total group of 23 patients who demonstrated p53 immunopositivity, sequencing studies identified mutations in p53 in ten patients. Nine of these cases (90%) were GSTM1 null. Of the 13 patients in whom no mutations were identified by sequencing, 11 (84.6%) were GSTM1 null.

Increased expression of p53 is likely during oxidative stress, since DNA damage is an early consequence of exposing cells to even physiological concentrations of H_2O_2, presumably because of intranuclear formation of $\cdot OH$. In our study some patients did not express p53 protein (though the p53 gene may carry mutations in some of these samples), others expressed persistent mutant protein or appeared to overexpress detectable wild-type protein (Sarhanis *et al.*, 1996). Expression of p53, detectable by immunohistochemistry, was significantly associated with GSTM1 null. We believe this observation reflects the role of GSTM1 in the detoxification of the products of oxidative stress (Strange, 1996). Thus, in the ovary, chronic failure to effectively detoxify the lipid and/or DNA products of the process of repair of the ovarian epithelium may result in damage to genes in the host cell. In some patients the p53 gene is also damaged, resulting in persistent expression of mutant protein. In other patients the oxidative stress causes damage to various genes, not including p53, resulting in overexpression of wild-type p53. These studies complement those showing that GST genotypes influence adduct formation and p53 mutational spectra in other tissues. It is important to emphasize, however, that the apparent protective effect of GST is not universal, as we found no relationship between GSTM1 genotype and p53 overexpression and mutations in ras and gsp in pituitary adenomas (Perrett *et al.*, 1995).

Concluding comments

Studies on the role of detoxifying enzymes such as the GSTs in mediating individual susceptibility to cancer form part of a growing literature on the relevance of allelism in a wide variety of genes on susceptibility to many pathologies. Indeed, given the high frequency of many GST alleles, it is likely that these polymorphisms exert a significant influence on susceptibility. The importance of the GST supergene family is indicated by studies using a variety of experimental approaches. Surprisingly, however, while we can confidently claim that some, if not all, GST genes encode enzymes that exert an important and presumably beneficial effect on cell activity, we can only guess at the true function of the members of this complex supergene family. Furthermore, it needs to be emphasized that the extent of altered risk associated with particular genotypes is generally not large, typically two- to threefold. Clearly, it is necessary to identify which other genes interact with the GSTs so that haplotypes associated with ten- to twentyfold increases in risk can be defined. These considerations form the basis for studies that simultaneously assess the influence of GSTs, cytochrome P450 and N-acetyl transferase polymorphisms on susceptibility. Future studies should take a variety of additional factors, including diet, into consideration, particularly where susceptibility genes in different populations are being compared. Age at diagnosis may also be important, as suggested by studies in patients with colon and breast cancers (Chenevix-Trench *et al.*, 1995; Ambrosone *et al.*, 1995). Gender and other hormonal factors are likely to exert a significant effect on expression (Hayes & Pulford, 1995). It is also worth emphasizing that future work will need to take into account interindividual differences in the level of induction of GST genes. Regulation of the expression of the GST genes is complex with tissue-specific changes having been identified during development (Strange, 1993), in response to physiological changes and after exposure to many drugs and chemicals (e.g. glucocorticoids, barbiturates, phenolic antioxidants) that appear to act via cis-acting elements (Prochaska & Talalay, 1988; Rushmore *et al.*, 1993). In some cases, inducing chemicals result from the catalytic activity of phase 1, cytochrome P450 enzymes, again emphasizing the complexity of unravelling the importance of individual polymorphisms and the need to study induction phenomena as already addressed in the case of CYP1A1 and other cytochrome P450 loci (Kellerman *et al.*, 1973, Nebert 1994).

Acknowledgements
We gratefully acknowledge the support of the Cancer Research Campaign, Medical Research Council, Arthritis and Rheumatism Council, Wellbeing (Royal College of Obstetrics and Gynaecologists) and North Staffordshire Hospital Centre Trust Fund. We also thank our colleague Dr Bill Farrell for much helpful advice.

References
Ahmad, H., Wilson, D.E., Fritz, R.R., Singh, S.V., Medh, R.D., Nagle, G.T., Awasthi, Y.C. & Kurosky, A. (1990) Primary and secondary analyses of glutathione S-transferase P1 from human placenta. *Arch. Biochem. Biophys.*, 287, 398-408

Alexandrie, A.-K, Ingelman Sundberg, M., Seidegard, J., Tornling, G. & Rannug, A. (1995) In: *Proceedings of the International ISSX Workshop on Glutathione S-transferases*. London, Taylor and Francis

Ali-Osman, F., Akande, A. & Mao, J., (1995) Molecular cloning, characterization and expression of novel functionally different human glutathione S-transferase-P-1 gene variant. In: *Proceedings of the International ISSX Workshop on Glutathione S-Transferase*. London,Taylor and Francis, pp.1061-3439

Ambrosone, C.B., Freudenheim, J.L., Graham, S., Marshall, J.R., Vena, J.E., Brasure, J.R., Laughlin, R., Nemoto, T., Michalek, A.M., Harrington, A., Ford, T.D. & Shields, P.G. (1995) Cytochrome P4501A1 and glutathione S-transferase (M1) genetic polymorphisms and postmenopausal breast cancer risk. *Cancer Res.*, 55, 3483-3485

Anttila, S., Luostarinen, L., Hirvonen, A., Elovaara, E., Karjalainen, A., Nurminen, T., Hayes, J.D., Vainio, H. & Ketterer, B. (1995) Pulmonary expression of glutathione S-transferase M3 in lung cancer patients: Association with GSTM1 polymorphism, smoking and asbestos exposure. *Cancer Res.*, 55, 3305-3309

Baez, S., Segura-Aguilar, J., Widersten, M., Johansson, A.-S. & Mannervik, B. (1997) Glutathione transferases catalyse the detoxification of oxidized metabolites (o-quinines) of catecholamines and may serve as an antioxidant system preventing degenerative cellular damage. *Biochem. J.*, 324, 25-28

Bell, D.A., Taylor, J.A., Paulson, D.F., Robertson, C.N., Mohler, J.L. & Lucier, G.W. (1992) Genetic risk and carcinogen exposure: a common inherited defect of the carcinogen-metabolism gene glutathione S-transferase M1 (GSTM1) that increases susceptibility to bladder cancer. *J. Natl Cancer Inst.*, 85, 1159-1164

Berhane, K., Widersten, M., Engstrom, A., Kozarich, J.W. & Mannervik, B. (1994) Detoxification of base propenals and other α, β-unsaturated aldehyde products of radical reactions and lipid peroxidation by human glutathione transferases. *Proc. Natl. Acad. Sci. USA*, 91, 1480-1484

Buetler, T.M. & Eaton, D.L. (1992) Glutathione S-transferases: amino acid sequence comparison, classification and phylogenetic relationship. *Environ. Carcinogenesis Ecotoxicol Rev.*, C10, 181-203.

Board, P.G. (1981) Biochemical genetics of glutathione S-transferase in man. *Am. J. Hum. Genet.*, 33, 36-43

Brockmöller, J., Kerb, R., Drakoulis, N., Staffeldt, B. & Roots, I. (1994) Glutathione S-transferase M1 and its variants A and B as host factors of bladder cancer susceptibility: a case-control study. *Cancer Res.*, 54, 4103-4111.

Campbell, E., Takahashi, Y., Abramovitz, M., Peretz, M. & Listowsky, I. (1990) A distinct human testis and brain class-mu glutathione-s-transferase: molecular cloning and characterization of a form present even in individuals lacking hepatic type-mu isoenzymes. *J. Biol. Chem.*, 265, 9188-9193

Chen, H., Sandler, D.P., Taylor, J.A., Shore, D.L., Liu, E., Bloomfield, C.D. & Bell, D.A. (1996) Increased risk for myelodysplastic syndromes in individuals with glutathione S-transferase theta 1 (GSTT1) gene defect. *Lancet*, 347, 295-297

Chen, L.Z & Board, P.G. (1987) Hgi A1 restriction fragment length polymorphism at the human glutathione S-transferase 2 locus. *Nucleic Acids Res.*, 15, 6306

Chenevix-Trench, G., Young, J., Coggan, M. & Board, P. (1995) Glutathione S-transferase M1 and T1 polymorphisms: susceptibility to colon cancer and age of onset. *Carcinogenesis*, 16, 1655-1657

Comstock, K.E., Sanderson, B.J.S., Claflin, G. & Henner, W.D. (1990) GST1 gene deletion determined by polymerase chain reaction. *Nucleic Acids Res.*, 18, 3670

Crotty B. (1994) Ulcerative colitis and xenobiotic metabolism. *Lancet*, 343, 35-38

Deakin, M., Elder, J., Hendrickse, C., Peckham, D., Baldwin, D., Pantin, C., Wild, N., Leopard, P., Bell, D.A., Jones, P., Duncan, H., Brannigan, K., Alldersea, J., Fryer, A.A. & Strange, R.C. (1996) Glutathione S-transferase GSTT1 genotypes and susceptibility to cancer: studies of interactions with GSTM1 in lung, oral, gastric and colorectal cancers. *Carcinogenesis*, 17, 881-884

DeJong, J.L., Chang, C., Wang-Peng, J., Knutsen, T. & Tu, C.-P.D (1988) The human liver glutathione transferase gene superfamily: expression and chromosome mapping of Hb subunit cDNA. *Nucleic Acids Res.*, 16, 8543-8554

DeJong, J.L., Mohandas, T. & Tu, C.-P.D. (1991) The human Hb (Mu)class glutathione S-transferases are encoded by a dispersed gene family. *Biochem. Biophys. Res. Commun.*, 180, 15-22

Del Boccio, G., Di Ilio, C., Alin, P., Jornvall, H. & Mannervik, B. (1987) Identification of a novel glutathione transferase in human skin homologous with class alpha glutathione transferase 2-2 in the rat. *Biochem. J.*, 244, 21-25

d'Errico, A., Taioli, E., Chen, X. & Vineis, P. (1996) Genetic metabolic polymorphisms and the risk of cancer: a review of the literature. *Biomarkers*, 1, 149-173

Duncan, H., Swan, C., Green, J., Jones, P., Brannigan, K., Alldersea, J., Fryer, A.A. & Strange, R.C. (1995) Susceptibility to ulcerative colitis and Crohn's disease: Interactions between glutathione S-transferase GSTM1 and GSTT1 genotypes. *Clin. Chim. Acta*, 240, 53-61

Eccles, D., Brett, L., Lessels, A., Gruber, L., Lane, D., Steel, C.M. & Leonard, R.C. (1992) Overexpression of the p53 protein and allele loss at 17p13 in ovarian carcinoma. *Br. J. Cancer*, 65, 40-45

Elexpuru-Camiruaga, J., Buxton, N., Kandula, V., Dias, V.S., Campbell, D., McIntosh, J., Broome, J., Jones, P., Inskip, A., Alldersea, J., Fryer, A.A. & Strange, R.C. (1995) Susceptibility to astrocytoma and meningioma: influence of allelism at glutathione S-transferase, GSTT1 and GSTM1 and cytochrome P450, CYP2D6 loci. *Cancer Res.*, 55, 4237-4239

Fryer, A.A., Zhao, L., Alldersea, J., Pearson, W.R. & Strange, R.C. (1993) Use of site-directed mutagenesis of allele-specific PCR primers to identify the GSTM1 A, GSTM1 B, GSTM1 A, B and GSTM1 null polymorphisms at the glutathione S-transferase, GSTM1 locus. *Biochem. J.*, 295, 313-315

Garcia-Closas, M., Kelsey, K.T., Wiencke, J.K. & Christiani, D.C. (1995) Nutrient intake as a modifier of the association between lung cancer and glutathione S-transferase μ deletion. *Proc. Am. Assoc. Cancer Res.*, 36, 281

Goodwin, A.K., Testa, J.R. & Hamilton, T.C. (1993) The biology of ovarian cancer development. *Cancer*, 71, 530-536

Greenblat, M.S., Bennett, W.P., Hollstein, M. & Harris, C.C. (1994) Mutations in the p53 tumour suppressor gene: clues to cancer etiology and molecular pathogenesis. *Cancer Res.*, 54, 4855-4878

Hall, A.G., Autzen, P., Cattan, A.R., Malcolm, A.J., Cole, M., Kernahan, J. & Reid, M.M. (1994) Expression of mu class glutathione S-transferase correlates with event-free survival in childhood acute lymphoblastic leukaemia. *Cancer Res.*, 54, 5251-5254

Hallier, E., Schroder, K.R., Asmuth, K., Dommermuth, A., Aust, B. & Goergens, H.W. (1994) Metabolism of dichloromethane (methylene chloride) to formaldehyde in human erythrocytes: influence of polymorphism of glutathione transferase theta (GST T1-1). *Arch. Toxicol.*, 68, 423-427

Hand, P.A., Inskip, A., Gilford, J., Alldersea, J., Elexpuru-Camiruaga, J., Hayes, J.D., Jones, P.W., Strange, R.C. & Fryer, A.A. (1996) Allelism at the glutathione S-transferase GSTM3 locus: interactions with GSTM1 and GSTT1 as risk factors for astrocytoma. *Carcinogenesis*, 17, 1919-1922

Harada, S., Nakamura, T. & Misawa, S. (1994) Polymorphism of pentanucleotide repeats in the 5' flanking region of the glutathione S-transferase (gst) pi gene. *Hum. Genet.*, 93, 223-224

Harries, L.W., Stubbins, M.J., Forman, D., Howard, G.C.W. & Wolf, C.R. (1997) Identification of genetic polymorphism at the GSTP1 locus and association with susceptibility to bladder, testicular and prostate cancer. *Carcinogenesis*, 18, 641-644

Hayes, J.D. & Pulford, D.J. (1995) The glutathione S-transferase supergene family: regulation of GST and the contribution of the isoenzymes to cancer chemoprotection and drug resistance. *Crit. Rev. Biochem. Mol. Biol.*, 30, 445-600

Hayes, J.D. & Strange, R.C. (1995) Potential contribution of the glutathione S-transferase supergene family to resistance to oxidative stress. *Free Radical Res. Commun.*, 22, 193-207

Heagerty, A.H.M., Fitzgerald, D., Smith, A., Bowers, B., Jones, P., Fryer, A.A., Zhao, L., Alldersea, J. & Strange, R.C. (1994) Glutathione S-transferase GSTM1 phenotypes and protection against cutaneous malignancy. *Lancet*, 343, 266-268

Heagerty, A., Smith, A., English, J., Lear, J., Perkins, W., Bowers, B., Jones, P., Gilford, J., Alldersea, J., Fryer, A.A. & Strange, R.C. (1996) Susceptibility to multiple cutaneous basal cell carcinomas: Significant interactions between glutathione S-transferase GSTM1 genotypes, skin type and male gender. *Br. J. Cancer*, 73, 44-48

Hirvonen, A., Husgafvel-Pursiainen, K., Anttila, S. & Vainio, H. (1993) The GSTM1 null genotype as a potential modifier for squamous cell carcinoma of the lung. *Carcinogenesis*, 14, 1479-1481

Inskip, A., Elexperu-Camiruaga, J., Buxton, N., Dias, P.S., MacIntosh, J., Campbell, D., Jones, P.W., Yengi, L., Talbot, A., Strange, R.C. & Fryer, A.A. (1995) Identification of polymorphism at the glutathione-S-transferase, GSTM3 locus: evidence for linkage with GSTM1*A. *Biochem. J.*, 312, 713-716

Jahnke, V., Matthias, C., Fryer, A.A. & Strange, R.C. (1996) Glutathione S-transferase and cytochrome P-450 polymorphism as risk factors for squamous cell carcinoma of the larynx. *Am. J. Surg.*, 172, 671-673

Kamisaka, K., Habig, W.H., Ketley, J.N., Arias, I.M. & Jakoby, W.B. (1975) Multiple forms of human glutathione S-transferase and their affinity for bilirubin. *Eur. J. Biochem.*, 60, 153-161

Karagas, M.R. (1994) Occurrence of cutaneous basal cell and squamous cell malignancies among those with a prior history of skin cancer. *J. Invest. Dermatol.*, 102, 10S-13S

Kato, S., Bowman, E.D., Harrington, A.M., Blomeke, B. & Shields, P.G. (1995) Human lung carcinogen-DNA adduct levels mediated by genetic polymorphisms *in vivo*. *J. Natl. Cancer Inst.*, 87, 902-907

Kellerman, G., Shaw, C.R. & Luyten-Kellerman, M. (1973) Aryl hydrocarbon hydroxylase inducibility and bronchogenic carcinoma. *N. Engl. J. Med.*, 289, 934-937

Kerb, R., Brockmöller, J., Cascorbi, I. & Roots, I. (1995) Glutathione S-transferase of class mu and theta as modulators of lung cancer susceptibility. In: *Proceedings of the International ISSX Workshop on Glutathione S-transferases*. London, Taylor Francis

Ketterer, B., Taylor, J., Meyer, D., Pemble, S., Coles, B., ChuLin, X. & Spencer, S. (1993) Some functions of glutathione transferases. In: Tew, K.,

Mannervik, B., Mantle, T.J., Pickett, C.B. & Hayes, J.D., eds, *Structure and Function of Glutathione Transferases*. Boca Raton, Florida; CRC Press; pp.15-27

Kumar, A., Das, B.C. & Shorma, J.K. (1994) Bam H1 restriction fragment length polymorphism (RFLP) at the human gst3 gene locus. *Hum. Genet.*, 94, 107-108

Lafuente, A., Pujol, F., Carretero, P., Perez Villa, J. & Cuchi, A. (1993) Human glutathione S-transferase mu (GSTmu) deficiency as a marker for susceptibility to bladder and larynx cancer among smokers. *Cancer Lett.*, 68, 49-54

Lear, J.T., Heagerty, A.H.M., Smith, A., Bowers, B., Payne, C.R., Smith, C.A.D., Jones, P.W., Gilford, J., Yengi, L., Alldersea, J., Fryer, A.A. & Strange, R.C. (1996) Multiple cutaneous basal cell carcinomas: glutathione S-transferase (GSTM1, GSTT1) and cytochrome P450 (CYP2D6, CYP1A1) polymorphisms influence tumour numbers and accrual. *Carcinogenesis*, 17, 1891-1896

Lin, H.J., Han, C.Y., Bernstein, D.A., Hsiao, W., Lin, B.K. & Hardy, S. (1994) Ethnic distribution of the glutathione S-transferase mu 1-1 (GSTM1) null genotype in 1473 individuals and application to bladder cancer susceptibility. *Carcinogenesis*, 15, 1077-1081

Mannervik, B. & Widersten, M. (1995) Human glutathione S-transferases: classification, tissue distribution, structure, and functional properties. In: *Advances in Man in Drug Metabolism*. Luxembourg, European Commission.

McWilliams, J.E., Sanderson, B.J.S., Harris, E.L., Richert-Boe, K.E. & Henner, W.D. (1995) Glutathione S-transferase M1 deficiency is associated with a moderate increase in risk of developing lung cancer. *Proc. Am. Assoc. Cancer Res.*, 36, 121

Mukhtar, H. & Elmets, C.A. (1996) Photocarcinogenesis: mechanisms, models and human health implications. *Photochem. Photobiol.*, 63, 356-357

Nakachi, K., Imai, K., Hayashi, S. & Kawajiri, K. (1993) Polymorphisms of the CYP1A1 and glutathione S-transferase genes associated with susceptibility to lung cancer in relation to cigarette dose in a Japanese population. *Cancer Res.*, 53, 2994-2999

Nakajima, T., Elovaara, E., Anttila, S., Hirvonen, A., Camus, A.-M., Hayes, J.D., Ketterer, B. & Vainio, H. (1995) Expression and polymorphism of glutathione S-transferase in human lungs: risk factors in smoking-related lung cancer. *Carcinogenesis*, 16, 707-711

Nazar-Stewart, V., Motulsky, A.G., Eaton, D.L., White, E., Hornung, S.K., Leng, Z.-T., Stapleton, P. & Weiss, N.S. (1993) The glutathione S-transferase μ polymorphism as a marker for susceptibility to lung carcinoma. *Cancer Res.*, 53, 2313-2318

Nebert, D.W. (1994) Drug-metabolizing enzymes in ligand-modulated transcription. *Biochem. Pharmacol.*, 47, 25-37

Nelson, H.H., Wiencke, J.K., Christiani, D.C., Cheng, T.J., Zuo, Z.F., Schwartz, B.S., Lee, B.K., Spitz, M.R., Wang, M. & Xu, X. (1995) Ethnic differences in the prevalence of the homozygous deleted genotype of glutathione S-transferase theta. *Carcinogenesis*, 16, 1243-1245

Norppa, H., Hirvonen, A., Jarventaus, H., Uukula, M., Tasa, G., Ojajarvi, A. & Sorsa, M. (1995) Role of GSTT1 and GSTM1 genotypes in determining individual sensitivity to sister chromatid exchange induction by diepoxybutane in cultured human lymphocytes. *Carcinogenesis*, 16, 1261-1264

Ollier, W., Davies, E., Snowden, N., Alldersea, J., Fryer, A.A., Jones, P. & Strange, R.C. (1996) Association of homozygosity for glutathione S-transferase GSTM1 null alleles with the Ro+/La-autoantibody profile in patients with systemic lupus erythematosus. *Arthritis Rheum.*, 39, 1763-1764

Pearson, W.R., Vorachek, W., Xu, S., Berger, R., Hart, I., Vannais, D. & Patterson, D. (1993) Identification of class-mu glutathione S-transferase genes GSTM1-GSTM5 on chromosome 1p13. *Am. J. Hum. Genet.*, 53, 220-233

Pemble, S., Schroeder, K.R., Spencer, S.R., Meyer, D.J., Hallier, E., Bolt, H.M., Ketterer, B. & Taylor, J.B. (1994) Human glutathione S-transferase theta (GSTT1): cDNA cloning and the characterization of a genetic polymorphism. *Biochem. J.*, 300, 271-276

Perera, F.P. (1996) Molecular epidemiology: insights into cancer susceptibility, risk assessment, and prevention. *J. Natl. Cancer Inst.*, 88, 496-509

Perrett, C.W., Clayton, R.N., Pistorello, M., Boscaro, M., Scanarini, M., Bates, A., Buckley, N., Jones, P., Fryer, A.A., Gilford, J., Alldersea, J. & Strange, R.C. (1995) GSTM1 and CYP2D6 genotype frequencies in patients with pituitary tumours: effects on p53, ras and gsp. *Carcinogenesis*, 16, 1643-1645

Prochaska, H.J. & Talalay, P. (1988) Regulatory mechanisms of monofunctional and bifunctional anticarcinogenic enzyme inducers in murine liver. *Cancer Res.*, 48, 4776-4782

Ross, V.L. & Board, P.G. (1993) Molecular cloning an heterologous expression of an alternatively spliced human mu class glutathione S-transferase transcript. *Biochem. J.*, 294, 373-380

Ross, V.L., Board, P.G. & Webb, G.C. (1993) Chromosomal mapping of the human mu class glutathione S-transferases to 1p13. *Genomics*, 18, 87-91

Rushmore, T.H., Nguyen, T. & Pickett, C.B. (1993) ARE and XRE mediated induction of glutathione S-transferase Ya subunit gene. In: Tew, K.D., Pickett, C.B., Mantle, T.J., Mannervik, B. & Hayes, J.D., eds, *Structure and Function of Glutathione Transferases*. Boca Raton, Florida; CRC Press; pp.119-128

Ryberg, D., Kure, E., Lystad, S., Skaug, V., Stangeland, L., Mercy, I., Børresen, A.-L. & Haugen, A. (1994) p53 mutations in lung tumours: relationship to putative susceptibility markers for cancer. *Cancer Res.*, 54, 1551-1555

Sarhanis, P., Redman, C., Perrett, C., Brannigan, K., Clayton, R.N., Hand, P., Musgrove, C., Suarez, V., Jones, P, Fryer, A.A., Farrell, W.E. & Strange, R.C. (1996) Epithelial ovarian cancer: influence of polymorphism at the glutathione S-transferase GSTM1 and GSTT1 loci on p53 expression. *Br. J. Cancer*, 74, 1757-1761

Schmieder, G.J., Yoshikawa, T., Mata, S.M., Streilein, J.W. & Taylor, J.R. (1992) Cumulative sunlight exposure and the risk of developing skin cancer in Florida. *J. Dermatol. Surg. Oncol.*, 18, 517-522

Schroeder, K.R., Hallier, E., Meyer, D.J., Wibel, F.A., Muller, A.M.F. & Bolt, H.M. (1996) Purification and characterization of a new glutathione S-transferase class theta form from human erythrocytes. *Arch. Toxicol.*, 70, 559-566

Schroeder, K.R., Wibel, F.A., Reich, S., Dannappel, D., Bolt, H.M. & Hallier, E. (1995) Glutathione S-transferase (GST) theta polymorphism influences background SCE rate. *Arch. Toxicol.*, 69, 505-507

Seidegard, J., Pero, R.W., Markowitz, M.M., Roush, G., Miller, D.G. & Beattie, E.J. (1990) Isoenzyme(s) of glutathione transferase (class mu) as a marker for the susceptibility to lung cancer: a follow-up study. *Carcinogenesis*, 11, 33-36

Seidegard, J., Vorachek, W.R., Pero, R.W. & Pearson, W.R. (1988) Hereditary differences in the expression of the human glutathione S-transferase activity on trans-stilbene oxide are due to a gene deletion. *Proc. Natl. Acad. Sci. USA*, 85, 7293-7297

Singhal, S.S., Zimniak, P., Awasthi, S., Piper, J.T., He, N., Teng, J.I., Petersen, D.R. & Awasthi, Y.C. (1994) Several closely related glutathione S-transferase isoenzymes catalysing conjugation of 4-hydroxynonenal are differentially expressed in human tissues. *Arch. Biochem. Biophys.*, 311, 242-250

Smith, G., Stanley, L.A., Sim, E., Strange, R.C. & Wolf, C.R. (1995) Metabolic polymorphisms and cancer susceptibility. *Cancer Surveys*, 25, 27-67

Sofaer, J. (1993) Crohn's disease: the genetic contribution. *Gut*, 34, 869-871

Strange, R.C. (1993) The glutathione S-transferase GSTM1 locus and cancer susceptibility, In: Tew, K., Mannervik, B., Mantle, T.J., Pickett, C.B. & Hayes, J.D., eds, *Structure and Function of Glutathione Transferases*. Boca Raton, Florida; CRC Press; pp.160-171

Strange, R.C. (1996) Glutathione S-transferases and cancer susceptibility. In: Vermeulen, N.P.E., Mulder,G.J., Nieuwenhuyse,H., Peters,W.H.M. & van Bladeren, P.J., eds, *Glutathione S-transferases: Structure, Function and Clinical Implications*. London, Taylor and Francis, pp. 239-248

Strange, R.C., Faulder, C.G., Davis, B.A., Brown, J.A.H., Hopkinson, D.A. & Cotton, W. (1984a) The human glutathione S-transferases: studies on the distribution of the GST1, GST2 and GST3 isoenzymes. *Biochem. Soc. Trans.*, 12, 285-286

Strange, R.C., Faulder, C.G., Davis, B.A., Brown, J.A.H., Hopkinson, D.A. & Cotton, W. (1984b) The human glutathione S-transferases: studies on the tissue distribution and genetic variation of the GST1, GST2 and GST3 isoenzymes. *Ann Hum. Genet.*, 48, 11-20

Strange, R.C., Fryer, A.A., Matharoo, B., Zhao, L., Broome, J., Campbell, D., Jones, P., Cervello-Pastor, I. & Singh.R. (1992) The glutathione S-transferases: comparison of isoenzyme expression in normal and astrocytoma brain. *Biochim. Biophys. Acta*, 1139, 222-228

Strange, R.C., Matharoo, B., Faulder, G.C., Jones, P., Cotton, W., Elder, J.B. & Deakin, M. (1991) The human glutathione S-transferases: a case-control study of the incidence of the GST1 0 phenotype in patients with adenocarcinoma. *Carcinogenesis*, 12, 25-28

Suzuki, T., Coggan, M., Shaw, D.C. & Board, P. (1987) Electrophoretic and immunological analysis of human glutathione S-transferase isozymes. *Ann Hum. Genet.*, 51, 95-106

Suzuki, T., Johnston, P.N. & Board, P.G. (1993) Structure and organization of the human alpha class glutathione S-transferase genes and related pseudogenes. *Genomics*, 18, 680-686

Szarka, C.E., Pfeiffer, G.R., Hum, S.T., Everley, L.C., Balshem, A.M., Moore, D.F., Litwin, S., Goosenberg, E.B., Frucht, H., Engstrom, P.F. & Clapper, M.L. (1995) Glutathione S-transferase activity and glutathione S-transferase mu expression in subjects with risk for colorectal cancer. *Cancer Res.*, 55, 2789-2793

Taylor, J.B., Oliver, J., Sherrington, R. & Pemble, S.E. (1991) Structure of human glutathione S-transferase class mu genes. *Biochem. J.*, 274, 587-593

Tew, K.D. (1994) Glutathione-associated enzymes in anticancer drug resistance. *Cancer Res.*, 54, 4313-4320

Warwick, A.P, , Sarhanis, P., Redman, C.W.E., Pemble, S., Taylor, J., Ketterer, B., Jones, P., Alldersea, J., Gilford, J., Yengi, L., Fryer, A.A. & Strange, R.C. (1994) Theta class glutathione S-transferase GSTT1 genotypes and susceptibility to cervical neoplasia: interactions with GSTM1, CYP2D6 and smoking. *Carcinogenesis*, 15, 2841-2845

Wiencke, J.K., Kelsey, K.T., Lamela, R.A. & Toscano Jr, W.A. (1990) Human glutathione S-transferase deficiency as a marker of susceptibility to epoxide-induced cytogenetic damage. *Cancer Res.*, 50, 1585-1590

Yengi, L., Inskip, A., Gilford, J., Alldersea, J., Bailey, L., Smith, A., Lear, J.T., Heagerty, A.H.M., Bowers, B., Hand, P., Hayes, J.D., Jones, P.W., Strange, R.C. & Fryer A.A. (1996) Polymorphism at the glutathione S-transferase GSTM3 locus: interactions with cytochrome P450 and glutathione S-transferase genotypes as risk factors for multiple basal cell carcinoma. *Cancer Res.*, 56, 1974-1977

Zhao, L., Alldersea, J., Fryer, A.A., Tighe, A., Ollier, B., Thomson, W., Jones, P. & Strange, R.C. (1994) Polymorphism at the glutathione S-transferase

GSTM1 locus: a study of the frequencies of the GSTM1 A, B, A/B and null phenotypes in Nigerians. *Clin. Chim. Acta*, 225, 85-88

Zhong, S., Howie, A.F., Ketterer, B., Taylor, J.B., Hayes, J.D., Beckett, G.J., Wathen, C.G., Wolf, C.R. & Spurr, N.K. (1991) Glutathione S-transferase mu locus: use of genotyping and phenotyping assays to assess association with lung cancer susceptibility. *Carcinogenesis*, 12, 1533-1537

Zhong, S., Wolf, C.R. & Spurr, N.K. (1993) Chromosomal assignment and linkage analysis of the human glutathione S-transferase mu gene (GSTM1) using intron specific polymerase chain reaction. *Hum. Genet.*, 90, 435-439

Zhong, S., Wyllie, A.H., Barnes, D., Wolf, C.R. & Spurr, N.K. (1994) Relationship between GSTM1 genetic polymorphism and susceptibility to bladder, breast and colon cancer. *Carcinogenesis*, 14, 1821-1824

Zimniak, P., Nanduri, B., Pikula, S., Bandorowiez-Pikula, J., Singhal, S.S., Srivastava, S.K., Awasthi, S. & Awasthi, Y.C. (1994) Naturally-occurring human glutathione S-transferase GSTP1-1 isoforms with isoleucine and valine in position 104 differ in enzymatic properties. *Eur. J. Biochem.*, 244, 893-899

Corresponding author
R.C. Strange
Clinical Biochemistry Research Group,
School of Postgraduate Medicine,
Keele University,
North Staffordshire Hospital,
Stoke-on-Trent, Staffordshire, ST4 7QB,
United Kingdom

Metabolic Polymorphisms and Susceptibility to Cancer
W. Ryder
IARC Scientific Publications No. 148
International Agency for Research on Cancer, Lyon, 1999

Chapter 20. Polymorphic NATs and cancer predisposition

A. Hirvonen

The acetylation polymorphism, discovered 40 years ago, holds a special place as one of the first described examples of a pharmacogenetic defect affecting xenobiotic biotransformation capacity in human populations. The genetically determined N-acetyltransferase activity is involved in activation/inactivation reactions of numerous xenobiotics. Therefore, it has been suggested that slow acetylator status may modify the individual responses to various chemicals. In humans, two genes, *NAT1* and *NAT2*, are responsible for N-acetyltransferase activity. To date several allelic variants of both *NAT1* and *NAT2* have been detected, and it has been suggested that some of them modify individual susceptibility to cancer. Slow NAT2 acetylation capacity has been suggested as conferring increased risk of bladder, breast, liver and lung cancers, and decreased risk of colon cancer, whereas a prominent change in the *NAT1* gene, putatively associated with increased NAT1 activity, has been suggested as increasing the risk of bladder and colon cancer and decreasing that of lung cancer. While three of the NAT2 variants have been shown to account for most of the slow *NAT2* acetylator genotypes in Caucasians, less complete data are available on how the *NAT1* variants modify NAT1 activity *in vivo*. This review discusses present knowledge on NAT polymorphisms, particularly in relation to individual cancer predisposition.

Functions and substrates for N-acetyltransferases

The N-acetylation polymorphism causes interindividual variations in biotransformation of various xenobiotics with a primary aromatic amine or a hydrazine structure (Evans, 1992; Hein et al., 1993). NAT2 (Blum et al., 1990), which was until recently thought to be the only polymorphic NAT, is responsible for the well-known inherited interindividual variation in the ability to acetylate substrates such as the arylamine drugs procainamide and sulphamethazine, the arylamine carcinogen benzidine, and some hydrazine drugs such as isoniazid and hydralazine (Evans, 1992; Hein et al., 1993). Initially, individual acetylator status was determined with isoniazid or sulfamethazine as a test substrate mirroring the NAT2-related acetylation capacity (Evans & White, 1964). Subsequently, Grant et al. (1984) introduced the now well established (Butler et al., 1992; Fuhr et al., 1996) and broadly used caffeine test. Caffeine is an innocuous, well-tolerated *in vivo* substrate, and the ratio of its secondary metabolites, 5-acetylamino-6-formylamino-3-methyluracil (AFMU) and 1-methylxanthine (1X) in urine, also specifically reveal the NAT2 acetylation capacity. Using the above test substrates, the NAT2 slow acetylator frequency has been shown to range worldwide from about 10% to more than 90% (Kadlubar et al., 1992). Recently, another human N-acetyltransferase, NAT1 (Blum et al., 1990), which is widely expressed in tissues (Hearse & Weber, 1973) and cultured cells (Coroneos et al., 1992), has also been found to be polymorphic (Vatsis & Weber, 1993). The substrate specificity of NAT1 is distinct from that of NAT2: NAT1 preferentially metabolizes 4-aminobenzoic acid and 4-aminosalicylic acid.

The NATs are involved in the metabolism of numerous carcinogens, such as acetoxy esters, arylamines, heterocyclic amines (mostly the N-hydroxy derivatives) and 4-aminobiphenyl (Hein et al., 1993; Probst et al., 1992; Kadlubar et al., 1992; Vineis et al., 1994). NAT2 polymorphically acetylates arylamines, including well-known bladder carcinogens, to arylamides (Hearse & Weber, 1973). N-acetyltransferase competes with

N-hydroxylation, which transforms arylamines into active carcinogens.

Molecular and biochemical characterization of the NAT polymorphisms

The acetylation polymorphism was discovered during the 1950s through the observation of interindividual variability in the metabolism of isoniazid (Evans, 1989). The first biochemical investigations established that impaired elimination of isoniazid, observed in more than 50% of Caucasians, was due to a reduction in the rate at which it was enzymatically N-acetylated in the liver (Evans & White, 1964). By the administration of this drug and the measure of ratios of acetylated to non-acetylated metabolites, researchers were able to classify subjects as rapid and slow acetylators. This reaction, now known to be mediated by the cytosolic NAT2 enzyme, involves transfer of acetate from acetyl coenzyme A (CoASAc) to primary aromatic amine and hydrazine functional groups to yield acetamides and hydrazides. Subsequent *in vivo* and *in vitro* studies have shown that the disposition of a variety of arylamine and hydrazine drugs and xenobiotics is affected by the same genetic defect (Evans, 1989; Evans 1992; Hein *et al.*, 1993).

However, any model for aromatic amine acetylation in man must also take into account the existence of two apparently distinct classes of substrates for acetylation. The first class, the so-called 'polymorphic' substrates (such as isoniazid, sulfamethazine and procainamide), display patterns of elimination which correlate with the classically defined acetylator phenotype, and can indeed be used as metabolic probes for phenotype determination. The second class, the so-called 'monomorphic' substrates (such as p-aminobenzoic acid and p-aminosalicylic acid), are highly acetylated both *in vivo* and *in vitro*, and yet these acetylation rates were until recently thought to be completely independent of the acetylator phenotype.

On the basis of immunochemical studies in the rabbit model for the human acetylation polymorphism (Patterson *et al.*, 1980) it had been assumed that: (1) the same isozyme of NAT was responsible for acetylating both monomorphic and polymorphic substrates; (2) slow acetylation in humans was likely to involve a qualitative

rather than a quantitative difference in the NAT protein responsible for mediating the enzymatic reaction. In order to investigate these possibilities more directly, strategies were developed to undertake the cloning and characterization of genes encoding human NAT enzyme(s). Using cytosolic fractions from human liver as a starting material, a series of chromatographic and electrophoretic procedures enabled partial purification of a protein capable of N-acetylating the polymorphic substrate sulfamethazine (Grant *et al.*, 1989). This protein was used for the development of a specific polyclonal antiserum and for sequence determination of selected tryptic peptides, allowing verification of the identity of the protein as a human NAT based on amino acid homology with peptide sequences derived from purified rabbit NAT (Andres *et al.*, 1987). The antiserum was used in *in vivo/in vitro* correlation studies to demonstrate that livers from individuals of the slow acetylator phenotype contained markedly reduced, but still detectable, levels of immunoreactive NAT protein (Grant *et al.*, 1990a), suggesting a quantitative rather than a qualitative difference in the enzyme between rapid and slow acetylators.

Meanwhile, Andres *et al.* (1987) used purified rabbit NAT obtained by means of the published purification scheme to obtain a polyclonal serum recognizing the rabbit enzyme, and synthesized a degenerate oligonucleotide probe derived from the rabbit NAT partial amino acid sequence. The combination of these reagents enabled the cloning of a cDNA encoding a rabbit NAT (Blum *et al.*, 1989a), and made it possible to show that the genetic defect in slow acetylators of this enzyme resulted from deletion of the entire gene encoding the enzyme, completely preventing its expression (Blum *et al.*, 1989b). In the course of investigations originally designed to characterize the pineal gland serotonin N-acetyltransferase a similar approach was used to clone a cDNA for rabbit NAT and to verify the observations with respect to the mechanism for the rabbit acetylation polymorphism (Sasaki *et al.*, 1991).

With these rabbit cDNA probes, orthologous NAT genes were cloned from genomic DNA of heterozygously rapid acetylator humans (Blum *et al.*, 1990) and cDNAs corresponding to their expressed transcripts (Oshako & Deguchi, 1990).

In humans, three NAT gene loci were shown to exist, one of which (*NATP*) contains multiple premature termination codons and is thus expected to be a non-expressed pseudogene. The two expressed genes, *NAT1* and *NAT2*, are both located on chromosome 8 (pter-q11) but are separated by at least 25 kb. The 870 bp intronless protein coding regions of *NAT1* and *NAT2* share 87% nucleotide sequence identity and encode 290 amino acid proteins which are 81% identical. The transcript for *NAT1* is encoded in a single exon, while that for *NAT2* arises from a 5' non-coding exon containing the coding and 3' regions (Ebisawa & Deguchi, 1991). The cloned genomic segments (Blum *et al.*, 1990) and the cDNAs (Oshako & Deguchi, 1990) may each be expressed in transient mammalian cell culture to yield fully functional enzyme proteins with the capacity to *N*-acetylate a variety of aromatic substrates.

Indeed, the results of such expression studies provided the first evidence that human acetylation polymorphism is regulated at the *NAT2* gene locus. The expressed product of the *NAT2* gene displays electrophoretic and kinetic properties (Blum *et al.*, 1990; Oshako & Deguchi, 1990; Grant *et al.*, 1991) that are very similar to those of the two human liver NAT2 isoforms whose content is markedly reduced in phenotypically slow acetylators (Grant *et al.*, 1990a). NAT2 shows kinetic sensitivity for polymorphic substrates whose disposition is affected by acetylator phenotype in human populations; reduction in the quantity of NAT2 in livers of slow acetylators thus impairs the elimination of such compounds from the body.

The involvement of the *NAT2* gene locus in the human acetylation polymorphism has subsequently been established unequivocally by the discovery and characterization of variant *NAT2* alleles whose presence is correlated with the acetylator phenotype, determined using isoniazid, sulfamethazine or caffeine as metabolic probes (Deguchi *et al.*, 1990; Oshako & Deguchi, 1990; Blum *et al.*, 1991; Hickman & Sim, 1991; Vatsis *et al.*, 1991). Southern analyses of human genomic DNA isolated from phenotypically rapid and slow acetylators had suggested early on that major genetic alterations, i.e., gene deletion, as observed in slow acetylator rabbits, were unlikely to account for a significant portion of the observed mutations in human populations. Thus, although at the protein level the human acetylation polymorphism resembles that in the rabbit, the underlying genetic basis is different in the two species. In addition, NAT2 protein is completely absent in livers from slow acetylator rabbits, while in the majority of slow acetylator humans a residual NAT2 enzyme activity can still be detected (Grant *et al.*, 1990a).

NAT1, on the other hand, is also expressed in human liver but selectively metabolizes monomorphic substrates whose disposition was thought to be unaffected by acetylator phenotype (Grant *et al.*, 1991). The product of the *NAT1* gene shows kinetic selectivity of compounds, such as *p*-aminosalicylic acid, whose predisposition is unrelated to the classically defined acetylation polymorphism governed by the *NAT2* gene locus. Indeed, both *in vitro* (Cribb *et al.*, 1991; Grant *et al.*, 1991; Grant *et al.*, 1992a) and *in vivo* (Grant *et al.*, 1992b) studies have demonstrated that the expression of *NAT1* is independent of *NAT2* expression. However, it would appear from the studies cited above that *NAT1* expression may also be highly variable in human populations. Preliminary work on developing a new *in vivo* test for variations in NAT1 function in humans (Grant *et al.*, 1992b) suggested that NAT1 activity is not normally distributed in a healthy population and that variant alleles at the *NAT1* gene locus can indeed be detected.

These findings may be of great clinical and toxicological importance, since certain chemicals may be *N*-acetylated to a significant degree by both NAT1 and NAT2. These include the carcinogenic aromatic amines 2-aminofluorene, benzidine, 4-aminophenyl, 4,4-dichloroaniline and 2-naphthylamine (Grant *et al.*, 1991; Grant *et al.*, 1992b; Hein *et al.*, 1992a,b; Lakshmi *et al.*, 1995; Zenser *et al.*, 1996) and the investigational cancer chemotherapeutic agent dinaline (4-amino-*N*-[2'-aminophenyl] benzamide) (Grant *et al.*, 1990b). It is therefore conceivable that concurrent variations in *NAT1* and *NAT2* may be independent contributing factors for predisposition to chemical-induced toxities. It is most important to clearly delineate not only such patterns of variation in NAT1 and NAT2 activity in human populations but also to more precisely define the catalytic specificities of these two enzymes for various aromatic amine substrates. The recent development of simple systems for the high-level expression of recombinant human NAT1 and NAT2 in *E. coli* (Dupret & Grant, 1992a) will undoubtedly be of value in such structure-function studies of the human *N*-acetyltransferase. This system has already been used in site-directed mutagenesis experiments to identify Cys[68] of NAT2 as the amino acid residue whose sulfhydryl group directly participates in the acetyl transfer reaction (Dupret & Grant, 1992a), and for the construction of NAT1/NAT2 protein chimeras to aid in mapping the regions of these enzymes which impart their distinct substrate selectivities (Dupret & Grant, 1992b; Dupret *et al.*, 1994).

Phenotype and genotype tests
Phenotype and genotype correlation and factors that induce or modify enzyme activity
As stated above, NAT1 and NAT2 are encoded at two distinct loci on chromosome 8p21.3-23.1 along with *NATP*, a pseudogene that does not encode a functional protein (Grant *et al.*, 1997). The new nomenclature of *NAT1* and *NAT2* alleles used subsequently in the present article is based on the consolidated classification system of Vatsis *et al.* (1995).

Seven *NAT1* alleles in human populations have been reported in the literature (Table 1) (Grant *et al.*, 1997). The *NAT1*4* allele is denoted as the wild type. A prominent change in one of the variants (*NAT1*10*), which possesses an alteration of the consensus polyadenylation signal (Vatsis & Weber, 1993), was recently associated with both higher NAT1 activity in bladder and colon tissue and DNA adduct levels in the colon tissues (Bell *et al.*, 1995a; Badavi *et al.*, 1995). Given that *NAT1* has been reported to be primarily responsible for the NAT activity in the human uroepithelium (Fredrickson *et al.*, 1994), these findings are of special interest in studies on the potential role of metabolic genotypes in individual bladder cancer risk.

Table 1. Variant alleles at the human *NAT1* gene locus[a]

Allele	Nucleotide change[b]											Amino acid change	Consequence	
	-344	-40	445	459	559	560	640	1075	1088	1091	1095		*In vitro*	*In vivo*
NAT1*4	C	A	G	G	C	G	T	*	T		C			Wild type
NAT1*3											A	None		Unknown
NAT1*5					Many							Many		Unknown
NAT1*10									A		A	None		↑NAT1?
NAT1*11	T	T	***A***	A			G	Δ9			A	Val^{149}Ile	↑V_{max}	↑NAT1
NAT1*14						***A***			A		A	Arg^{187}Gln	↓affinity	↓NAT1
NAT1*15						***T***						Arg^{187}Stop	no NAT1	↓NAT1
NAT1*16										+[AAA]	A	None		Unknown

[a] Adapted from Vatsis *et al.* (1994, 1995), Deitz *et al.* (1997), Doll *et al.* (1997), Grant *et al.* (1997), and Hughes *et al.* (1997).

[b] Only changes from the wild-type (*NAT1*4*) sequence (top line) are indicated. Nucleotide substitutions shown in bold italics change the amino acid indicated and have a functional consequence, those in regular italics change an amino acid with no or unknown effect on NAT1 function, and those in regular font are silent. The asterisk at position 1075 represents a trinucleotide repeat, 9 nucleotides of which are deleted in the *NAT1*11* allele.

The association between the *NAT1*10* allele and NAT1 activity *in vivo* has not been confirmed in subsequent studies. This may at least partly be explained by previous misclassifications of a recently described *NAT1*14* allele having $C^{560}A$ base substitution ($Arg^{187}Gln$), in combination with the $T^{1088}A$ and $C^{1095}A$ substitutions present in the *NAT1*10* allele (Table 1). This allele produces a defective NAT1 protein, leading to functional impairment in the metabolism of NAT1 selective substrates both *in vitro* and *in vivo* (Grant *et al.*, 1997). In *NAT1*3* allele only the latter substitution is present in comparison to the wild type

*NAT1*4* allele, whereas in the *NAT1*11* allele, $C^{-344}T$, $A^{-40}T$, $G^{459}A$ (no amino acid change), $T^{640}G$ ($Ser^{214}Ala$) and a 9 bp deletion between nucleotides 1065-1095 are found in addition. It was recently suggested that an allele *NAT1*17* differed from *NAT1*11* in that it also had $G^{445}A$ substitution ($Val^{149}Ile$). Subsequently, however, it has been agreed that *NAT1*11* also contains this substitution, and the *NAT1*17* designation will be used for some future new alleles (see Deitz *et al.*, 1997). Consequently, the previous finding that the $G^{445}A$ substitution ($Val^{149}Ile$) correlates with increased *N*-acetylation activity (Doll *et al.*, 1997)

Table 2. Variant alleles at the human *NAT2* gene locus[a]

Allele	Phenotype	Nucleotide change[b]							Amino acid change	Consequence	
		191	282	341	481	590	803	857		*In vitro*	*In vivo*
*NAT2*4*	Rapid	G	C	T	C	G	A	G		Wild type	
*NAT2*5A*	Slow			C	T				Ile^{114}Thr	↓V_{max}	↓NAT2
*NAT2*5B*	Slow			C	T		G		Lys^{268}Arg		
*NAT2*5C*	Slow			C			G				
*NAT2*6A*	Slow		T			A			Arg^{197}Gln	↓stability	↓NAT2
*NAT2*6B*	Slow					A					
*NAT2*7A*	Slow							A	Gly^{286}Glu	↓stability	↓NAT2
*NAT2*7B*	Slow		T					A		↑affinity	
*NAT2*12A*	Rapid						G		Lys^{268}Arg	None	None
*NAT2*12B*	Rapid		T				G				
*NAT1*13*	Rapid		T								
*NAT2*14A*	Slow	A							Arg^{64}Gln	↓stability	↓NAT2
*NAT2*14B*	Slow	A	T								
*NAT2*17*	Unknown				$A^{434}C$				Gln^{145}Pro	Unknown	Unknown
*NAT2*18*	Unknown							$A^{845}C$	Lys^{282}Thr	Unknown	Unknown

[a] Adapted from Vatsis *et al.* (1995) and Grant *et al.* (1997).

[b] Only changes from the wild-type (*NAT2*4*) sequence (top line) are indicated. Nucleotide substitutions shown in bold italics change the amino acid indicated and have a functional consequence, those in regular italics change an amino acid with no or unknown effect on NAT2 function, and those in regular font are silent. Thus substitutions at positions 191, 341, 590 and 857 are diagnostic for defective NAT2 function and hence for the slow acetylator phenotype.

is now expected to apply to the *NAT1*11* allele. In the *NAT1*15* allele, $C^{559}T$ substitution ($Arg^{187}Stop$) results in truncated protein and a total loss of NAT1 activity. In the *NAT1*5* allele many nucleotide substitutions are observed together with the $C^{1095}A$ substitution, whereas in the *NAT1*16* allele a three base-pair insertion between nucleotides 1086 and 1095 (resulting in no amino acid changes) is found in addition. The functional repercussions of these *NAT1* variants remain to be determined (Grant *et al.*, 1997).

As for the *NAT2*, in addition to the wild type allele *NAT2*4*, at least 23 different *NAT2* mutations have been found to date (Blum *et al.*, 1990; Oshako & Deguchi, 1990; Vatsis *et al.*, 1991; Bell *et al.*, 1993; Grant, 1993; Lin *et al.*, 1993; Ferguson *et al.*, 1994; Hein *et al.*, 1994; Lin *et al.*, 1994; Vatsis *et al.*, 1995). Seven of the nucleotide transitions (Table 2) (Grant *et al.*, 1997) lead to amino acid changes: $G^{191}A$ ($Arg^{64}Glu$) substitution in the *NAT2*14A* and *14B* alleles (detected particularly in people of African-American origin); $T^{341}C$ ($Ile^{114}Thr$) substitution in the *NAT2*5A*, *5B*, and *5C* alleles; $A^{434}C$ ($Gln^{145}Pro$) substitution in the *NAT2*17* allele; $G^{590}A$ ($Arg^{197}Gln$) substitution in the *NAT2*6A* and *6B* alleles; $A^{803}G$ ($Lys^{268}Arg$) substitution in the *NAT2*5B*, *5C*, *12A*, and *12B* alleles; $A^{845}C$ ($Lys^{282}Thr$) substitution in the *NAT2*18* allele; and $G^{857}A$ (Gly^{286} to Glu) substitution in the *NAT2*7A* and *7B* alleles. The remaining two C-to-T base substitutions in nt 282 in the alleles *NAT2*6A*, *7B*, *13* and *14B*, and in nt 481 in the alleles *NAT2*5A* and *5B*, exert no influence on the amino acid sequence.

Several reported allelic variants of *NAT2* result from certain combinations of the nine base substitutions listed above. Most of the variant alleles are known to show low acetylation capacity; the amino acid changes in NAT2 encoded by *NAT2*12A*, *12B*, and *13* alleles do not interfere with acetylation capacity, whereas the phenotypic consequences of the amino acid changes in NAT2 encoded by *NAT2*17* and *18* alleles are still unknown. Rapid acetylators have at least one wild-type *NAT2*4* allele, whereas slow acetylators have inherited two alleles associated with slow acetylation.

The *NAT2*5* alleles were not originally detected by RFLP analysis in a Japanese population (Deguchi *et al.*, 1990) but have more recently been observed in Chinese subjects; it appears that a large part of the interethnic difference in the frequency of the slow acetylator phenotype in the Caucasian and Oriental (especially Japanese) subjects (Evans, 1989) may be accounted for by a reduction in the frequency of *NAT2*5* in the latter group. *NAT2*6A* was observed both by cloning the gene (Blum *et al.*, 1991) and by detection of a restriction fragment length polymorphism (RFLP) (Deguchi *et al.*, 1990; Blum *et al.*, 1991; Ebisawa & Deguchi, 1991). *NAT2*7B* was cloned from a cDNA library (Oshako & Deguchi, 1990) and was originally thought to be restricted to Orientals (Vatsis *et al.*, 1991); this is now known not to be the case (Blum *et al.*, 1991; Hickman & Sim, 1991). *NAT2*13* was amplified from the hepatoma cell line Hep3B (Coroneos *et al.*, 1992) and has also been observed in human populations.

The mechanism by which some of these mutant alleles lead to reductions in NAT2 protein content in human liver has also been investigated. Deguchi *et al.* (1990) suggested that the *NAT2*6A* allele was associated with decreased NAT2-specific mRNA levels, implying a transcriptional defect. However, Blum *et al.* (1991) subsequently demonstrated, both in human liver and in a heterologous mammalian expression system, that the quantity of transcript produced from both *NAT2*5* and *NAT2*6A* was not different from that produced by *NAT2*4*. *NAT2*7B* also appeared to produce normal levels of transcript upon expression in mammalian cell culture (Oshako & Deguchi, 1990). In the *NAT2*5A* allele, both the $T^{341}C$ substitution resulting in $Ile^{114}Thr$ amino acid change and $C^{481}T$ substitution, which is silent, appear to be necessary to produce a mutant phenotype, suggesting a defect in translational level. On the other hand, in *NAT2*6A* the single $G^{590}A$ substitution, which leads to an $Arg^{197}Gln$ amino acid change, was sufficient to produce the mutant phenotype in cell culture by producing a protein with reduced stability (Blum *et al.*, 1991). However, the recent observation that the *NAT2*6B* allele, which also appears to contain only the above-mentioned nucleotide substitution, is associated with the rapid acetylator phenotype *in vivo*, underlines the need for further work to more precisely define the role of these genetic alterations in producing phenotypic variations in human populations. It will also be crucial to determine whether phenotypic differences exist among the *NAT2* allelic variants associated with slow acetylation, and whether these play a significant role in affecting predisposition to aromatic amine-induced toxicity. Fortuitously, all but one (position 341) of these nucleotide substitutions also lead to an alteration in a naturally occurring restriction endonuclease recognition sequence, providing a straightforward method to detect their occurrence in population studies (Deguchi *et al.*, 1990; Blum *et al.*, 1991; Hickman & Sim, 1991; Cascorbi *et al.*, 1995).

Accuracy, reproducibility and feasibility
Because of the large number of mutations identified in the *NAT2* gene, the use of phenotype has still been suggested as an important technique in studies on *NAT2* polymorphism. Undeniably, phenotyping can provide a simple overview of activity level without the necessity of checking for every possible mutation that has been identified (Mashimo *et al.*, 1992). In addition, discordance, when found, can indicate the possibility of a yet unidentified genetic mutation (Bell *et al.*, 1993). While phenotyping produces a continuous variable (with caffeine this is the urinary molar ratio of AAMU/1X or AFMU/1X), most investigators find conversion of this number to a dichotomous variable more convenient. Plotting the data on a log-probability scale gives a clear break between rapid and slow phenotype, as demonstrated recently by Butler *et al.* (1992), who used an antimode of 0.6 for the individual molar AFMU/1X ratios to differentiate between slow and fast acetylators. In other laboratories, different values of the antimode have also been used, e.g. 0.48 by Grant *et al.* (1984) and 0.85 by Braz Vieira de Silva Pontes *et al.* (1993). The numerical value of the antimode is thus obviously laboratory-dependent.

The phenotyping assay requires knowledge of the metabolites of the surrogate drug, caffeine. This information comes from an HPLC assay performed on a sample of urine collected during hour 4 to 5 after caffeine dosing. The use of an HPLC system that includes a diode array detector is important in order to minimize misclassification. The columns used in the assay seem, how-ever, to have significant variation in their performance level. Because of this, columns are purchased from the same lot number if at all possible. Despite this, there are some columns that give poor separation of caffeine metabolites and cannot be used.

The interindividual biological and procedural variability of the caffeine test may also contribute to the discrepancies. Although in general the caffeine test has been proved to be a sensitive method separating slow and fast acetylators by a clear bimodal distribution (Butler *et al.*, 1992; Fuhr *et al.*, 1996), Grant *et al.* (1984) reported an interday reproducibility of the AFMU/1X ratio of 11-14.5%, explaining discrepancies in the narrow range of the antimode but not of extremes. Discrepant cases tended to be more frequent among rapid genotypes of individuals older than the median age of 60 years. This may derive from slightly reduced hepatic or renal function in the elderly.

Recent studies showed that NAT1 may also contribute to AFMU formation. Vatsis & Weber (1993) reported an individual variability of NAT1 activity in lymphocytes due to mutations in the exon and post-translational region of the *NAT1* gene. Cribb *et al.* (1994) found a correlation between acetylation rate of the NAT1 substrate *p*-aminobenzoic acid and the AFMU/1X ratio among carriers of slow *NAT2* genotypes. Outliers of NAT2 genotype-phenotype correlation should thus be investigated also for *NAT1* polymorphism. Such an overlapping substrate specificity was shown for other NAT test substrates as well (Hein *et al.*, 1993).

At present the correlation of the *NAT1* alleles with the phenotype is still somewhat uncertain. In the first paper on the genotype-phenotype correlation (Bell *et al.*, 1995a) the *NAT1*10* allele was associated with higher NAT1 activity, whereas the *NAT1*3* and *NAT1*4* alleles were associated with the slow activity. The phenotype of the only person with *NAT1*11* allele was about intermediate to means of the *NAT1*10* and *NAT1*4*. This agrees with the observations relating the $G^{445}A$ substitution ($Val^{149}Ile$) with increased N-acetylation activity (Doll *et al.*, 1997). However, the association between the *NAT1*10* allele and NAT1 activity *in vivo* could not be confirmed in a couple of recent studies (Anne C. Deitz, personal communication). This may be due to the relative lability of the NAT1 enzyme or to falsely defining the putatively "real" slow allele, NAT1*14 as NAT1*10 in the studies; if the NAT1*14 frequency was slow in a given ethnic group there would be very little misclassification, whereas if it was high it would have a large impact on the outcome of the study.

Given the limitations of the *in vivo* phenotype studies discussed above, one may ask where the limit would be for rational phenotyping. In routine analysis there should be an equilibrium between cost, time required to obtain results, and accuracy. Recently there has been much debate on whether one should use phenotyping or genotyping analyses in molecular epidemiological studies on environmentally induced diseases. One of the main advantages of genotyping over phenotyping is, of course, that the use of probe drugs is avoided, and genotype data cannot be falsified by the disease under study, as has been suggested, e.g. in patients with diabetes mellitus (Mrozikiewicz *et al.*, 1994; Neugebauer *et al.*, 1994). Although it seems clear that lower costs and less time should also be required in order to obtain results with genotyping methods, such methods allowing complete detection of all mutations, e.g. carried at the NAT2 gene by one individual, are relatively expensive and several days are necessary to complete the analyses. This would not, of course, be feasible in clinical practice. Instead, it has been suggested that once the prevalence of the allelic variants in a given population is determined the use of analytical procedures designed to check the most frequent mutations could be used to simplify the analyses while keeping a high predictive capacity.

Cascorbi *et al.* (1995) discovered discrepancies between NAT2 genotype and phenotype in 6.7% of samples for both rapid genotype and slow phenotype or vice versa. Similar rates (6.8%) of nonconcordants were reported by Blum *et al.* (1991) and Hickman & Sim (1991), whereas somewhat lower rates, 2.5% and 4.2%, were reported by Graf *et al.* (1992) and Mrozikiewicz *et al.* (1994) respectively. Biological variability in phenotypic expression of certain genotypes may explain such cases, but extremes have been found which cannot be explained in this way. Strategies for detecting new mutations of unusual mutation-linkage patterns have been developed (Cascorbi *et al.*, 1995). The

two recently discovered A-to-T transversions (NAT2*17 and NAT2*18) found in one individual by Lin *et al.* (1994) exemplify the existence of other extremely rare mutations in the NAT2 gene. However, in the study by Cascorbi *et al.* (1995) in which all currently known mutations were characterized in a large sample of a Caucasian population, the sequencing of the NAT2 coding region confirmed the genotype as determined by PCR/RFLP analyses.

Moreover, on the basis of this analysis in 533 individuals, Cascorbi *et al.* (1995) could exclude the possibility that unexpected combination of mutations led to genotypes coding for an alternative phenotype. They were able to prove that the acetylation capacity of the NAT2*5A, NAT2*5C and NAT2*13 alleles, which had been characterized only *in vitro*, clearly coded for a slow acetylator type. Although NAT2*13 contained only a silent mutation, homozygous carriers and all carriers of combinations with other slow alleles presented a slow acetylation capacity. Moreover, it could be shown that homozygous carriers of the rapid NAT2*4 allele exhibited a significantly higher acetylation capacity than those with heterozygous genotypes. This gene-dose effect possibly has consequences for the susceptibility to cancer initiation mediated by toxification of arylamine carcinogens (Hein *et al.*, 1993). Different mean acetylation ratios of the major slow genotypes NAT2*5/*5 (*5 comprises *5A, *5B, and *5C) > NAT2*5/*6A > NAT2*6A/*6A demonstrate also significant differences in the *in vivo* acetylation capacities of the slow alleles NAT2*5 (especially *5B), *6A, *7B, and *13. In contrast, Hein *et al.* (1994) obtained a lower activity of NAT2*5A, *5B, or *5C alleles than NAT2*6A and *7B in bacterial expression systems, whereas NAT2*13 proved to have rapid activity. However, the expression of NAT2 alleles in *E. coli* does not completely reflect the expression in human hepatocytes.

It should also be pointed out that genotyping analyses are usually conducted with genomic DNA, and that two NAT2 genes are analysed at the same time. This could theoretically introduce a pitfall in genotyping studies, since the point mutations in the NAT2 gene can occur either in isolation or in combination. Therefore, a subject carrying two inactivating mutations could be either a rapid or a poor acetylator, depending on whether they were located in the same or different alleles respectively. To avoid such problems an *NAT2* genotyping method was developed that allows the detection of the seven point mutations and permits the separate analysis of each allele in every subject (Martínez *et al.*, 1995). On this basis it was deduced that, for the purpose of phenotype prediction, the analysis of mutations at $T^{341}C$ and $G^{590}A$ would be enough to obtain a good predictive capacity in the population studied.

Distribution of the phenotype and genotype in different populations

The basis for many ethnic variations in disease incidence and mortality may include differences in metabolic pathways as well as differences in

environmental and dietary exposure. Investigators have reported a wide range of values for acetylation activity in different groups (Lin *et al.*, 1994). The *NAT1* putative fast acetylator alleles are found in frequencies ranging from 15% to 25% in Caucasians, and up to 50% in Asians (Bell *et al.*, 1995b; Probst-Hensch *et al.*, 1996; Bouchardy *et al.*, 1998), whereas the *NAT2* slow acetylator alleles range from 5% in Japan to 90% in Egypt (Weber *et al.*, 1988). Table 3 contains a representative list of reports on NAT1 and NAT2 genotype or phenotype frequencies from different ethnic groups.

From the scarce population studies so far completed on *NAT1* it appears that *NAT1*4* and *NAT1*10* are the most prevalent alleles in

Table 3. Prevalence of NAT1 and NAT2 slow acetylator phenotypes and genotypes in various populations

	Caucasians	Chinese	Japanese	Koreans	Blacks	Hispanics	Indians	Filipinos	Malays
NAT1 genotype									
Bell *et al.* (1995b)	71 (112)[a]								
Probst-Hensch *et al.* (1996)	50 (484)								
Bouchardy *et al.* (1998)	57 (172)								
NAT2 phenotype									
Wolf *et al.* (1980)	51 (74)								
Cartwright *et al.* (1982)	57 (95)								
Evans *et al.* (1983)	60 (852)								
Ladero *et al.* (1985)	57 (157)								
Mommsen *et al.* (1985)	51 (100)								
NAT2 genotype									
Roots *et al.* (1992)	52 (101)								
Bell *et al.* (1993)	56 (372)					41 (128)			
Lin *et al.* (1993)	60 (100)	27 (70)	13 (98)	38 (96)		32 (148)			
	53 (76)								
Lin *et al.* (1994)		37 (100)	14 (79)				54 (61)	37 (100)	
Hirvonen *et al.* (1995)	51 (137)								
Zhao *et al.* (1995)		28 (187)					38 (139)		42 (146)
Agúndez *et al.* (1996)	54 (505)								
Brockmöller *et al.* (1996a)	58 (373)								
Cascorbi *et al.* (1996)	58 (278)								
Hunter *et al.* (1997)	58 (466)								
Bouchardy *et al.* (1998)	53 (172)								

[a] The numbers of subjects analysed are given in parentheses. Studies with small sample sizes are not included.

Caucasians (Bell *et al.*, 1995b; Probst-Hensch *et al.*, 1996; Bouchardy *et al.*, 1997). As for *NAT2*, the most prevalent alleles in a Japanese population are *NAT2*4* and *NAT2*6A*, whereas the *NAT2*5* alleles (most notably *5B*) predominate in Caucasians. Although *NAT2*5C*, *6A* and *13* are present at relatively low frequencies, their discovery provides an explanation for most of the phenotype-genotype discrepancies that were reported using genotyping methods designed only to detect *NAT2*5* and *6A* and classifying all other alleles as *NAT2*4* (Deguchi *et al.*, 1990; Blum *et al.*, 1991; Hickman & Sim, 1991; Vatsis *et al.*, 1991).

The predominance of the putative *NAT1* slow acetylator status associated genotype has been reported to be about 71% among British Caucasians (Bell *et al.*, 1995b), 57% among French Caucasians (Bouchardy *et al.*, 1998), and 50% among an American population consisting of Caucasians, African-Americans, and Latinos (Probst-Hensch *et al.*, 1996). The predominance of the *NAT2* slow acetylator genotype was found to be about 60% among Germans by analysing six or seven mutations (Lin *et al.*, 1993; Cascorbi *et al.*, 1995), 53% among American Caucasians by analysing six mutations (Lin *et al.*, 1993), and 63% among Polish (Mrozikiewicz *et al.*, 1994) and 51% among Finns by analysing the three most common mutations (Hirvonen *et al.*, 1995). In contrast, in Japanese or Chinese populations the rapid genotype is largely overrepresented (Mashimo *et al.*, 1992; Lin *et al.*, 1993; Rothman *et al.*, 1993). The lower frequency of slow acetylators (about 54%) among Caucasians of Spanish extraction (Agúndez *et al.*, 1996) may only partly reflect ethnic differences, as there are differences between the studies in the completeness of the genotyping method. Many earlier authors characterized the so-called mutations M1 ($C^{481}T$), M2 ($G^{590}A$) and M3 ($G^{857}A$) with allele-specific PCR. This method contains a higher risk of misclassification than RFLP, since two independent reactions are performed instead of one. Moreover, alleles *NAT2*5C*, *13* and *14B* were disregarded and misclassified as wild type. Since combinations of these alleles with other slow *NAT2* alleles have been shown to arise together in 8.5% of all genotypes (Cascorbi *et al.*, 1995) the slow acetylator frequency may be underestimated if mutations at nt positions 282 and either 803 or 341 are not considered.

Relevance of the enzyme in carcinogenesis in experimental models

Acetylator phenotype, as determined by the use of probe drugs, has been associated with many spontaneous and chemically induced diseases (Evans, 1989). N-acetylation of aromatic amine procarcinogens is generally considered to be a detoxifying mechanism, while competing N-oxidation by cytochrome P4501A2 (Guengerich & Shimada, 1991) produces reactive hydroxylamines that can be further metabolized to DNA-binding electrophiles. Such chemical-DNA adducts can increase rates of somatic mutation which, if they occur in genes controlling rates of cellular proliferation, may lead to a more highly malignant phenotype. Thus one might expect rapid acetylation to protect against aromatic amine-induced cancer, as appears to be the case for bladder cancer. However, in Ames *Salmonella typhimurium* mutagenicity tests, generally considered to be valid predictors of carcinogenic potential for a variety of chemicals, high levels of the endogenous bacterial acetyltransferase are required for the mutagenic potential of aromatic amines to be observed (Einistö *et al.*, 1991).

It is now clear that the acetyltransferases may also play an important role in metabolic activation pathways subsequent to P450-dependent N-oxidation. Such pathways may include direct O-acetylation of hydroxylamines to produce unstable acetoxy esters that spontaneously decompose, forming highly electrophilic arylnitrenium ions. Alternatively, consecutive N-acetylation and N-oxidation reactions may produce N-hydroxy-N-acetylarylamines (arylhydroxamic acids), which can undergo intramolecular N,O-acetyltransfer, again forming the acetoxy ester. Deacetylation of these compounds by microsomal deacetylases is also known to occur, and to play a modulatory role with respect to toxic responses observed after aromatic amine exposure in animals. Animal studies have previously demonstrated that O-acetylation and N,O-acetyltransfer may be mediated by NAT enzymes (Mattano *et al.*, 1989; Trinidad *et al.*, 1990). More recently, the ability of recombinant human *NAT1* and *NAT2* to perform such reactions has also been shown (Hein *et al.*, 1993). Indeed, new *Salmonella typhimurium* tester strains containing recombinant human *NAT1* and *NAT2* (Grant *et al.*, 1992a) should provide more accurate predictions of the carcinogenic potency of aromatic amines than those relying on metabolic activation by endogenous bacterial enzymes with significantly different catalytic specificities.

It is thus apparent that the ability of a given arylamine to be activated to potentially carcinogenic DNA-binding species and ultimately to produce tumours in a target tissue depends on both the relative tissue levels of NAT1, NAT2 and P4501A2 (each subject to genetic and/or environmentally regulated patterns of interindividual variation) and the catalytic selectivities of these enzymes for *N*-oxidation, *N*-acetylation, *O*-acetylation or *N,O*-acetyltransfer of the chemical in question.

Evidence supporting a role for NAT1 in metabolism of aromatic amines has been analysed in several studies. Expression of human NAT1 in mammalian and bacterial cells showed that NAT1 activates the bicyclic aromatic amines to compounds that can adduct to DNA, often more efficiently than does NAT2 (Grant *et al.*, 1992a,b; Minchin *et al.*, 1992; Probst *et al.*, 1992; Hein *et al.*, 1994). NAT1 and NAT2 are found in human colon and are thus available for the local activation of aromatic amines from tobacco or diet (Turesky *et al.*, 1991; Ilett *et al.*, 1994; Minchin, 1994). Colon cells possess higher activity for the conversion of NAT1-selective substrates than the NAT2-selective substrates (Ilett *et al.*, 1994). NAT1 is also expressed at high levels in the bladder mucosa, and involvement of the *NAT1*10* allele in the bioactivation of aromatic amines in bladder mucosa has been demonstrated. For example, DNA adduct levels of 4-aminobiphenyl were found to be twofold higher in individuals with the *NAT1*10* allele (Badavi *et al.*, 1995).

Evidence for role of NATs in carcinogenesis in humans: potential bias and confounders

Previous phenotyping studies as well as subsequent genotyping studies (see Table 4 for representative genotyping findings) have suggested a modifying role for *NAT* genotypes in all major cancer sites. Two main types of biological mechanism could explain a link between *N*-acetylation

and cancer. First, CYP-mediated *N*-hydroxylation of arylamines yields electrophilic intermediates that are inactivated by conjugation with glucuronide or acetylation by NATs (Weber *et al.*, 1988). In urinary bladder carcinogenesis, *N*-acetylation of arylamines represents a competing pathway for *N*-oxidation. The unconjugated *N*-hydroxy metabolites can enter the circulation, undergo renal filtration, and be transported to the urinary bladder (Kadlubar *et al.*, 1992). A number of previous phenotyping studies provided evidence that the NAT2 slow acetylator phenotype is a significant risk factor for the occurrence of bladder cancer, particularly if there is occupational exposure to arylamines (d'Errico *et al.*, 1996). Subsequent genotyping studies supported the important role of NAT2 slow acetylation status as a risk factor for arylamine-induced bladder cancer (Risch *et al.*, 1995; Brockmöller *et al.*, 1996; Golka *et al.*, 1996). There is, however, also the possibility that slow acetylators survive longer than rapid acetylators with bladder cancer (Evans *et al.*, 1983). Preliminary epidemiological data suggest that a prominent variant allele of *NAT1* (*NAT1*10*), associated with increased enzyme activity, is also a risk factor in smoking-related bladder cancer (Taylor *et al.*, 1995).

Another line of research is based on the hypothesis that fast acetylators are at increased risk for cancers at other sites than bladder due to the activation of procarcinogens such as heterocyclic amines. Exposure to heterocyclic amines is fairly common (Turesky *et al.*, 1991); these potent mutagens and rodent carcinogens are formed when meat and fish are cooked at household temperatures. The heterocyclic amines are poor substrates for *N*-acetylation in human liver, but they readily undergo hepatic *N*-oxidation and subsequent *N*-glucuronidation, resulting in conjugated *N*-hydroxy metabolites that can be transported to the colonic lumen. In colonic mucosa, the *N*-hydroxy derivatives are good substrates for *O*-acetylation, which results in reactive *N*-acetoxy-arylamines that are capable of forming covalent DNA adducts (Kadlubar *et al.*, 1992). The association between the *NAT1* fast acetylator trait and colorectal tumours could be due to enhanced *O*-acetylation of aromatic amines in cigarette smoke or of heterocyclic amines in cooked meat, because both smoking and a high intake of red meat have

		NAT1		**NAT2**	
Cancer site	Genotype	% (n)	OR (95% CI)	% (n)	OR (95% CI)
Bladder					
Cascorbi et al. (1994)	Slow				
Controls				61 (460)	1.0
Cases				66 (160)	1.3 (0.9-1.8)
Brockmöller et al. (1996)	Slow				
Controls				58 (373)	1.0
Cases				62 (374)	1.2 (0.8-1.7)
Breast					
Ambrosone et al. (1996)	Slow				
Controls (premenopausal)				57 (114)	1.0
Cases (premenopausal)				57 (119)	0.9 (0.7-2.0)
Controls (postmenopausal)				53 (213)	1.0
Cases (postmenopausal)				57 (185)	1.3 (0.8-1.9)
Hunter et al. (1997)	Slow				
Controls				57 (466)	1.0
Cases				57 (466)	1.0 (0.7-1.2)
Colon					
Bell et al. (1995b)	Fast				
Controls		29 (112)	1.0	45 (112)	1.0
Cases		44 (202)	1.9 (1.2-3.1)	48 (202)	1.1 (0.7-1.8)
Probst-Hensch et al. (1996)	Fast				
Controls		50 (484)	1.0	47 (484)	1.0
Cases		50 (441)	1.0 (0.8-1.4)	48 (441)	1.1 (0.8-1.4)
Liver					
Agúndez et al. (1996)	Slow				
Controls				54 (258)	1.0
Cases				68 (100)	1.8 (1.1-3.0)
Lung					
Cascorbi et al. (1996)	Slow				
Controls				42 (657)	1.0
Cases				44 (389)	1.1 (0.7-1.7)
Bouchardy et al. (1998)	Slow				
Controls		56 (170)	1.0	53 (170)	1.0
Cases		66 (148)	1.9 (1.1-3.2)	57 (148)	1.1 (0.7-1.8)

Table 4. Cancer risk associated with the *NAT* genotypes[a]

[a] Studies with small sample sizes or not reporting OR values are not included.

previously been associated with colorectal cancer (Giovannucci et al., 1994). The role of NAT1 activity is less clear if heterocyclic amines are the aromatic amine compounds of primary relevance to human colorectal cancer. Some data indicate that, among the acetyltransferases, NAT2 is more important than NAT1 for bioactivation of heterocyclic amines *in vitro* (Minchin et al., 1992;

Yanagawa et al., 1994; Wild et al., 1995; Yokoi et al., 1995).

Rapid acetylators were suggested to be at higher risk of developing cancer of the colon in several phenotyping studies (reviewed by d'Errico et al., 1996), and two recent genotyping studies have led to similar conclusions (Probst-Hecnsch et al., 1995; Gil & Lechner, 1998).

Moreover, preliminary epidemiological data suggest that the NAT1*10 allele is also a risk factor in smoking-related colon cancer (Bell et al., 1995b).

The N-acetylation phenotype has also been widely studied in relation to susceptibility to breast cancer and lung cancer. Several case-control studies compared the prevalence of the slow acetylator phenotype in breast cancer patients with its prevalence in controls, with mixed results (Bulovskaya et al., 1978; Philip et al., 1987; Ladero et al., 1987, Webster et al., 1989; Ilett et al., 1990). Similarly, a recent genotyping study indicated an increased risk of breast cancer for slow acetylators who smoked 20 or more cigarettes per day (Ambrosone et al., 1995), but two subsequent studies provided little evidence of an association between NAT2 genotype and breast cancer (Hunter et al., 1997; Millikan et al., 1998).

Other studies have evaluated the utility of acetylation as a risk marker for pulmonary malignancies and liver cancer. A set of four phenotyping studies yielded inconclusive results about the potential association between NAT2 acetylator status and lung cancer risk (Burgess & Trafford, 1985; Philip et al., 1988; Roots et al., 1988; Ladero et al., 1991). Neither did the subsequent genotyping studies give any conclusive evidence (Martínez et al., 1995; Cascorbi et al., 1996a; Bouchardy et al., 1998). However, the potential role of NAT genotypes as modifiers of individual responses to environmental agents was supported by three recent studies; the NAT2 slow acetylator genotype presented an increased risk of mesothelioma (Hirvonen et al., 1996), NAT1 genotype associated with higher activity increased the risk of smoking-related lung cancer (Bouchardy et al., 1998), and the NAT2 slow acetylator genotype increased the risk of hepatocellular carcinoma (Agúndez et al., 1996).

N-acetylation may therefore be an important detoxification step in environmental exposures, comparable to that of glutathione conjugation. The combination of the NAT1 and NAT2 susceptible genotypes may appear to be a particularly unfavourable genotype composition in arylamine exposures. In agreement with this, the recently observed association between increased risk (OR = 1.9, 95% CI = 1.2-3.6) of colorectal cancer and the fast NAT1 acetylator allele

(NAT1*10) was most apparent (OR = 2.8, 95% CI = 1.4-5.7) among fast NAT2 acetylators (Bell et al., 1995b). This underlines the importance of the establishment of combined impact of all relevant genes for a given exposure employing carefully selected cases and controls from homogenous populations (Hirvonen, 1997).

The importance of combined genotypes in environmental exposures is further demonstrated by some of the recent studies. The GSTM1 null genotype has been associated with significantly higher aromatic DNA-adduct levels in bus maintenance workers with the NAT2 slow acetylator genotype compared to those with the GSTM1 gene (Hou et al., 1995). In a similar study, non-smoking bus drivers with the NAT2 slow acetylator genotype and the GSTM1 null genotype were shown to have the highest levels of both DNA adducts and cytogenetic damage (Norppa et al., 1996). Moreover, the aminobiphenyl-haemoglobin adduct levels have been shown to be most elevated in smokers possessing this combination of the genotypes compared to smokers with other combinations (Yu et al., 1995). Further addressing the potential importance of the individual acetylation capacity, the carcinogenic DNA adduct levels in the mucosa of the urinary bladder were found to be highest in arylamine-exposed individuals who had inherited both the slow NAT2 acetylator genotype and the rapid NAT1 acetylation-associated (NAT1*10) allele (Badawi et al., 1995).

To conclude, the molecular epidemiology of NAT-related predisposition to cancer promises to be a fruitful area of research, provided that the potential biases and confounders discussed above are carefully controlled in the studies.

References

Agúndez, J.A.G., Olivera, M., Martínez, C., Ladero, J.M. & Benítez, J. (1996) Identification and prevalence study of 17 allelic variants of the human NAT2 gene in a white population. Pharmacogenetics, 6, 423-428

Andres, H.H., Vogel, R.S., Tarr, G.E., Johnson, L. & Weber, W.W. (1987) Purification, physiochemical, and kinetic properties of liver acetyl-CoA:arylamine N-acetyltransferase from rapid acetylator liver. Mol. Pharmacol., 31, 446-456

Ambrosone, C.B., Freudenheim, J.L., Graham, S., Marshall, J.R., Vena, J.R., Brasure, J.R., Michalek, A.M., Laughlin, R., Nemoto, T., Gillenwater, K.A. Harrington, A. & Shields, P.G. (1995) Cigarette smoking, N-acetyltransferase 2 genetic polymorphisms, and breast cancer risk. *JAMA*, 276, 1494-1501

Badawi, A., Hirvonen, A., Bell, D.A., Lang, N. & Kadlubar, F.F. (1995) Role of aromatic amine acetyltransferases NAT1 and NAT2 in carcinogen-DNA adduct formation in the human urinary bladder. *Cancer Res.*, 55, 5230-5237

Bell, D., Taylor, J.A., Butler, M.A., Stephens, E.A., Wiest, J., Brubaker, L.H., Kadlubar, F.F. & Lucier, G.W. (1993) Genotype/phenotype discordance for human arylamine N-acetyltransferase (NAT2) reveals a new slow acetylator allele common in African-Americans. *Carcinogenesis*, 14, 1689-1692

Bell, D.A., Badavi, A., Lang, N., Ilett, K.F., Kadlubar, F.F. & Hirvonen A. (1995a) Polymorphism in the NAT1 polyadenylation signal: association of NAT1*10 allele with higher N-acetylation activity in bladder and colon tissue samples. *Cancer Res.*, 55, 5226-5229

Bell, D.A., Stephens, D.A., Castranio, T., Umbach, D.M., Watson, M., Deakin, M., Elder, J., Hendrickse, C., Duncan, H. & Strange, R.C. (1995b) Polyadenylation polymorphism in the acetyltransferase 1 gene (NAT1) increases risk of colorectal cancer. *Cancer Res.*, 55, 3537-3542

Blum, M., Grant, D.M., Demierre, A. & Meyer, U.A. (1989a) Nucleotide sequence of a full-length cDNA for arylamine N-acetyltransferase from rabbit liver. *Nucleic Acids Res.*, 17, 3589

Blum, M., Grant, D.M., McBride, O.W., Heim, M. & Meyer, U.A. (1989b) N-acetylation pharmacogenetics: a gene deletion causes absence of arylamine N-acetyltransferase in liver of slow acetylator rabbits. *Proc. Natl. Acad. Sci. USA*, 86, 9554-9557

Blum, M., Grant, D.M., McBride, W., Heim, M. & Meyer, U.A. (1990) Human arylamine N-acetyltransferase genes: isolation, chromosomal localization, and functional expression. *DNA Cell. Biol.*, 9, 193-203

Blum, M., Demierre, A., Grant, D.M., Heim, M. & Meyer, U.A. (1991) Molecular mechanism of slow acetylation of drugs and carcinogens in humans. *Proc. Natl. Acad. Sci. USA*, 88, 5237-5241

Bouchardy, C., Mitrunen, K., Wikman, H., Husgafvel-Pursiainen, K., Dayer, P., Benhamou, S. & Hirvonen, A. (1998) N-acetyltransferase NAT1 and NAT2 genotypes and lung cancer risk. *Pharmacogenetics*, 8, 291-298

Braz Vieira de Silva Pontes, Z., Vincent-Viry, M., Gueguen, R., Gatteau, M.M. & Siest, G. (1993) Acetylation phenotypes and biological variation in a French Caucasian population. *Eur. J. Clin. Biochem.*, 31, 59-67

Brockmöller, J., Cascorbi, I., Kerb, R. & Roots, I. (1996) Combined analysis of inherited polymorphisms in arylamine N-acetyltransferase 2, glutathione S-transferases M1 and T1, microsomal epoxide hydrolase, and cytochrome P450 enzymes as modulators of bladder cancer risk. *Cancer Res.*, 56, 3915-3925

Bulovskaya, L.N., Krupkin, R.G., Bochina, T.A., Shipkova, A.A. & Pavlova, M.V. (1978) Acetylator phenotype in patients with breast cancer. *Oncology*, 35, 185-188

Burgess, E.J. & Trafford, A.P. (1985) Acetylator phenotype in patients with lung carcinoma - a negative report. *Eur. J. Respir. Dis.*, 67, 17-19

Butler, M.A., Lang, N.P., Yong, J.F., Caporaso, N.E., Vineis, P., Hayes, R.B., Teitel, C.H., Massengill, J.P., Lawsen, M.F. & Kadlubar, F.F. (1992) Determination of CYP1A2 and NAT2 phenotypes in human population by analysis of caffeine urinary metabolites. *Pharmacogenetics*, 2, 116-127

Cartwright, R.A., Glashan, R.W., Rogers, H.J., Ahmad, R.A., Barham-Hall, D., Higgins, E. & Kahn, M.A. (1982) Role of N-acetyltransferase phenotypes in bladder carcinogenesis: a pharmacogenetic epidemiological approach to bladder cancer. *Lancet*, 2, 842-846

Cascorbi, I., Drakoulis, N., Brockmöller, J., Mauer, A., Mrozikiewicz, P. & Roots, I. (1994)

Polymorphism of the human arylamine N-acetyltransferase (NAT2) gene in German bladder cancer patients [abstract]. *Naunyn-Schmiedeberg's Arch. Pharmacol.*, Suppl. 349, R 132

Cascorbi, I., Drakoulis, N., Brockmöller, J., Maurer, A., Sperling, K. & Roots, I. (1995) Arylamine N-acetyltransferase (NAT2) mutations and their allelic linkage in unrelated Caucasian individuals: correlation with phenotypic. *Am. J. Hum. Genet.*, 57, 581-592

Cascorbi, I., Brockmöller, J., Mrozikiewicz, P.M., Bauer, S., Loddenkemper, R. & Roots, I. (1996) Homozygous rapid arylamine N-acetyltransferase (NAT2) genotype as a susceptibility factor for lung cancer. *Cancer Res.*, 56, 3961-3966

Coroneos, E., Hickman, D., Risch, A., Kelly, S.L. & Sim, E. (1992) Arylamine N-acetyltransferase in cultured cell lines. *J. Basic Clin. Physiol. Pharmacol.*, 3 (Suppl.), 228

Cribb, A.E., Grant, D.M., Miller, M.A. & Spielberg, S.P. (1991) Expression of monomorphic arylamine N-acetyltransferase (NAT1) in human leucocytes. *J. Pharmacol. Exp. Therap.*, 259, 1241-1246

Cribb, A.E., Isbrucker, R., Levatte, T., Tsui, B., Gillespie, C.T. & Renton, K.W. (1994) Acetylator phenotyping: the urinary caffeine metabolite ratio in slow acetylators correlates with a marker of systemic NAT1 activity. *Pharmacogenetics*, 4, 166-170

Deguchi, T., Mashimo, M. & Suzuki T. (1990) Correlation between acetylator phenotypes and genotypes of polymorphic arylamine N-acetyltransferase in human liver. *J. Biol. Chem.*, 265, 12757-12760

Deitz, A.C., Doll, M.A. & Hein, D.W. (1997) A restriction fragment length polymorphism assay that differentiates human N-acetyltransferase-1 (NAT1) alleles. *Anal. Biochem.*, 253, 219-224

d'Errico, A., Taioli, E., Chen, X & Vineis P. (1996) Genetic polymorphisms and the risk of cancer: a review of the literature. *Biomarkers*, 1, 149-173

Doll, M.A., Jiang, W., Deitz, A.C., Rustan, T.D. & Hein, D.W. (1997) Identification of a novel allele at the human NAT1 acetyltransferase locus. *Biochem. Biophys. Res. Commun.*, 233, 584-591

Dupret, J-M. & Grant, D.M. (1992a) Site-directed mutagenesis of recombinant human arylamine N-acetyltransferase expressed in E. coli: evidence for direct involvement of Cys[68] in the catalytic mechanism of polymorphic human NAT2. *J. Biol. Chem.*, 267, 7381-7385

Dupret, J.-M. & Grant D.M. (1992b) Investigation of structure-function relationships of human arylamine N-acetyltransferases NAT1 and NAT2 by functional expression of NAT1/NAT2 protein chimeras in E. coli. *J. Basic Clin. Physiol. Pharmacol.*, 3 (Suppl.), 193

Dupret, J.-M., Goodfellow, G.H., Janezic, S.A. & Grant, D.M. (1994) Structure-function studies of human arylamine N-acetyltransferases NAT1 and NAT2. *J. Biol. Chem.*, 269, 26830-26835

Ebisawa, T. & Deguchi, T. (1991) Structure and restriction fragment length polymorphism of genes for human liver arylamine N-acetyltransferase. *Biochem. Biophys. Res. Comm.*, 177, 1252-1257

Einistö, P., Watanabe, M., Ishidate, M. & Nohmi, T. (1991) Mutagenicity of 30 chemicals in *Salmonella typhimurium* strains possessing different nitroreductase or O-acetyltransferase activities. *Mutat. Res.*, 259, 95-102

Evans, D.A. (1992) N-acetyltransferase. In: Kalow, W., ed, *Pharmacogenetics of Drug Metabolism*. New York, Pergamon Press, pp. 95-178

Evans, D.A.P. (1989) N-acetyltransferase. *Pharmacol. Ther.*, 42, 157-234

Evans, D.A.P., Eze, L.C. & Whitney, E.J. (1983) The association of the slow acetylator phenotype with bladder cancer. *J. Med. Genet.*, 20, 330-333

Evans, D.A.P., Manley, K.A. & McKusick, V.A. (1960) Genetic control of isoniazid metabolism in man. *Br. Med. J.*, 2, 285-491

Evans D.A.P. & White, T.A. (1964) Human acetylation polymorphism. *J. Lab. Clin. Med.*, 63, 394-403

Ferguson, R.J., Doll, M.A., Rustan, T., Baumstark, B.R. & Hein, D.W. (1994) Syrian hamster monomorphic N-acetyltransferase (NAT1) alleles: amplification, cloning, sequencing, and expression in E. coli. *Pharmacogenetics*, 4, 82-90

Fredrickson, S.M., Messing, E.M., Reznikoff, C.A. & Swaminathan, S. (1994) Relationship between *in vivo* acetylator phenotypes and cytosolic N-acetyltransferase and O-acetyltransferase activities in human uroepithelial cells. *Cancer Epidemiol. Biomarkers Prev.*, 3, 25-32

Fuhr, U., Rost, K.L., Engelhardt, R., Sachs, M., Liermann, Belloc, C., Beaune, P., Janezic, S., Grant, D., Meyer, U.A. & Staib H. (1996) Evaluation of caffeine as a test drug for CYP1A2, NAT2 and CYP2E1 phenotyping in man by *in vivo* versus *in vitro* correlations. *Pharmacogenetics*, 6, 159-176

Gil, J.P. & Lechner, M.C. (1998) Increased frequency of wild-type arylamine-N-acetyltransferase allele *NAT2*4* homozygotes in Portuguese patients with colorectal cancer. *Carcinogenesis*, 19, 37-41

Giovannucci, E., Rimm, E.B., Stampfer, M.J., Hunter, D., Rosner, B., Willett, W.C., & Speizer, F.E. (1994) A prospective study of cigarette smoking and risk of colorectal adenoma and colorectal cancer in US men. *J. Natl. Cancer Inst.*, 86, 183-191

Golka, K., Prior, V., Blaszkewicz, M., Cascorbi, I., Schöps, W., Kierfeld, G., Roots, I. & Bolt, H.M. (1996) Occupational history and genetic N-acetyltransferase polymorphism in urothelial cancer patients of Leverkusen, Germany. *Scand. J. Work Environ. Health.*, 22, 332-338

Graf, T., Broly, F., Hoffmann, F., Probst, M., Meyer, U.A. & Howald, H. (1992) Prediction of phenotype for acetylation and for debrisoquine hydroxylation by DNA-tests in healthy human volunteers. *Eur. J. Clin. Pharmacol.*, 43, 399-403

Grant, D.M. (1993) Molecular genetics of the N-acetyltransferases. *Pharmacogenetics*, 3, 45-50

Grant, D.M., Tang, B.K. & Kalow, W. (1984) A simple test for acetylator phenotype using caffeine. *Br. J. Clin. Pharmacol.*, 17, 459-464

Grant, D.M., Lottspeich, F. & Meyer, U.A. (1989) Evidence for two closely related isozymes of arylamine N-acetyltransferase in human liver. *FEBS Lett.*, 244, 203-207

Grant, D.M., Mörike, K., Eichelbaum, M. & Meyer, U.A. (1990a) Acetylation pharmacogenetics: the slow acetylator phenotype is caused by decreased or absent arylamine N-acetyltransferase in human liver. *J. Clin. Invest.*, 85, 968-972

Grant, D.M., Vollmer, K.-O. & Meyer, U.A. (1990b) *In vitro* metabolism of dinaline and acetyldinaline by human liver. *12th European Workshop on Drug Metabolism.* Basel, Switzerland. 147

Grant, D.M., Blum, M., Beer, M. & Meyer, U.A. (1991) Monomorphic and polymorphic human arylamine N-acetyltransferases: a comparison of liver isozymes and expressed products of two cloned genes. *Mol. Pharmacol.*, 39, 184-191

Grant, D.M., Josephy, P.D., Lord, H.L. & Morrison, L.D. (1992a) *Salmonella typhimurium* strains expressing human arylamine N-acetyltransferases: metabolism and mutagenic activation of aromatic amines. *Cancer Res.*, 52, 3961-3964

Grant, D.M., Vohra, P., Avis, Y. & Ima, A. (1992b) Detection of a new polymorphism of human arylamine N-acetyltransferase NAT1 using p-aminosalicylic acid as an *in vivo* probe. *J. Basic Clin. Physiol. Pharmacol.*, 3, Suppl.), 244

Grant, D.M., Hughes, N.C., Janezic, S.A., Goodfellow, G.H., Chen, H.J., Gaedigk, A., Yu, V.L. & Grewal, R. (1997) Human acetyltransferase polymorphisms. *Mutat. Res.*, 376, 61-70

Guengerich, F.P. & Shimada, T. (1991) Oxidation of toxic and carcinogenic chemicals by human cytochrome P450 enzymes. *Chem. Res. Toxicol.*, 4, 391-407

Hearse, D.J. & Weber, W.W. (1973) Multiple N-acetyltransferases and drug metabolism. Tissue distribution, characterization and significance of mammalian N-acetyltransferase. *Biochem. J.*, 132, 519-526

Hein, D.W., Doll, M.A., Rustan, T.D., Gray, K., Feng, Y., Ferguson, R.J. & Grant, D.M. (1993) Metabolic activation and deactivation of arylamine carcinogens by recombinant human NAT1 and polymorphic NAT2 acetyltransferases. *Carcinogenesis*, 14, 1633-1638

Hein, D.W., Doll, M.A., Rustan, T.D. & Ferguson, R.J. (1995) Metabolic activation of N-hydroxyarylamines and N-hydroxyarylamides by 16 recombinant human *NAT2* allozymes: effects of 7 specific *NAT2* nucleic acid substitutions. *Cancer Res.*, 55, 3531-3536

Hein, D.W., Rustan, T.D. & Grant, D.M. (1992a) Human liver polymorphic (NAT2) and monomorphic (NAT1) N-acetyltransferase isozymes catalyse metabolic activation of N-hydroxyarylamine and N-hydroxy-N-acetyl-arylamine proximate carcinogens. *FASEB J.*, 6, A1274

Hein, D.W., Rustan, T.D., Doll, M.A., Bucher, K.D., Ferguson, R.J., Feng, Y., Furman, E.J. & Gray, K. (1992b) Acetyltransferases and susceptibility to chemicals. *Toxicol. Lett.*, 64/65, 123-130

Hein, D.W., Rustan, T.D., Ferguson, R.J. & Doll, M.A. (1994) Metabolic activation of aromatic and heterocyclic N-hydroxyarylamines by wild-type and mutant recombinant human NAT1 and NAT2 acetyltransferases. *Arch. Toxicol.*, 68, 129-133

Hickman, D. & Sim, E. (1991) N-acetyltransferase polymorphism: comparison of phenotype and genotype in humans. *Biochem. Pharmacol.*, 42, 1007-1014

Hirvonen, A. (1997) Combinations of susceptible genotypes and individual responses to toxicants. *Environ. Health Perspect.*, 105, 755-758

Hirvonen, A., Pelin, K., Tammilehto, L., Karjalainen, A., Mattson, K. & Linnainmaa, K. (1995) Inherited *GSTM1* and *NAT2* defects as con-

current risk modifiers for asbestos-associated human malignant mesothelioma. *Cancer Res.*, 55, 2981-2983

Hirvonen, A., Saarikoski, S., Linnainmaa, K., Koskinen, K., Husgafvel-Pursiainen, K. & Vainio, H. (1996) *GST* and *NAT* genotypes and asbestos-associated pulmonary disorders. *J. Natl. Cancer Inst.*, 88, 1853-1856

Hou, S.-M., Lambert, B. & Hemminki, K. (1995) Relationship between hprt mutant frequency, aromatic DNA adducts and genotypes for *GSTM1* and *NAT2* in bus maintenance workers. *Carcinogenesis*, 16, 1913-1917

Hughes, N.C., Janezic, S.A., McQueen, K.L., Jewett, M.A.S., Castranio, T., Bell, D.A. & Grant, D.M. (1997) Identification and characterization of variant alleles of human acetyltransferase *NAT1* with defective function using p-aminosalicylate as an *in vivo* and *in vitro* probe. *Pharmacogenetics*, 8, 55-66

Hunter, D.J., Hankinson, S.E., Hough, H., Gertig, D.M., Garcia-Closas, M., Spiegelman, D., Manson, J.E., Colditz, G.A., Willett, W.C., Speizer, F.E. & Kelsey, K. (1997) A prospective study of *NAT2* acetylation genotype, cigarette smoking, and risk of breast cancer. *Carcinogenesis*, 18, 2127-2132

Ilett, K.F., David, B.M., Detchon, P., Castleden, W.M. & Kwa, R. (1987) Acetylator phenotype in colorectal carcinoma. *Cancer Res.*, 47, 1466-1469

Ilett, K.F., Detchon, P., Ingram, D.M. & Castleden W.M. (1990) Acetylation phenotype is not associated with breast cancer. *Cancer Res.*, 50, 6649-6651

Ilett, K.F., Ingram, D.M., Carpenter, D.S., Teitel, C.H., Lang, N.P., Kadlubar, F.F. & Minchin, R.F. (1994) Expression of monomorphic and polymorphic N-acetyltransferases in human colon. *Biochem. Pharmacol.*, 47, 914-917

Kadlubar, F.F., Butler, M.A., Kaderlik, K.R., Chou, H.C. & Lang, N.P. (1992) Polymorphisms for aromatic amine metabolism in humans: relevance for human carcinogenesis. *Environ. Health Perspect.*, 98, 69-74

Kelly, S. & Sim, E. (1994) Arylamine N-acetyltransferase in Balb/c mice: identification of a novel mouse isoenzyme by cloning and expression *in vitro*. *Biochem. J.*, 302, 347-535

Ladero, J.M., Fernandez, M.J., Palmeiro, R., Munoz, J.J., Jara, C., Lazaro, C. & Perez-Manga, G. (1987) Hepatic acetylator polymorphism in breast cancer. *Oncology*, 44, 341-344

Ladero, J.M., Gonzalez, J.F., Benitez, J., Vargas, E., Fernandez, M.J., Baki, W. & Diaz-Rubio, M. (1991) Acetylator polymorphism in human colorectal carcinoma. *Cancer Res.*, 51, 2098-2100

Ladero, J.M., Kwok, C.K., Jara, F., Fernandez, M.J., Dilmi, A.M., Tapia, D. & Uson, A.C. (1985) Hepatic acetylator polymorphism in bladder cancer patients. *Ann. Clin. Res.*, 17, 97-99

Lakshmi, V.M., Bell, D.A., Watson, M., Zenser, T.V. & Davis, B.B. (1995) N-acetylbenzidine and N,N'-diacetylbenzidine formation by rat and human liver slices exposed to benzidine. *Carcinogenesis*, 16, 1565-1571

Lin, H., Han, C.-Y., Lin, B.K. & Hardy, S. (1993) Slow acetylator mutations in the human polymorphic N-acetyltransferase gene in 786 Asians, Blacks, Hispanics, and Whites: application to metabolic epidemiology. *Am. J. Hum. Genet.*, 52, 827-834

Lin, H., Han, C.-Y., Lin, B.K. & Hardy, S. (1994) Ethnic distribution of slow acetylator mutations in the polymorphic N-acetyltransferase (*NAT2*) gene. *Pharmacogenetics*, 4, 125-134

Martínez, C., Agúndez, J.A.G., Olivera, M., Martín, R., Ladero, J.M. & Benítez, J. (1995) Lung cancer and mutations at the polymorphic *NAT2* gene locus. *Pharmacogenetics*, 5, 207-214

Mashimo, M., Suzuki, T., Abe, M. & Deguchi, T. (1992) Molecular genotyping of N-acetylation polymorphism to predict phenotype. *Hum. Genet.*, 90, 139-142

Mattano, S.S., Land, S., King, C.M. & Weber, W.W. (1989) Purification and biochemical characterization of hepatic arylamine N-acetyltransferase from

rapid and slow acetylator mice: identity with arylhydroxamine acid N,O-acetyltransferase and N-hydroxy-arylamine O-acetyltransferase. *Mol. Pharmacol.*, 35, 599-609

Millikan, R.C., Pittman, G.S., Newman, B., Tse, C.-K.J., Selmin, O., Rockhill, B., Savitz, D.S., Moorman, P.G. & Bell, D.A. (1988) Cigarette smoking, N-acetyltransferases 1 and 2, and breast cancer risk. *Cancer Epidemiol. Biomarkers Prev.*, 7, 371-378

Minchin, R.F. (1994) Expression of monomorphic and polymorphic N-acetyltransferases in human colon. *Biochem. Pharmacol.*, 47, 914-915

Minchin, R.F., Reeves, P.T., Teitel, C.H., McManus, M.E., Mojarrabbi, B., Ilett, K.F. & Kadlubar, F.F. (1992) N- and O-acetylation of aromatic and heterocyclic amine carcinogens in by human monomorphic and polymorphic acetyltransferase expressed in cos-1 cells. *Biochem. Biophys. Res. Commun.*, 185, 839-844

Mommsen, S., Barford, N.M. & Aagaard, J. (1985) N-acetyltransferase phenotypes in the urinary bladder carcinogenesis of a low risk population. *Carcinogenesis*, 6, 199-201

Mrozikiewicz, P.M., Drakoulis, N. & Roots, I. (1994). Polymorphic arylamine N-acetyltransferase (NAT2) genes in children with insulin-dependent diabetes mellitus. *Clin. Pharm. Ther.*, 56, 626-634

Neugebauer, S., Baba, T., Watanabe, T., Ishizaki, T. & Kurokawa, K. (1994) The N-acetyltransferase (NAT) gene: an early risk marker for diabetic nephropathy in Japanese type 2 diabetes patients? *Diabet. Med.*, 11, 783-788

Norppa, H. (1997) Cytogenetic markers of susceptibility: influence of polymorphic carcinogen metabolizing enzymes. *Environ. Health Perspect.*, 105 (Suppl.), 829-835

Oshako, S. & Deguchi, T. (1990) Cloning and expression of cDNAs for polymorphic and monomorphic arylamine N-acetyltransferases from human liver. *J. Biol. Chem.*, 265, 4630-4634

Patterson, E., Radtke, H. & Weber, W.W. (1980) Immunochemical studies of rabbit *N*-acetyltransferases. *Mol. Pharmacol.*, 17, 367-373

Philip, P.A., Fitzgerald, D.L., Cartwright, R.A., Peake, M.D. & Rogers, H.J. (1988) Polymorphic acetylation capacity in lung cancer. *Carcinogenesis.*, 9, 491-493

Philip, P.A., Rogers, H.J., Mills, R.R., Rubens, R.D. & Cartwright, R.A. (1987) Acetylator status and its relationship to breast cancer and other diseases of the breast. *Eur. J. Cancer Clin. Oncol.*, 23, 1701-1706

Probst, M., Blum, M., Fasshauer, I., D'Orazio, D., Meyer, U. & Wild D. (1992) The role of human acetylation polymorphism in the metabolic activation of the food carcinogen 2-amino-3-methylimidazo[4,5-f]quinoline (IQ). *Carcinogenesis*, 13, 1713-1717

Probst-Hensch, N.M., Haile, R.W., Ingles, S.A., Longnecker, M.P., Han, C.-Y., Lin, B.K., Lee, D.B., Sakamoto, G.T., Frankl, H.D., Lee, E.R. & Lin, H.J. (1995) Acetylation polymorphism and prevalence of colorectal adenomas. *Cancer Res.*, 55, 2017-2020

Probst-Hensch, N.M., Haile, R.W., Li, D.S., Sakamoto, G.T., Louie, A.D., Lin, B.K., Frankl, H.D., Lee, E.R. & Lin, H.J. (1996) Lack of association between the polyadenylation polymorphism in the *NAT1* (acetyltransferase 1) gene and colorectal adenomas. *Carcinogenesis*, 17, 2125-2129

Risch, A., Wallace, D.M.A., Bathers, S. & Sim, E. (1995) Slow *N*-acetylation genotype is a susceptibility factor in occupational and smoking- related bladder cancer. *Hum. Mol. Gen.*, 4, 231-236

Roots, I., Drakoulis, N., Ploch, M., Heinemeyer, G., Loddenkemper, R., Minks, T., Nitz, M., Otte, F. & Koch, M. (1988) Debrisoquine hydroxylation phenotype, acetylation phenotypes, and ABO blood groups as genetic host factors of lung cancer risk. *Klin. Wochenschr.*, 66 (Suppl. XI), 87-97

Rothman, N., Hayes, R.B., Bi, W., Caporaso, N., Broly, F., Woosley, R.L., Yin, S., Feng, P., You, X. &

Meyer, U.A. (1993) Correlation between *N*-acetyltransferase activity and *NAT2* genotype in Chinese males. *Pharmacogenetics*, 3, 250-255

Sasaki, Y., Oshako, S. & Deguchi. T. (1991) Molecular and genetic analyses of arylamine N-acetyltransferase polymorphism of rabbit liver. *J. Biol. Chem.*, 266, 13243-13250

Taylor, J.A., Umbach, D., Stephens, E., Paulson, D., Robertson, C., Mohler, J.L. & Bell, D.A. (1995) Role of *N*-acetylation polymorphism at *NAT1* and *NAT2* in smoking-associated bladder cancer. *Proc. Am. Assoc. Cancer Res.*, 36, 282

Trinidad, A., Hein, D.W., Rustan, T.D., Ferguson, R.J., Miller, L.S., Bucher, K.D., Kirlin, W.G., Ogolla, F. & Andrews, A.F. (1990) Purification of hepatic polymorphic arylamine *N*-acetyltransferase from homozygous rapid acetylator inbred hamster: identity with polymorphic *N*-hydroxylamine-*O*-acetyltransferase. *Cancer Res.*, 50, 7942-7949

Turesky, R.J., Lang, N.P., Butler, M.A., Teitel, C.H. & Kadlubar, F.F. (1991) Metabolic activation of carcinogenic heterocyclic aromatic amines by human liver and colon. *Carcinogenesis*, 12, 1839-1845

Vatsis, K.P., Martell, K.J. & Weber, W.W. (1991) Diverse point mutations in the human gene for polymorphic *N*-acetyltransferase. *Proc. Natl. Acad. Sci. USA*, 88, 6333-6337

Vatsis, K.P. & Weber, W.W. (1993) Structural heterogeneity of Caucasian *N*-acetyltransferase at the *NAT1* gene locus. *Arch. Biochem. Biophys.*, 301, 71-76

Vatsis, K.P., Weber, W.W., Bell, D.A., Dupret, J.-M., Evans, D.A.P., Grant, D.M., Hein, D.W., Lin, H.J., Meyer, U.A., Relling, M.V., Sim, E., Suzuki, T. & Yamazoe, Y. (1995) Nomenclature for *N*-acetyltransferases. *Pharmacogenetics*, 5, 1-17

Vineis, P., Bartsch, H., Caporaso, N., Harrington, A.M., Kadlubar, F.F., Landi, M.T., Malaveille, C., Shields, P., Skipper, P., Talaska, G. & Tannenbaum, S.R. (1994) Genetically based *N*-acetyltransferase metabolic polymorphism and low-level environmental exposure to carcinogens. *Nature*, 369, 154-156

Weber, W.W., Mattano, S.S. & Levy, G.N. (1988) Acetylator pharmacogenetics and aromatic amine-induced cancer. In: King, C.M., Romano, J. & Schuezle, D., eds, *Carcinogenic and Mutagenic Responses to Aromatic Amines and Nitroarenes*. New York, Elsevier Science Publishing Co., Inc., pp. 115-123

Webster, D.J.T., Flook, D., Jenkins, J., Hutchings, A. & Routledge, P.A. (1989) Drug acetylation in breast cancer. *Br. J. Cancer*, 60, 236-237

Wild, D., Fesrs, W., Michel, S., Lord, H.L. & Josephy, P.D. (1995) Metabolic activation of heterocyclic aromatic amines catalysed by human arylamine N-acetyltransferase isozymes (NAT1 and NAT2) expressed in *Salmonella typhimurium*. *Carcinogenesis*, 16, 643-648

Wolf, H., Lower, G.M. & Bryan, G.T. (1980) Role of N-acetyltransferase phenotype in human susceptibility to bladder carcinogenic arylamines. *Scand. J. Urol. Nephrol.*, 14, 161-165

Yanagawa, Y., Sawada, M., Deguchi, T., Gonzalez, F.J. & Kamataki, T. (1994) Stable expression of human CYP1A2 and N-acetyltransferases in Chinese hamster CHL cells: mutagenic activation of 2-amino-3-methylimidazo[4,5-*f*]quinoline and 2-amino-3,8-dimethylimidazo[4,5-*f*-quino-xaline. *Cancer Res.*, 54, 3422-3427

Yokoi, T., Sawada, M. & Kamataki, T. (1995) Polymorphic drug metabolism: studies with recombinant Chinese hamster cells and analyses in human populations. *Pharmacogenetics*, 5, S65-S69

Yu, M.C., Ross, R.K., Chan, K., Henderson, B.E., Skipper, P.L., Tannenbaum, S.R. & Goetzee, G.A. (1995) Glutathione S-transferase M1 genotype affects aminobiphenyl-haemoglobin adduct levels in White, Black and Asian smokers and non-smokers. *Cancer Epidemiol. Biomarkers Prev.*, 4, 861-864

Zenser, T.V., Lakshmi, V.M., Rustan, T.D., Doll, M.A., Deitz, A.C., Davis, B.B. & Hein, D.W. (1996) Human N-acetylation of benzidine: role of NAT1 and NAT2. *Cancer Res.*, 56, 3941-3947

Zhao, B., Lee, E.J.D., Wong, J.Y.Y., Yeoh, P.N. & Gong, N.H. (1995) Frequency of mutant CYP1A1, NAT2 and GSTM1 alleles in normal Indians and Malays. *Pharmacogenetics*, 5, 275-280

A. Hirvonen
Finnish Institute of Occupational Health,
Department of Industrial Hygiene and Toxicology,
FIN-00250 Helsinki, Finland

Metabolic Polymorphisms and Susceptibility to Cancer
W. Ryder
IARC Scientific Publications No. 148
International Agency for Research on Cancer, Lyon, 1999

Chapter 21. Additional polymorphisms and cancer

Michael J. Stubbins and C. Roland Wolf

The purpose of this Chapter is to investigate as many of the less-studied genes as possible in relation to their importance in cancer susceptibility. For example, within the cytochrome P450 superfamily there are genes whose protein product is solely responsible for the detoxification of specific carcinogens. For a number of these genes, although genetic polymorphisms have not been identified, defined phenotypic polymorphisms have been demonstrated in specific populations. Other examples are given in which functional metabolic polymorphisms have been elucidated yet pertinent experiments for the determination of cancer risk have not been performed. The status of work relating to the genes in question is summarized and areas demanding future study are highlighted.

Cancer is a multifactorial disease, and susceptibility is, in part, modulated by interindividual variation in the expression of enzymes involved in the activation/detoxification of carcinogenic compounds (Wolf, 1990; Smith *et al.*, 1995). When studying the contribution of metabolic polymorphisms to cancer susceptibility it is important to identify as many variables in this type of analysis as possible, so as to reduce the number of confounding factors. The present volume has dealt with polymorphisms in genes that encode drug-metabolizing enzymes and with the way in which these polymorphisms relate to cancer susceptibility. This section concentrates on the possible importance of metabolic polymorphisms in human genes that have received only limited study, for which detailed analyses are not possible. We have aimed to cover each enzyme in sufficient detail to give an outline of the results that have been obtained and of the prospects for future work. It should be noted, however, that many polymorphic genes which do not encode drug-metabolizing enzymes nevertheless influence carcinogenesis (e.g. DNA repair enzymes, p53). Allelic variants of these genes represent an important area for future study (Wolf, 1990).

The cytochrome P450 superfamily of enzymes
Members of the cytochrome P450 CYP2B subfamily
The human CYP2B subfamily comprises three genes: CYP2B6, CYP2B7 and a CYP2B7-like pseudogene (CYP2B7P) that lacks the 3'-untranslated region and

perhaps also exon 9 (Hoffman *et al.*, 1995). Of these three genes, the CYP2B7 and CYP2B7P genes are known to be functionally inactive, and the CYP2B6 gene produces the only functionally active protein (Yamano *et al.*, 1989). All three genes are localized to a cluster in close proximity to the human CYP2A and CYP2F genes on chromosome 19q12-13.2 (Fig. 1) (Hoffman *et al.*, 1995). The CYP2B subfamily is characterized by the response of these genes to induction by phenobarbital.

There have been few reports concerning the non-functional CYP2B7 gene, although it is known that expression of the CYP2B7 protein is restricted to the lung (Nhamburo *et al.*, 1989). CYP2B6 protein, which is predominantly expressed in human liver and exhibits considerable variation, is undetectable in some individuals (Forrester *et al.*, 1992; Burke *et al.*, 1994). This can be partly related to exposure to anticonvulsive drugs. It has been shown that mRNAs from members of the CYP2A and CYP2B gene families are subject to alternative splicing (Miles *et al.*, 1989, 1990). Indeed, three alternatively spliced CYP2B6 mRNAs have been reported (Miles *et al.*, 1989, 1990), all of which are unable to produce a functional CYP2B6 protein. In all liver samples tested the alternatively spliced CYP2B6 variants have been identified in addition to the correctly spliced, full-length transcript (Miles *et al.*, 1989, 1990). The level of aberrantly spliced mRNA is subject to individual variability, and can constitute a high proportion of the total mRNA formed. This therefore

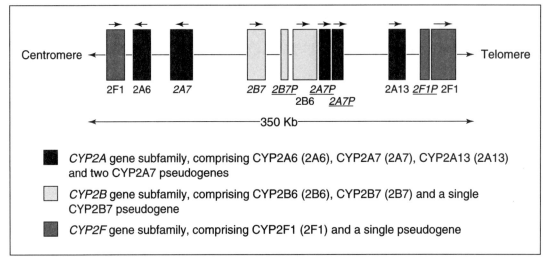

Figure 1. Structural organization of the CYP2 family of genes on human chromosome 19. A cluster of genes from the CYP2A, CYP2B and CYP2F subfamilies is shown, spanning 350 kb of genomic DNA. The directions of transcription are indicated by arrows. Non-functional genes are represented in italics, and pseudogenes are underscored and italicized. Telomere and centromere directions are also indicated. (Redrawn from Fernandez-Salguego *et al.*, 1995; Hoffman *et al.*, 1995)

represents a potentially extremely important factor in the modulation of CYP2B6 protein levels. The same applies to several other P450 genes but has not been studied in detail (Miles *et al.*, 1989; Miles *et al.*, 1990; Ding *et al.*, 1995).

Smith *et al.* (1993) showed that CYP2B6 is induced by barbiturates such as phenobarbital, and *in vitro* experiments have shown that CYP2B6 activates several substrates, including 6-aminochrysene and nicotine (Mimura *et al.*, 1993), as well as being responsible for the specific metabolism of the anti-cancer drugs cyclophosphamide and ifosfamide (Chang *et al.*, 1993). The importance of CYP2B6 in the metabolism of these and other xenobiotics may seem surprising, given that typical levels of CYP2B6 expression are approximately only 1% of the total hepatic P450 expression. However, its central role in the metabolism of these drugs means that interindividual differences in CYP2B6 levels may have severe clinical effects. As yet there is no evidence that genetic polymorphisms at the CYP2B6 locus play a role in determining differences in protein levels or activity.

Members of the cytochrome P450 CYP2C subfamily
The human CYP2C subfamily of cytochrome P450 isozymes comprises four members, localized to a gene cluster spanning over 500 kb of genomic DNA on chromosome 10q24, and arranged in the

following order: CYP2C18, CYP2C19, CYP2C9 and CYP2C8 from centromere to telomere (Fig. 2) (Gray *et al.*, 1995). A fifth gene, CYP2C10, has also been reported (Umbenhauer *et al.*, 1987), but recent evidence indicates that its separate classification based on a divergent 3'-non-coding region has arisen due to a cloning artefact (Gray *et al.*, 1995; Stubbins *et al.*, 1996). All CYP2C genes are composed of 9 exons and share a high level of sequence homology, both at the amino acid (88.7-95.7%) and nucleotide level (82.6-93.9%) (de Morais *et al.*, 1993; Goldstein & de Morais., 1994).

CYP2C8
Several CYP2C8 cDNAs have been cloned from human liver cDNA libraries (Nelson *et al.*, 1996) using probes from both the rat CYP2C6 cDNA (Kimura *et al.*, 1987) and the rabbit progesterone-21-hydroxylase P450 1 cDNA (Okino *et al.*, 1987). CYP2C8 is expressed in significant amounts in human liver and is subject to considerable interindividual variation in expression level (Forrester *et al.*, 1992). CYP2C8 metabolizes a large number of compounds, including benzo[*a*]pyrene, carbamazapine, 7-ethoxy-coumarin, testosterone, benzphetamine, retinol and retinoic acid (Leo *et al.*, 1989; Yun *et al.*, 1992; Kerr *et al.*, 1994). Purified CYP2C8 protein is more active than either CYP2C9 or CYP3A4 in activat-

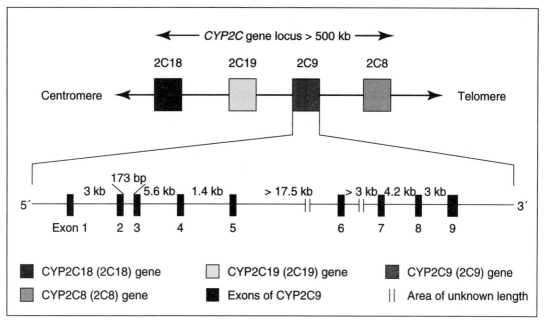

Figure 2. The structural organization of the *CYP2C* gene locus and the intron/exon structure of the *CYP2C9* gene are illustrated. Approximate intron sizes are indicated above each intron, and the telomere and centromere directions are also indicated (Gray *et al.*, 1995; de Morais *et al.*, 1993).

ing benzo[*a*]pyrene to mutagenic products in *Salmonella typhimurium*, indicating that CYP2C8 may play a role in the genotoxicity of benzo[*a*]pyrene in human liver (Yun *et al.*, 1992). However, the enzymes that play a predominant role in the metabolism of this compound have proved difficult to identify. In view of the role of CYP2C8 in the metabolism of benzo[*a*]pyrene, a tobacco smoke carcinogen, coupled with the fact that polymorphisms in other P450 isozymes have been linked to susceptibility to various types of cancer, it is interesting to speculate whether a polymorphism in the CYP2C8 gene would have any effect on cancer susceptibility.

Interestingly, cDNA-expressed CYP2C8 is also the principal (and possibly the only) enzyme responsible for the 6α-hydroxylation of the anti-cancer drug taxol to its principal human metabolite and detoxification product, 6α-hydroxytaxol (Rahman *et al.*, 1994). Taxol ("paclitaxel") is currently used in the treatment of refractory ovarian and breast cancer (Rahman *et al.*, 1994).

Several variant CYP2C8 cDNA sequences have been reported, but it has not yet been determined whether these represent true CYP2C8 alleles.

Given the important substrates that CYP2C8 is known to metabolize, if these cDNAs were to represent true alleles of CYP2C8 it would be of obvious importance to ascertain the frequencies of such alleles in the general population and the phenotypic consequences of possessing them in terms of CYP2C8 substrate metabolism. Other evidence suggests that there is an appreciable variation in the levels of CYP2C8 protein expression in human liver (Wrighton *et al.*, 1987), but a genetic basis for this variation has not been identified. Given that genetic polymorphisms have now been identified at the CYP2C9, CYP2C18 and CYP2C19 gene loci, it seems likely that the CYP2C8 gene is polymorphically expressed. In view of the fact that CYP2C8 is, as yet, the only isozyme known to be capable of metabolizing taxol, this is an important enzyme for future study in relation to cancer susceptibility.

CYP2C9

CYP2C9 was first described as the P450 responsible for the 4'-hydroxylation of the anti-epileptic drug *S*-mephenytoin, although recent work involving the use of recombinant CYP2C proteins

Table 1. Differences in published CYP2C9/2C10 cDNA sequences

No.	Source of CYP2C9 sequence Ω	Sites of nucleotide differences											
		4	6	63	144	175	239	280	281	358	359	417	475
1	2C9 Romkes et al., 1991 †M61857	Leu CTT	Val GTC	Pro CCT	Arg CGT	Cys TGC	Phe TTT	Ser TCT	Glu GAA	Tyr TAC	Ile ATT	Gly GGC	Gly GGA
2	2C9 Yasumori et al., 1987 †D00173	Leu CTT	Val GTC	Pro CCG	Arg CGT	Cys TGC	Phe TTT	Ser TCT	Glu GAA	Tyr TAC	Ile ATT	Gly GGC	Gly GGA
3	2C9 Meehan et al., 1988 §	Leu CTT	Val GTC	Pro CCT	Cys TGT	Tyr TAC	Leu CTT	Ser TCT	Glu GAA	Tyr TAC	Ile ATT	Gly GGC	Gly GGA
4	2C9 Kimura et al., 1987 †Y00498	Leu* CTT	Val* GTC	Pro CCT	Cys TGT	Cys TGC	Phe TTT	Ser TCA	Stop TAA	Tyr TAC	Ile ATT	Gly GGC	Gly GGA
5	2C9 Ged et al., 1988 †M21940	‡	‡	‡	Arg CGT	Cys TGC	Phe TTT	Ser TCA	Glu GAA	Cys TGC	Ile ATT	Gly GGC	Gly GGA
6	2C9 Romkes et al., 1991 †M61855	Leu CTT	Val GTC	Pro CCT	Arg CGT	Cys TGC	Phe TTT	Ser TCT	Glu GAA	Tyr TAC	Leu CTT	Gly GGC	Gly GGT
7	2C10 Umbenhauer et al., 1987 †M15331	Leu CTT	Val GTC	Pro CCT	Arg CGT	Cys TGC	Phe TTT	Ser TCA	Glu GAA	Cys TGC	Ile ATT	Asp GAC	Gly GGA

Ω Of the 7 sequences proposed as CYP2C9 alleles shown in the above table, only sequence 1 was identified as a true allele in both Caucasians and Orientals (CYP2C9*1). Of the remaining sequences, none have been identified as they are presented here. Of sequences 3 and 4 which possess arginine at codon 144 (CYP2C9*2), none of the remaining changes have been identified. Similarly, although sequence 6 which contains leucine at codon 359 has been identified as a CYP2C9 allele (CYP2C9*3), the subsequent difference at codon 475 has not been identified.

* = previously reported as Ile (4) and Ser (6) respectively.
† = accession number for GenBank EMBL database.
‡ = cDNA not sequenced over this region.
§ = this cDNA sequence was rechecked and found to be as reported.

[ ] = 100% sequence homology between all CYP2C9 cDNAs.

[ ] = homology between two CYP2C9 cDNA sequences.

[ ] = alteration seen in one cDNA only.

has shown that CYP2C9 and associated allelic variants have very low catalytic activity towards this compound, and that this drug, now obsolete, is efficiently metabolized by CYP2C19 (Goldstein et al., 1994). However, CYP2C9 is responsible for the metabolism of a number of other clinically important drugs, including tolbutamide, phenytoin, diclofenac, mefanamic acid, S-warfarin, D 1-tetrahydrocannabinol, piroxicam, tenoxicam, tienilic acid, naproxen and ibuprofen (Relling et al.,

Table 2. cDNA sequences identified as CYP2C9 alleles in 100 Caucasian individuals (reproduced from Stubbins *et al.* 1996)

Codon	63	144	175	239	281	358	359	417
*CYP2C9*1*	Pro	Arg	Cys	Phe	Glu	Tyr	Ile	Gly
	(CCT)	(CGT)	(TGC)	(TTT)	(GAA)	(TAC)	(ATT)	(GGC)
*CYP2C9*2*	Pro	**Cys**	Cys	Phe	Glu	Tyr	Ile	Gly
	(CCT)	**(TGT)**	(TGC)	(TTT)	(GAA)	(TAC)	(ATT)	(GGC)
*CYP2C9*3*	Pro	Arg	Cys	Phe	Glu	Tyr	**Leu**	Gly
	(CCT)	(CGT)	(TGC)	(TTT)	(GAA)	(TAC)	**(CTT)**	(GGC)

1990; Page *et al.*, 1991; Rettie *et al.*, 1992; Goldstein & de Morais, 1994 and references therein; Miners *et al.*, 1995). In most individuals, CYP2C9 is the major CYP2C protein expressed in liver (Goldstein & de Morais, 1994), and a number of CYP2C9 cDNA clones have been isolated by several laboratories. To date, six distinct CYP2C9 cDNA sequences have been reported, which differ by nine single base substitutions (Table 1) (Kimura *et al.*, 1987; Yasumori *et al.*, 1987; Ged *et al.*, 1988; Meehan *et al.*, 1988; Romkes *et al.*, 1991).

The metabolism of tolbutamide and phenytoin by CYP2C9 is the major pathway of elimination of these drugs (Veronese *et al.*, 1991). Phenotyping studies have identified rare individuals with an impaired capacity to metabolize both tolbutamide and phenytoin (Kutt *et al.*, 1964; Scott & Poffenbarger, 1979; Vasko *et al.*, 1980; Vermeij *et al.*,

1988; Page *et al.*, 1991), indicating that there may be a genetic polymorphism at the CYP2C9 gene locus. Recently, PCR-based genotyping assays have elucidated the genetic basis for the CYP2C9 polymorphism in both Caucasian and Oriental populations (Wang *et al.*, 1995; Stubbins *et al.*, 1996; Sullivan-Klose *et al.*, 1996). Three alleles have been identified in Caucasians: CYP2C9*1, CYP2C9*2 and CYP2C9*3 (Table 2) (Stubbins *et al.*, 1996; Sullivan-Klose *et al.*, 1996). Of these, only CYP2C9*1 and CYP2C9*3 have been identified in Orientals (Wang *et al.*, 1995; Sullivan-Klose *et al.*, 1996). The frequencies of the various CYP2C9 alleles in various ethnic groups are summarized in Table 3.

CYP2C9*1 is the most common allele in all populations studied to date, with an allele frequency of 0.79-0.86 in Caucasians, 0.985 in African-Americans, and 0.97-0.98 in Orientals. A

Table 3. CYP2C9 genotyping studies shown with relative allele frequencies, study population and study size

Study name	Population (size)	Allele frequencies		
		CYP2C9*1	CYP2C9*2	CYP2C9*3
Wang et al., 1995	Oriental (135)	0.98	0	0.02
Stubbins et al., 1996	Caucasian (100)	0.79	0.125	0.085
Sullivan-Klose et al., 1996	Caucasian (100)	0.86	0.08	0.06
	African-American (100)	0.985	0.01	0.005
	Taiwanese (98)	0.974	0	0.026
Inoue et al., 1997	Caucasian (45)	0.86	0.11	0.03
	Japanese (39)	0.98	0	0.02

C → T nucleotide substitution at codon 144 in CYP2C9*1 leads to an Arg → Cys amino acid substitution creating CYP2C9*2 (Table 2). CYP2C9*2 has an allele frequency of 0.08-0.125 in Caucasians and 0.01 in African-Americans, but appears to be absent in Orientals (Table 3). An A → C substitution at codon 359 of CYP2C9*1 results in the conversion of Ile → Leu, creating CYP2C9*3 (Table 2). CYP2C9*3 occurs with an allele frequency of 0.03-0.085 in Caucasians, 0.005 in African-Americans and approximately 0.02 in Orientals (Table 3).

Preliminary evidence from the heterologous expression of each allelic variant in mammalian cells suggested that both CYP2C9*2 and CYP2C9*3 had altered abilities to metabolize CYP2C9 substrates (Kaminsky et al., 1993; Veronese et al., 1993). However, there are indications that it is the CYP2C9*3 allele which confers the "poor metabolizer" phenotype when present in homozygous form. Evidence from various laboratories has suggested that the homozygous CYP2C9*3 allele has poor catalytic activity for the oxidations of tolbutamide and phenytoin (Spielberg et al., 1996; Sullivan-Klose et al., 1996). Haining et al. (1996), using a baculovirus-mediated cDNA expressed CYP2C9, showed that this variant had a fivefold lower Vmax and a fivefold higher Km for S-warfarin. The observed activity differences may be explained by the localization of Ile359 in a region of the protein which has been associated with substrate binding (SRS 5) (Gotoh, 1992).

In addition, Sullivan-Klose et al. (1996) found that a patient diagnosed as a poor metabolizer of tolbutamide was homozygous for CYP2C9*3, lending more weight to the hypothesis that it is the CYP2C9*3 allele which confers the poor metabolizer phenotype. A second individual, exhibiting intermediate metabolism for tolbutamide, was heterozygous for CYP2C9*3. In contrast, preliminary results from our laboratory and those of Bhasker et al. (1997) suggest that there is no apparent correlation of genotype with the hydroxylation of phenytoin, tolbutamide, torasemide and diclofenac in human liver microsomes, although a cDNA-expressed variant containing Arg144/Leu359 has an almost fourfold higher Km than the Arg144/Ile359 or Cys144/Ile359 forms (Bhasker et al., 1997).

Only one study (London et al., 1996) has been presented on the association of CYP2C9 genotype with cancer susceptibility. It was based on the fact that CYP2C9 is known to play a role in the metabolism of the tobacco smoke carcinogen, benzo[a]pyrene, and on the possibility that an altered capacity to metabolize or detoxify this compound may alter an individual's predisposition to lung cancer. The investigators studied the frequency of the CYP2C9*2 allele in 329 incident cases of lung cancer (152 African-American and 177 Caucasian) and 700 population controls (239 African-American and 461 Caucasian). Their findings indicate that there is a slight but not statistically significant increase in the risk of developing lung cancer for both African-American and Caucasian populations. Further studies are needed to clarify the role of the CYP2C9 polymorphism in cancer susceptibility.

CYP2C18

The CYP2C18 cDNA was cloned from a human liver cDNA library screened with a cDNA for rat liver P450IIC13 (CYP2C13) and an oligonucleotide probe for human CYP2C8 (Romkes et al., 1991). Recombinant CYP2C18 is unable to metabolize most of the compounds known to be substrates for CYP2C9 and CYP2C19 and, although CYP2C18 is known to have some activity towards the CYP2C9 substrates tolbutamide and tienilic acid, no specific CYP2C18 substrates have yet been identified. In human liver the expression levels of CYP2C18 protein are appreciably lower than those of any of the other CYP2C proteins, and CYP2C18 mRNA is found at a level approximately seven to eight times lower in human liver than either CYP2C8 or CYP2C9 (Furuya et al., 1991). In the epidermis, however, the relative expression of the different CYP2C isoforms is reversed, with CYP2C18 representing the most abundant CYP2C enzyme at both the protein and mRNA level (Zaphiropoulos, 1997).

Two allelic variants of CYP2C18 have been isolated from the same cDNA library, differing by only a single nucleotide and resulting in a Met → Thr substitution at codon 385. A further variant CYP2C18 cDNA, containing six silent nucleotide differences and a single amino acid substitution (Phe219 → Leu), was isolated by PCR analysis of genomic DNA using primers generated from

CYP2C9 (Furuya *et al.*, 1991). Recently, a single base pair change has been identified in the 5'-flanking region of the CYP2C18 gene, which has an allele frequency of 21.4% in an Oriental population (Tsuneoka *et al.*, 1996). The incidence of this variant was found to be linked with the low-activity alleles of the polymorphic CYP2C19 gene (Tsuneoka *et al.*, 1996). In addition, a new non-functional CYP2C18 allele (2C18m1) has recently been identified in a Japanese population (Komai *et al.*, 1996). A T → A point substitution at position 204 of exon 2 results in an amino acid change from Tyr68 to a Stop codon. This produces an inactive truncated protein, only 67 amino acids in length (Komai *et al.*, 1996). In the same study a small Japanese population (n = 40) was genotyped for the presence of this allele, yielding an allele frequency of 0.275 for CYP2C18m1 (Komai *et al.*, 1996).

Detailed studies have not yet been performed for this P450 isoform. The phenotypic consequences of these variations in CYP2C18 sequence are, therefore, unknown.

It appears that alternative splicing may also play a role in the regulation of the CYP2C18 gene. In addition to observations from our own laboratory, a recent report has shown that not only is CYP2C18 the most abundant CYP2C protein found in human epidermis, but it is subject to a high degree of alternative splicing (Zaphiropoulos, 1997). By RT-PCR, several CYP2C18 mRNA species have been identified in the epidermis. In addition to the normal mRNA composed of nine exons, species lacking exons 4 or 5, exons 4, 5 and 6, and exons 4, 5, 6 and 7 were also detected. Alternative splicing has already been documented as a possible regulatory mechanism for the expression of cytochrome P450 genes CYP2B6 and CYP2A7 (Miles *et al.*, 1989, 1990; Yamano *et al.*, 1989; Ding *et al.*, 1995), and the same appears to be true for CYP2C18. The phenotypic consequences of possessing an alternatively spliced form of CYP2C18 in terms of drug metabolism are the subject of current investigation.

CYP2C19

The CYP2C19 cDNA was originally cloned from a human liver cDNA library screened with a cDNA for rat liver P450IIC13 and an oligonucleotide probe for human CYP2C8 (Romkes *et al*, 1991).

CYP2C19 has been identified as the major human S-mephenytoin 4'-hydroxylase (Goldstein *et al.*, 1994), but it is also responsible for the metabolism of a number of other commonly prescribed drugs, including omeprazole (Andersson *et al.*, 1992), proguanil (Ward *et al.*, 1991), certain barbiturates (Adedoyin *et al.*, 1994; Küpfer & Branch, 1985), citalopram (Sindrup *et al.*, 1993) and diazepam (Bertilsson *et al.*, 1989). A genetic polymorphism in the metabolism of S-mephenytoin is well documented (Küpfer & Preisig, 1984; Wedlund *et al.*, 1984; Wilkinson *et al.*, 1989), individuals having been classified as either poor metabolizers (PMs) or extensive metabolizers (EMs) of the drug. Individuals classed as EMs hydoxylate S-mephenytoin quickly, whilst the R-enantiomer remains in the body to be slowly eliminated. In PM individuals, both R-mephenytoin and S-mephenytoin tend to accumulate, leading to overdose toxicities following ordinary doses (Kalow, 1986). There are marked interethnic differences in PM frequency, ranging from 2-5% in Caucasians to 18-23% in Japanese (Nakamura *et al.*, 1985; Wilkinson *et al.*, 1989). The PM phenotype is inherited as an autosomal recessive trait (Inaba *et al.*, 1986; Ward *et al.*, 1987).

The major genetic defect leading to the PM phenotype is a single-base pair (G → A) substitution in exon 5 of CYP2C19 (CYP2C19m1) which introduces an alternative splice site and leads to aberrant splicing of the CYP2C19 mRNA from codon 215 (de Morais *et al.*, 1994a). Consequently, a premature stop codon is introduced 20 amino acids downstream of the splice site, leading to a truncated and non-functional protein (de Morais *et al.* 1994a). CYP2C19m1 accounts for approximately 80% of defective alleles in both Caucasian and Japanese populations.

A second gene-inactivating allele (CYP2C19m2) has recently been identified in Japanese populations (de Morais *et al.*, 1994b), where a G → A base substitution in exon 4 creates a premature stop codon at amino acid 212 (de Morais *et al.*, 1994b). In combination, CYP2C19m1 and CYP2C19m2 account for almost all Japanese PMs. The CYP2C19m2 allele has not, however, been identified in Caucasians, indicating the presence of one or more additional gene-inactivating CYP2C19 alleles. Indeed, preliminary findings by Ferguson *et al.* (1996) have identified a new rare mutant CYP2C19 allele (CYP2C19m3) in Caucasians, but this allele has not been extensively characterized. Xiao *et al.* (1997) compared the frequency of CYP2C19 alleles in two Chinese ethnic groups. Their findings indicate that CYP2C19 allele frequencies differ in Han and Bai Chinese populations, the former having a higher proportion of PMs and heterozygous EMs than the Bai population. In addition, a single individual phenotyped as a PM of *S*-mephenytoin was found to be heterozygous for CYP2C19m1 and a new allele (CYP2C19m4) with an amino acid substitution at codon 433 (Arg → Trp). Amino acid 433 lies in the haem-binding region of the protein and may produce an inactive protein (Xiao *et al.*, 1997).

In spite of the considerable interest in CYP2C19 the polymorphisms at this gene locus have not been significantly studied in relation to cancer susceptibility. The metabolic activation of tobacco compounds is known to be mediated by several P450 enzymes, but the precise metabolic pathways involved are still unclear. In this respect the role of CYP2C19 has not yet been determined, despite the fact that no tobacco smoke procarcinogens have been reported to be CYP2C19 substrates. In fact, only a few studies have so far been performed, the first of which (Ayesh & Idle, 1985) indicated no link between CYP2C19 activity and lung cancer, although it was performed on a very small population. More recently, a weak association has been reported between non-aggressive bladder cancer and high CYP2C19 activity (Kaisary *et al.*, 1987). Finally, work by Benhamou *et al.* (1997) confirmed the lack of association between CYP2C19 activity and lung cancer. In a study of 129 lung cancer patients and 159 controls (all male Caucasians), no significant interaction was observed between CYP2C19 activity and lung cancer susceptibility.

To our knowledge, no studies have yet been presented on the frequencies of the non-functional CYP2C19m1 or CYP2C19m2, or on the recently discovered CYP2C19m3 or m4 alleles in cancer populations. Such work may be of some importance, given recent evidence that yeast-expressed CYP2C19 has a major role to play in the accumulation of the proximate mutagen benzo(a)pyrene-7,8-dihydrodiol (Gautier *et al.*, 1996).

Members of the cytochrome P450 CYP2E gene suibfamily

The human CYP2E subfamily of P450 monooxygenases comprises a single gene, CYP2E1, localized to chromosome 10q24.3-qter (Song *et al.*, 1986; Kolble *et al.*, 1993). The CYP2E1 gene spans approximately 11.4 kb of genomic DNA and has a promoter region containing a basal transcription element (BTE) and several hepatocyte nuclear factor (HNF1) binding sites (Ingelman-Sundberg *et al.*, 1995). In rodent models the expression of CYP2E1 is regulated developmentally, hormonally and via mRNA and protein stabilization by the interplay of several distinct functional mechanisms (Gonzalez, 1990). Although human CYP2E1 gene expression is not as well characterized, at least some of the features of regulation in humans are thought to be similar to those of rodents (Perrot *et al.*, 1989).

CYP2E1

CYP2E1 has been the subject of much scientific attention due to its ubiquitous role in the metabolism and activation of an array of solvent carcinogens (which also act to induce its expression) such as N-nitrosamines, benzene, styrene, carbon tetrachloride, ethylene glycol and, most importantly, ethanol (Bartsch & Montesano, 1984; Hong & Yang, 1985; Wrighton *et al.*, 1986, 1987b; Yoo et al., 1988; Guengerich & Shimada, 1988; Guengerich *et al.*, 1991). CYP2E1 metabolizes and is induced by ethanol and catalyses its conversion to acetaldehyde (Gonzalez, 1988). As such, CYP2E1 has been implicated in the pathogenesis of a number of alcohol-related diseases, including alcoholism, cirrhosis and cancers of the oral cavity, nasopharynx, oesophagus, breast and stomach (Driver & Swan 1987; Yang *et al.*, 1990; Kato *et al.*, 1995; Lucas *et al.*, 1995; Hildesheim *et al.*, 1997). CYP2E1 is also responsible for the metabolism of a number of endogenous compounds, such as acetone and acetal. Furthermore, acetone has been proposed to be an endogenous CYP2E1 substrate (Koop & Casazza, 1985). Interindividual differences in both the catalytic activities (up to fiftyfold variation) and protein levels of CYP2E1 have been reported (Wrighton *et al.*, 1986; Yoo *et al.*, 1988).

Currently, there is much confusion about the role of various polymorphisms in the CYP2E1 gene in relation to cancer susceptibility. Several

Table 4. CYP2E1 genotyping studies for the *Rsa* I and *Dra* I RFLPs

Population	Population type	*Rsa* I - C2 (n)		*Dra* I - C (n)		Reference
African-American	Control	0.01	(252)	0.08	(228)	Stephens *et al.*, 1994
African-American	Control	0.02	(174)	na		Kato *et al.*, 1993
European-American	Control	0.04	(898)	0.11	(284)	Stephens *et al.*, 1994
European-American	Control	0.02	(214)	na		Kato *et al.*, 1993
Taiwanese	Control	0.28	(240)	0.24	(238)	Stephens *et al.*, 1994
Japanese	Control	0.19	(404)	na		Hayashi *et al.*, 1991
Japanese	Control	0.27	(98)	na		Kato *et al.*, 1993
Japanese	Control	na		0.26	(112)	Uematsu *et al.*, 1991a
Swedish	Control	0.05	(404)	0.10	(412)	Persson *et al.*, 1993
Finnish	Control	0.01	(242)	0.11	(242)	Hirvonen *et al.*, 1993
Japanese	Control	na		0.29	(152)	Uematsu *et al.*, 1994
Japanese	Lung cancer	na		0.25*	(182)	Uematsu *et al.*, 1994
Japanese	Digestive tract cancers	na		0.36	(90)	Uematsu *et al.*, 1994
Japanese	Control	0.203	(612)	na		Oyama *et al.*, 1997
Japanese	NSCLC	0.307	(126)	na		Oyama *et al.*, 1997
Chinese	Control	0.21	(320)	0.24	(320)	Hildesheim *et al.*, 1997
Chinese	Nasopharyngeal cancer	0.23	(364)	0.25	(364)	Hildesheim *et al.*, 1997
German Caucasian	Controls	0.029	(175)	0.087	(121)	Matthias *et al.*, 1998
German Caucasian	Oral/pharyngeal cancer	0.029	(122)	0.076	(118)	Matthias *et al.*, 1998
German Caucasian	Laryngeal cancer	0.035	(257)	0.076	(229)	Matthias *et al.*, 1998

n   Number of individuals studied.

*   Althought the overall frequency of the Dra I allele in the lung cancer population is not significantly changed, the frequency of individuals heterozygous for this allele is dramatically   increased from 28.9% to 46.2%.

NSCLC   Non-small-cell lung cancer.

variant sequences have been identified within this gene. RFLPs have been detected for *Taq* 1 (McBride *et al.*, 1987), *Rsa* I (Uematsu *et al.*, 1991a) and *Msp* I (Uematsu *et al.*, 1991c) in intronic sequences. Interestingly, *Pst* I and *Rsa* I RFLPs identify two further variant sequences in the 5′ untranslated region, and furthermore the *Rsa* I RFLP has been associated with an alteration in the transcriptional activation of the gene. It has been suggested that this base pair change leads to an altered interaction of the promoter region with the transcription factor HNF-1 (Watanabe *et al.*, 1990; Hayashi *et al.*, 1991). Finally, *Rsa* I and *Dra* I identify two additional variant sequences in introns 5 and 6 respectively (Uematsu *et al.*, 1991a,b).

Significant interethnic variation has been reported in the frequency of the RFLPs in the CYP2E1 gene (Table 4). For example, in control populations the *Dra* I RFLP, caused by a T → A transversion in intron 6, is present at an allele frequency of 0.08-0.11 in Caucasians and African-Americans (Persson *et al.*, 1993; Hirvonen *et al.*, 1993; Stephens *et al.*, 1994; Matthias *et al.*, 1998), but is present at a frequency of 0.24-0.29 in Oriental populations (Uematsu *et al.*, 1991a; Stephens *et al.*, 1994; Uematsu *et al.*, 1994; Hildesheim *et al.*, 1997) (Table 4). The same is true of the *Rsa* I RFLP, the frequency range being 0.01-0.05 in African-Americans and Caucasian controls (Hirvonen *et al.*, 1993; Kato *et al.*, 1993; Persson *et al.*, 1993; Stephens *et al.*, 1994; Matthias *et al.*,

1998) and 0.19-0.28 in Oriental populations (Hayashi *et al.*, 1991; Kato *et al.*, 1993; Stephens *et al.*, 1994; Hildesheim *et al.*, 1997; Oyama *et al.*, 1997) (Table 4). There have been contradictory and inconclusive reports associating this allele with susceptibility to lung cancer and exposure to smoking (Uematsu *et al.*, 1994); these results need further clarification (Table 4). A large case-control study was recently carried out by Matthias *et al.* (1998) to investigate polymorphisms in a number of drug- metabolizing enzymes and susceptibility to tobacco-related cancers of the aerodigestive tract. Their findings indicated no association of CYP2E1 genotypes with these cancers. Finally, the *Rsa* I polymorphism has been associated with susceptibility to nasopharyngeal cancer (Hildesheim *et al.*, 1997) in a population of non-smokers, where possession of homozygous c2 alleles conferred a 9.3-fold increased risk of disease in comparison with individuals homozygous for the c1 allele (Hildesheim *et al.*, 1997).

There has also been a report of a higher frequency of the *Dra* I RFLP in other alcohol- related diseases (Lucas *et al.*, 1996): in a study of 260 controls and 511 alcoholics, an increase was found in its frequency from 0.079 in controls to 0.141 in alcoholics without clinical symptoms and to 0.125 in alcoholics with clinical symptoms.

Recently, two new CYP2E1 gene variants have been described with differences in the coding sequence of the gene (Hu *et al.*, 1997). CYP2E1*2 contains a G → A substitution at nucleotide 1168, converting Arg76 → His, whilst CYP2E1*3 contains a G → A substitution in exon 8, converting Val389 → Ile. The corresponding cDNAs have been cloned and expressed in COS-1 cells, and levels of CYP2E1 mRNA, protein and rate of chlorzoxazone hydroxylation have been measured. The results of this analysis suggest that whilst CYP2E1*3 has almost identical properties to the wild-type cDNA, CYP2E1*2 only produces roughly one third of the protein expression and one third of the catalytic activity compared to the wild-type enzyme, whilst yielding similar amounts of mRNA (Hu *et al.*, 1997). Screening a total population of 198 individuals indicated that these variants were rare, only two of 78 Chinese control subjects being homozygous for CYP2E1*2, and only one of 42 Italian alcoholic cirrhosis subjects possessing a heterozygous

CYP2E1*3 allele (Hu *et al.*, 1997). Further studies are needed to clarify the extent of the associations of the CYP2E1 polymorphisms with cancer susceptibility.

The highly functionally conserved nature of CYP2E1 indicates that it may have an important endogenous role in addition to its functions in the metabolism of xenobiotics. Lee *et al.* (1996) generated a mouse line lacking Cyp2e1 expression. The Cyp2e1 knockout mice were found to be fertile and did not exhibit any physical abnormalities, indicating that the Cyp2e1 gene is not required for mammalian development and normal physiology. Differences between these knockout animals and wild-type mice only became apparent following treatment with the analgesic acetaminophen (paracetamol). In this case the mice lacking Cyp2e1 expression appeared to be less sensitive to the hepatotoxic effects of this drug than those possessing the Cyp2e1 enzyme. These results tend to indicate that Cyp2e1 is the principal enzyme responsible for the activation of acetaminophen to its active, hepatotoxic metabolite. Mice lacking the enzyme would be protected from the toxic effects of this drug since they would be unable to form the toxic metabolite (Lee *et al.*, 1996).

The association of CYP2E1 with cancer susceptibility is still unclear. This situation can only be resolved by more intensive studies.

Members of the cytochrome P450 CYP3A gene subfamily

The CYP3 gene cluster is located on chromosome 7q22-qter (Spurr *et al.*, 1989). It encodes at least four highly homologous genes for which cDNAs have previously been reported: CYP3A3 (P450HLp, or hPCN2) (Molowa *et al.*, 1986), CYP3A4 (NF10, NF25 and hPCN1) (Beaune *et al.*, 1986; Gonzalez *et al.*, 1988; Bork *et al.*, 1989), which is expressed postnatally in all human livers, CYP3A5 (hPCN3, or P450HLp2) (Aoyama *et al.*, 1989; Schuetz *et al.*, 1989), and CYP3A7 (P450HFL33) (Komori *et al.*, 1989a,b). Two CYP3A proteins have also been purified from human adult and fetal liver respectively: CYP3A4 (P450NF) and CYP3A7 (P450HFLa) (Guengerich *et al.*, 1986; Kitada *et al.*, 1987). The different gene products of the CYP3 locus are involved in a wide number of reactions, including human liver oxidation of nifedipine (Guengerich *et al.*, 1986a), quinidine (Guengerich *et al.*, 1986b) and midazolam (Kronbach *et al.*, 1989), the 2- and 4-hydroxylation of 17β-estradiol (Guengerich *et al.*, 1986a; Ball *et al.*, 1990), the 6β-hydroxylation of testosterone, the metabolism of cyclosporin A (Kronbach *et al.*, 1988; Aoyama *et al.*, 1989), aldrin epoxidation and several other reactions involving dihydroxypyrimidine compounds. Enzymes from the CYP3 family (predominantly CYP3A4) are major components of the total hepatic P450 content and can be induced by glucocorticoids, phenobarbital-like compounds and macrolide antibiotics (Wrighton *et al.*, 1985). CYP3A3, CYP3A4, CYP3A5 and CYP3A7 share over 85% sequence homology at the amino acid level and are encoded by relatively large genes, a single gene spanning approximately 30 kb of genomic DNA (Hashimoto *et al.*, 1993; Kolars *et al.*, 1994).

Members of this subfamily not only constitute the major P450s in human liver but are also expressed in extrahepatic tissues. By far the major CYP3A protein in human liver is CYP3A4, whereas CYP3A5 is the major form found in the stomach (Kolars *et al.*, 1994). By Northern Blot analysis, only CYP3A4 has been detected throughout the length of the digestive tract, but using reverse transcriptase-polymerase chain reaction (RT-PCR) analysis, both CYP3A4 and CYP3A5 mRNA species have been detected, whilst CYP3A7 has been consistently found only in the liver (Kolars *et al.*, 1994). It was recently demonstrated that the use of RT-PCR could detect CYP3A3/4 and CYP3A5, but not CYP3A7 mRNA, in human placenta (Hakkola *et al.*, 1996).

Polycyclic aromatic hydrocarbons (PAHs) are some of the most potent chemical carcinogens known, and accordingly much effort has been given to the study of the metabolism of the PAH carcinogen benzo(a)pyrene (BaP) in human liver. However, until relatively recently no consensus had been reached on which definitive P450 isozymes were responsible for the major route of metabolism of BaP - that of 3-hydroxylation (Hall *et al.*, 1989). With a view to easing the degree of speculation surrounding this matter, Yun (1992) studied a panel of 21 human liver microsomal samples. The findings indicated that in samples exhibiting high BaP 3-hydroxylation activity, this

could be attributed to members of the P450 2C and 3A gene families. The data are supported by work with inhibitory chemicals and antibodies and by the high correlation between rates of BaP 3-hydroxylation and nifedipine oxidation - a marker for CYP3A4 activity. Since CYP3A4 is known to be the major P450 isozyme expressed in adult human liver (Forrester *et al.*, 1992) it would appear to play a significant role in BaP 3-hydroxylation in this organ. Because it has been shown that members of the CYP3A subfamily of P450 isozymes are important in the metabolism of BaP, it is important to summarize the evidence that a genetic mechanism is responsible for the wide interindividual variation in the metabolism of a number of CYP3A family substrates. For example, the well-characterized substrate nifedipine (a calcium channel blocker) has been shown in various studies to exhibit wide individual variation in its disposition (Kleinbloesem *et al.*, 1984); 17% of the Dutch population studied was classified as phenotypically deficient in the first step of nifedipine metabolism.

Exposure to the potent carcinogen aflatoxin B1 (AFB1) is strongly correlated with the incidence of liver cancer in many areas of Africa and Asia. Activation of AFB1 to metabolites having mutagenic properties is known to involve members of the CYP3A family of enzymes (Aoyama *et al.*, 1990; Forrester *et al.*, 1990b). Using vaccinia virus-expressed human hepatic CYP3A3 and CYP3A4, it has been demonstrated that both of these isozymes activate AFB1 to mutagenic metabolites (assessed by the production of His revertants of *Salmonella typhimurium* in the Ames test) and additionally catalyse the conversion of AFB1 to DNA-bound derivatives (Aoyama *et al.*, 1990). It should be noted, however, that although CYP3A family members probably play an important role in AFB1 activation, several other cytochrome P450 forms have the capacity to activate this toxin (Forrester *et al.*, 1990b).

CYP3A3

The CYP3A3 and CYP3A4 genes are highly homologous, sharing 97% amino acid sequence homology (Table 5) (Gonzalez *et al.*, 1988). It has been suspected for some time that CYP3A3 is either a variant allele of CYP3A4 or a cloning artefact, and is not the product of an entirely separate

Table 5. Published differences in *CYP3A3/CYP3A4* cDNA sequences

Allele	Sites of nucleotide amino acid differences																Source of sequence
	3	72	92	105	106	164	187	193	200	203	224	225	252	279/280	392	431	
CYP3A3	CTC / Leu	TGG / Trp	CTA / Leu	CGC / Arg	GAG / Glu	CGA / Arg	TCA / Ser	GTC / Val	CAG / Gln	CTT / Leu	ACA / Thr	GTC / Val	GCT / Ala	CAT AAG / His Lys	TGG / Trp	ATA / Ile	*CYP3A3*
#NF10¥	CTC / Leu	TGG / Trp	ACA / Thr	CGG / Arg	AGG / Arg	GCA / Ala	ACA / Thr	ATC / Ile	CAA / Gln	TTT / Phe	ATC / Ile		TC T / Ser	CAG / Gln	TGG / Trp	ACA / Thr	Bork (1989) †J04449
#NF25‡¥	CTC / Leu	TGG / Trp	ACA / Thr	CGG / Arg	AGG / Arg	GCA / Ala	ACA / Thr	ATC / Ile	CAA / Gln	TTT / Phe	ACA / Thr	GTC / Val	TCT / Ser	CAG / Gln	TGG / Trp	ATA / Ile	Beaune (1986) †M14096
#hPCN1‡**	CTC / Leu	TGG / Trp	ACA / Thr	CGG / Arg	AGG / Arg	GCA / Ala	ACA / Thr	ATC / Ile	CAA / Gln	TTT / Phe	ACA / Thr	GTC / Val	TCT / Ser	CAG / Gln	GTG / Val	ATA / Ile	Gonzalez (1988) †M18907

\# = All expressed in yeast (Peyronneau *et al.*, 1993); ¥ = Different clones from the same cDNA library;
‡ = Functionally equivalent alleles; † = accession number for GenBank EMBL database;
**Clone hPCN1 was found to be identical to another clone isolated by Spurr *et al.*, 1989 (†X12387).

gene. CYP3A3 shares a number of common substrates with CYP3A4, including the endogenous steroids progesterone and androstenedione (Aoyama *et al.*, 1989), as well as a number of commonly prescribed drugs - nifedipine, erythromycin, lidocaine, cyclosporin and tamoxifen (Kronbach *et al.*, 1989; Schuetz *et al.*, 1994). In fact, no unique substrates have been identified for CYP3A3, and it will be interesting to ascertain whether CYP3A3 is either an allelic variant of CYP3A4, a separate gene product, or an artefact of cloning. Until this question has been resolved, no association can be made between CYP3A3 and cancer susceptibility.

CYP3A4

CYP3A4 encodes a 52 kDa protein responsible for the metabolism of a wide variety of substrates including nifedipine, a dihydropyrimidine calcium antagonist and vasodilator (Guengerich *et al.*, 1986), erythromycin, troleandomycin, quinidine, cyclosporin A, 17α-ethynylestradiol, lido-

caine and diltiazem (Peyronneau *et al.*, 1993, and references therein). The level of expression of CYP3A4 has been studied in human liver samples and has been shown to vary up to sixtyfold (Forrester *et al.*, 1992). Several cDNA clones related to CYP3A4 have been isolated (Table 5): NF25 (Beaune *et al.*, 1986) and NF10 (Bork *et al.*, 1989) were both isolated by using polyclonal and monoclonal antibodies raised against P450NF to screen the same human liver cDNA library, while hPCN1 (Gonzalez *et al.*, 1988) was isolated from another cDNA library using the rat P450PCN1 as a probe. There are only three amino acid differences between these three cDNA sequences (Table 5).

All three CYP3A4 variants have been expressed in *S. cerevisiae*, and substrate binding affinities and catalytic activities have been calculated for a range of substrates (Peyronneau *et al.*, 1993). In terms of binding affinities, it was found that the two amino acid differences (Trp392 and Thr431 in NF25 → Val392 and Ile431 in hPCN1 (Table 5)) have no effect on substrate binding with the substrates erythralosamine 2'-monobenzoate (2'-MBEM), cyclosporin and dihydroergotamine, but in the cases of testosterone and erythralosamine small but significant differences in substrate binding were detected. In contrast however, P450 NF10, which differs from both NF25 and hPCN1 by a single amino acid deletion immediately adjacent to the splice acceptor site of intron 7 (Ile224 replaces Thr224-Val225), was produced as a denatured form (P450 NF10 always showed a reduced CO-binding spectrum with an absorption maximum around 420 nm, characteristic of a denatured P450), and no detectable difference spectra were produced in good agreement with the hypothesis of a denatured protein unable to bind haem (Peyronneau et al., 1993). In catalytic activity studies using nifedipine, lidocaine, quinidine and testosterone, no catalytic activity could be detected for P450 NF10, as expected because of the lack of absorption at 450 nm of the protein. Yeast microsomes containing P450 NF25 and hPCN1, however, displayed typical and comparable CYP3A4 catalytic activities towards all the tested substrates, although P450 hPCN1 was always found to be slightly less active than P450 NF25 by a factor of ~1.5 (Peyronneau et al., 1993).

Due to the proximity of the single amino acid deletion in P450 NF10 to the intron 7/exon 8 boundary, this variant could be the result of alternative mRNA splicing - a mechanism that has already been shown to affect the expression of several cytochrome P450 genes (Miles et al., 1989, 1990; Ding et al., 1995). In many cases, although the aberrantly spliced mRNA can be translated into a truncated protein, its haem-binding capacity is lost and therefore the protein cannot function as a P450 monooxygenase (Kimura et al., 1989). For example, the transcript of human CYP2B6 is also alternatively spliced, and at least three mRNA species are derived from this gene (Miles et al., 1989, 1990). Preliminary results from our own laboratory suggest that the NF10 cDNA sequence either does not exist in a Scottish Caucasian population or that it is a very rare allele. It would therefore be unable to account for the large interindividual variation in the metabolism of nifedipine. These results, however, do not preclude the possibility of a genetic polymorphism in the CYP3A4 gene, and further investigation is needed to ascertain whether such a polymorphism exists and, if it does, its association with cancer susceptibility.

CYP3A5

The CYP3A5 gene encodes a 502 amino acid, 57.1 kDa protein which shares 84% amino acid and 89% nucleotide sequence homology with CYP3A4. CYP3A5 was reported to be expressed in 10-20% of human livers (Aoyama et al., 1989). Intriguingly, it has been reported that CYP3A5 is present in a statistically significantly higher percentage of children and adolescents as compared with the remaining population (Wrighton et al., 1990). The full-length CYP3A5 cDNA was cloned from a human liver library constructed from RNA extracted from a liver known to express only CYP3A5 probed with a P450 hPCN1 probe (Aoyama et al., 1989). Enzymatic assays involving the use of recombinant vaccinia virus-expressed CYP3A4 and CYP3A5 in HepG2 cells have shown that both enzymes are similarly active in the oxidation of nifedipine. Both enzymes also catalysed the 6β-hydroxylation of the steroid hormones testosterone, progesterone and androstenedione, but CYP3A4 exhibited expressed activity that was several times higher than that of CYP3A5. In addition it was noted that several minor steroid oxidation products were formed (e.g. 15β-hydroxytestosterone) by the expressed CYP3A4 but not by CYP3A5, indicating that CYP3A5 is a more highly regiospecific monooxygenase catalyst with steroid substrates (Aoyama et al., 1989). Differences were also noted in the metabolism of cyclosporine: two hydroxylated metabolites and one demethylated metabolite were formed by CYP3A4, whereas only one metabolite was formed by CYP3A5. It can be concluded that CYP3A5 is differentially expressed in the adult human population and has overlapping substrate specificity with CYP3A4 in terms of steroid and drug substrates (Aoyama et al., 1989).

Evidence for the extrahepatic expression of CYP3A5 is now rapidly accumulating. Haehner et al. (1996) determined the expression of mRNAs corresponding to CYP3A3, CYP3A4, CYP3A5 and CYP3A7 in human kidney by RT-PCR. All kidneys examined expressed CYP3A5 protein and contained the corresponding mRNA. CYP3A4 mRNA was detected in 40% of the kidney samples, and

70% of those that contained detectable CYP3A4 mRNA also expressed detectable levels of the corresponding protein. Therefore, in contrast to hepatic tissue, where CYP3A4 is ubiquitously expressed, in renal tissue it is the CYP3A5 protein that is the universally expressed member of the CYP3A subfamily. A similar situation appears to be true in human lung, where, by immunohistochemistry and RT-PCR analysis, CYP3A5 has been identified as the predominant CYP3A form, with CYP3A4 only present in 20% of individuals (Anttila et al., 1997). Using similar techniques, the relative expression of CYP3A isoforms in human colonic tissue has been investigated (Gervot et al., 1996). By immunoblot and iso-electric focusing experiments, CYP3A5 was identified as the principal CYP3A protein present in human colon, whilst by RT-PCR the CYP3A5 mRNA was also found to be the most abundant CYP3A mRNA (Gervot et al., 1996).

A role for CYP3A5 in the variability of nifedipine oxidation cannot be precluded, but a possible mechanism has yet to be established. In addition, the mechanism of regulation of the CYP3A5 gene is still uncertain and remains an important focus for future study.

The alcohol and aldehyde dehydrogenase enzymes

Although alcohol consumption has been established as a risk factor for the development of oesophageal cancer, the mechanisms by which alcohol induces this high-mortality cancer have not yet been determined. In all likelihood, as is the case for the majority of diseases, there will be a complex interplay of both genetic and environmental factors in the etiology of this one. Two families of enzymes may be of particular importance in the metabolism of alcohol. Polymorphic expression of both alcohol and aldehyde dehydrogenases (ADH and ALDH) is well documented; both alcohol and acetaldehyde are implicated in the pathogenesis of liver, breast and colon cancers, and of cancers of the larynx, pharynx and oesophagus in humans. In man, five members of the ADH family have been characterized, two of which are polymorphic (ADH2 and ADH3) (Smith et al., 1986; Bosron et al., 1986). In addition there are five ALDH genes, the mitochondrial ALDH2 gene being subject to a well-defined, dominant

genetic defect in approximately 50% of Orientals (this defect is rarely seen in other ethnic groups) (Crabb et al., 1989; Ehrig et al., 1990). The ALDH2 gene encodes an enzyme that is critical for the elimination of acetaldehyde generated by the consumption of alcohol. The polymorphism in ALDH2 is highly prevalent and the mutant allele ALDH2*2 is inactive. Yokoyama et al. (1996) have carried out a study focusing on patients with oesophageal squamous cell carcinoma. They examined DNA from a small group of alcoholics (40 cases with oesophageal SCC and 55 controls) and non-alcoholic drinkers (29 cases and 28 controls) and concluded that there was a substantially higher risk of developing oesophageal cancer in those individuals who possessed the ALDH2*2 gene in both of the groups tested (alcoholics and non-alcoholic drinkers). If substantiated, these results would suggest that because people who possess a mutant ALDH2*2 allele have a high concentration of blood acetaldehyde after drinking alcohol, acetaldehyde (a recognized animal carcinogen) plays a role in the pathogenesis of alcohol-related oesophageal cancer in humans (Yokoyama et al., 1996). It is possible that individuals who possess the mutant ALDH2*2 allele may decrease their risk of developing the cancer if they decrease their alcohol consumption.

Katsuki et al. (1996) utilized a mutant strain of Long-Evans rats (Long-Evans cinamon rats (LEC)) to investigate the metabolism of ethanol, having previously established that these rats displayed spontaneous hepatitis and liver cancer and died of acute ethanol intoxication after being fed a liquid diet containing 5% ethanol. The concentration of ethanol in the blood of the LEC rats was higher than that in Wistar rats, indicating that ethanol oxidation was impaired in the LEC rats. However, while the expression of CYP2E1 was the same as in the Wistar rats, both ADH and ALDH activities were remarkably suppressed in LEC rat liver. When the decrease in the activity of the ADH enzyme was further investigated it was found that a 9 CA repeat insertion and a point mutation were present in the first intron of a class I ADH gene. These results suggest a more important role for the ADH (and possibly ALDH) genes in the susceptibility to alcohol-related disease than for CYP2E1, but they need to be substantiated by more detailed genetic analysis in humans.

In the case of ethanol metabolism it is obvious that an individual's susceptibility to cancer is determined by a complex interplay of factors. For any individual a detailed analysis of the CYP2E1, ALDH and ADH genes is needed, together with detailed genotype-phenotype correlations, if a meaningful measure of susceptibility to alcohol-related cancers is to be made.

Microsomal epoxide hydroxylase

Microsomal epoxide hydrolase (mEH) is involved in Phase I metabolism, and is capable of catalysing the hydrolysis a wide variety of highly reactive epoxide intermediates to produce more water-soluble trans-dihydrodiol derivatives (Hassett et al., 1994). This enzyme is widely distributed, being present in most cell types and tissues, and is highly inducible (Oesch, 1973; Omiecinski et al., 1993). Epidemiological studies have shown that mEH activity in the liver, lung and peripheral blood leukocytes is subject to a fiftyfold interindividual variation in white populations (Omiecinski et al., 1993; Hassett et al., 1997).

Interestingly, two allelic variants of mEH have been reported to date (Hassett et al., 1994). Both mutant alleles arise because of discrete point mutations which lead to amino acid changes: Tyr113 → His and His139 → Arg (Hassett et al., 1994). The conversion of Tyr113 → His has been reported to increase mEH activity by 25%, whilst the His139 → Arg substitution has been shown to decrease mEH activity by up to 40% (Hassett et al., 1994). The result of these polymorphisms is therefore to produce four metabolic phenotypes in the population - fast, normal, slow and very slow hydrolase activities, dependant on the specific genotypic combination. However, from transient transfection studies using constructed cDNAs of the different mEH alleles it appears that the amino acid substitutions may affect protein stability (Hassett et al., 1994). Hassett et al. (1997) showed that hepatic mEH enzyme activity and corresponding mEH protein content exhibited approximately eightfold interindividual variation, but this variation was poorly correlated with mEH RNA levels. Using genotyping assays to screen for the two alleles, they found that the polymorphisms did not exclusively predict mEH phenotype in the tissue samples examined. These results tend to indicate that there are as yet unidentified factors that influence mEH protein levels and activity. The factors may be genetic but may also involve protein stability or differences in the translational efficiency of the polymorphic mRNA transcripts.

Few data have been presented which indicate that the polymorphisms in mEH can affect susceptibility to cancer. It should be noted that mEH has been implicated in both protection against and potentiation of the effects of chemical carcinogens. Of particular interest is the fact that substrates for this enzyme include procarcinogenic epoxide metabolites of polycyclic aromatic hydrocarbons, and as such the polymorphism identified could have an important role in determining the susceptibility of an individual to cancer. Only one study has set out to prove a link between the mEH polymorphisms and a disease phenotype. A recent investigation into the association between the mEH polymorphisms and susceptibility to lung disease was carried out by Smith and Harrison (1997). The results indicated a fourfold to fivefold increase in the frequency of the very slow phenotype in populations suffering from either chronic obstructive pulmonary disorder or emphysema, when compared with controls. In addition a slight but non-significant increase in the frequency of the very slow phenotype in lung cancer patients was reported. However, this study involved only 50 individuals and needs to be substantiated by more detailed case-control studies.

Myeloperoxidase

Myeloperoxidase (MPO) is a glycosylated lysosomal enzyme located in the azurophilic (primary) granules of polymorphonuclear neutrophils (PMNs) and monocytes, where it comprises 3-5% of the total cell protein (Weil et al., 1987). It is a haemoprotein that functions as an oxidative antimicrobial agent by catalysing the generation of hypochlorous acid (HOCl, a potent microbicide) and other reactive oxygen species from hydrogen peroxide and chloride anions during phagocytosis. The highly toxic compounds generated by such reactions contribute significantly to the overall cytotoxic function of PMNs (Selsted et al., 1993). MPO gene expression is restricted to the myeloid lineage and is highest in bone marrow precursors, peaking at the promyelocyte stage (Fouret *et al.*, 1989).

The human MPO gene has been cloned and characterized. It has been shown to span 10 kb of genomic DNA on chromosome 17q11-q21 (Weil *et al.*, 1987) and to consist of 12 exons (Chang *et al.*, 1986; Johnson *et al.*, 1987; Kizaki *et al.*, 1994; Morishita *et al.*, 1987; Yamada *et al.*, 1987; Weil *et al.*, 1987). Structural analyses have shown that the MPO gene encodes a 745 amino acid, 83 kDa precursor polypeptide that is posttranslationally processed to yield a 13.5 kDa light chain and a 59 kDa heavy chain subunit. The MPO holoenzyme exists as a tetramer composed of two heavy and two light chain subunits, with a combined size of 150 kDa (Andrew *et al.*, 1981; Anderson *et al.*; 1982; Morishita *et al.*, 1987; Olsen *et al.*, 1984). Exposure to environmental insults, including tobacco smoke, stimulates the recruitment of neutrophils into human lung tissue (Humminghake *et al.*, 1990) with the local release of MPO (London *et al.*, 1997; Schmekel *et al.*, 1990). MPO activates various carcinogens associated with tobacco smoking, among them benzo[*a*]pyrene (Mallet *et al.*, 1991) and aromatic amines (Kadlubar *et al.*, 1992). A lack of this enzyme may therefore have serious consequences for an individual's susceptibility to cancer.

A deficiency of MPO can be either acquired or congenital. The congenital condition affects between 1 in 2000 and 1 in 4000 individuals in the USA (Parry *et al.*, 1981). A genetic basis for congenital MPO deficiency has been elucidated (Nauseef *et al.*, Kizaki *et al.*, 1994). The genetic defect consists of a point mutation at codon 569 (R569W), converting arginine (CGG) to tryptophan (TGG). It has been predicted that this amino acid substitution affects posttranslational processing of the protein and the folding and/or stability of the encoded protein (Kizaki *et al.*, 1994). Acquired MPO deficiency is a common feature of certain myeloid and lymphoid leukaemias (Bendix-Hensen *et al.*, 1983) as well as of myelodysplastic syndromes (Bendix-Hensen *et al.*, 1986).

As regards the acquired form of MPO deficiency, a single base pair (G → A) polymorphism in the 5' untranslated region of the gene was originally identified by Austin *et al.* (1993) as a somatic mutation found in acute myelocytic leukaemia bone marrow cells but not in normal bone marrow cells. Subsequently, it was discovered that this mutation was actually a polymorphism in an Alu repeat of the promoter region of the gene (Piedrafita *et al.*, 1996). The polymorphism is situated in a cluster of hormone response elements 463 bp upstream of the MPO gene (-463G/A), and the two alleles have been termed Sp (-463G) and N (-463A). This region of the Alu repeat contains an exact match for the 10 bp consensus core binding site for the SP1 transcription factor (TGAGGC_GGGT) only in individuals possessing the Sp (-463G) allele. Piedrafita *et al.* (1996) also demonstrated that the possession of each allele had functional significance *in vitro*, as demonstrated by transcription reporter gene assays, where the presence of the SP1 element (Sp allele) increased the transcription of a reporter gene 25-fold. This would lead to decreased transactivation in individuals possessing the N allele (Piedrafita *et al.*, 1996). Indeed, although the original classification of this polymorphism as a mutation was incorrect, both studies investigating the association of acute myeloid leukemia (AML) with MPO have shown an increase in the prevalence of the homozygous SpSp genotype in AML cases (Austin *et al.*, 1993; Piedrafita *et al.*, 1996). A further study (Reynolds *et al.*, 1997) has shown that the homozygous SpSp genotype is correlated with increased MPO mRNA levels in primary myeloid leukemia cells and that this higher expressing SpSp genotype is overrepresented in defined subtypes of leukaemia, suggesting that higher levels of MPO are associated with an increased risk for these subtypes. Further work is needed, but these lines of evidence support the hypothesis of a link between MPO expression and AML.

Preliminary data have shown that this polymorphism may also affect susceptibility to lung cancer (London *et al.*, 1997). In an age- and sex-matched study involving 703 controls (244 African-Americans and 459 Caucasians) and 339 lung cancer patients (157 African-Americans and 182 Caucasians) it was found that Caucasians with the homozygous N genotype (approximately 8% of the population) were at 70% reduced risk of lung cancer, while African-Americans with the same genotype (9.4%) were at 39% reduced risk of lung cancer (London *et al.*, 1997). These preliminary results need to be substantiated by further studies.

NAD(P)H:quinone oxidoreductase

NAD(P)H:quinone oxidoreductase (NQO1) (EC.1.6.99.2), also termed DT-diaphorase, is a ubiquitously expressed homodimeric flavoenzyme for which two roles have been proposed: (1) to protect cells from the toxic effects of quinones, quinone amines and their precursors (Lind *et al.*, 1982; Jaiswal, 1991); and (2) to carry out the bioactivation of certain procarcinogens (Traver *et al.*, 1992). The enzyme is characterized by its ability to catalyse the two electron reduction of quinones such as mitomycin C (Siegel *et al.*, 1990a) and diaziquone (Siegel *et al.*, 1990b), and of other anticancer agents (Ernster, 1967; Traver *et al.*, 1992; Gasdaska *et al.*, 1995). It differs from other quinone reductases in being able to use either NADH or NADPH as a cofactor (Edwards *et al.*, 1980). The reductive activation of several quinone-containing antitumour agents by NQO1 causes DNA damage to cells, either by alkylation or by oxidative stress, and leads to cell toxicity (Riley *et al.*, 1992; Workman, 1994).

The human NQO1 gene has been cloned and found to consist of six exons spanning 20 kb of genomic DNA (Jaiswal *et al.*, 1988) on chromosome 16q2.2 (Rosvold *et al.*, 1995; Schulz *et al.*, 1997). This gene encodes a protein of 273 amino acids (Jaiswal, 1991). The role of NQO1 in cellular protection is supported by the findings that NQO1 activity is greater in tumour tissue than in normal tissue of the same origin (Schor *et al.*, 1983; Schlager *et al.*, 1990), and that NQO1 specifically prevents the formation of benzo[*a*]pyrene quinone-DNA adducts generated by CYP1A1 and P450 reductase (Joseph *et al.*, 1994).

Traver *et al.* (1992) demonstrated that variation in NQO1 enzyme activity was related to sequence differences at the NQO1 locus. They identified a C → T point mutation in the coding region of the NQO1 gene in a human colon cancer cell line (BE cells) which lacked NQO1 enzyme activity but had high levels of gene expression. This single base substitution (C609 → T) occurs in exon 6 of the gene, causing the conversion of Pro187 → Ser (Traver *et al.*, 1992; Rosvold *et al.*, 1995). Three phenotypes are possible in terms of NQO1 activity: (a) individuals homozygous for the Pro187 → Ser mutation completely lack NQO1 activity; (b) individuals heterozygous at this gene locus experience an approximately threefold decrease in quinone reductase activity; and (c) individuals possessing homozygous Pro187 alleles retain wild-type NQO1 activity (Kuehl *et al.*, 1995).

Rosvold *et al.* (1995) ascertained that the identified C609 → T NQO1 mutation was, in fact, a polymorphism present at a frequency of 0.13 in the general population. The Ser187 variant was consequently classified as a true allele of NQO1 and was termed the null allele because of its lack of activity (Schulz *et al.*, 1997). Having determined that the Ser187 polymorphism was a true allele of NQO1, Rosvold *et al.* (1995) screened a population of 150 lung cancer patients for this polymorphism. The frequency of the NQO1 null allele varied from 0.13 in the Centre d'Etude Polymorphisme Humain (CEPH) reference panel (n = 82), to 0.22 in the lung cancer patient group (n = 150), indicating that this polymorphism was possibly of particular importance in the susceptibility of individuals to lung cancer .

Rosvold *et al.* (1995) carried out the same type of analysis on an additional small Caucasian population (n = 77) in which individuals had no previous history of cancer. When the population was stratified according to smoking status an intriguing result was obtained. As with the lung cancer patients and the CEPH population, a shift from a null allele frequency of 0.14 in the non-smoking group (n = 37) to a frequency of 0.26 for the smokers (n = 40) was observed. This finding must be substantiated with a larger number of individuals in a study specifically designed to investigate the effect in question.

These results, however, contrast with those found in a recent study conducted in Mexican-Americans and African-Americans (Wiencke *et al.*, 1997). In this study, an increase in the frequency of the Pro187 genotype was observed in 177 lung cancer patients from both ethnic backgrounds, when compared with 297 control individuals. Furthermore, it was found that the Pro187 genotype was twice as common among African-Americans than among Mexican-Americans (Wiencke *et al.*, 1997). Overall, the results indicate that this polymorphism, in common with a number of the other metabolic polymorphisms mentioned in this Chapter, is subject to significant interethnic variation. Further studies are needed to verify the role of each genotype in respect of cancer susceptibility in each ethnic group.

Schulz et al. (1997) investigated the association of this polymorphism with urological malignancies in a German population. Their findings are very similar to those of Rosvold et al. (1995) in lung cancer patients. In 260 control individuals the frequency of the null allele was found to be 0.133, whereas in 131 patients with renal cell carcinoma it was 0.191 and in 99 patients with urothelial cell carcinoma it was 0.182. These results, taken together with those of Rosvold et al. (1995), support the hypothesis that this polymorphism, and hence insufficient NQO1 activity, may be an important factor in determining an individual's susceptibility to cancer.

In the latter stages of benzene metabolism, NQO1 is responsible for the conversion of the highly haematotoxic and genotoxic benzoquinones to less toxic hydroxy metabolites (Ross, 1996). Rothman et al. (1997) investigated whether decreased NQO1 activity could predispose an individual to benzene poisoning, a diagnosis strongly associated with the subsequent development of haematological malignancies and non-malignant related disorders. In a Chinese population of 49 benzene-exposed workers, the frequency of individuals homozygous for the NQO1 null allele was 0.41, and this was subsequently found to be almost double the frequency (23) in 48 control individuals who were not exposed to benzene. In addition to calculating the frequency of the NQO1 polymorphism this study measured the frequency of CYP2E1 polymorphisms and obtained an estimate of CYP2E1 enzyme activity on the basis of the fractional excretion of chlorzoxazone. Taken together, the results indicated that, although the CYP2E1 genotype did not influence the risk of benzene poisoning, subjects with both a rapid clearance of chlorzoxazone and homozygous NQO1 null alleles had a risk of benzene poisoning which was increased by a factor of 7.6 in comparison with individuals having a slow clearance of chlorzoxazone and possessing either of the two remaining NQO1 genotypes.

Further studies are needed if we are to be able to clearly evaluate the role of the NQO1 polymorphism in cancer susceptibility. In view of the observation that this polymorphism is of particular importance in conjuction with exposure to certain chemicals (e.g. tobacco smoke, benzene) it may prove to be relevant to cancer susceptibility only when an individual is exposed to such chemicals.

Sulfotransferases

Although sulfation has been recognized for over a hundred years as an important conjugation reaction, interest in the sulfotransferase (ST) family of enzymes has expanded only during the last ten years (Coughtrie et al., 1996). It has become increasingly clear that sulfation is an important mechanism in the modulation of both endogenous and exogenous bioactive and possibly carcinogenic molecules. In general the addition of a sulfate moiety decreases the biological activity of a compound and increases its polarity, thereby facilitating excretion from the body (Falany et al., 1991). However, the STs are also capable of activating aromatic amines, benzylic alcohols of polycyclic aromatic hydrocarbons and many other carcinogens (reviewed in Miller, 1994). STs fall into two major classes, the phenol sulfotransferases (PSTs), which include the estrogen ST (EST) and the hydroxysteroid (or alcohol) sulfotransferases (HSTs). STs catalyse the transfer of the sulfate moiety from the active donor molecule 3'-phosphoadenosine 5'-phosphosulfate (PAPS) to an appropriate acceptor compound, forming a sulfate ester (Jones et al., 1993).

Five human cytosolic STs have been characterized: an EST, an HST and three PSTs. Interindividual variation in human ST expression has been reported (Weinshilboum et al., 1997). Two isoforms of PST have been characterized in human tissues: a thermostable (often termed phenol-metabolizing) form and a thermolabile (often termed monoamine-metabolizing) form, which differ in their substrate specificity, inhibitor sensitivity, thermal stability and regulation (Raftogianis et al., 1996 and references therein). The association of polymorphisms in sulfotransferase genes with susceptibility to cancer has not been studied in great detail, but new RFLPs and allelic variants have recently been identified

(Jones *et al.*, 1995, 1996; Wood *et al.*, 1996; Zhu *et al.*, 1996). It will be interesting to see if any of these polymorphisms relate to cancer susceptibility, given that the enzymes are capable of bioactivating a wide range of carcinogenic compounds.

Conclusions

The use of PCR-based assays to determine an individual's genotype with respect to polymorphism in specific drug-metabolizing enzymes affords a specific insight into the field of susceptibility to various genetically based diseases, including cancer. This Chapter has outlined recent work on some of the less extensively studied enzymes involved in drug metabolism, and has considered what additional studies are required in order to draw more accurate conclusions on individual susceptibility to cancer. As molecular biology and automation continue to develop more accurate and faster techniques for this type of analysis it should prove possible to screen even larger disease and control populations with a view to clarifying some of the preliminary observations mentioned here.

We have described metabolic polymorphisms that have not been discussed in other sections of the book. Almost by definition the present Chapter deals with polymorphisms, often recently identified, which have not been studied in detail with respect to genotype-phenotype correlations or to disease susceptibility. Indeed the phenotypic consequences of allelic variants have not, in certain areas, been established. One aim of this section is to identify further genes for future susceptibility studies. It is important to note that polymorphisms in genes not involved in carcinogen metabolism, which are vital elements in tumour initiation and progression, such as those of repair enzymes, are virtually unstudied in relation to susceptibility to cancers that do not exhibit a strong familial trait. This also represents an important area for future study.

References

Adedoyin, A., Prakash, C., O'Shea, D., Blair, I.A. & Wilkinson, G.R. (1994) Stereoselective disposition of hexobarbital and its metabolites: relationship to the S-mephenytoin polymorphism in Caucasian and Chinese subjects. *Pharmacogenetics*, 4, 27-38

Andersen, M.R., Atkin, C.L. & Eyre, H.L. (1982) Intact form of myeloperoxidase from normal human neutrophils. *Arch.Biochem.Biophys.*, 214, 273-283

Andersson, T., Regardh, C.G., Lou, Y.C., Zhang, Y., Dahl, M.L. & Bertilsson, L. (1992) Polymorphic hydroxylation of S-mephenytoin and omeprazole metabolism in Caucasian and Chinese subjects. *Pharmacogenetics*, 2, 25-31

Andrews, P.C. & Krinsky, N.I. (1981) The reductive cleavage of myeloperoxidase in half, producing enzymatically active hemi-myeloperoxidase. *J. Biol. Chem.*, 256, 4211-4218

Anttila, S., Hukkanen, J., Hakkola, J., Stjernvall, T., Beaune, P.H., Edwards, R.J., Boobis, A.R., Pelkonen, O. & Raunio, H. (1997) Expression and localisation of CYP3A4 and CYP3A5 in human lung. *Am. J. Respir. Cell Mol. Biol.*, 16, 242-249

Aoyama, T., Yamano, S., Waxman, D.J., Lapenson, D.P., Meyer, U.A., Fischer, V., Tyndale, R., Inaba, T., Kalow, W., Gelboin, H.V. & Gonzalez, F.J. (1989) Cytochrome P-450 hPCN3, a novel cytochrome P-450 IIIA gene product that is differentially expressed in adult human liver. cDNA and deduced amino acid sequence and distinct specificities of cDNA-expressed hPCN1 and hPCN3 for the metabolism of steroid hormones and cyclosporine. *J. Biol. Chem.*, 264, 10388-10395

Aoyama, T., Yamano, S., Guzelian, P.S., Gelboin, H.V. & Gonzalez, F.J. (1990) Five of 12 forms of vaccinia virus-expressed human hepatic cytochrome P450 metabolically activate aflatoxin B1. *Proc.Natl. Acad. Sci. USA*, 87, 4790-4793

Austin, G.E., Lam, L., Zaki, S.R., Chan, W.C., Hodge, T., Hou, J., Swan, D., Zhang, W., Racine, M., Whitsett, C. & Brown, B. (1993) Sequence comparison of putative regulatory DNA of the 5-flanking region of the myeloperoxidase gene in normal and leukaemic bone marrow cells. *Leukemia*, 7, 1445-1450

Ayesh, R. & Idle, J.R. (1985) Evaluation of drug oxidation phenotypes in the biochemical epidemiology of lung cancer risk. In: Boobis, A.R.,

Cladwell, J., De Matteis, F. & Elcombe, C.R., eds, *Microsomes and Drug Oxidations*. London, Taylor & Francis, pp. 340-346

Ball, S.E., Forrester, L.M., Wolf, C.R. & Back, D.J. (1990) Differences in the cytochrome P-450 isoenzymes involved in the 2-hydroxylation of estradiol and 17α- ethinylestradiol. Relative activities of rat and human liver enzymes. *Biochem. J.*, 267, 221-226

Bartsch, H. & Montesano, R. (1984) Relevance of nitrosamines to human cancer. *Carcinogenesis*, 5, 1381-1393

Beaune, P.H., Umbenhauer, D.R., Bork, R.W., Lloyd, R.S. & Guengerich, F.P. (1986) Isolation and sequence determination of a cDNA clone related to human cytochrome P-450 nifedipine oxidase. *Proc. Natl. Acad. Sci. USA*, 83, 8064-8068

Bendix-Hensen, K. (1986) Myeloperoxidase-deficient polymorphonuclear leukocytes (VII): Incidence in untreated myeloproliferative disorders. *Scand.J. Haematol.*, 36, 3-7

Bendix-Hensen, K. & Nielson, H.K. (1983) Myeloperoxidase-deficient polymorphonuclear leukocytes (I): incidence in untreated myeloid leukaemia, lymphoid leukaemia, and normal humans. *Scand.J. Haematol.*, 30, 415-419

Benhamou, S., Bouchardy, C. & Dayer, P. (1997) Lung cancer risk in relation to mephenytoin hydroxylation activity. *Pharmacogenetics*, 7, 157-159

Bertilsson, L., Henthorn, T.K., Sanz, E., Tybring, G., Sawe, J. & Villen, T. (1989) Importance of genetic factors in the regulation of diazepam metabolism: relationship to S-mephenytoin, but not debrisoquin, hydroxylation phenotype. *Clin. Pharmacol. Ther.*, 45, 348-355

Bhasker, C.R., Miners, J.O., Coulter, S. & Birkett, D.J. (1997) Allelic and functional variability of cytochrome P4502C9. *Pharmacogenetics*, 7, 51-58

Bork, R.W., Muto, T., Beaune, P.H., Srivastava, P.K., Lloyd, R.S. & Guengerich, F.P. (1989) Characterization of mRNA species related to human liver cytochrome P-450 nifedipine oxidase and the regulation of catalytic activity. *J. Biol. Chem.*, 264, 910-919

Bosron, W.F. & Li, T.K. (1986) Genetic polymorphism of human liver alcohol and aldehyde dehydrogenases, and their relationship to alcohol metabolism and alcoholism. *Hepatology*, 6, 502-510

Burke, M.D., Thompson, S., Weaver, R.J., Wolf, C.R. & Mayer, R.T. (1994) Cytochrome P450 specificities of alkoxyresorufin O-dealkylation in human and rat liver. *Biochem. Pharmacol.*, 48, 923-936

Chang, K.S., Trujillo, J.M., Cook, R.G. & Stass, S.A. (1986) Human myeloperoxidase gene: molecular cloning and expression in leukemia cells. *Blood*, 68, 1411-1414

Chang, T.K., Weber, G.F., Crespi, C.L. & Waxman, D.J. (1993) Differential activation of cyclophosphamide and ifosphamide by cytochromes P-450 2B and 3A in human liver microsomes. *Cancer Res.*, 53, 5629-5637

Coughtrie, M.W.H. (1996) Sulfation catalysed by the human cytosolic sulfotransferases - chemical defence or molecular terrorism? *Hum. Exp. Toxicol.*, 15, 547-555

Crabb, D.W., Edenberg, H.J., Bosron, W.F. & Li, T.K. (1989) Genotypes for aldehyde dehydrogenase deficiency and alcohol sensitivity. The inactive ALDH2(2) allele is dominant. *J. Clin. Invest.*, 83, 314-316

de Morais, S.M., Schweikl, H., Blaisdell, J. & Goldstein, J.A. (1993) Gene structure and upstream regulatory regions of human CYP2C9 and CYP2C18. *Biochem. Biophys. Res. Commun.*, 94, 194-201

de Morais, S.M., Wilkinson, G.R., Blaisdell, J., Nakamura, K., Meyer, U.A. & Goldstein, J.A. (1994a) The major genetic defect responsible for the polymorphism of S-mephenytoin metabolism in humans. *J. Biol. Chem.*, 269, 15419-15422 de Morais, S.M., Wilkinson, G.R., Blaisdell, J., Meyer, U.A., Nakamura, K. & Goldstein, J.A. (1994b) Identification of a new genetic defect responsible for the polymorphism of (S)-mephenytoin metabolism in Japanese. *Mol. Pharmacol.*, 46, 594-598

Ding, S., Lake, B.G., Friedberg, T. & Wolf, C.R. (1995) Expression and alternative splicing of the cytochrome P-450 CYP2A7. *Biochem. J.*, 306, 161-166

Driver, H.E. & Swan, R.F. (1987) Alcohol and human cancer: a review. *Anticancer Res.*, 7, 309-320.

Edwards, Y.H., Potter, J. & Hopkinson, D.A. (1980) Human FAD-dependent NAD(P)H diaphorasel. *Biochem. J.*, 187, 429-436

Ehrig, T., Bosron, W.F. & Li, T.K. (1990) Alcohol and aldehyde dehydrogenase. *Alcohol*, 25, 105-116

Ernster, L. (1967) DT-diaphorase. *Methods Enzymol.*, 10, 309-317

Falany, C.N. (1991) Molecular enzymology of human liver cytosolic sulfotransferases. *Trends Pharmacol. Sci.*, 12, 255-259

Ferguson, R.J., De Morais, S.M.F., Benhamou, S., Bouchardy, C., Blaisdell, J., Wilkinson, G.R., Linko, P., Dayer, P. & Goldstein, J.A. (1996) A novel genetic defect of human CYP2C19 responsible for poor metabolism of S-mephenytoin. Presented at ISSX (San Diego, CA)

Forrester, L.M. & Wolf, C.R. (1990a) Genetic susceptibility to environmental insults. In: Cohen, R.D., Lewis, B., Alberti, K.G.M.M. & Denman, A.M., eds, *The Metabolic and Molecular Basis of Acquired Disease*. London, Baillière Tindall, pp. 3-18

Forrester, L.M., Neal, G.E., Judah, D.J., Glancey, M.J. & Wolf, C.R. (1990b) Evidence for involvement of multiple forms of cytochrome P-450 in aflatoxin B1 metabolism in human liver. *Proc. Natl. Acad. Sci. USA*, 87, 8306-8310

Forrester, L.M., Henderson, C.J., Glancey, M.J., Back, D.J., Park, B.K., Ball, S.E., Kitteringham, N.R., McLaren, A.W., Miles, J.S., Skett, P. & Wolf, C.R. (1992) Relative expression of cytochrome P450 isoenzymes in human liver and association with the metabolism of drugs and xenobiotics. *Biochem. J.*, 281, 359-368

Fouret, P., du Bois, R.M., Bernaudin, J.F., Takahashi, H., Ferrans, V.J. & Crystal, R.G. (1989) Expression of the neutrophil elastase gene during human bone marrow cell differentiation. *J. Exp. Med.*, 169, 833-840

Furuya, H., Meyer, U.A., Gelboin, H.V. & Gonzalez, F.J. (1991) Polymerase chain reaction-directed identification, cloning, and quantification of human CYP2C18 mRNA. *Mol. Pharmacol.*, 40, 375-382

Gasdaska, P.Y., Fisher, H. & Powis, G. (1995) An alternatively spliced form of NQO1 (DT-diaphorase) messenger RNA lacking the putative quinone substrate binding site is present in human normal and tumour tissues. *Cancer Res.*, 55, 2542-2547

Gautier, J.-C., Lecoeur, S., Cosme, J., Perret, A., Urban, P., Beaune, P. & Pompon, D. (1996) Contribution of human cytochrome P450 to benzo(a)pyrene and benzo(a)pyrene-7,8-dihydrodiol metabolism, as predicted from heterologous expression in yeast. *Pharmacogenetics*, 6, 489-499

Ged, C., Umbenhauer, D.R., Bellew, T.M., Bork, R.W., Srivastava, P.K., Shinriki, N., Lloyd, R.S. & Guengerich, F.P. (1988) Characterization of cDNAs, mRNAs, and proteins related to human liver microsomal cytochrome P-450 (S)-mephenytoin 4'-hydroxylase. *Biochemistry*, 27, 6929-6940

Gervot, L., Carriere, V., Costet, P., Cugnenc, P.H., Berger, A., Beaune, P.H. & Dewaziers, I. (1996) CYP3A5 is the major cytochrome-P450 3A expressed in human colon and colonic cell lines. *Environ. Toxicol. Pharmacol.*, 2, 381-388

Goldstein, J.A. & De Morais, S.M. (1994a) Biochemistry and molecular biology of the human CYP2C subfamily. *Pharmacogenetics*, 4, 285-299

Goldstein, J.A., Faletto, M.B., Romkes, S.M., Sullivan, T., Kitareewan, S., Raucy, J.L., Lasker, J.M. & Ghanayem, B.I. (1994b) Evidence that CYP2C19 is the major (S)-mephenytoin 4'-hydroxylase in humans. *Biochemistry*, 33, 1743-1752

Gonzalez, F.J. (1988) The molecular biology of cytochrome P450s. *Pharmacol. Rev.*, 40, 243-288

Gonzalez, F.J. & Nebert, D.W. (1990) Evolution of the P450 gene superfamily. *Trends Genet.*, 6, 182-186

Gonzalez, F.J., Schmid, B.J., Umeno, M., Mcbride, O.W., Hardwick, J.P., Meyer, U.A., Gelboin, H.V. & Idle, J.R. (1988) Human P450PCN1: sequence, chromosome localization, and direct evidence through cDNA expression that P450PCN1 is nifedipine oxidase. *DNA*, 7, 79-86

Gotoh, O. (1992) Substrate recognition sites in cytochrome P450 family 2 (CYP2) proteins inferred from comparative analyses of amino acid and coding nucleotide sequences. *J. Biol. Chem.*, 267, 83-90

Gray, I.C., Nobile, C., Muresu, R., Ford, S. & Spurr, N.K. (1995) A 2.4-megabase physical map spanning the CYP2C gene cluster on chromosome 10q24. *Genomics*, 28, 328-332

Guengerich, F.P., Kim, D.-H. & Iwasaki, M. (1991) Role of human cytochrome P-450 IIE1 in the oxidation of many low-molecular-weight cancer suspects. *Chem. Res. Toxicol.*, 4, 168-179

Guengerich, F.P., Martin, M.V., Beaune, P.H., Kremers, P., Wolff, T. & Waxman, D.J. (1986a) Characterization of rat and human liver microsomal cytochrome P-450 forms involved in nifedipine oxidation, a prototype for genetic polymorphism in oxidative drug metabolism. *J. Biol. Chem.*, 261, 5051-5060

Guengerich, F.P., Muller, E.D. & Blair, I.A. (1986b) Oxidation of quinidine by human liver cytochrome P-450. *Mol. Pharmacol.*, 30, 287-295

Guengerich, F.P. & Shimada, T. (1991) Oxidation of toxic and carcinogenic chemicals by human cytochrome P-450 enzymes. *Chem. Res. Toxicol.*, 4, 391-407

Haehner, B.D., Gorski, J.C., Vandenbranden, M., Wrighton, S.A., Janardan, S.K., Watkins, P.B. & Hall, S.D. (1996) Bimodal distribution of renal cytochrome-p450 3a activity in humans. *Mol. Pharmacol.*, 50, 52-59

Haining, R.L., Hunter, A.P., Veronese, M.E., Trager, W.F. & Rettie, A.E. (1996) Allelic variants of human cytochrome P450 2C9: baculovirus-mediated expression, purification, structural characterization, substrate stereoselectivity and prochiral selectivity of the wild-type and I359L mutant forms. *Arch. Biochem. Biophys.*, 333, 447-458

Hakkola, J., Pasanen, M., Hukkanen, J., Pelkonen, O., Maenpaa, J., Edwards, R.J., Boobis, A.R. & Raunio, H. (1996) Expression of xenobiotic-metabolizing cytochrome P450 forms in human full-term placenta. *Biochem. Pharmacol.*, 51, 403-411

Hall, M., Forrester, L.M., Parker, D.K., Grover, P.L. & Wolf, C.R. (1989) Relative contribution of various forms of cytochrome P450 to the metabolism of benzo[a]pyrene by human liver microsomes. *Carcinogenesis*, 10, 1815-1821

Hashimoto, H., Toide, K., Kitamura, R., Fujita, M., Tagawa, S., Itoh, S. & Kamataki, T. (1993) Gene structure of CYP3A4, an adult-specific form of cytochrome P450 in human livers, and its transcriptional control. *Eur. J. Biochem.*, 218, 585-595

Hassett, C., Aicher, L., Sidhu, J.S. & Omiecinski, C.J. (1994) Human microsomal epoxide hydrolase: genetic polymorphism and functional expression *in vitro* of amino acid variants. *Hum. Mol. Genet.*, 3, 421-428

Hassett, C., Lin, J., Carty, C.L., Laurenzana, E.M. & Omiecinski, C.J. (1997) Human hepatic microsomal epoxide hydrolase: comparative analysis of polymorphic expression. *Arch. Biochem. Biophys.*, 337, 275-283

Hayashi, S., Watanabe, J. & Kawajiri, K. (1991) Genetic polymorphisms in the 5'-flanking region change transcriptional regulation of the human cytochrome P450IIE1 gene. *J. Biochem.Tokyo*, 110, 559-565

Hildesheim, A., Anderson, L., Chen, C.-J., Cheng, Y.-J. Brinton, L.A., Daly, A.K., Reed, C.D., Chen, I.-H., Caporaso, N.E., Hsu, M.-M., Chen, J.-Y., Idle, J.R., Hoover, R.N., Yang, C.-S. & Chhabra, S.K. (1997) CYP2E1 genetic polymorphisms and risk of nasopharyngeal carcinoma in Taiwan. *J. Natl. Cancer Inst.*, 89, 1207-1212

Hirvonen, A., Husgafvel-Pursiainen, K., Anttila, S., Kavjalainen, A. & Vainio, H. (1993) The human CYP2E1 gene and lung cancer: Dra I and Rsa I restriction fragment length polymorphism in a Finnish study population. *Carcinogenesis*, 14, 85-88

Hoffman, S.M.G., Fernandez-Salguero, P., Gonzalez, F.J. & Mohrenweiser, H.W. (1995) Organization and evolution of the cytochrome P450 *CYP2A-2B-2F* subfamily gene cluster on human chromosome 19. *J. Mol. Evol.*, 41, 894-900

Hong, J. & Yang, C.S. (1985) The nature of microsomal *N*-nitrosodimethylamine demethylase and its role in carcinogen activation. *Carcinogenesis*, 6, 1805-1809

Hu, Y., Oscarson, M., Johansson, I., Yue, Q.Y., Dahl, M.L., Tabone, M., Arinco, S., Albano, E. & Ingelman-Sundberg, M. (1997) Genetic polymorphism of human CYP2E1 - characterization of 2 variant alleles. *Mol. Pharmacol.*, 51, 370-376

Humminghake, G.W. & Crystal, R.G. (1990) Cigarette smoking and lung destruction: acculmulation of neutrophils in the lungs of cigarette smokers. *Am. Rev. Respir. Dis.*, 128, 833-838

Inaba, T., Jurima, M. & Kalow, W. (1986) Family studies of mephenytoin hydroxylation deficiency. *Am. J. Hum. Genet.*, 38, 768-772

Ingelman-Sundberg, M. & Johansson, I. (1995) The molecular genetics of the human drug-metabolizing cytochrome P450s. In: Pacifici,

G.M. & Fracchia, G.N., eds, *Advances in Drug Metabolism in Man.* Luxembourg, European Commission, pp.543-586

Inoue, K., Yamazaki, H., Imiya, K., Akasaka, S., Guengerich, F.P. & Shimada, T. (1997) Relationship between *CYP2C9* and *2C19* genotypes and tolbutamide methyl hydroxylation and *S*-mephenytoin 4'-hydroxylation activities in livers of Japanese and Caucasian populations. *Pharmacogenetics*, 7, 103-113

Jaiswal, A.K. (1991) Human NAD(P)H:quinone oxidoreductase (*NQO1*) gene structure and induction by dioxin. *Biochemistry*, 30, 10647-10653

Jaiswal, A.K., McBride, O.W., Adesnik, M. & Nebert, D.W. (1988) Human dioxin-inducible cytosolic NAD(P)H:Menadione oxidoreductase. *J. Biol. Chem.*, 263, 13572-13578

Johnson, K.R., Nauseef, W.M., Care, A., Wheelock, M.J., Shane, S., Hudson, S., Koeffler, H.P., Selsted, M.E., Miller, C.W. & Rovera, G. (1987) Characterization of cDNA clones for human myeloperoxidase: Predicted amino acid sequence and evidence for multiple mRNA species. *Nucleic Acids Res.*, 15, 2013-2028

Jones, A.L., Roberts, R.C. & Coughtrie, M.W.H. (1993) The human phenolsulfotransferase polymorphism is determined by the level of expression of the enzyme protein. *Biochem. J.*, 296, 287-290

Jones, A.L., Hagen, M., Coughtrie, M.W., Roberts, R.C. & Glatt, H. (1995) Human platelet phenol-sulfotransferases: cDNA cloning, stable expression in V79 cells and identification of a novel allelic variant of the phenol-sulfating form. *Biochem. Biophys. Res. Commun.*, 208, 855-862

Jones, A.L., Roberts, R.C. & Coughtrie, M.W. (1996) Detection of a SacI restriction fragment length polymorphism at the human phenol-sulphotransferase locus. *Clin. Genet.*, 49, 164-165

Joseph, P. & Jaiswal, A.K. (1994) NAD(P)H:-quinone oxidoreductase (DT diaphorase) specifically prevents the formation of benzo[*a*]pyrene quinone-DNA adducts generated by cytochrome P4501A1 and P450 reductase. *Proc. Natl. Acad. Sci. USA*, 91, 8413-8417

Kadlubar, F.F., Butler, M.A., Kaderlik, K.R., Chou, H.C. & Lang N.P. (1992) Polymorphisms for aromatic amine metabolism in humans: relevance for human carcinogenesis. *Environ. Health Perspect.*, 98, 69-74

Kaisary, A., Smith, P., Jacqz, E., McAllister, C.B., Wilkinson, G.R., Ray, W.A. & Branch, R.A. (1987) Genetic predisposition to bladder cancer: ability to hydroxylate debrisoquine and mephenytoin as risk factors. *Cancer Res.*, 47, 5488-5493

Kalow, B. (1986) The genetic defect of mephenytoin hydroxylation. *Xenobiotica*, 16, 379-389

Kaminsky, L.S., de Morais, S.M.F., Faletto, M.B., Dunbar, D.A. & Goldstein, J.A. (1993) Correlation of human cytochrome P4502C substrate specificities with primary structure: warfarin as a probe. *Mol. Pharmacol.*, 43, 234-239

Karam, W.G. & Chiang, J.Y. (1992) Polymorphisms of human cholesterol 7 alpha-hydroxylase. *Biochem. Biophys. Res. Commun.*, 185, 588-595

Kato, S., Onda, M., Matsukura, N., Tokunaga, A., Tajiri, T., Kim, D.Y., Tsuruta, H., Matsuda, N., Yamashita, K. & Shields, P.G. (1995) Cytochrome P4502E1 (CYP2E1) genetic polymorphism in a case-control study of gastric cancer and liver disease. *Pharmacogenetics*, 5, 141-144

Kato, S., Shields, P.G., Caporaso, N.E., Hoover, R.N., Trump, B.F., Sugimura, H., Weston, A. & Harris, C.C. (1992) Cytochrome P450IIE1 genetic polymorphisms, racial variation, and lung cancer risk. *Cancer Res.*, 52, 6712-6715

Katsuki, S., Kato, J., Nakajima, M., Inui, N., Sasaki, K., Kohgo, Y. & Niitsu, Y. (1996) Analysis of ca repeats in first intron of class-I ADH gene in Long-Evans cinnamon rats developing fatal intoxication after ethanol intake. *Alcoholism - Clin. Exp. Res.*, 20, A33-A35

Kerr, B.M., Thummel, K.E., Wurden, C.J., Klein, S.M., Kroetz, D.L., Gonzalez, F.J. & Levy, R.H. (1994) Human liver carbamazepine metabolism. Role of CYP3A4 and CYP2C8 in 10,11-epoxide formation. *Biochem. Pharmacol.*, 47, 1969-1979

Kimura, H., Sogawa, K., Sakai, Y. & Fujii, K.Y. (1989) Alternative splicing mechanism in a cytochrome P-450 (P-450PB-1) gene generates the two mRNAs coding for proteins of different functions. *J. Biol. Chem.y*, 264, 2338-2342

Kimura, S., Pastewka, J., Gelboin, H.V. & Gonzalez, F.J. (1987) cDNA and amino acid sequences of two members of the human P450IIC gene subfamily. *Nucleic Acids Res.*, 15, 10053-10054

Kitada, M., Kamataki, T., Itahashi, K., Rikihisa, T. & Kanakubo, Y. (1987) P-450 HFLa, a form of cytochrome P-450 purified from human fetal livers, is the 16 alpha-hydroxylase of dehydroepiandrosterone 3-sulfate. *J. Biol. Chem.*, 262, 13534-13537

Kizaki, M., Miller, C.W., Selsted, M.E. & Koeffler, H.P. (1994) Myeloperoxidase (MPO) gene mutation in hereditary MPO deficiency. *Blood*, 83, 1935-1940

Kleinbloesem, C.H., van, B.P., Faber, H., Danhof, M., Vermeulen, N.P. & Breimer, D.D. (1984) Variability in nifedipine pharmacokinetics and dynamics: a new oxidation polymorphism in man. *Biochem. Pharmacol.*, 33, 3721-4

Kolars, J.C., Lown, K.S., Schmiedlin, R.P., Ghosh, M., Fang, C., Wrighton, S.A., Merion, R.M. & Watkins, P.B. (1994) CYP3A gene expression in human gut epithelium. *Pharmacogenetics*, 4, 247-259

Kolble, K. (1993) Regional mapping of short tandem repeats on human chromosome 10: cytochrome P450 gene CYP2E, D10S196, D10S220, and D10S225. *Genomics*, 18, 702-704

Komai, K., Sumida, K., Kaneko, H. & Nakatsuka, I. (1996) Identification of a new non-functional CYP2C18 allele in Japanese: substitution of T204 to A in exon 2 generates a premature stop codon. *Pharmacogenetics*, 6, 117-119

Komori, M., Nishio, K., Fujitani, T., Ohi, H., Kitada, M., Mima, S., Itahashi, K. & Kamataki, T. (1989a) Isolation of a new human fetal liver cytochrome P450 cDNA clone: evidence for expression of a limited number of forms of cytochrome P450 in human fetal livers. *Arch. Biochem. Biophys.*, 272, 219-225

Komori, M., Nishio, K., Ohi, H., Kitada, M. & Kamataki, T. (1989b) Molecular cloning and sequence analysis of cDNA containing the entire coding region for human fetal liver cytochrome P-450. *J. Biochem.Tokyo*, 105, 161-163

Koop, D.R. & Casazza, J.P. (1985) Identification of ethanol-inducible P-450 isozyme 3a as the acetone and acetol monooxygenase of rabbit microsomes. *J. Biol. Chem.*, 260, 13607-13612

Kronbach, T., Fischer, V. & Meyer, U.A. (1988) Cyclosporine metabolism in human liver: identification of a cytochrome P-450III gene family as the major cyclosporine-metabolizing enzyme explains interactions of cyclosporine with other drugs. *Clin. Pharmacol.Ther.*, 43, 630-635

Kronbach, T., Mathys, D., Umeno, M., Gonzalez, F.J. & Meyer, U.A. (1989) Oxidation of midazolam and triazolam by human liver cytochrome P450IIIA4. *Mol. Pharmacol.*, 36, 89-96

Kuehl, B.L., Paterson, J.W., Peacock, J.W., Paterson, M.C. & Rauth, A.M. (1995) Presence of a heterozygous substitution and its relationship to DT-diaphorase activity. *Br. J. Cancer*, 72, 555-561

Küpfer, A. & Branch, R.A. (1985) Stereoselective mephobarbital hydroxylation cosegregates with mephenytoin hydroxylation. *Clin. Pharmacol. Ther.*, 38, 414-418

Küpfer, A. & Preisig, R. (1984) Pharmacogenetics of mephenytoin: a new drug hydroxylation polymorphism in man. *Eur. J. Clin. Pharmacol.*, 26, 753-759

Kutt, H., Wolk, M., Scherman, R. & McDowell, F. (1964) Insufficient parahydroxylation as a cause of diphenylhydantoin toxicity. *Neurology*, 14, 542-548

Lee, K.D., Baek, S.J. & Shen, R.F. (1994) Cloning and characterization of the human thromboxane synthase gene promoter. *Biochem. Biophys. Res. Commun.*, 201, 379-387

Lee, S.S., Buters, J.T., Pineau, T., Fernandez-Salguero, P. & Gonzalez, F.J. (1996) Role of CYP2E1 in the hepatotoxicity of acetaminophen. *J. Biol. Chem.*, 271, 12063-12067

Leo, M.A., Lasker, J.M., Raucy, J.L., Kim, C.I., Black, M. & Lieber, C.S. (1989) Metabolism of retinol and retinoic acid by human liver cytochrome P450IIC8. *Arch. Biochem. Biophys.*, 269, 305-312

Lind, C., Hochstein, P. & Ernster, L. (1982) DT-diaphorase as a quinone reductase: a cellular control device against semiquinone and superoxide radical formation. *Arch. Biochem. Biophys.*, 216, 178-185

Lind, C., Cadenas, E., Hochstein, P. & Ernster, L. (1990) DT-diaphorase: Purification, properties and function. *Methods Enzymol.*, 186, 287-301

London, S.J., Daly, A.K., Leathart, J.B.S., Navidi, W.C. & Idle, J.R. (1996) Lung cancer risk in relation to the *CYP2C9*1/CYP2C9*2* genetic polymorphism among African-Americans and Caucasians in Los Angeles County, California. *Pharmacogenetics*, 6, 527-533

London, S.J., Lehman, T.A. & Taylor, J.A. (1997) Myeloperoxidase genetic polymorphism and lung cancer risk. *Cancer Res.*, 57, 5001-5003

Lucas, D., Menez, C., Floch, F., Gourlaouen, Y., Sparfel, O., Joannet, I., Bodenez, P., Jezequel, J., Gouerou, H., Berthou, F., Bardou, L.G. & Menez, J.F. (1996) Cytochromes P4502E1 and P4501A1 genotypes and susceptibility to cirrhosis or upper aerodigestive tract cancer in alcoholic caucasians. *Alcohol - Clin. Exp. Res.*, 20, 1033-1037

Lucas, D., Menez, C., Girre, C., Berthou, F., Bodenez, P., Joannet, I., Hispard, E., Bardou, L.G. & Menez, J.F. (1995) Cytochrome P450 2E1 genotype and chlorzoxazone metabolism in healthy and alcoholic Caucasian subjects. *Pharmacogenetics*, 5, 298-304

Mallet, W.G., Mosebrook, D.R. & Trush, M.A. (1991) Activation of (+)-trans-7,8-dihydroxy-7,8-dihydrobenzy[*a*]pyrene to diolepoxides by human polymorphonuclear leukocytes or myeloperoxidase. *Carcinogenesis*, 12, 521-524

Matthias, C., Bockmühl, U., Jahnke, V., Jones, P.W., Hayes, J.D., Alldersea, J., Gilford, J., Bailey, L., Bath, J., Worrall, S.F., Hand, P., Fryer, A.A. & Strange, R.C. (1998) Polymorphism in cytochrome P450 CYP2D6, CYP1A1, CYP2E1 and glutathione S-transferase, GSTM1, GSTM3, GSTT1 and susceptibility to tobacco-related cancers: studies in upper aerodigestive tract cancers. *Pharmacogenetics*, 8, 91-100

McBride, O.W., Umeno, M., Gelboin, H.V. & Gonzalez, F.J. (1987) A *Taq* I polymorphism in the human *P450IIE1* gene on chromosome 10 (*CYPZE*). *Nucleic Acids Res.*, 15, 10071

Meehan, R.R., Gosden, J.R., Rout, D., Hastie, N.D., Friedberg, T., Adesnik, M., Buckland, R., van, H.V., Fletcher, J., Spurr, N.K., Sweeney, J. & Wolf, C.R. (1988) Human cytochrome P-450 PB-1: a multigene family involved in mepheny-toin and steroid oxidations that maps to chromosome 10. *Am. J. Hum. Genet.*, 42, 26-37

Miles, J.S., McLaren, A.W. & Wolf, C.R. (1989) Alternative splicing in the human cytochrome P450IIB6 gene generates a high level of aberrant messages. *Nucleic Acids Res.*, 17, 8241-8255

Miles, J.S., McLaren, A.W., Gonzalez, F.J. & Wolf, C.R. (1990) Alternative splicing in the human cytochrome P450IIB6 gene: use of a cryptic exon within intron 3 and splice accep-tor site within exon 4. *Nucleic Acids Res.*, 18, 189

Miller, J.A. (1994) Recent studies on the meta-bolic activation of chemical carcinogens. *Cancer Res.*, 54, S1879-S1881

Mimura, M., Baba, T., Yamazaki, H., Ohmori, S., Inui, Y., Gonzalez, F.J., Guengerich, F.P. & Shimada, T. (1993) Characterization of cytochrome P-450 2B6 in human liver micro-somes. *Drug Metab. Dispos.*, 21, 1048-1056

Miners, J.O., Rees, D.L., Valente, L., Veronese, M.E. & Birkett, D.J. (1995) Human hepatic cytochrome P450 2C9 catalyses the rate-limiting pathway of torsemide metabolism. *J. Pharmacol. Exp. Ther.*, 272, 1076-1081

Molowa, D.T., Schuetz, E.G., Wrighton, S.A., Watkins, P.B., Kremers, P., Mendez, P.G., Parker, G.A. & Guzelian, P.S. (1986) Complete cDNA sequence of a cytochrome P-450 inducible by glu-cocorticoids in human liver. *Proc. Natl. Acad. Sci. USA*, 83, 5311-5315

Morishita, K., Kubota, N., Asano, S., Kaziro, Y. & Nagata, S. (1987) Molecular cloning and charac-terization of cDNA for human myeloperoxidase. *J. Biol. Chem.*, 262, 3844-3851

Nakamura, K., Goto, F., Ray, W.A., McAllister, C.B., Jacqz, E., Wilkinson, G.R. & Branch, R.A. (1985) Interethnic differences in genetic poly-morphism of debrisoquin and mephenytoin hydroxylation between Japanese and Caucasian populations. *Clin. Pharmacol.Ther.*, 38, 402-408

Nelson, D.R., Koymans, L., Kamataki, T., Stegeman, J.J., Feyereisen, R., Waxman, D.J., Waterman, M.R., Gotoh, O., Coon, M.J., Estabrook, R.W., Gunsalus, I.C. & Nebert, D.W. (1996) P450 superfamily - update on new sequences, gene-mapping, accession numbers and nomenclature. *Pharmacogenetics*, 6, 1-42

Nhamburo, P.T., Gonzalez, F.J., McBride, O.W., Gelboin, H.V. & Kimura, S. (1989) Identification of a new P450 expressed in human lung: com-plete cDNA sequence, cDNA-directed expression, and chromosome mapping. *Biochemistry*, 28, 8060-8066

Oesch, F. (1973) Mammalian epoxide hydrases: inducible enzymes catalysing the inactivation of carcinogenic and cytotoxic metabolites derived from aromatic and olefinic compounds. *Xenobiotica*, 3, 305-340

Okino, S.T., Quattrochi, L.C., Pendurthi, U.R., McBride, O.W. & Tukey, R.H. (1987) Characterization of multiple human cytochrome P-450 1 cDNAs. The chromosomal localization of the gene and evidence for alternate RNA splicing. [Erratum published in *J. Biol. Chem.*, 1988, 263(5), 2576.] *J. Biol. Chem.*, 262, 16072-16079

Olsen, R.L. & Little, C. (1984) Studies on the subunits of human myeloperoxidase. *Biochem. J.*, 220, 701-709

Omiecinski, C.J., Aicher, L., Holubkov, R. & Checkoway, H. (1993) Human peripheral lymphocytes as indicators of microsomal epoxide hydrolase activity in liver and lung. *Pharmacogenetics*, 3, 150-158

Oyama, T., Kawamoto, T., Mizoue, T., Sugio, K., Fodama, Y., Mitsusomi, T. & Uasumoto, K. (1997) Cytochrome P450 2E1 polymorphism as a risk factor for lung cancer: in relation to p53 gene mutation. *Anticancer Res.*, 17, 583-587

Page, M.A., Boutagy, J.S. & Shenfield, G.M. (1991) A screening test for slow metabolizers of tolbutamide. *Br. J. Clin. Pharmacol.*, 31, 649-654

Parry, M.F., Root, R.K., Metcalf, J.A., Delaney, K.K., Kaplow, L.S. & Richard, W.J. (1981) Myeloperoxidase deficiency: prevalence and clinical significance. *Ann. Intern. Med.*, 95, 293-301

Perrot, N., Nalpas, B., Yang, C.S. & Beaune, P.H. (1989) Modulation of cytochrome P450 isozymes in human liver by ethanol and drug intake. *Eur. J. Clin. Invest.*, 19, 549-555

Persson, I., Johansson, I., Bergling, H., Dahl, M.L., Seidegard, J., Rylander, R., Rannug, A., Hogberg, J. & Sundberg, M.I. (1993) Genetic polymorphism of cytochrome P4502E1 in a Swedish population. Relationship to incidence of lung cancer. *FEBS Lett.*, 319, 207-211

Peyronneau, M.A., Renaud, J.P., Jaouen, M., Urban, P., Cullin, C., Pompon, D. & Mansuy, D. (1993) Expression in yeast of three allelic cDNAs coding for human liver P-450 3A4. Different stabilities, binding properties and catalytic activities of the yeast-produced enzymes. *Eur. J. Biochem.*, 218, 355-361

Piedrafita, F.J., Molander, R., Vansant, G., Orlova, E.A., Pfahl M. & Reynolds, W.F. (1996) An Alu element in the myeloperoxidase promoter contains a composite SP1-thyroid hormone-retinoic acid response element. *J. Biol. Chem.*, 271, 14412-14420

Raftogianis, R.B., Her, C. & Weinshilboum, R.M. (1996) Human phenol sulfotransferase pharmacogenetics: *STP1** gene cloning and structural characterization. *Pharmacogenetics*, 6, 473-487

Rahman, A., Korzekwa, K.R., Grogan, J., Gonzalez, F.J. & Harris, J.W. (1994) Selective biotransformation of taxol to 6 alpha-hydroxytaxol by human cytochrome P450 2C8. *Cancer Res.*, 54, 5543-5546

Relling, M.V., Aoyama, T., Gonzalez, F.J. & Meyer, U.A. (1990) Tolbutamide and mephenytoin hydroxylation by human cytochrome P450s in the CYP2C subfamily. *J. Pharmacol. Exp. Ther.*, 252, 442-447

Rettie, A.E., Korzekwa, K.R., Kunze, K.L., Lawrence, R.F., Eddy, A.C., Aoyama, T., Gelboin, H.V., Gonzalez, F.J. & Trager, W.F. (1992) Hydroxylation of warfarin by human cDNA-expressed cytochrome P-450: a role for P-4502C9 in the etiology of (S)-warfarin-drug interacti0ons. *Chem. Res. Toxicol.*, 5, 54-59

Reynolds, W.F., Chang, E., Douer, D., Ball, E.D. & Kanda, V. (1997) An allelic association implicates myeloperoxidase in the etiology of acute promyelocytic leukaemia. *Blood*, 90, 2730-2737

Riley, R.J. & Workman, P. (1992) DT-diaphorase and cancer chemotherapy. *Biochem. Pharmacol.* 43, 1657-1669

Romkes, M., Faletto, M.B., Blaisdell, J.A., Raucy, J.L. & Goldstein, J.A. (1991) Cloning and expression of complementary DNAs for multiple members of the human cytochrome P450IIC subfamily [Erratum published in *Biochemistry*, 1993, 32(5), 1390.] *Biochemistry*, 30, 3247-3255

Ross, D. (1996) Metabolic basis of benzene toxicity. *Eur. J. Haematol. Suppl.*, 60, 111-118

Rosvold, E.A., McGlynn, K.A., Lustbader, E.D. & Buetow, K.H. (1995) Identification of an NAD(P)H:quinone oxidoreductase polymorphism and its association with lung cancer and smoking. *Pharmacogenetics*, 5, 199-206

Rothman, N., Smith, M.T., Hayes, R.B., Traver, R.D., Hoener, B.-A., Campleman, S., Li, G.-L., Dosemeci, M., Linet, M., Zhang, L., Xi, L., Wacholder, S.,. Lu, W., Meyer, K.B., Titenko-Holland, N., Stewart, J.T., Yin, S. & Ross, D. (1997) Benzene poisoning, a risk factor for haematological malignancy, is associated with the NQO1 609C T mutation and rapid fractional excretion of chlorzoxazone. *Cancer Res.*, 57, 2839-2842

Schlager, J.J. & Powis, G. (1990) NAD(P)H:-(quinone acceptor) oxidoreductase in human normal and tumour tissue: effects of cigarette smoking and alcohol. *Int. J. Cancer*, 45, 403-409

Schor, N.A. & Cornelisse, C.J. (1983) Biochemical and quantitative histochemical study of reduced pyridine nucleotide dehydrogenation by human colonic carcinomas. *Cancer Res.*, 43, 4850-4855

Schmekel, B., Karlsson, S.E., Linden, M., Sundstrom, C. Tegner, H. & Venge, P. (1990) Myeloperoxidase in human lung lavage. I. A marker of local neutrophil activity. *Inflammation*, 14, 447-454

Schuetz, J.D., Molowa, D.T. & Guzelian, P.S. (1989) Characterization of a cDNA encoding a new member of the glucocorticoid-responsive cytochromes P450 in human liver. *Arch. Biochem. Biophys.*, 274, 355-365

Schuetz, J.D., Beach, D.L. & Guzelian, P.S. (1994) Selective expression of cytochrome P450 CYP3A mRNAs in embryonic and adult human liver. *Pharmacogenetics*, 4, 11-20

Schulz, W.A., Krummeck, A., Rösinger, I., Eickelmann, P., Neuhaus, C., Ebert, T., Schmitz-Dräger, B.J. & Sies, H. (1997) Increased frequency of a null-allele for NAD(P)H:quinone oxidoreductase in patients with urological malignancies. *Pharmacogenetics*, 7, 235-239

Scott, J. & Poffenbarger, P.L. (1979) Pharmacogenetics of tolbutamide metabolism in humans. *Diabetes*, 28, 41-51

Selsted, M.E., Miller, C.W., Novotny, M.J., Morris, W.L. & Koeffler, H.P. (1993) Molecular analysis of myeloperoxidase deficiency shows heterogeneous patterns of the complete deficiency state manifested at the genomic, mRNA, and protein levels. *Blood*, 82, 1317-1322

Siegel, D., Gibson, N.W., Preusch, P.C. & Ross, D. (1990a) Metabolism of mitomycin C by DT-diaphorase: role in mitomycin C-induced DNA damage and cytotoxicity in human colon carcinoma cells. *Cancer Res.*, 50, 7483-7489

Siegel, D., Gibson, N.W., Preusch, P.C. & Ross, D. (1990b) Metabolism of diaziquone by NAD(P)H:(quinone acceptor) oxidoreductase (DT-dipaphorase): role in diaziquone-induced DNA damage and cytotoxicity in human colon carcinoma cells. *Cancer Res.*, 50, 7293-7300

Sindrup, S.H., Brosen, K., Hansen, M.G., Aaes, J.T., Overo, K.F. & Gram, L.F. (1993) Pharmacokinetics of citalopram in relation to the sparteine and the mephenytoin oxidation polymorphisms. *Ther. Drug Monit.*, 15, 11-17

Smith, C.A.D. & Harrison, D.J. (1997) Association between polymorphism in gene for microsomal epoxide hydrolase and susceptibility to emphysema. *Lancet*, 350, 630-633

Smith, G., Harrison, D.J., East, N., Rae, F., Wolf, H. & Wolf, C.R. (1993) Regulation of cytochrome P450 gene expression in human colon and breast tumour xenografts. *Br. J. Cancer*, 68, 57-63

Smith, G., Henderson, C.J., Parker, M.G., White, R., Bars, R.G. & Wolf, C.R. (1993) 1,4-Bis[2-(3,5-dichloropyridyloxy)]benzene, an extremely potent modulator of mouse hepatic cytochrome P-450 gene expression. *Biochem. J.*, 289, 807-813

Smith, G., Stanley, L.A., Sim, E., Strange, R.C. & Wolf, C.R. (1995) Metabolic polymorphisms and cancer susceptibility. *Cancer Surv.*, 25, 27-65

Smith, M. (1986) Genetics of human alcohol and aldehyde dehydrogenases. *Adv. Hum. Genet.*, 15, 249-290

Song, B.J., Gelboin, H.V., Park, S.S., Yang, C.S. & Gonzalez, F.J. (1986) Complementary DNA and protein sequences of ethanol-inducible rat and human cytochrome P-450s. Transcriptional and post-transcriptional regulation of the rat enzyme [Erratum published in *J. Biol. Chem.*, 1987, 262(18), 8940.] *J. Biol. Chem.*, 261, 16689-16697

Spielberg, S., McCrea, J., Cribb, A., Rushmore, T., Waldman, S., Bjomsson, T., Lo, M.-W. & Goldberg, M. (1996) A mutation in *CYP2C9* is responsible for decreased metabolism of losartan. *Clin. Pharmacol. Ther.*, 59, 215

Spurr, N.K., Gough, A.C., Stevenson, K. & Wolf, C.R. (1989) The human cytochrome P450 CYP3 locus: assignment to chromosome 7q22-qter. *Hum. Genet.*, 81, 171-174

Stephens, E.A., Taylor, J.A., Kaplan, N., Yang, C.H., Hsieh, L.L., Lucier, G.W. & Bell, D.A. (1994) Ethnic variation in the CYP2E1 gene: polymorphism analysis of 695 African-Americans, European-Americans and Taiwanese. *Pharmacogenetics*, 4, 185-192

Stubbins, M.J., Harries, L.W., Smith, G., Tarbit, M.H. & Wolf, C.R. (1996) Genetic analysis of the human cytochrome P450 *CYP2C9* locus. *Pharmacogenetics*, 6, 429-439

Sullivan-Klose, T.H., Ghanayem, B.I., Bell, D.A., Zhang, Z.-Y., Kaminsky, L.S., Shenfield, G.M., Miners, J.O., Birkett, D.J. & Goldstein, J.A. (1996) The role of the *CYP2C9*-Leu359 allelic variant in the tolbutamide polymorphism. *Pharmacogenetics*, 6, 341-349

Traver, R.D., Tetsuro, H., Danenberg, K.D., Stadlbauer, T.H.W., Danenberg, P.V., Ross, D. & Gibson, N.W. (1992) NAD(P)H:quinone oxidoreductase gene expression in human colon carcinoma cells: characterization of a mutation which modulates DT-diaphorase activity and mitomycin sensitivity. *Cancer Res.*, 52, 797-802

Tsuneoka, Y., Matsuo, Y., Okuyama, E., Watanabe, Y. & Ichikawa, Y. (1996) Genetic analysis of the cytochrome P-45OIIC18 (CYP2C18) gene and a novel member of the CYP2C subfamily. *FEBS Lett.*, 384, 281-284

Uematsu, F., Kikuchi, H., Ohmachi, T., Sagami, I., Motomiya, M., Kamataki, T., Komori, M. & Watanabe, M. (1991a) Two common RFLPs of the human CYP2E gene. *Nucleic Acids Res.*, 19, 2803

Uematsu, F., Kikuchi, H., Motomiya, M., Abe, T., Sagami, I., Ohmachi, T., Wakui, A., Kanamaru, R. & Watanabe, M. (1991b) Association between restriction fragment length polymorphism of the human cytochrome P450IIE1 gene and susceptibility to lung cancer. *Jpn. J. Cancer Res.*, 82, 254-256

Uematsu, F., Kikuchi, H., Abe, T., Motomiya, M., Ohmachi, T., Sagami, I. & Watanabe, M. (1991c) MspI polymorphism of the human CYP2E gene. *Nucleic Acids Res.*, 19, 5797

Uematsu, F., Kikuchi, H., Motomiya, M., Abe, T., Ishioka, C., Kanamaru, R., Sagami, I. & Watanabe, M. (1992) Human cytochrome *P450IIE1* gene: *Dra* I polymorphism and susceptibility to cancer. *Tohoku J. Exp. Med.*, 168, 113-117

Uematsu, F., Ikawa, S., Kikuchi, H., Sagami, I., Kanamaru, R., Abe, T., Satoh, K., Motomiya, M. & Watanabe, M. (1994) Restriction fragment length polymorphism of the human CYP2E1 (cytochrome P450IIE1) gene and susceptibility to lung cancer: possible relation to low smoking exposure. *Pharmacogenetics*, 4, 58-63

Uibo, R., Aavik, E., Peterson, P., Perheentupa, J., Aranko, S., Pelkonen, R. & Krohn, K.J. (1994) Autoantibodies to cytochrome P450 enzymes P450scc, P450c17, and P450c21 in autoimmune polyglandular disease types I and II and in isolated Addison's disease. *J. Clin. Endocrinol. Metab.*, 78, 323-328

Umbenhauer, D.R., Martin, M.V., Lloyd, R.S. & Guengerich, F.P. (1987) Cloning and sequence determination of a complementary DNA related to human liver microsomal cytochrome P-450 S-mephenytoin 4-hydroxylase. *Biochemistry*, 26, 1094-1099

Vasko, M.R., Bell, R.D., Daly, D.D.& Pippenger, C.E. (1980) Inheritance of phenytoin hypometabolism: a kinetic study of one family. *Clin. Pharmacol. Ther.*, 27, 96-103

Vermeij, P., Ferrari, M.D., Buruma, O.J., Veenema, H. & de Wolff, F.A. (1988) Inheritance of poor phenytoin parahydroxylation capacity in a Dutch family. *Clin. Pharmacol. Ther.*, 44, 588-593

Veronese, M.E., Mackenzie, P.I., Doecke, C.J., McManus, M.E., Miners, J.O. & Birkett, D.J. (1991) Tolbutamide and phenytoin hydroxylations by cDNA-expressed human liver cytochrome P4502C9. *Biochem. Biophys. Res. Commun.*, 175, 1112-1118

Veronese, M.E., Doecke, C.J., Mackenzie, P.I., McManus, M.E., Miners, J.O., Rees, D.L., Gasser, R., Meyer, U.A. & Birkett, D.J. (1993) Site-directed mutation studies of human liver cytochrome P-450 isoenzymes in the CYP2C subfamily. *Biochem. J.*, 289, 533-538

Wang, S.L., Huang, J., Lai, M.D. & Tsai, J.J. (1995) Detection of CYP2C9 polymorphism based on the polymerase chain reaction in Chinese. *Pharmacogenetics*, 5, 37-42

Ward, S.A., Goto, F., Nakamura, K., Jacqz, E., Wilkinson, G.R. & Branch, R.A. (1987) S-mephenytoin 4-hydroxylase is inherited as an autosomal-recessive trait in Japanese families. *Clin. Pharmacol.Ther.*, 42, 96-99

Ward, S.A., Helsby, N.A., Skjelbo, E., Brosen, K., Gram, L.F. & Breckenridge, A.M. (1991) The activation of the biguanide antimalarial proguanil co-segregates with the mephenytoin oxidation polymorphism - a panel study. *Br. J. Clin. Pharmacol.*, 31, 689-692

Watanabe, J., Hayashi, S., Nakachi, K., Imai, K., Suda, Y., Sekine, T. & Kawajiri, K. (1990) PstI and RsaI RFLPs in complete linkage disequilibrium at the CYP2E gene. *Nucleic Acids Res.*, 18, 7194

Wedlund, P.J., Aslanian, W.S., McAllister, C.B., Wilkinson, G.R. & Branch, R.A. (1984) Mephenytoin hydroxylation deficiency in Caucasians: frequency of a new oxidative drug metabolism polymorphism. *Clin. Pharmacol. Ther.*, 36, 773-780

Weil, S.C., Rosner, G.L., Reid, M.S., Chisholm, R.L., Farber, N.M., Spitznael, J.K. & Swanson, M.S. (1987) cDNA cloning of human myeloperoxidase: Decrease in myeloperoxidase mRNA upon induction of HL-60 cells. *Proc. Natl. Acad. Sci. USA*, 84, 2057-2061

Wiencke, J.K., Spitz, M.R., McMillan, A. & Kelsey, K.T. (1997) Lung cancer in Mexican-Americans and African-Americans is associated with the wild-type genotype of the NAD(P)H:quinone oxidoreductase polymorphism. *Cancer Epidemiol. Biomarkers Prev.*, 6, 87-92

Weinshilboum, R.M., Otterness, D.M., Aksoy, I.A., Wood, T.C., Her, C. & Raftogianis, R. B. (1997) Sulfation and sulfotransferases 1: Sulfotransferase molecular biology: cDNAs and genes. *FASEB J.*, 11, 3-14

White, P.C. & New, M.I. (1988) Molecular genetics of congenital adrenal hyperplasia. *Baillieres Clin. Endocrinol. Metab.*, 2, 941-965

Wilkinson, G.R., Guengerich, F.P. & Branch, R.A. (1989) Genetic polymorphism of S-mephenytoin hydroxylation. *Pharmacol. Ther.*, 43, 53-76

Winqvist, O., Gustafsson, J., Rorsman, F., Karlsson, F.A. & Kampe, O. (1993) Two different cytochrome P450 enzymes are the adrenal antigens in autoimmune polyendocrine syndrome type I and Addison's disease. *J. Clin. Invest.*, 92, 2377-2385

Wolf, C.R. (1990) Metabolic factors in cancer susceptibility. *Cancer Surv.*, 9, 437-474

Wood, T.C., Her, C., Aksoy, I., Otterness, D.M. & Weinshilboum, R.M. (1996) Human dehydroepiandrosterone sulfotransferase pharmacogenetics: quantitative Western analysis and gene sequence polymorphisms. *J. Ster. Biochem. Mol. Biol.*, 59, 467-478

Workman, P. (1994) Enzyme-directed bioreductive drug development revisited: a commentary on recent progress and future prospects with emphasis on quinone anticancer agents and quinone metabolizing enzymes, particularly DT-diaphorase. *Oncol. Res.*, 6, 461-475

Wrighton, S.A., Maurel, P., Schuetz, E.G., Watkins, P.B., Young, B. & Guzelian, P.S. (1985) Identification of the cytochrome P-450 induced by macrolide antibiotics in rat liver as the glucocorticoid responsive cytochrome P-450p. *Biochemistry*, 24, 2171-2178

Wrighton, S.A., Thomas, P.E., Molowa, D.T., Haniu, M., Shivley, J.E., Maines, S.L., Watkins, P.B., Parker, G., Mendez-Picon, G., Lewin, W. & Guzelian, P.S. (1986) Characterization of ethanol-inducible human liver N-nitrosodimethylamine demethylase. *Biochemistry*, 25, 6731-6735

Wrighton, S.A., Thomas, P.E., Willis, P., Maines, S.L., Watkins, P.B., Levin, W. & Guzelian, P.S. (1987a) Purification of a human liver cytochrome P-450 immunochemically related to several cytochromes P-450 purified from untreated rats. *J. Clin. Invest.*, 80, 1017-1022

Wrighton, S.A., Thomas, P.E., Ryan, D.E. & Lewin, W. (1987b) Purification and characterization of ethanol-inducible human hepatic cytochrome P-450HLj. *Arch. Biochem. Biophys.*, 258, 292-297

Wrighton, S.A., Brian, W.R., Sari, M.A., Iwasaki, M., Guengerich, F.P., Raucy, J.L., Molowa, D.T. & Vandenbranden, M. (1990) Studies on the expression and metabolic capabilities of human liver cytochrome P450IIIA5 (HLp3). *Mol. Pharmacol.*, 38, 207-213

Xiao, Z.-S., Goldstein, J.A., Xie, H.-G., Blaisdell, J., Wang, W., Jiang, C.-H., Yan, F.-X., He, N., Huang, S.-L., Xu, Z.-H. & Zhou, H.-H. (1997) Differences in the incidence of the *CYP2C19* polymorphism affecting the *S*-mephenytoin phenotype in Chinese Han and Ban populations and identification of a new rare *CYP2C19* mutant allele. *J. Pharmacol. Exp. Ther.*, 281, 604-609

Yamada, M., Hur, S.J., Hashinaka, K., Tsuneoka, K., Saeki, T., Nishio, C., Sakiyama, F. & Tsunasawa, S. (1987) Isolation and characterization of a cDNA coding for human myeloperoxidase. *Arch. Biochem. Biophys.*, 255, 147-155

Yamano, S., Nhamburo, P.T., Aoyama, T., Meyer, U.A., Inaba, T., Kalow, W., Gelboin, H.V., McBride, O.W. & Gonzalez, F.J. (1989) cDNA cloning and sequence and cDNA-directed expression of human P450 IIB1: identification of a normal and two variant cDNAs derived from the CYP2B locus on chromosome 19 and differential expression of the IIB mRNAs in human liver. *Biochemistry*, 28, 7340-7348

Yang, C.S., Jeong-Sook, V.H., Ishizaki, H. & Hong, Y. (1990) Cytochrome P450 IIE1 roles in nitrosamine metabolism and mechanism of regulation. *Drug Metab. Rev.*, 22, 147-159

Yasumori, T., Kawano, S., Nagata, K., Shimada, M., Yamazoe, Y. & Kato, R. (1987) Nucleotide sequence of a human liver cytochrome P-450 related to the rat male specific form. *J. Biochem. Tokyo*, 102, 1075-1082

Yokoyama, A., Muramatsu, T., Ohmori, T., Higuchi, S., Hayashida, M. & Ishii, H. (1996) Oesophageal cancer and aldehyde dehydrogenase-2 genotypes in Japanese males. *Cancer Epidemiol. Biomarkers Prev.*, 5, 99-102

Yoo, J.S., Guengerich, F.P. & Yang, C.S. (1988) Metabolism of N-nitrosodialkylamines by human liver microsomes. *Cancer Res.*, 48, 1499-1504

Yun, C.H., Shimada, T. & Guengerich, F.P. (1992) Roles of human liver cytochrome P4502C and 3A enzymes in the 3-hydroxylation of benzo(a)pyrene. *Cancer Res.*, 52, 1868-1874

Zaphiropoulos, P.G. (1997) Exon skipping and circular RNA formation in transcripts of the human cytochrome P-450 2C18 gene in epidermis and of the rat androgen binding protein gene in testis. *Mol. Cell. Biol.*, 17, 2985-2993

Zhu, X., Veronese, M.E., Iocco, P. & McManus, M.E. (1996) cDNA cloning and expression of a new form of human aryl sulfotransferase. *Int. J. Biochem. Cell Biol.*, 28, 565-571

Corresponding author
Michael J. Stubbins
GLP Clinical Genotyping Laboratory,
Glaxo Wellcome Research and Development,
Building 2, GC25, Park Road, Ware,
Hertfordshire, SG12 0DP, United Kingdom

Metabolic Polymorphisms and Susceptibility to Cancer
W. Ryder
IARC Scientific Publications No. 148
International Agency for Research on Cancer, Lyon, 1999

Chapter 22. Interactions between detoxifying enzyme polymorphisms and susceptibility to cancer

Anthony A. Fryer and Peter W. Jones

Many case-control studies on the role of detoxifying enzyme polymorphisms in susceptibility to cancer have identified significant associations, though few have identified effects with sufficient strength to be useful clinically. Odds ratios of 2-3 are the usual finding. Therefore, combinations of risk alleles are increasingly studied in the hope of identifying haplotypes with sufficient biological impact (odds ratio >15) to warrant further study in a clinical setting. The study of interactions between different detoxifying enzyme loci should be based on biological sense, for example the classical view of two-step xenobiotic detoxification, overlapping substrate specificities, detoxification of molecules derived from the same pathological insult (e.g. detoxification of nitrosamines and polycyclic aromatic hydrocarbons in cigarette smoke) or simultaneous regulation of expression. The rationale behind these mechanisms is discussed.

Considerable amounts of data have focused on the interaction between CYP1A1 and GSTM1, particularly in Japanese patients with lung cancer. In this regard there is accumulating evidence suggesting that the combination of GSTM1 null/CYP1A1 rare alleles, particularly in combination with smoking, confers highly significant increased risk. However, there is now some debate on the importance of these data in terms of chemical detoxification, since certain studies suggest that the CYP1A1 polymorphisms that have been investigated do not influence function or expression of the gene. Indeed, the influence of CYP2D6 genetic variation is also disputed, suggesting that these polymorphisms may be acting more as linkage markers than by influencing chemical carcinogenesis themselves. What is clear from the many studies on interactions between detoxifying enzyme polymorphisms is the comparative lack of supporting data on synergism between these genes.

Given the inevitable increase in the complexity of studies, a basic explanation of the statistical approaches to the assessment of interactions is included in this Chapter. A more detailed statistical/epidemiological assessment is given elsewhere in the book. Since there is an increasing reluctance of journals to publish case-control studies describing the (usually moderate) influence of detoxifying enzyme polymorphisms, it is important that scientists understand what statistical approach is appropriate and address the issue from a novel and clinically significant angle. This is likely to involve multiple genes and subgroup analysis of some kind.

We focus below on interactions between detoxifying enzyme polymorphisms and their significance in mediating susceptibility to cancer. Our aim is to discuss reasons why combinations of genotypes should be assessed and to review studies where significant interactions have been reported. Finally, some examples of our experience in the statistical analysis of interactions are presented.

Since the initial studies that identified a possible link between aryl hydrocarbon hydroxylase inducibility and bronchogenic carcinoma (Kellermann et al., 1973) the number of reports showing correlations between polymorphism in carcinogen-metabolizing enzymes and susceptibility to disease has increased dramatically. Many of the earlier case-control studies focused on individual loci of the glutathione S-transferase (GST), cytochrome P450 (CYP) or N-acetyl transferase (NAT) supergene families, often in relatively small numbers of patients (d'Errico et al., 1996). Over the past few years, however, studies have become increasingly complex, covering particular subgroups of patients within a disease group in an attempt to assess more specifically the influence of a genotype. Thus the effects of polymorphism have been examined in postmenopausal women with breast cancer (Ambrosone *et al.*, 1995) or in low-consumption tobacco users with lung cancer (Nakachi *et al.*, 1993). End points other than susceptibility (using a case-control approach) to the disease in question have also been considered. For instance, prognostic indicators such as the severity/aggressiveness of disease (re lung cancer - Anttila *et al.*, 1994; Goto *et al.*, 1996; re colorectal cancer - Bell *et al.*, 1995b; re skin cancer - Lear *et al.*, 1997b), the age of onset (re lung cancer - Alexandrie *et al.*, 1994) and the development of multiple tumours (re skin cancer - Lear *et al.*, 1996; Yengi *et al.*, 1996) are increasingly being investigated. More commonly, a number of detoxifying gene loci are being simultaneously assessed in case groups in which consideration is being given to the potential combined effect of genotypes. These analyses, often only possible in large case groups because of the rarity of some genotypes, are the subject of the present Chapter.

Why interactions?

The rationale for studying interactions between different detoxifying enzyme loci depends on several assumptions, among them the following: the classical view of two-step xenobiotic detoxification demonstrated *in vivo;* overlapping substrate specificities; detoxification of molecules derived from the same pathological insult (e.g. detoxification of reactive oxygen species or repair of the products of damage induced by reactive oxygen species); and simultaneous regulation of expression.

The central dogma of two-step detoxification proposed by Nebert *et al.* (1996) states that exogenous or endogenous toxic compounds are detoxified in an initial phase 1 activation reaction followed by a phase 2 conjugation reaction that renders the resultant compound more water-soluble and, therefore, more easily excreted. Phase 1 reactions, usually involving the introduction of atomic oxygen, are catalysed by members of the cytochrome P450 supergene family, and generate an active oxygenated intermediate. This intermediate then acts as a substrate for phase 2 enzymes such as the glutathione S-transferases, N-acetyl transferases, sulfotransferases or UDP-glucuronyl transferases, which add polar moieties to the active oxygen. Since the oxygenated intermediate is often more reactive and potentially more carcinogenic than the starting chemical, coordinated expression of phase 1 and phase 2 genes is likely to be critical. For example, *in vivo* metabolism of

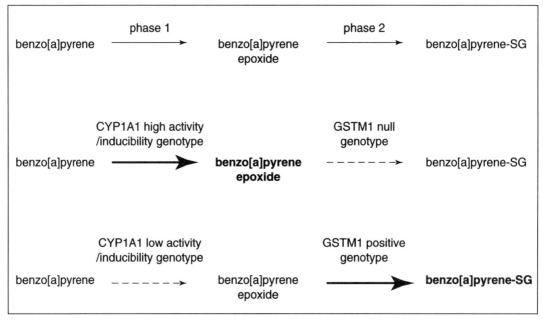

Figure 1. The effect of polymorphism at phase 1 and phase 2 loci on metabolism of benzo[a]pyrene.

benzo[a]pyrene, a polycyclic aromatic hydrocarbon (PAH), is thought to follow this process, the parent compound being metabolized by cytochrome P450 enzymes such as CYP1A1 to benzo[a]pyrene epoxide, a substrate for mu class GST enzymes (Ketterer *et al.*, 1993). It is reasonable to hypothesize, therefore, that risk of tobacco-related diseases may be mediated by individual ability to metabolize tobacco-derived PAHs. In particular, genetic variation in both phase 1 and 2 enzymes may influence this process as indicated in Fig .1.

Thus, patients with high inducibility/activity variants at CYP1A1 together with the GSTM1 null genotype would be at higher risk than either of the risk genotypes alone due to accumulation of the reactive epoxide intermediate.

Furthermore, synergistic effects between detoxifying enzymes are also possible when the same chemical is metabolized by more than one polymorphic enzyme. For example, nitrosamines are substrates for CYP2D6 and CYP2E1 (Hung *et al.*, 1997; Camus *et al.*, 1993; Penman *et al.*, 1993) and epoxides are utilized by GSTM1 and GSTT1 (Ketterer *et al.*, 1993; Hayes & Pulford, 1995). Interactions between phase 1 and 2 enzymes are also worthy of study on this basis. Thus, dichloromethane is metabolized in humans by

two pathways: oxidation by a CYP-dependent pathway or conjugation with glutathione by the theta class GST (Hallier *et al.*, 1994).

The detoxification of molecules derived from the same pathological insult (e.g. detoxification of separate carcinogens in cigarette smoke) may result in synergism between detoxifying enzymes. Thus, the role of GST, NAT and CYP enzymes in protection against the deleterious effects of oxidative stress or chemicals in cigarette smoke may result in synergism either by effects on the same or separate mutational events (Fig. 2).

For example, cigarette smoke contains numerous potentially carcinogenic compounds, such as nitrosamines and PAHs. Nitrosamines are metabolized by CYP2D6 and CYP2E1 (Hung *et al.*, 1997; Camus *et al.*, 1993; Penman *et al.*, 1993); CYP2E1 in mice is induced by tobacco smoke (Seree *et al.*, 1996). In addition, PAHs are substrates for CYP1A1 and GSTM1 (Raunio *et al.*, 1995b; Ketterer *et al.*, 1993), suggesting that polymorphism in any combination of these genes may influence cumulative risk. Similarly, substrates for GSTM1 and GSTT1 include the products of damage to DNA (e.g. DNA hydroperoxides) induced by reactive oxygen species (Hayes & Strange, 1995). Furthermore, while CYP1A1 has largely been studied in the con-

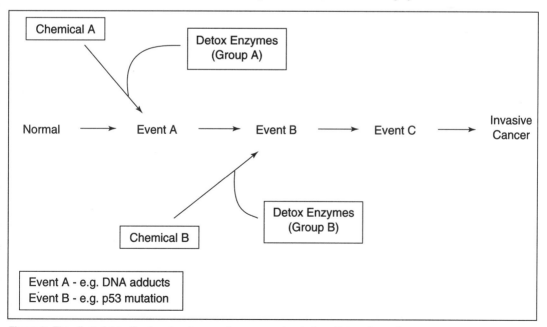

Figure 2. The effect of detoxification of endogenous/exogenous chemicals on the carcinogenic process.

text of environmental pollutants (e.g. PAHs), there is evidence that its products participate in defence against oxidative stress (Smith *et al.*, 1995; Nebert, 1994). In the case of carcinoma of the oral cavity, tobacco and alcohol consumption appear additive as risk factors (Hung *et al.*, 1997). Thus, in addition to genes involved in metabolism of tobacco-derived carcinogens, CYP2E1 is potentially important in the metabolism of ethanol with the concomitant production of free radicals (Ingelman-Sundberg *et al.*, 1993), thereby offering a potential mechanism for the synergistic effects of these habits (Hung *et al.*, 1997).

Finally, recent evidence (Nebert *et al.*, 1993) suggests that the expression of some transcription factors may result in up-regulation of the expression of several genes. Thus, a battery of genes including CYP1A1 and CYP1A2, aldehyde dehydrogenase and some GSTs are coordinately induced via the Ah receptor mechanism. In addition to this activation through binding to xenobiotic responsive elements (XRE) in the upstream region of these genes, antioxidant responsive elements (ARE) have also been identified in the GST alpha genes (Rushmore *et al.*, 1991), suggesting that the coordinated expression of genes involved in defence against oxidative stress may be important.

Interactions associated with increased risk of cancer

The first observation to be made in the study of interactions between detoxifying enzyme loci is that there is a surprising lack of supporting data. Although the case for interactions is strong, data from many studies have failed to identify interactions between genes which are more significant than either of the main effects alone. For example, a comprehensive study by Brockmöller *et al.* (1996) on eight genes (NAT2, epoxide hydrolase, GSTM1, GSTT1, CYP2D6, CYP2C19, CYP1A1, CYP2E1) and seven characteristics of patients (gender, age, smoking, occupation, differentiation, invasiveness, tumour type) identified no significant synergistic interactions. The reason for this is unclear, although a failure to identify *in vivo* substrates and a question mark over the functional relevance of some allelic variants may be significant. The key case-control studies on interactions and susceptibility to disease are summarized in Table 1.

Interactions between phase 1 and phase 2 enzymes

(i) CYP1A1/2

Possibly because of the quantity of information available on the products of the gene loci, many of the data on interactions relate to the combined effect of polymorphism in GSTM1 and CYP1A1, gene loci whose products metabolize PAHs. Thus, studies in 85 Japanese squamous cell lung cancer patients and 170 matched controls showed the combined CYP1A1 val/val/GSTM1 null genotype conferred a remarkably high risk of lung cancer (Hayashi *et al.*, 1992), particularly in low-dose cigarette smokers (odds ratio = 41.0) (Nakachi *et al.*, 1993). In contrast, Kihara *et al.* (1995), working with 118 patients with squamous or small cell lung cancer, suggested the effect of the combined genotype demonstrated a dose-dependent increase in risk, giving increases in risk of up to twenty-twofold for the GSTM1 null/CYP1A1 m2m2 combination in patients with heaviest cigarette consumption. These studies are more difficult to reproduce in Caucasians due to the significantly lower frequency of CYP1A1 mutant alleles (m2m2 frequency <2%) compared to Japanese populations (m2m2 frequency >10%). Data from Anttila *et al.* (1994) and Alexandrie *et al.* (1994), however, demonstrated this combination to be influential in Caucasians in particular subgroups determined by tumour site and age of diagnosis, respectively. The basis for this phenomenon is suggested by studies showing the GSTM1 null genotype to be associated with high inducibility of CYP1A1 gene transcription (Vaury *et al.*, 1995). Since the CYP1A1 m2 allele may influence inducibility (Petersen *et al.*, 1991), effects of the Ile/Val polymorphism in CYP1A1 may arise out of the known linkage disequilibrium between these polymorphisms and/or the increased activity of Val/Val homozygotes that has been suggested (Kawajiri *et al.*, 1993; Kiyohara *et al.*, 1996). However, the issue of the functional significance of either of these CYP1A1 polymorphisms remains open to debate: some studies reveal no functional difference between the *CYP1A1-Ile* and *CYP1A1-Val* alleles (Zhang *et al.*, 1996) and only moderate increases in inducibility associated with the CYP1A1 m2 allele (Landi *et al.*, 1994). These data support the classical two-phase view of detoxification of an environmentally-derived car-

Table 1. Summary of case-control studies examining the effect of multiple detoxifying enzyme polymorphisms

Genes studied	Disease group	Subgroup (if any)	No. cases/controls	Significant interaction(s)	OR (95% CI) vs other combinations	OR (95% CI) vs low-risk genotype	Synergistic	Reference
GSTM1, GSTT1, CYP2D6	Astrocytoma		109/408	GSTT1 null and CYP2D6 PM	3.70 (0.71-20.0)	ND	No	Elexpuru-Caminuaga et al, 1995
GSTM1, GSTT1, GSTM3	Astrocytoma		102/300	GSTT1 null and GSTM3 AA	1.98 (1.08-3.63)	ND	No	Hand et al, 1996
GSTM1, GSTT1, CYP2D6	Basal cell Ca		737/563	None	-	-	-	Heagerty et al, 1996
GSTM1, GSTT1, NAT2, CYP2D6, CYP2C19, CYP1A1,CYP2E1, EH	Bladder Ca		374/373	GSTM1 null and NAT2 slow acetylator	1.48 (NK)	NK	No	Brockmoller et al, 1996
CYP1A1, GSTM1	Breast Ca	Postmenopausal	161/217	None	-	-	-	Ambrosone et al, 1995
GSTM1, CYP1A1	Breast Ca		58/NK	None reported	-	-	-	Kato et al, 1996
GSTM1, GSTT1	Breast Ca		77/127	None	-	-	-	Chem et al, 1996
GSTM1, CYP2D6	Cervical Ca		77/190	None	-	-	-	Warwick et al, 1994a
GSTM1, GSTT1, CYP2D6	Cervical Ca		68/167	None	-	-	-	Warwick et al, 1994b
GSTM1, GSTT1	Colon Ca		132/200	None reported	-	-	-	Chenevix-Trench et al, 1995
GSTM1, NAT2	Colon Ca	Current smokers	447/487	GSTM1 null and NAT2 fast acetylator	ND	10.33 (1.94-55.04)	NK	Probst-Hensch et al, 1995
NAT2, CYP1A2	Colon Ca		75/205	NAT2 rapid and CYP1A2 rapid (phenotypes)	2.91 (1.38-6.11)	ND	NK	Lang et al, 1994
GSTM1, GSTT1	Colorectal Ca		252/577	None	-	-	-	Deakin et al, 1996
GSTM1, GSTT1	Colorectal Ca		103/126	None reported	-	-	-	Katoh et al, 1996
CYP2D6, NAT2	Epileptics		93/243	None reported	-	-	-	Borlak et al, 1994
CYP2E1, NQO1	Haematological		50/50	NK	-	-	-	Rothman et al, 1996
CYP2D6, NAT2	Hepatocellular		100/258	CYP2D6 EM and NAT2 slow acetylator	ND	0.38 (0.23-0.63)	NK	Agundez et al, 1996
GSTM1, CYP2E1	Hepatocellular		30/150	None	-	-	-	Yu et al, 1995
GSTM1, GSTT1	Hepatocellular	Aflatoxin exposed	32/73	GSTM1 null and GSTT1 null	-	-	-	Chen et al, 1996
CYP1A1, GSTM1	Lung Ca	Light smokers	85/170	CYP1A1val/val and GSTM1 null	ND	41.00 (8.68-193.61)	NK	Nakachi et al, 1993

Table 1 (Contd). Summary of case-control studies examining the effect of multiple detoxifying enzyme polymorphisms

Genes	Cancer	Subgroup	Cases/Controls	Genotype combination				Reference
CYP1A1, GSTM1	Lung Ca	Heavy smokers	118/331	CYP1A1m2m2 and GSTM1 null	ND	21.9 (4.68-112.7)	NK	Kihara et al, 1995
CYP1A1, GSTM1	Lung Ca	SCC, <66 years old	36/329	CYP1A1m2 allele and GSTM1 null	3.0 (1.2-7.2)			Alexandrie et al, 1994
GSTM1, CYP1A1	Lung Ca		298/385	GSTM1 null and CYP1A1 m1m2+m2m2	Not given	Not given	Yes	Garcia-Closas et al, 1996
GSTM1, CYP1A1, CYP2D6, EH	Lung Ca		93/98	None reported				Caporaso et al, 1996
GSTM1, GSTT1	Lung Ca		108/577	None				Deakin et al, 1996
GSTM1, GSTP1	Lung Ca	Mostly NSCLC	133/297	GSTM1 null and GSTP1 AG+GG	1.96 (1.26-3.06)	ND	No	Ryberg et al, 1997
GSTM1, GSTT1, CYP2E1	Lung Ca		52/48	None reported				El-Zein et al, 1997
GSTM1, GSTT1, CYP2D6	Meningioma		48/408	GSTT1 null and CYP2D6 PM	6.67 (0.95-41.7)	ND	No	Elexpuru-Camiruaga et al, 1995
GSTM1, NAT2	Mesothelioma	Asbestos-related	44/270	GSTM1 null and NAT2 slow acetylator	2.7 (1.4-5.2)	3.6 (1.3-9.6)	NK	Hirvonen et al, 1995
GSTM1, GSTT1, NAT2	Pulmonary disorders	Asbestos-related	76/69	GSTM1 null and NAT2 slow acetylator	3.0 (1.3-6.9)	5.1 (1.6-17.6)	NK	Hirvonen et al, 1996
GSTM1, CYP1A1	Oral Ca		66/Not given	None reported				Lazarus et al, 1996
GSTM1, GSTT1	Oral Ca		40/577	None				Deakin et al, 1996
GSTM1, GSTT1	Head and neck Ca		161/152	None				McWilliams et al, 1996
GSTM1, GSTT1, GSTM3, CYP2D6, CYP1A1, CYP2E1	Laryngeal Ca		269/216	None				Janke et al, 1996
GSTM1, GSTT1	Ovarian Ca		84/325	None				Sarhanis et al, 1996
GSTM1, GSTT1	SLE	Ro+ve/La-ve	12/569	GSTM1 null and GSTT1 null	6.20 (ND)	ND	NK	Ollier et al, 1996
GSTM1, GSTT1	Stomach Ca		139/126	None reported				Katoh et al, 1996
GSTM1, CYP1A1	Stomach Ca		156/NK	None reported				Kato et al, 1996
GSTM1, GSTT1	Stomach Ca		136/577	None				Deakin et al, 1996
GSTM1, GSTT1	Ulcerative colitis		245/373	None reported				Duncan et al, 1995
GSTM1, CYP1A1	Urothelial Ca		83/101	None reported				Katoh et al, 1995

cinogen, the reactive intermediate being the true carcinogen (Nebert *et al.*, 1996). Thus, high inducibility of the CYP1A1 m2m2 genotype in combination with an inability to metabolize the reactive, oxygenated intermediate (GSTM1 null genotype) would result in the build-up of the intermediate, thereby increasing cancer risk. Support for the view that the combined genotype results in increased carcinogenic potential is shown in studies by Ichiba *et al.* (1994) demonstrating a 60% increase in median aromatic DNA adduct levels in Swedish chimney sweeps with the combined GSTM1 null/CYP1A1 m1m1 genotype. Further, Kawajiri *et al.* (1996), looking at the relationship between the combined genotype and mutations in p53 in a group of Japanese non-small-cell lung cancer patients, demonstrated that the combination of homozygosity for CYP1A1 rare alleles (m2m2 or val/val) and GSTM1 null conferred a remarkably high risk (odds ratios 9.24 and 8.17 respectively) of p53 mutations in smokers. Similar results were obtained with mutations in *Ki-Ras*. These studies were extended (Goto *et al.*, 1996) in order to examine the effect of the combined genotype on indicators of prognosis in lung cancer patients, using survival time as an outcome measure. Data from this study supported the effect of the combined genotype, indicating that the mean survival time for lung cancer patients with the combined GSTM1 null/CYP1A1 m1m2+m2m2 was significantly lower than for other genotype combinations (log rank test, p = 0.017, *df* = 3). Thus three-year survival rates for the respective genotype combinations were: GSTM1 positive/CYP1A1 m1m1, 66.4%; GSTM1 null/-CYP1A1 m1m1, 54.6%; GSTM1 positive/CYP1A1 m1m2+m2m2, 45.7%; GSTM1 null/CYP1A1 m1m2+m2m2, 36.6%. However, it is not clear whether the effect of the combined genotypes is due to the additive effects of the individual genotypes or whether the two genotypes are indeed synergistic. Although the data on the role of the CYP1A1/GSTM1 combination in mediating susceptibility to lung cancer appears consistent, particularly in Japanese, no such interaction was detected in breast cancer (Ambrosone *et al.*, 1995) and we have not identified this effect in several cancers, including cutaneous basal cell carcinoma (BCC) (Yengi *et al.*, 1996).

Although we did not identify interactions between GSTM1 and CYP1A1 in cutaneous BCC (Lear *et al.*, 1996), we found a significant interaction between CYP1A1 m1m1 and GSTM3 AA (Yengi *et al.*, 1996), providing further support for the view that the combination of CYP1A1 and a mu class GST influences susceptibility. Both GSTM3 (Yengi *et al.*, 1996) and CYP1A1 (Raunio *et al.*, 1995b) are expressed in skin. Further, data showing that UV-oxidized tryptophan binds to the CYP1A1 ligand-dependent Ah receptor transcription factor and that UV induces CYP1A1 expression in skin suggest a role for allelism at this locus in skin carcinogenesis (Rannug *et al.*, 1987; Gonzalez, 1995). The consequences of the 3'-downstream mutation is compatible with data showing GSTM1 null is associated with high inducibility of CYP1A1 transcription (Vaury *et al.*, 1995) and implies that CYP1A1 m1m1 provides less effective detoxification on exposure to carcinogens (Nebert, 1994; Raunio *et al.*, 1995b). This is interesting in the context of causative mechanisms, since BCC is not thought to be smoking-related, suggesting that the substrates may be endogenous UV-induced chemicals, such as reactive oxygen species.

We have recently identified an interactive effect between CYP1A1 and GSTT1 with tumour site in cutaneous BCC (Lear *et al.*, 1997a). To our knowledge this is the first identified interaction between these polymorphisms. These data suggest that individuals deficient in the ability to repair oxidative stress-induced damage to DNA and/or lipids are genetically predisposed to BCC and are more likely to develop trunk tumours. Since UV constitutes an oxidative stress (Emerit, 1992), GSTT1 null individuals may be more susceptible to UV-induced BCC following relatively little UV exposure resulting in an increased number of tumours at a younger age and the development of lesions on intermittently exposed sites such as the trunk. However, in contrast to the situation with GSTT1 null, no GSTM1 null effect was identified, complementing data showing that the products of these loci have some differences in substrate specificities (Norppa *et al.*, 1995).

A phenotypic approach in patients with colorectal cancer has identified important interactions between CYP1A2 and NAT2 which are related to dietary ingestion of heterocyclic amines

(Lang *et al.* 1994), although the genetic basis of variation in CYP1A2 activity is unclear.

(ii) CYP2D6

Data on interactions with CYP2D6 genotypes and phase 2 enzymes is sparse. Roots *et al.* (1992), using phenotyping assays, showed that CYP2D6 metabolism of debrisoquine was significantly lower in lung cancer patients with low mu class GST activity towards *trans*-stilbene epoxide compared with those with high activity. This effect is difficult to explain and further work is required to investigate the phenomenon. We, however, have not observed any genotypic interaction between polymorphism in CYP2D6 and GST in several case groups and controls (cervical neoplasia, astrocytoma and meningioma, cutaneous basal cell carcinoma) (Warwick *et al.*, 1994a,b; Elexpuru-Camiruaga *et al.*, 1995; Heagerty *et al.*, 1996) even when one or both of the single-gene polymorphisms were shown to be important. One study has addressed the role of polymorphism at CYP2D6 and NAT simultaneously in patients with epilepsy (Borlak *et al.*, 1994) and shown that particular alleles at both gene loci influence susceptibility, although the role of the combined genotype was not discussed, possibly due to the relatively small case group (n=93) and the infrequency of the poor metabolizer NAT and CYP2D6 risk genotypes (both less than 10%). It is important to note that, currently, there are relatively few data on the functional ability of CYP2D6 to metabolize carcinogens (Crespi *et al.*, 1991).

(iii) CYP2E1

A small study of CYP2E1 and GSTM1 genotyping in patients with hepatocellular carcinoma (Yu *et al.*, 1995) did not identify significant interactions between the two loci, although the number of cases studied was very small (n = 30) and therefore insufficiently powerful to identify all but the most dramatic effects. El-Zein *et al.* (1997) studied CYP2E1, GSTM1 and GSTT1 polymorphisms in lung cancer patients but the case group included adenocarcinoma and squamous cell carcinoma patients and was not sufficiently large (52 cases, 48 controls) to detect interactive effects. In the larger study by Brockmöller *et al.* (1996), no significant interactive effects involving CYP2E1 were identified in bladder cancer patients.

Although polymorphisms have been identified in other CYP genes, for instance CYP2C19 and CYP2A6, there are few data on interactions involving these loci, except for the negative findings involving CYP2C19 in bladder cancer patients as described by Brockmöller *et al.*(1996).

Interactions between phase 2 enzymes

(i) Mu class GST

Within the glutathione S-transferase supergene family some isoforms demonstrate overlap in substrate specificities. Much of the interest in GST in the context of disease susceptibility has centred on polymorphism in the GSTM1 gene. GSTM1 is one of five mu genes (M1-M5) on chromosome 1 (Pearson *et al.*, 1993) whose products demonstrate overlap in substrate specificities (Comstock *et al.*, 1994; Hayes & Pulford, 1995), implying that the protein products of one mu class locus will compensate functionally for the absence of other family members. Indeed, studies in lung cancer suggest coordinated expression of some mu class genes; thus, *GSTM1*0* homozygotes express less GSTM3 than subjects with other GSTM1 genotypes (Anttila *et al.*, 1995). The mechanism for this observation is unknown but may be related to the finding that GSTM3 is also polymorphic with two alleles, *GSTM3*A* and *GSTM3*B* (Inskip *et al.*, 1995). Importantly, *GSTM3*B* is in linkage disequilibrium with *GSTM1*A* and contains in intron 6 a recognition motif for the YY1 transcription factor which regulates gene expression from intragenic sites (Becker *et al.*, 1994). The widely expressed YY1 factor influences the expression of many genes (Becker *et al.*, 1994), suggesting that *GSTM3*A* and *GSTM3*B* may be expressed at different levels and that GSTM3 genotypes confer different efficiencies in the metabolism of carcinogens. Support for this view comes from studies in our laboratory in patients with cutaneous BCC (Yengi *et al.*, 1996). Among cases with 2-35 primary tumours we used the Poisson regression model to study the association between genotype and number of lesions. The GSTM1 and GSTM3 genotypes alone were not associated with an increased number of tumours, but the combination of GSTM3 AA with GSTM1 null was significantly associated with increased tumour numbers (Yengi *et al.*, 1996). Presumably, individuals with GSTM3 AA and GSTM1 null are less able to metabolize the products of the oxidative stress associated with UV exposure. These data complement studies showing lower levels of immunohistochemical positivity for GSTM3 in the lungs of subjects with GSTM1 null (Anttila et al., 1995; Nakajima et al., 1995) and suggest a similar effect in skin. This may reflect the linkage of GSTM3*B with GSTM1*A (Inskip et al., 1995) and the consequent association of GSTM3*A with the other GSTM1 alleles, the majority of which are GSTM1*0. This would suggest that absence of the GSTM1*A allele may be a better risk marker than homozygous GSTM1*0, because of the stronger linkage with GSTM3*A. This view is further supported by data of Brockmöller et al. (1996) showing that the effect of GSTM1 on bladder cancer risk was more marked in patients lacking the GSTM1*A allele than in those lacking both expressed alleles (odds ratio 1.6 vs. 1.9).

Ryberg et al. (1997) examined the possibility of interaction between the newly described GSTP1 polymorphism (Ali-Osman et al., 1997; Harries et al., 1996) and GSTM1 genotypes and the influence on adduct levels and lung cancer risk. Of the four genotype combinations (GSTM1 null/GSTP1 AA, GSTM1 null/GSTP1 AG+GG, GSTM1 positive/GSTP1 AA, GSTM1 positive/GSTP1 AG+GG), the highest adduct levels were observed in patients with the GSTM1 null/GSTP1 AG+GG haplotype, who had significantly higher adduct levels than in all other genotype combinations (P = 0.011). However, although this genotype combination accounted for approximately 60% of the χ^2 value in case-control comparisons, no synergistic effect on lung cancer risk could be confirmed.

(ii) Theta class GST
The concept of increased susceptibility in patients with the GSTM1/GSTT1 double null genotype is attractive in the context of protection against oxidative stress, since both gene products metabolize the products of damage induced by reactive oxygen species (Hayes & Strange, 1995). However, although some studies have examined both genotypes in a number of pathologies including colon cancer (Deakin et al., 1996), we are not aware of any report of a significant interaction between these gene polymorphisms. We identified an increased proportion of individuals null at both

GSTM1 and GSTT1 in epithelial ovarian cancer (Sarhanis et al., 1996) and photosensitive systemic lupus erythematosus (Ollier et al., 1996), but these effects may be due to the increased frequencies of the individual genotypes alone. Similarly, Chen et al. (1996) have recently assessed the role of GSTM1 null and GSTT1 null genotypes as mediators of risk of hepatocellular carcinoma in patients exposed to aflatoxin. This study suggested the possibility of an interaction, although the case group was small (32 cases and 73 controls) and both genotypes alone significantly influenced the levels of aflatoxin-albumin adducts. We found no evidence of interaction between GSTM1 null and GSTT1 null in patients with meningioma and astrocytoma (Elexperu-Camiruaga et al., 1996), even though GSTT1 null alone was shown to be influential, further supporting the view that while these enzymes both utilize epoxide as substrates they differ in the particular epoxides they preferentially detoxify (Norppa et al., 1995).

(iii) NAT
Further promising candidates for susceptibility are the phase II N-acetyltransferase genes NAT1 and NAT2 which encode enzymes that can utilize carcinogenic aryl- and heterocyclic amines found in cigarette smoke, environmental pollution and cooked food (e.g. 2-naphthylamine, 2-amino-3-methylimidazo-[4,5-f]quinoline) (Sinha et al., 1994; Lang et al., 1994; Kadlubar et al., 1992). NAT2 activity varies widely in human populations, about 55% of Caucasians demonstrating little or no activity and being classed as slow acetylators. Individuals with NAT2 rapid phenotypes appear to be at increased risk of colon cancer following exposure to heterocyclic amines in cooked foods, while slow acetylators are at increased risk of arylamine-induced bladder cancer (Risch et al., 1995; Lang et al., 1994). NAT1 gene is also polymorphic (Bell et al., 1995b), high-risk NAT1 genotypes being associated with susceptibility to bladder and colon cancers. Similarly, the frequency of homozygosity for GSTM1*0 is increased in bladder and colon cancer patients (Bell et al., 1995a,b), suggesting that a combined GSTM1/NAT1/2 genotype may influence bladder cancer risk. Recently, Brockmöller et al. (1996) showed that individuals deficient in

both enzymes were at higher risk of bladder cancer than the individual genotypes, though it 'did not exceed the effect expected if GSTM1 and NAT2 acted independently as risk factors'. This possibility of a combined effect on bladder cancer risk is further supported by Gabbani *et al.* (1996), who showed that coke oven workers with the combined GSTM1 null/NAT2 slow acetylator genotype demonstrated increased urinary mutagenicity. There is some preliminary evidence of a possible interaction between GSTM1 null and NAT2 rapid acetylator genotypes in colon cancer (Probst-Hensch *et al.*, 1995), but larger case groups are needed to confirm this. However, further evidence in favour of a combined effect comes from studies in asbestos-related malignant mesothelioma (Hirvonen *et al.*, 1995): in patients with high exposure to asbestos the risk attributed to GSTM1 and NAT2 genotypes alone was increased by factors of 2.3 and 3.7 respectively, whereas it was increased by a factor of 7.4 for the combined genotype. Data describing associations between the combined GSTM1 null/NAT2 slow acetylator genotypes and increased DNA adduct levels are conflicting. Thus, some studies have shown a positive effect (Hou *et al.*, 1995) while others have failed to show any association (Nielsen *et al.*, 1996). Even where the frequency of subjects with the combined genotype is greater in cases than controls it is essential to confirm that the effect is synergistic, since there is also evidence that these gene products may have separate effects on cancer risk (Hirvonen *et al.*, 1994).

Interactions between phase 1 enzymes

No significant interactions between phase 1 enzymes have been identified despite the fact that CYP2D6 and CYP2E1 show some overlap in substrate specificities. Head and neck cancer is a particularly attractive candidate for the study of interactions between phase 1 enzymes since cigarette smoke and alcohol, both recognized risk factors, contain substrates for CYP1A1 (PAH), CYP2E1 (nitrosamines, alcohol) and CYP2D6 (nitrosamines). We, however, have not detected any significant association of allelic variation at any of these loci, either alone or in combination, with tumours of the oral cavity, pharynx or larynx, although, as mentioned above, some of the

problems of identifying interactions involving CYP1A1 or CYP2E1 in Caucasians may arise from the rarity of mutant alleles in these populations compared with Japanese.

Statistical analysis of interactions

Difficulty in analysing combined genotypes often arises from the size of the case groups under consideration (Smith & Day, 1984). Thus, for assessment of GSTM1 null and GSTT1 null genotypes, with an equal number of cases and controls, an odds ratio of 2.0, 80% power and a two-sided significance level of 95%, 148 and 186 subjects would be required in each group respectively. The same power, odds ratio and significance level for the interactive term would require 307 cases and controls. With rare genotype combinations such as CYP2D6 PM/GSTT1 null, the number of cases and controls would be 2172, making these studies unlikely unless the odds ratio were considerably higher than that indicated above or the proportion of controls to cases unequal (although there is likely to be little advantage if this proportion is greater than 3:1). In either case, small frequencies require the use of statistical packages capable of dealing with small or sparse data sets.

With regard to the approach to be used, if one or both of the individual genotype frequencies is significantly different in the case group, the identification of a significantly different proportion of subjects with the combined genotype is not sufficient to establish an interactive effect since the strength of the main effect or effects may drive the proportion to significance. Thus, when we identified a significant association of both GSTT1 null and CYP2D6 PM genotypes in patients with both astrocytoma and meningioma (Elexperu-Camiruaga *et al.*, 1996) it was tempting to speculate that these were synergistic. This possibility was supported by data linking exposure to halomethanes in some industrial processes to risk of these tumours, particularly since, as described above, dichloromethane is metabolized in humans by both CYP- and GST-mediated pathways (Hallier *et al.*, 1994; Ploemen *et al.*, 1997). Although the number of patients with the combined genotype was, as expected, significantly increased in the case group compared with controls, this was due to the increased frequencies of the individual genotypes.

The interpretation of the significance of inter-actions may be simplified if the two factors involved are first tested for independence. Thus, if factors A and B are found to be independent within both the case and control groups using chi-square tests, the interactive effect can be predicted exactly by using the estimates of the effects of the two factors alone since:

$$P(A \text{ and } B) = P(A) \times P(B), \text{ when A and B are independent}$$

Under these conditions, the odds ratio for the combined genotype will approximate to the product of the odds ratios of the single factors. This is demonstrated in the example described above for the influence of CYP2D6 PM and GSTT1 null on susceptibility to astrocytoma and meningioma.

If, however, one or both factors are known to be dependent in the cases or controls (or both), as would be true for GSTM1 null and GSTM3 AA genotypes, then the interactive term must be tested in the presence of the main effects since it is not possible to predict P(A and B) from P(A) and P(B). Breslow & Day (1980) define a true interactive effect as being possible only when P(A and B) is different from what would be expected from P(A) and P(B) and where P(A and B) for the cases is different from P(A and B) for the controls:

$$\text{i.e. } P(A \text{ and } B) \neq P(A) \times P(B) \text{ in cases and/or controls}$$

$$\text{and } P(A \text{ and } B)_{cases} \neq P(A \text{ and } B)_{controls}$$

Under these conditions, the two factors are likely to be synergistic in their contribution to overall risk.

Both independent and dependent situations can be addressed by use of logistic regression analysis. For example, if the combined term (A+B) as well as the two individual factors A and B are significantly more common in the case group than in the controls, the dependence status of the two components can be assessed by including the main effects in the model with the combined term. If the significance of the combined term disappears in the presence of the main effects, the individual factors are independent and therefore not synergistic. For example, using logistic regression analysis, the proportion of individuals with both GSTM3 AA and GSTT1 null (model including the interaction term only) in our astrocytoma case group (Hand *et al.*, 1996) was significantly greater than in the controls (p = 0.023). In the presence of the main effects (model including the interaction term, GSTM3 AA alone and GSTT1 null alone), the significance of the combined genotype (interaction term) disappeared, suggesting the factors to be independent and the significance of the combined effect to be driven by the strength of the GSTT1 null effect.

If, however, logistic regression analysis demonstrates that the significance of the combined term remains in the presence of the main effects, this suggests that there is a true interactive effect and that the factors are synergistic. This is demonstrated by the comparison of the proportions of subjects with skin type 1 and GSTM1 null in patients with single (n = 640) and multiple (n = 304) cutaneous BCC. Using logistic regression, with correction for age and gender, the contribution to risk of multiple tumours is as follows:

Model	p	χ^2	Odds ratio	95% CI
GSTM1 null alone	0.4641	0.54	1.12	0.82-1.53
Skin type 1 alone	0.2576	1.28	1.32	0.81-2.13
GSTM1 null + skin type 1	0.0019	9.65	3.07	1.51-6.21
GSTM1 null + skin type 1 (in the presence of the main effects; GSTM1 null alone and skin type 1 alone)	0.0097	6.69	3.93	1.39-11.09

Thus, the combined term remains significant in the presence of the main effects and suggests that this is a true interaction. This is confirmed by χ^2 tests in the single and multiple BCC group:

2x2 table of GSTM1 null and skin type 1 in single BCC: p = 0.0064 χ^2 = 7.43

2x2 table of GSTM1 null and skin type 1 in multiple BCC: p = 0.262 χ^2 = 1.26

indicating that the two factors are independent in the multiple BCC group but not in single BCC.

The problem of correcting for confounding factors can also be addressed using logistic regression analysis. We have used this approach to assess the influence of genotypes and patient characteristics in cases of astrocytoma and meningioma (Elexperu-Camiruaga et al., 1996). As various factors (GSTM1, GSTT1, CYP2D6, gender, age) were studied the influence on susceptibility of each factor alone and in combination was studied by logistic regression analysis. Combinations of genotypes and characteristics were studied in the presence of the main effects and only those where the interactive term was more significant than either of the main effects were included. For example, the combination GSTT1 null + GSTM1 null was considered in the presence of the main effects (GSTT1 null and GSTM1 null). Since age and gender were significant confounding factors, analysis of the influence of genotypes and other patient characteristics were corrected for these factors. In this way the effect of possible confounding factors is minimized. A further approach is to use matched data sets. For example, for each case, a control matched for age and gender can be used to control the effect of these potentially confounding factors (Breslow & Day, 1980), although patient recruitment is more time-consuming. Correction for age may be important, particularly in genetic analyses of relatively common cancers such as BCC, since some may suggest that a control group containing patients with a younger mean age than the cases may contain a number of cases 'waiting to happen' (i.e. those who will become cases by the time they reach the same age group as the cases). A difference in genotype frequencies between cases and controls may consequently be masked. Further, if a specific genotype is associated with altered survival, correction for age

may be important, particularly in the study of cancers normally presenting in the sixth decade onwards (e.g. oral, colorectal, gastric, lung and non-melanoma skin cancers).

A further important consideration in the analysis is the link between association and causality. Campbell & Machin (1992) suggest that certain additional questions should be asked to provide a stronger argument that the relationship between, in this case, polymorphism and disease, is causal. For example, there is likely to be a significant association between sales of sunscreens and the seasonal incidence of sunburn, although few would advocate that the application of sunscreens increases the incidence of sunburn. Campbell & Machin (1992) suggest that the following points should be addressed:

Have other studies in different populations led to similar conclusions?

Are the results biologically plausible?

Are the subjects with heaviest exposure at greater risk than those with lightest exposure?

Does the disease incidence in a population increase or decrease following increasing or decreasing exposure to a risk factor?

The larger the relative risk, the more convincing the result.

The inclusion of many variables in some studies requires consideration of correction for multiple analyses, an area of which many groups are becoming increasingly aware. In this regard it is important to distinguish between exploratory and confirmatory studies. In the former a number of candidate genes whose influence is postulated on the basis of related supporting evidence may be selected. In this case, testing for multiple analyses is less important since its intention is not to identify factors with a definitive role but those worthy of further study in confirmatory studies. The causality issue is therefore less critical in exploratory studies. In confirmatory analyses, only candidates showing promise in exploratory studies are assessed. This does not have to be done in particularly large study groups as long as the sample size provides sufficient statistical power, but a cohort of patients separate from that of the exploratory study is required and the results have to be significant enough to remain important after correction for multiple analyses (e.g. Bonferoni correction).

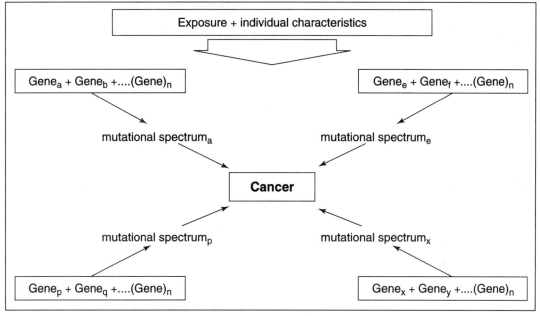

Figure 3. The mechanism by which genes interact to increase cancer risk.

Concluding remarks

Although many reviews have discussed the role of polymorphism in carcinogen-metabolizing enzymes in relation to susceptibility to disease, few have made reference to the combined effects of genotypes, possibly because of the comparative newness of the field. The interactions between GSTM1 and CYP1A1 are discussed briefly in the more general review by Raunio *et al.* (1995a), although much of the work in this area has appeared subsequently. Studies of the effects of individual polymorphisms have generally indicated moderate increases in risk (approximately threefold), suggesting that the investigation of multiple loci is necessary to allow identification of clinically significant at-risk groups. It is likely, therefore, that studies of multiple loci will increase and/or include other covariates such as exposure or patient characteristics. In our recent analyses of the role of carcinogen-metabolizing enzymes in susceptibility to cutaneous basal cell carcinoma we studied five gene loci (GSTM1, GSTM3, GSTT1, CYP2D6, CYP1A1) and ten patient characteristics (age, gender, smoking status, skin type, hair colour, eye colour, tumour numbers, tumour site, occupation, social class), and obtained several outcome measures in over 800 patients (Yengi *et al.*, 1996; Lear *et al.*, 1996). Thus, individual susceptibility to multifactorial diseases such as cancer is likely to be dependent on various haplotypes, each associated with different mutational spectra (Fig. 3).

Unravelling these different molecular routes presents major difficulties, and there is clearly a critical requirement for collaboration between scientists, clinicians, epidemiologists and statisticians in the design and execution of meaningful projects.

Acknowledgments

We are grateful to the Cancer Research Campaign, West Midlands Health Authority Locally Organized Research Scheme, North Staffordshire Hospital Trust Funds and Schering Health Care for financial support.

References

Agundez, J.A.S., Olivera, M., Ladero, J.M., Rodriguez-Lescure, A., Ledesma, M.C., Diaz-Rubio, M., Meyer, U.A. & Benitez, J. (1996) Increased risk for hepatocellular carcinoma in NAT2-slow acetylators and CYP2D6-rapid metabolizers. *Pharmacogenetics*, 6, 501-512

Alexandrie, A.K., Sundberg, M.I., Seidegard, J., Tornling, G. & Rannug, A. (1994) Genetic susceptibility to lung cancer with special emphasis on CYP1A1 and GSTM1: a study on host factors in relation to age at onset, gender and histological cancer types. *Carcinogenesis*, 15, 1785-1790

Ali-Osman, F., Akande, O., Antoun, G., Mao, J.-X. & Buolamwini, J. (1997) Molecular cloning, characterization, and expression in *Escherichia coli* of full-length cDNAs of three human glutathione S-transferase pi gene variants. *J. Biol. Chem.*, 272, 10004-10012

Ambrosone, C.B., Freudenheim, J.L., Graham, S., Marshall, J.R., Vena, J.E., Brasure, J., R., Laughlin, R., Nemoto, T., Michalek, A.M., Harrington, A., Ford, T.D. & Shields, P.G. (1995) Cytochrome P4501A1 and glutathione S-transferase (M1) genetic polymorphisms and postmenopausal breast cancer risk. *Cancer Res.*, 55, 3483-3485

Anttila, S., Hirvonen, A., Husgafvel-Pursiainen, K., Karjalainen, A., Nurminen, T. & Vainio, H. (1994) Combined effect of CYP1A1 inducibility and GSTM1 polymorphism on histological type of lung cancer. *Carcinogenesis*, 15, 1133-1135

Anttila, S., Luostarinen, L., Hirvonen, A., Elovaara, E., Karjalainen, A., Nurminen, T., Hayes, J.D., Vainio, H. & Ketterer, B. (1995) Pulmonary expression of glutathione S-transferase M3 in lung cancer patients: association with GSTM1 polymorphism, smoking, and asbestos exposure. *Cancer Res.*, 55, 3305-3309

Becker, K.G., Jedlicka, P., Templeton, N.S., Liotta, L. & Ozato, K. (1994) Characterization of hUCRBP (YY1, NF-E1, δ): a transcription factor that binds the regulatory regions of many viral and cellular genes. *Gene*, 150, 259-266

Bell, D.A., Badawi, A.F., Lang, N.P., Ilett, K.F., Kadlubar, F.F. & Hirvonen, A. (1995a) Polymorphism in the N-acetyltransferase 1 (NAT1) polyadenylation signal: association of NAT1*10 allele with higher N-acetylation activity in bladder and colon tissue. *Cancer Res.*, 55, 5226-5229

Bell, D.A., Stephens, E.A., Castranio, T., Umbach, D.M., Watson, M., Deakin, M., Elder, J., Hendrickse, C., Duncan, H. & Strange, R.C. (1995b) Polyadenylation polymorphism in the acetyltransferase 1 gene (NAT1) increases risk of colorectal cancer. *Cancer Res.*, 55, 3537-3542

Borlak, J.T., Harsany, V., Schneble, H. & Haegele, K.D. (1994) pNAT and CYP2D6 gene polymorphism in epileptic patients. *Biochem. Pharmacol.*, 48, 1717-1720

Breslow, N.E. & Day, N.E. (1980) In: *Statistical Methods in Cancer Research, Volume 1 - The Analysis of Case-control Studies*. Lyon, IARC Scientific Publications No.32

Brockmöller, J., Cascorbi, I., Kerb, R. & Roots, I. (1996) Combined analysis of inherited polymorphisms in arylamine N-acetyltransferase 2, glutathione S-transferases M1 and T1, microsomal epoxide hydrolase, and cytochrome P450 enzymes as modulators of bladder cancer risk. *Cancer Res.*, 56, 3915-3925

Campbell, M.J. & Machin, D. (1992) *Medical Statistics; a Commonsense Approach*. Second Edition. Chichester, John Wiley & Sons

Camus, A.M., Geneste, O., Honkakoski, P., Bereziat, J.C., Henderson, C.J., Wolf, C.R., Bartsch, H. & Lang, M.A. (1993) High variability of nitrosamine metabolism among individuals: role of cytochromes P450 2A6 and 2E1 in the dealkylation of N-nitrosodimethylamine and N-nitrosodiethylamine in mice and humans. *Mol. Carcinogenesis*, 7, 268-275

Caporaso, N., Falk, R., Tucker, M.A., Shaw, G.L., Frame, J., Poland, A., Song, J., Struewing, J. & Modi, B. (1996) Genetic susceptibility markers in a hospital-based case-control study of lung cancer. *Proc. Am. Assoc. Cancer Res.*, 37, 258-259

Chen, C.J., Yu, M.W., Liaw, Y.F., Wang, L.W., Chiamprasert, S., Matin, F., Hirvonen, A, Bell, D.A. & Santella, R.M. (1996) Chronic hepatitis B carriers with null genotypes of glutathione S-transferase M1 and T1 polymorphisms who are exposed to aflatoxin are at increased risk of hepatocellular carcinoma. *Am. J. Hum. Genet.*, 59, 128-134

Chenevix-Trench, G., Young, J., Coggan, M. & Board, P. (1995) Glutathione S-transferase M1 and T1 polymorphisms: susceptibility to colon cancer and age of onset. *Carcinogenesis*, 16, 1655-1657

Chern, H.D., Huang, C.S., Wang, H.J., Wang, M. & Chang, K.T. (1996) Glutathione S-transferase M1 and T1 polymorphisms: Susceptibility to breast cancer in Taiwan. *Proc. Am. Assoc. Cancer Res.*, 37, 106

Comstock, K.E., Widersten, M., Hao, X.Y., Henner, W.D. & Mannervik, B. (1994) A comparison of the enzymatic and physicochemical properties of human glutathione transferase M4-4 and three other human Mu class enzymes. *Arch. Biochem. Biophys.*, 311, 487-495

Crespi, C.L., Penman, B.W., Gelboin, H.V. & Gonzalez, F.J. (1991) A tobacco smoke-derived nitrosamine, 4-(methylnitrosamino)-1-(3-pyridyl)-1-butanone, is activated by multiple human cytochrome P450s including the polymorphic human cytochrome P4502D6. *Carcinogenesis*, 12, 1197-1201

Deakin, M., Elder, J., Hendrickse, C., Peckham, D., Baldwin, D., Pantin, C., Wild, N., Leopard, P., Bell, D.A., Jones, P., Duncan, H., Brannigan, K., Alldersea, J., Fryer, A.A. & Strange, R.C. (1996) Glutathione S-transferase GSTT1 genotypes and susceptibility to cancer: studies of interactions with GSTM1 in lung, oral, gastric and colorectal cancers. *Carcinogenesis*, 17, 881-884

d'Errico, A., Taioli, E., Chen, X. & Vineis, P. (1996) Genetic metabolic polymorphisms and the risk of cancer: a review of the literature. *Biomarkers*, 1, 149-173

Duncan, H., Swan, C., Green, J., Jones, P., Brannigan, K., Alldersea, J., Fryer, A.A. & Strange, R.C. (1995) Interactions between glutathione S-transferase GSTM1 and GSTT1 genotypes and susceptibility to ulcerative colitis and Crohn's disease. *Clin. Chim. Acta*, 240, 53-61

Elexperu-Camiruaga, J., Buxton, N., Kandula, V., Dias, P.S., Campbell, D., McIntosh, J., Broome, J., Jones, P., Inskip, A., Alldersea, J., Fryer, A.A. &

Strange, R.C. (1996) Susceptibility to astrocytoma and meningioma: influence of allelism at glutathione S-transferase, GSTT1 and GSTM1 and cytochrome P450, CYP2D6 loci. *Cancer Res.*, 55, 4237-4239

El-Zein, R.A., Zwischenberger, J.B., Abdel-Rahman, S.Z., Sankar, A.B. & Au, W.W. (1997) Polymorphism of metabolising genes and lung cancer histology: prevalence of CYP2E1 in adenocarcinoma. *Cancer Letters*, 112, 71-78

Emerit, I. (1992) Free radicals and ageing of the skin. *EXS*, 62, 328-341

Garcia-Closas, M., Kelsey, K.T., Wienke, J.K. & Christiani, D.C. (1996) Lung cancer susceptibility and glutathione-S-transferase μ deletion (GSTM1). *Proc. Am. Assoc. Cancer Res.*, 37, 260

Gonzalez, F. (1995) Role of cytochrome P450 1A1 in skin cancer. In: Mukhtar, H., ed, *Skin Cancer: Mechanisms and Human Relevance*. Boca Raton, Florida; CRC press; pp. 89-97

Goto, I., Yoneda, S., Yamamoto, M., & Kawajiri, K. (1996) Prognostic significance of germ line polymorphisms of the *CYP1A1* and glutathione S-transferase genes in patients with non-small cell lung cancer. *Cancer Res.*, 56, 3725-3730

Hallier, E., Schroder, K.R., Asmuth, K., Dommermuth, A., Aust, B. & Goergens, H.W. (1994) Metabolism of dichloromethane (methylene chloride) to formaldehyde in human erythrocytes: influence of polymorphism of glutathione transferase theta (GST T1-1). *Arch. Toxicol.*, 68, 423-427

Hand, P.A., Inskip, A., Gilford, J., Alldersea, J., Elexpuru-Camiruaga, J., Hayes, J.D., Jones, P.W., Strange, R.C. & Fryer, A.A. (1996) Allelism at the glutathione S-transferase GSTM3 locus: interactions with GSTM1 and GSTT1 as risk factors for astrocytoma. *Carcinogenesis*, 17, 1919-1922

Harries, L.W., Stubbins, M.J., Forman, D. & Wolf, C.R. (1997) Identification of genetic polymorphism at the glutathione S-transferase pi locus and association with susceptibility to bladder, testicular and prostate cancer. *Carcinogenesis*, 18, 641-644

Hayashi, S.I., Watanabe, J. & Kawajiri, K. (1992) High susceptibility to lung cancer analysed in terms of combined genotypes of CYP1A1 and mu-class glutathione S-transferase genes. *Jpn. J. Cancer Res.*, 83, 866-870

Hayes, J.D. & Pulford, D.J. (1995) The glutathione S-transferase supergene family. Regulation of GST and the contribution of the isoenzymes to cancer chemoprotection and drug resistance. *Crit. Rev. Biochem. Mol. Biol.*, 30, 445-600

Hayes, J.D. & Strange, R.C. (1995) Potential contribution of the glutathione S-transferase supergene family to resistance to oxidative stress. *Free Radical Res.*, 22, 193-207

Heagerty, A., Smith, A., English, J., Lear, J., Perkins, W., Bowers, B., Jones, P., Gilford, J., Alldersea, J., Fryer, A.A. & Strange, R.C. (1996) Susceptibility to multiple cutaneous basal cell carcinomas: significant interactions between glutathione S-transferase GSTM1 genotypes, skin type and male gender. *Br. J. Cancer*, 73, 44-48

Hirvonen, A., Nylund, L., Kociba, P., Husgafvel-Pursiainen, K. & Vainio, H. (1994) Modulation of urinary mutagenicity by genetically determined carcinogen metabolism in smokers. *Carcinogenesis*, 15, 813-815

Hirvonen, A., Pelin, K., Tammilehto, L., Karjalainen, A., Mattson, K. & Linnainmaa, K. (1995) Inherited GSTM1 and NAT2 defects as concurrent risk modifiers in asbestos-related human malignant mesothelioma. *Cancer Res.*, 55, 2981-2983

Hirvonen, A., Saarikoski, S.T., Linnainmaa, K., Koskinen, K., Husgafvel-Pursianen, K., Mattson, K. & Vainio, H. (1996) Glutathione S-transferase and N-acetyltransferase genotypes and asbestos-associated pulmonary disorders. *J. Natl. Cancer Inst.*, 88, 1853-1865

Hou, S.M., Lambert, B. & Hemminki, K. (1995) Relationship between hprt mutant frequency, aromatic DNA adducts and genotypes for GSTM1 and NAT2 in bus maintenance workers. *Carcinogenesis*, 16, 1913-1917

Hung, H.-C., Chuang, J., Chien, Y.-C., Chern, H.-D., Chiang, C.-P., Kuo, Y.-S., Hildesheim, A. & Chen, C.-J. (1997) Genetic polymorphisms of CYP2E1, GSTM1, and GSTT1: environmental factors and risk of oral cancer. *Cancer Epidemiol. Biomarkers Prev.*, 6, 901-905

Ichiba, M., Hagmar, L., Rannug, A., Hogstedt, B., Alexandrie, A.K., Carstensen, U. & Hemminki, K. (1994) Aromatic DNA adducts, micronuclei and genetic polymorphism for CYP1A1 and GST1 in chimney sweeps. *Carcinogenesis*, 15, 1347-1352

Ingelman-Sundberg, M., Johansson, I., Yin, H., Terelius, Y., Eliasson, E., Clot, P. & Albano, E. (1993) Ethanol-inducible cytochrome P4502E1: genetic polymorphism, regulation, and possible role in the etiology of alcohol-induced liver disease. *Alcohol*, 10, 447-452

Inskip, A., Elexperu-Camiruaga, J., Buxton, N., Dias, P.S., MacIntosh, J., Campbell, D., Jones, P.W., Yengi, L., Talbot, J.A., Strange, R.C. & Fryer, A.A. (1995) Identification of polymorphism at the glutathione S-transferase, GSTM3 locus: evidence for linkage with *GSTM1*A*. *Biochem. J.*, 312, 713-716

Jahnke, V., Matthias, C., Fryer, A.A. & Strange, R.C. (1996) Glutathione S-transferase and cytochrome P-450 polymorphism as risk factors for squamous cell carcinoma of the larynx. *Am. J. Surg.*, 172, 671-673

Kadlubar, F., Butler, M.A., Kaderlik, K., Chou, H. & Lang, N. (1992) Polymorphisms of aromatic amine metabolism in humans: relevance for human carcinogenesis. *Environ. Health Persp.*, 98, 69-74

Kato, S., Onda, M., Matsukura., N., Tokunaga, A., Matsuda, N., Higuchi, K., Furukawa, K., Yamashita, K. & Shields, P.G. (1996) Cytochrome p450 1A1 (CYP1A1) and glutathione S-transferase M1 (GSTM1) genetic polymorphisms for gastric and breast cancer. *Proc. Am. Assoc. Cancer Res.*, 37, 259

Katoh, T. & Bell, D.A. (1996) Glutathione S-transferase M1 and T1 genetic polymorphism and susceptibility to gastric and colorectal adenocarcinoma. *Proc. Am. Assoc. Cancer Res.*, 37, 257-258

Katoh, T., Inatomi, H., Nagaoka, A. & Sugita, A. (1995) Cytochrome P4501A1 gene polymorphism and homozygous deletion of the glutathione S-transferase M1 gene in urothelial cancer patients. *Carcinogenesis*, 16, 655-657

Kawajiri, K., Eguchi, H., Nakachi, K., Sekiya, T. & Yamamoto, M. (1996) Association of CYP1A1 germ line polymorphisms with mutations of the p53 gene in lung cancer. *Cancer Res.*, 56, 72-76

Kawajiri, K., Nakachi, K., Imai, K., Watanabe, J. & Hayashi, S. (1993) The CYP1A1 gene and cancer susceptibility. *Crit. Rev. Oncol. Hematol.*, 14, 77-87

Kellermann, G., Shaw, C.R. & Luyten-Kellermann, M. (1973) Aryl hydrocarbon hydroxylase inducibility and bronchogenic carcinoma. *N. Engl. J. Med.*, 289, 934-939

Ketterer, B., Taylor, J., Meyer, D., Pemble, S., Coles, B., Chulin, X. & Spencer, S. (1993) Some functions of glutathione transferases. In: Tew, K., Mannervik, B., Mantle, T.J., Pickett, C.B. & Hayes, J.D., eds, *Structure and Function of Glutathione Transferases*. Boca Raton, Florida; CRC Press; pp. 15-27

Kihara, M., Kihara, M. & Noda, K. (1995) Risk of smoking for squamous and small cell carcinomas of the lung modulated by combinations of CYP1A1 and GSTM1 gene polymorphisms in a Japanese population. *Carcinogenesis*, 16, 2331-2336

Kiyohara, C., Hirohata, T. & Inutsuka, S. (1996) The relationship between aryl hydrocarbon hydroxylase and polymorphisms of the CYP1A1 gene. *Jpn. J. Cancer Res.*, 87, 18-24

Landi, M.T., Bertazzi, P.A., Shields, P.G., Clark, G., Lucier, G.W., Garte, S.J., Cosma, G. & Caporaso, N.E. (1994) Association between CYP1A1 genotype, mRNA expression and enzymatic activity in humans. *Pharmacogenetics*, 4, 242- 246

Lang, N.P., Butler, M.A., Massengill, J., Lawson, M., Stotts, R.C., Hauer-Jensen, M. & Kadlubar, F.F. (1994) Rapid metabolic phenotypes for acetyl-transferase and cytochrome P4501A2 and putative exposure to food-borne heterocyclic amines increase the risk for colorectal cancer or polyps. *Cancer Epidemiol. Biomarkers Prev.*, 3, 675-682

Lazarus, P., Ren, Q., Strudwick, S., Muscat, J., Stern, J. & Schantz, S. (1996) GSTM1 and CYP1A1 polymorphisms and oral cavity cancer risk. *Proc. Am. Assoc. Cancer Res.*, 37, 107

Lear, J.T., Heagerty, A.H.M., Smith, A., Bowers, B., Rowland Payne, C., Smith, C.A.D., Jones, P.W., Gilford, J., Yengi, L., Alldersea, J., Fryer, A.A. & Strange, R.C. (1996) Multiple cutaneous basal cell carcinomas: glutathione S-transferase (GSTM1, GSTT1) and cytochrome P450 (CYP2D6, CYP1A1) polymorphisms influence tumour numbers and accrual. *Carcinogenesis*, 17, 1891-1896

Lear, J.T., Smith, A., Bowers, B., Heagerty, A.H.M., Jones, P.W., Gilford, J., Alldersea, J., Strange, R.C. & Fryer, A.A. (1997a) Tumour site in cutaneous basal cell carcinoma: influence of glutathione S-transferase, GSTT1 and cytochrome P450, CYP1A1 genotypes and their interactions. *J. Invest. Dermatol.*, 108, 519-522

Lear, J.T., Smith, A.G., Heagerty, A.H.M., Bowers, B., Jones, P.W., Gilford, J., Alldersea, J., Strange, R.C. & Fryer, A.A. (1997b) Truncal site and detoxifying enzyme polymorphisms significantly reduce time to presentation of next cutaneous basal cell carcinoma. *Carcinogenesis*, 18, 1499-1503

McWilliams, J.E., Cohen, J.I. & Henner, W.D., (1996) Glutathione S-transferase M1 and T1 deficiencies and head and neck cancer risk. *Proc. Am. Assoc. Cancer Res.*, 37, 107

Nakachi, K., Imai, K., Hayashi, S. & Kawajiri, K. (1993) Polymorphisms of the CYP1A1 and glutathione S-transferase genes associated with susceptibility to lung cancer in relation to cigarette dose in a Japanese population. *Cancer Res.*, 53, 2994-2999

Nakajima, T., Elovaara, E., Anttila, S., Hirvonen, A., Camus, A.M., Hayes, J.D., Ketterer, B. & Vainio, H. (1995) Expression and polymorphism of glutathione S-transferase in human lungs: risk factors in smoking-related lung cancer. *Carcinogenesis*, 16, 707-711

Nebert, D.W. (1994) Drug-metabolizing enzymes in ligand-modulated transcription. *Biochem. Pharmacol.* 47, 25-37

Nebert, D.W., McKinnon, R.A. & Puga, A. (1996) Human drug-metabolizing enzyme polymorphisms: effect on risk of toxicity and cancer. *DNA Cell Biol.*, 15, 273-280

Nebert, D.W., Puga, A. & Vasiliou, V. (1993) Role of the Ah receptor and the dioxin-inducible [Ah] gene battery in toxicity, cancer, and signal transduction. *Ann. NY Acad. Sci.*, 685, 624-640

Nielsen, P.S., de Pater, N., Okkels, H. & Autrup, H. (1996) Environmental air pollution and DNA adducts in Copenhagen bus drivers - effect of GSTM1 and NAT2 genotypes on adduct levels. *Carcinogenesis*, 17, 1021-1027

Norppa, H., Hirvonen, A., Jarventaus, H., Uuskula, M., Tasa, G., Ojajarvi, A. & Sorsa, M. (1995) Role of GSTT1 and GSTM1 genotypes in determining individual sensitivity to sister chromatid exchange induction by diepoxybutane in cultured human lymphocytes. *Carcinogenesis*, 16, 1261-1264

Ollier, W.E.R., Davies, E., Snowden, N., Alldersea, J., Fryer, A.A., Jones, P. & Strange, R.C. (1996) Association of homozygosity for glutathione S-transferase GSTM1 null alleles with the Ro+/La-autoantibody profile in patients with systemic lupus erythematosus. *Arthritis Rheum.*, 39, 1763-1764

Pearson, W.R., Vorachek, W.R., Xu, S.J., Berger, R., Hart, I., Vannais, D. & Patterson, D. (1993) Identification of class-mu glutathione transferase genes GSTM1-GSTM5 on human chromosome 1p13. *Am. J. Hum. Genet.*, 53, 220-233

Penman, B.W., Reece, J., Smith, T., Yang, C.S., Gelboin, H.V., Gonzalez, F.J. & Crespi, C.L. (1993) Characterization of a human cell line expressing high levels of cDNA-derived CYP2D6. *Pharmacogenetics*, 3, 28-39

Petersen, D.D., McKinney, C.E., Ikeya, K., Smith, H.H., Bale, A.E., McBride, O.W. & Nebert, D.W. (1991) Human CYP1A1 gene: cosegregation of the enzyme inducibility phenotype and an RFLP. *Am. J. Hum. Genet.*, 48, 720-725

Ploemen, J.P., Wormhoudt, L.W., Haenen, G.R., Oudshoom, M.J., Commandeur, J.N., Vermeulen, N.P., de Waziers, I., Beune, P.H., Watabe, T. & van Bladeren, P.J. (1997) The use of human *in vitro* metabolic parameters to explore the risk assessment of hazardous compounds: the case of ethylene dibromide. *Toxicol. Appl. Pharmacol.*, 143, 56-69

Probst-Hensch, N.M., Haile, R.W., Ingles, S.A., Longnecker, M.P., Han, C.Y., Lin, B.K., Lee, D.B., Sakamoto, G.T., Frankl, H.D., Lee, E.R. & Lin, H.J. (1995) Acetylation polymorphism and prevalence of colorectal adenomas. *Cancer Res.*, 55, 2017-2020

Rannug, A., Rannug, U., Rosenkranz, H.S., Winquist, L., Westerholm, R., Agurell, E. & Grafstrom, A.K. (1987) Certain photooxidised derivatives of tryptophan bind with very high affinity to the Ah receptor and are likely to be endogenous signal substances. *J. Biol. Chem.*, 262, 15422-15427

Raunio, H., Husgafvel-Pursiainen, K., Anttila, S., Hietanen, E., Hirvonen, A. & Pelkonen, O. (1995a) Diagnosis of polymorphisms in carcinogen-activating and inactivating enzymes and cancer susceptibility-a review. *Gene*, 159, 113-121

Raunio, H., Panasen, M., Maenpaa, J., Hakkola, J. & Pelkonen, O. (1995b) Expression of extrahepatic cytochrome P450 in humans. In: Pacifici, G.M. &. Fracchia, G.N., eds, *Advances in Drug Metabolism in Man.* Brussels, European Commission, Directorate-General of Science, Research and Development; pp. 233-287

Risch, A., Wallace, D.M., Bathers, S. & Sim, E. (1995) Slow N-acetylation genotype is a susceptibility factor in occupational and smoking related bladder cancer. *Hum. Mol. Genet.*, 4, 231-236

Roots, I., Brockmöller, J., Drakoulis, N. & Loddenkemper, R. (1992) Mutant genes of cytochrome P-450IID6, glutathione S-transferase class Mu, and arylamine N-acetyltransferase in lung cancer patients. *Clin. Invest.*, 70, 307-319

Rothman., N., Traver, R.D., Smith, M.T., Hayes, R.B., Li, G.-L., Campleman, S., Dosemeci, M., Zhang, L., Linet, M., Wacholder, S., Yin, S.-N. & Ross, D. (1996) Lack of NAD(P)H:quinone oxi-doreductase activity (NQ01) is associated with increased risk of benzene hematotoxicity. *Proc. Am. Assoc. Cancer Res.*, 37, 258

Rushmore, T.H., Morton, M.R. & Pickett, C.B. (1991) The antioxidant responsive element. Activation by oxidative stress and identification of the DNA consensus sequence required for functional activity. *J. Biol. Chem.*, 266, 11632-11639

Ryberg, D., Skaug, V., Hewer, A., Phillips, D.H., Harries, L.W., Wolf, C.R., Ogreid, D., Ulvik, A., Vu, P. & Haugen, A. (1997) Genotypes of the glu-tathione transferase M1 and P1 and their signifi-cance for lung DNA adduct levels and cancer risk. *Carcinogenesis*, 18, 1285-1289

Sarhanis, P., Redman, C., Perrett, C., Brannigan, K., Clayton, R.N., Hand, P., Musgrove, C., Suarez, V., Jones, P., Fryer, A.A., Farrell, W.E. & Strange, R.C. (1996) Epithelial ovarian cancer: influence of polymorphism at the glutathione S-transferase GSTM1 and GSTT1 loci on p53 expression. *Br. J. Cancer*, 74, 1757-1761

Seree, E.M., Villard, P.H., Re, J.L., De Meo, M., Lacarelle, B., Attolini, L., Dumenil, G., Catalin, J., Durand, A. & Barra, Y. (1996) High inducibility of mouse renal CYP2E1 gene by tobacco smoke and its possible effect on DNA single strand breaks. *Biochem. Biophys. Res. Commun.*, 219, 429-434

Sinha, R., Rothman, N., Brown, E.D., Mark, S.D., Hoover, R.N., Caporaso, N.E., Levander, O.A., Knize, M.G., Lang, N.P. & Kadlubar, F.F. (1994) Pan-fried meat containing high levels of hetero-cyclic aromatic amines but low levels of poly-cyclic aromatic hydrocarbons induces cytochrome P4501A2 activity in humans. *Cancer Res.*, 54, 6154-6159

Smith, P.G. & Day, N.E. (1984) The design of case-control studies: the influence of confound-ing and interaction effects. *Int. J. Epidemiol.*, 13, 356-365

Smith, G., Stanley, L.A., Sim, E., Strange, R.C. & Wolf, C.R. (1995) Metabolic polymorphisms and cancer susceptibility. *Cancer Surveys*, 25, 27-65

Vaury, C., Laine, R., Noguiez, P., de Coppet, P., Jaulin, C., Praz, F., Pompon, D. & Amor-Gueret, M. (1995) Human glutathione S-transferase M1 null genotype is associated with a high inducibil-ity of cytochrome P450 1A1 gene transcription. *Cancer Res.*, 55, 5520-5523

Warwick, A.P., Redman, C.W., Jones, P.W., Fryer, A.A., Gilford, J., Alldersea, J. & Strange, R.C. (1994a) Progression of cervical intraepithelial neoplasia to cervical cancer: interactions of cytochrome P450 CYP2D6 EM and glutathione S-transferase GSTM1 null genotypes and cigarette smoking. *Br. J. Cancer*, 70 , 704-708

Warwick, A.P., Sarhanis, P., Redman, C., Pemble, S., Taylor, J.B., Ketterer, B., Jones, P., Alldersea, J., Gilford, J., Yengi, L., Fryer, A.A. & Strange, R.C. (1994b) Theta class glutathione S-transferase GSTT1 genotypes and susceptibility to cervical neoplasia: interactions with GSTM1, CYP2D6 and smoking. *Carcinogenesis*, 15, 2841-2845

Yengi, L., Inskip, A., Gilford, J., Alldersea, J., Bailey, L., Smith, A., Lear, J.T., Heagerty, A.H., Bowers, B., Hand, P., Hayes, J.D., Jones, P.W., Strange, R.C. & Fryer, A.A. (1996) Polymorphism at the glutathione S-transferase locus GSTM3: interactions with cytochrome P450 and glu-tathione S-transferase genotypes as risk factors for multiple cutaneous basal cell carcinoma. *Cancer Res.*, 56, 1974-1977

Yu, M.-W., Gladek-Yarborough, A., Chiamprasert, S., Santella, R.M., Liaw, Y.-F. & Chen, C.-J. (1995) Cytochrome P450 2E1 and glutathione S-trans-ferase M1 polymorphisms and susceptibility to hepatocellular carcinoma. *Gastroenterol.*, 109, 1266-1273

Zhang, Z.Y., Fasco, M.J., Huang, L., Guengerich, F.P. & Kaminsky, L.S. (1996) Characterization of purified human recombinant cytochrome P4501A1-Ile462 and -Val462: assessment of a role for the rare allele in carcinogenesis. *Cancer Res.*, 56, 3926-3933

Corresponding author
Anthony A. Fryer
Clinical Biochemistry Research Group,
Centre for Cell and Molecular Medicine,
University of Keele, North Staffordshire Hospital,
Stoke-on-Trent, Staffordshire, ST4 7PA, United Kingdom

Metabolic Polymorphisms and Susceptibility to Cancer
W. Ryder
IARC Scientific Publications No. 148
International Agency for Research on Cancer, Lyon, 1999

Chapter 23. Review of studies of selected metabolic polymorphisms and cancer

Angelo d'Errico, Núria Malats, Paolo Vineis and Paolo Boffetta

In this Chapter we analyse the design and results of the epidemiological studies on the following metabolic polymorphisms: CYP1A1, CYP1A2, CYP2D6, CYP2E1, GSTM1, GSTM3, GSTT1, NAT1 and NAT2. We evaluate all the studies investigating the association between these polymorphisms, alone or combined, and the occurrence of cancer at different sites, and we perform meta-analyses of the available results for the combinations of polymorphisms and cancers with a relatively large number of studies.

We also examine studies concerning the association between the prevalence of each polymorphism and the occurrence of outcomes other than cancer which are biomarkers of target dose (DNA and protein adducts), cytogenetic damage (sister chromatid exchange, chromosomal aberration and micronuclei) or genetic mutation (Ames test, mutations in hprt locus, mutations in oncogenes and tumour-suppressor genes). We define these studies as cross-sectional or transitional.

At the end of this Chapter are plots of publication bias assessment and graphs depicting the meta-analyses. The Annex comprises tables relating to the design and results of the studies.

Materials and methods

Epidemiological studies published until May 1997 were retrieved by means of Medline and Cancerlit. Three types of study are distinguished:
- case-control studies, which evaluate possible differences in the prevalence of polymorphisms between cancer cases and controls or between subgroups of them (e.g. smokers);
- case-case studies, in which the prevalence of polymorphisms is compared between different subgroups of cancer cases;
- cross-sectional studies, comparing frequencies or levels of markers of target dose and cytogenetic or genetic damage between subjects carrying different polymorphisms.

In order to compare the designs of case-control studies we collected information on the following categories:
- number and type of cases;
- number and type of controls;
- response rates;
- phenotyping and genotyping techniques;
- assessment of exposures potentially interacting with the polymorphism;
- assessment of variables characterizing sub-populations of cancer cases and controls;
- any therapies administered to cancer cases and controls before the phenotyping/genotyping test;
- frequency of the polymorphism in controls;
- power of the study.

The design of case-cases studies has been analysed by collecting information on the same categories as for case-control studies, except, of course, where reference is made to controls.

For cross-sectional studies we collected information on:
- number and type of subjects screened to ascertain the prevalence of polymorphisms;
- type of analysis performed to measure the prevalence of the outcome of interest in the subjects sampled;
- phenotyping and genotyping techniques;
- assessment of exposures potentially interacting with the polymorphism;
- assessment of variables characterizing sub-populations of subjects;
- any therapies administered to subjects before the phenotyping/genotyping test;
- frequency of the polymorphism in controls.

The meaning of each category of information collected is discussed briefly below.

CASES

Information is reported on the number and ethnicity of cases, whether they are incident or prevalent, and whether the diagnosis of cancer was confirmed histologically (or cytologically). In this review we decided to consider cases to be prevalent unless stated otherwise. The choice of incident rather than prevalent cases is preferable because, in the latter, the distribution of polymorphisms could be affected by various factors whose importance increases with the time elapsed since diagnosis:

• a certain polymorphism could be associated with survival among cases;

• cases could change their phenotype with the progression of the disease because of metabolic impairment, as has been observed in advanced stages of different types of cancer;

• phenotype could be modified by treatment with drugs, either acting as substrates of these enzymes and inducing them, or interfering in the metabolism of the substance used as a probe for phenotyping subjects.

The histological confirmation of diagnosis is an important tool for reducing diagnostic misclassification and evaluating the association of the polymorphism with different histologies of a particular cancer.

CONTROLS

This section contains information concerning number and ethnicity of controls, whether they were drawn from the general population of healthy subjects or selected among hospital patients, and the variables by which they were matched to cases.

The choice of healthy controls is preferable because in hospital controls the frequency of a specific phenotype/genotype could be associated with the occurrence of the disease that led to hospitalization.

Controls were most frequently matched to cases by gender, age, ethnicity, place of residence and smoking status. Importantly, while in cohort studies matching is a tool to prevent a variable from being a confounder, in case-control studies

this is not true; in fact, especially if a confounding variable is strongly associated with the exposure in the source population, matching controls to cases by that variable could introduce confounding in the data, even if it is absent in the source population, biasing the crude estimate towards the null value (Rothman et al., 1986). For this reason we consider that confounding has been removed only if a matching variable has been controlled by stratified or multivariate analysis.

RESPONSE RATES

Information on response rates is an important feature because a low response rate could imply selection bias: responders could represent a peculiar subgroup of cases or controls in the source population. For example, if phenotyping requires administering drugs with possible adverse reactions, such as debrisoquine, it is possible that a higher proportion of poor metabolizers (PMs), who are more likely to have experienced side-effects, will refuse to participate, causing under-representation of PMs among the controls (Shaw et al., 1995). Lower response rates can be expected among controls, especially among outpatients and healthy controls, who are not under the direct influence of clinicians and feel freer than cases to refuse participation.

PHENOTYPING AND GENOTYPING

Since techniques for genotyping are quite standardized we report only the names of such techniques.

For phenotyping we collected information related to:

• name and dosage of the substance administered;

• kind of analysis performed;

• metabolic ratio, when relevant, i.e. the ratio of the parent compound to a specific metabolite, representing the criterion for separating phenotypic categories.

Error in metabolic phenotyping can be caused by variability in the dosage of the substance administered, in subject compliance, and in techniques of sampling collection and storage. It may also result from exposure to drugs or other factors able to inhibit or induce enzyme activity (Brosen et al., 1987) and from measurement errors.

Genotyping is affected by errors related to DNA analysis techniques, such as contamination during the analysis, false priming in PCR assays (Heim & Mayer, 1991) and detection of a pseudogene.

The measurement error in the characterization of both phenotypes and genotypes is given by the accuracy of the test, i.e. its sensitivity and specificity, defined respectively as the proportion of susceptibles correctly classified and the proportion of non-susceptibles correctly classified as such. The prevalence of the polymorphism in a population influences the bias introduced by misclassification in the measure of effect: sensitivity is important when a polymorphism is widespread (over 85%), since small decreases cause the misclassification of many subjects, while a decrease in specificity produces little bias. Conversely, when the prevalence is very low (under 15%), even small variation in specificity may cause important changes in the odds ratio (OR), while variation in sensitivity does not greatly affect the value of the OR (Rothman et al., 1993).

EXPOSURES

Some studies assessed the exposure of subjects to some environmental carcinogens (tobacco smoke, alcohol, aflatoxin) and occupational carcinogens (PAHs, asbestos, aromatic amines, etc.). Metabolic polymorphisms are supposed to encode enzymes interacting with certain carcinogenic substances, activating or inactivating them. For this reason, differences in cancer risk between subjects carrying different phenotypes/genotypes should, theoretically, occur only if they have been exposed to such carcinogens, being equal to zero among unexposed subjects. If we did not assess the presence of an exposure that could interact with a polymorphism in a population under study, we would find a risk for carrying the polymorphism which would be the average of the ORs among unexposed subjects (assumed to be = 1) and exposed subjects. This would mask the true risk linked to the polymorphism, evaluable only in the presence of that exposure. Statistically, therefore, such exposures cannot be treated as confounders but need to be considered as effect modifiers of the association between metabolic polymorphisms and cancer risk. Consequently, in the analysis of design, we attributed to a study the assessment of the role of a certain exposure only

if the interaction with the polymorphism was evaluated through stratification or by testing for interaction in multivariate analysis.

COVARIATES

Age, gender, ethnicity, cancer histology and other variables are reported which have been controlled for in data analysis, being potential confounders or effect modifiers of the association between a polymorphism and cancer risk. Although it is not known whether some of these variables act as confounders or effect modifiers, we decided to report those variables for which at least the potential confounding role has been controlled for through adjustment of risk estimates.

Regarding ethnicity in particular, subjects involved in studies conducted in Australia, Brazil, the USA, and London and Paris areas were considered to be of mixed ethnicity unless otherwise stated, because in these areas non-Caucasian minorities represent a consistent proportion of the population. Subjects enrolled in studies performed in Europe (except London and Paris) and in the Mediterranean area were considered to be Caucasians, even if this was not explicitly stated to be the case.

THERAPY

Information about therapy administered to the subjects in the studies is reported because of the possible interference of drug treatment or other therapies (chemotherapy, radiotherapy, surgery) with polymorphic enzyme activity.

PREVALENCE OF POLYMORPHISMS

The prevalence is reported of polymorphisms among the controls in each study: it provides an estimate of the prevalence of polymorphisms in the population from which controls are drawn. This measure permits evaluation of the differences in the distribution of a polymorphism among different populations. Differences in the prevalence of polymorphisms have been reported in particular among populations of different ethnic origin; NAT2 slow acetylator polymorphism, for example, occurs in less than 10% of Asian populations but in about 50% of Caucasian populations. This sort of difference can have a confounding effect that needs to be controlled for in data analysis. Nevertheless, this problem can also occur among populations of the same ethnicity in which the prevalence of a polymorphism is not homogeneous. Let us suppose that we perform a case-control study on 1000 cases and 1000 controls of the same ethnicity and that the prevalence of a certain polymorphism is found to be 40% among controls and 40% among cases; the OR for carrying the polymorphism is 1.00 (0.84-1.20). Now let us imagine that the population from which cases and controls are drawn is composed of three genetic subpopulations, representing different proportions of the general population and showing different prevalences of the polymorphism, as indicated below:

Population	Proportion	Polymorphism prevalence
1	40%	50%
2	20%	40%
3	40%	30%
Total	100%	40%

If, in such a situation, the proportion of the three genetic subpopulations is unbalanced between cases and controls, confounding can occur such that the risk estimate is biased, as in the table below.

Note that the frequencies of the polymorphism observed among the controls in each subpopulation are different (population 1, p = 0.25; population 2, p = 0.36; population 3, p = 0.13) but compatible with the theoretical frequencies listed above in the subpopulations.

In this example the crude OR is 1.00 whereas the adjusted value is 1.31 (1.07-1.59), indicating a significantly higher risk associated with the polymorphism.

Note that such a situation is extreme if the prevalence of a polymorphism is high, as in the above example, but becomes more probable if the prevalence is 10% or below.

How can we assess whether such a genetic stratification exists?

It is important to assess if the prevalence of a polymorphism is different among different populations of the same ethnicity; for example we can compare prevalences found in Caucasian populations in different countries in order to decide if the observed fluctuations in prevalence are due to random variations or whether Caucasian ethnicity is composed of different subpopulations having different prevalences. If we find that the prevalence is significantly different in different populations of the same ethnic group it becomes necessary to assess if our population is genetically homogeneous or composed of a mosaic of subpopulations with different prevalences of the polymorphism. This problem is expected to be especially important in countries such as Australia, Canada, and the USA, where the population of Caucasian ethnicity is actually a mosaic of populations recently migrated from all the European and Mediterranean countries; for this reason, estimates from studies performed in these countries could be biased by a residual confounding that would be very difficult to ascertain. Nevertheless, the existence of unknown genetic sub-populations could produce distortion of risk estimates in other countries, especially where a consistent internal migration has taken place.

Population	–	Cases	+	–	Controls	+	(%)	OR
1	80	200	120	140	300	160	(53)	1.31 (0.91-1.89)
2	140	250	110	310	500	190	(38)	1.28 (0.94-1.74)
3	380	550	170	150	200	50	(25)	1.34 (0.93-1.94)
Total	600	1000	400	600	1000	400	(40)	1.31 (1.07-1.59)*

Note: the presence of a certain polymorphism is reported as + and its absence as -.

*Mantel-Haenszel adjusted OR.

STATISTICAL ANALYSIS

ORs for case-control studies were extracted from published papers or computed from crude and stratified data, when available. The frequency of metabolic polymorphisms was compared between cases and controls by means of the χ^2 test, expressing the strength of association between a certain phenotype/genotype and cancer status as an OR. Meta-analysis was performed for any association using both fixed and random effect models; fixed effects were computed using a variance-based method involving confidence intervals, as described by Greenland (1987), random effects by the method of DerSimonian & Laird (1986), using published formulae (Fleiss & Gross, 1991); it was performed on crude ORs and, when estimates where available, on ORs stratified by features of study design (incident/prevalent cases, hospital/healthy controls, genotyping/phenotyping), by exposure to environmental and occupational carcinogens, or by covariates such as ethnicity, age and gender; it was computed for only those polymorphisms investigated in a substantial number of studies, in particular GSTM1, GSTT1, CYP1A1 (Msp I, Exon 7, AA), CYP2E1 (5'-flanking region, Dra I), NAT2 and CYP2D6. Whenever a cell of a 2 × 2 table contained a number of subjects = 0, in order to obtain an odds ratio to include in the meta-analysis a value of 0.5 has been added to each cell.

In order to ascertain the presence of publication bias in meta-analysis, which would result in a higher probability for small studies of displaying a risk in excess, we plotted a measure of estimate (the natural logarithm of the OR) on the x axis and a measure of the precision of the estimate (the inverse of the variance of each study, also defined as weight) on the y axis. The presence of a publication bias has been evaluated on the basis of the asymmetry of such a plot on the x axis, because studies having higher variance would present higher natural logarithms of the OR.

To reduce the possibility of error in assessing publication bias by a simple visual examination, we performed a linear regression, using the inverse of variance (weight) as the independent variable and the natural logarithm of the ratio OR/meta-OR as the dependent variable in order to test if they were significantly inversely correlated at a p value <0.1. In the absence of asym-

metry ORs are normally distributed around the meta-OR, their distribution being equivalent to a sampling distribution of means, and so the natural logarithm of the ratio OR/meta-OR represents the standard normal deviate (SND). In the absence of publication bias the regression line runs through the origin of the SND: for this reason we also tested whether the constant included the origin of the SND at a p-value <0.1 (Egger *et al.*, 1997).

The power of the studies has been computed as the probability of finding a statistically significant association between a certain phenotype/genotype and cancer status, assuming that the true OR = 2 and that the proportion of the relevant phenotype/genotype in the population is the same as in the controls, and that the α-risk is 0.05. Estimates of the power of the studies have been obtained by using the POWER 2 software of R. Shore of the Department of Environmental Epidemiology, New York University Medical School, based on the method of Fleiss *et al.*(1980).

In case-case and cross-sectional studies the prevalence of polymorphisms in different subgroups of subjects was also compared by means of the χ^2 test, but for these studies the probability that the frequency of a polymorphism differs between subgroups has been expressed mainly as a p-value, since the choice of a referent category is not straightforward.

GSTM1

The design of the case-control and case-case studies of GSTM1 are summarized in Annex Table 1.

BLADDER CANCER: CASE-CONTROL STUDIES
Design

We identified 12 case-control studies investigating the association between GSTM1 polymorphism and the occurrence of bladder cancer. The analysis of study design showed that:
- five studies had at least a group of incident cases and seven used prevalent cases;
- eight studies used a healthy control group with which to compare polymorphism frequency in cases;
- none of the studies reported response rates;
- moreover in two it was not possible to determine the ethnicity of the subjects;
- genotyping was performed in 11 studies;

- exposure to tobacco-smoking was assessed in five studies for cases and controls and in two studies for cases only; occupational exposure was assessed in four studies;
- the covariates most frequently considered included: age in five studies, gender in four, ethnicity in eleven, cancer histology in seven, tumour grade in five and tumour stage in two;
- information about therapy was reported in one study;
- statistical power greater than 80% (for an OR equal to or greater than 2 and $\alpha = 0.05$) was attained in five studies.

Results *(Annex Table 4)*

In ten of twelve studies the overall OR exceeded 1.00; of the five studies considering smoking exposure, three showed an excess risk among smokers, while in the two studies reporting data on occupation there were ORs above 1.00 for exposed subjects.

Risks for histologies other than transitional cell carcinoma (TCC) were reported in only one study because the vast majority of bladder cancer is normally represented by TCC; this study revealed an OR above 1.00 for other histologies. All five studies reporting estimates concerning TCC found ORs above 1.00.

ORs over 1.00 were found in nine of eleven studies based on genotyping and in the only one based on phenotyping.

Stratification or restriction by ethnicity showed ORs above 1.00 for Caucasians in eight of nine studies, while for Asians the risk linked to GSTM1null was in excess in two of three studies, and for African-Americans this was true in both of the studies considered.

Only one study reported risks stratified by gender and age, showing an OR higher in males than in females; the risk seemed higher in younger than older subjects.

Concerning interactions between metabolic polymorphisms in determining risk of bladder cancer, a significant interaction was reported between CYP2D6 and GSTM1, revealing a significantly higher risk for 2D6 extensive metabolizers (EM), who also carry GSTM1null polymorphism, compared to 2D6 poor metabolizers (PM) who were positive for GSTM1. In one study a significant interaction was revealed between the NAT2 and

GSTM1 polymorphisms. Comparison of the prevalence of GSTM1 between subgroups of cancer patients indicates that this polymorphism is not significantly associated with grade or stage of bladder cancer.

Meta-analysis *(Annex Graphs 4, 5)*

Meta-analysis of risk estimates was performed on 11 studies: the study by Brockmöller *et al.* (1996) was not included because it added few cases and controls to that of Brockmöller *et al.* (1994) and gave less detailed results.

Meta-analysis of overall ORs, giving an OR = 1.57 (1.36-1.81), revealed that estimates were too heterogeneous to be pooled.

Stratification by ethnicity showed that for Caucasians the estimates lacked homogeneity (OR = 1.54 (1.32-1.80)). Such heterogeneity disappeared when studies based on genotyping were selected (OR = 1.50 (1.28-1.76)) but reappeared when, among these, the subset of estimates concerning incident cases only was considered. Heterogeneity persisted in studies based on genotyping and, among these, in the subset of estimates concerning incident cases only. A meta-analysis of the studies based on genotyping, incident cases and population controls left only two studies giving a meta-OR = 1.33 (0.89-1.98).

Selecting estimates for Caucasian smokers, we pooled three studies and obtained an OR = 1.58 (1.23-2.05); this did not seem much different from the value obtained by pooling the two available estimates for Caucasian non-smokers, OR = 1.61 (0.95-2.73); however, it should be noted that the latter confidence interval is wide and includes unity. A meta-analysis performed on four studies for ORs concerning only TCC histology among Caucasians gave an OR = 1.68 (1.30-2.19). When one study based on phenotyping was eliminated the meta-OR was reduced to 1.57 (1.18-2.08).

Meta-analysis for Asians gave a meta-OR = 1.77 (1.09-2.91); the three studies combined in the analysis were based on genotyping and used population controls, but only one of them concerned incident cases, so it was not possible to ascertain if the selection of the studies having this feature would have changed the result of the pooled estimate. Only one of these studies took into account cancer histology and none considered smoking exposure.

Meta-analysis for African-Americans in two studies based on genotyping yielded a pooled OR = 1.52 (0.69-3.37).

Risk estimates concerning subjects occupationally exposed to bladder carcinogens were obtained in a study on Caucasians and another on Asians, both based on genotyping and prevalent cases; meta-analysis of these estimates gave an OR = 1.49 (0.79-2.83).

LUNG CANCER: CASE-CONTROL STUDIES
Design
We found 22 case-control studies on the association between GSTM1 polymorphism and lung cancer.

- 18 used incident cases and three used prevalent cases, while the ethnicity of the subjects was unknown in 3 studies;
- 18 used at least a group of healthy controls;
- two reported response rates, ranging from 41.4% to 80%;
- genotyping was performed in 19 studies;
- exposure to tobacco smoking was assessed for cases and controls in 15 studies, occupational exposure in four studies, and alcohol exposure in one; moreover in one study the overall exposure to environmental and occupational carcinogens was assessed by means of the total DNA-adducts level;
- the covariates most frequently considered were age in nine studies, gender in 11, ethnicity in 19, and cancer histology in 14;
- information on therapy was reported in five studies;
- statistical power greater than 80% (for an OR equal to or greater than 2 and $\alpha = 0.05$) was attained in 11 of 21 studies (including the results obtained by Seidegard et al. (1986, 1990) considered as a single study).

Results   (Annex Table 3)
Among the 21 studies on GSTM1 and lung cancer an OR above 1.00 was obtained in 17 risk estimates for subjects carrying the GSTM1null polymorphism.

Among the 14 studies considering smoking exposure, the OR for GSTM1null in smokers exceeded 1.00 in ten studies. Among studies in which at least two levels of smoking exposure were considered, excess risk estimates were found in seven of eight studies on heavy smokers and in five of eight on light smokers.

Risk for occupationally exposed subjects was reported in only one study, which showed an increased risk for carriers of GSTM1null who were exposed to asbestos.

We considered the three most frequent types of cancer histology: squamous cell carcinoma, (SQ), small cell carcinoma (SC) and adenocarcinoma (AD). ORs were above 1.00 in 11 of 14 studies for SQ, in seven of nine for SC and in eight of 12 for AD.

Only four studies reported risks stratified by age separately: in two the risk was higher for younger patients than for older ones, while in the other two it was higher for older patients.

Stratification or restriction by gender was performed in six studies: for males all six showed an excess risk for GSTM1null polymorphism, while for females four showed risks above 1.00.

Stratification or restriction by ethnicity showed that ten of 13 studies found risks above 1.00 for Caucasians; all six studies on Asians found ORs above 1.00, while the only available study on African-Americans reported an excess risk linked to GSTM1null.

In two studies a significant interaction between GSTM1null and CYP1A1 Exon7 MM polymorphisms was reported in Asians; in one of two others with Asian subjects there was a significant interaction between GSTM1null and CYP1A1 MspI MM polymorphisms, while in a Caucasian population no significant interaction was demonstrated between GSTM1null and MspI MM+WM.

Meta-analysis   (Graphs 1-3)
Meta-analysis of data was performed on 21 studies. A meta-OR = 1.34 (1.21-1.48) was obtained but the estimates lacked homogeneity.

The pooled analysis of ORs reported for Caucasians (13 studies) gave an OR = 1.21 (1.06-1.39) and this also lacked homogeneity. Heterogeneity among estimates for Caucasians also persisted in studies based on genotyping, while for estimates based on genotyping and incident cases we obtained a homogeneous result (OR = 1.20 (1.03-1.41)); the risk increased when only healthy controls were considered, with OR = 1.30 (1.08-1.56). Meta-analysis of the two phenotype-based studies on Caucasians gave an OR = 1.69

(1.01-2.83). On selecting only risk estimates for Caucasian smokers we obtained a meta-OR = 1.22 (0.96-1.54); the selection from these of ORs based on genotyping and incident cases (five studies) gave an OR = 1.12 (0.87-1.45). Slightly higher but also non-significant meta-ORs came from pooled analyses on light and heavy smokers performed in three studies which were also based on genotyping and incident cases.

Among genotype-based studies, stratification by cancer histology showed no association of GSTM1null with AD, while both meta-ORs for SQ and SC were higher than the corresponding meta-OR for combined histologies. Risk estimates for SQ and SC were further increased when only ORs based on incident cases were selected (OR = 1.40 (1.01-1.95) and OR = 1.86 (1.16-2.97) respectively). It was not possible to investigate the interaction between smoking and different histologies because only one study reported an OR for SC among smokers.

Meta-analysis restricted to Asian subjects in six studies gave a meta-OR = 1.45 (1.23-1.70); a higher value (OR = 1.61 (1.28-2.02)) was obtained with restriction to Asian smokers. The pooled risk for light smokers (OR = 1.24 (0.87-1.77)) was much lower than that for heavy smokers (OR = 1.89 (1.37-2.60)), suggesting that susceptibility to lung cancer linked to GSTM1null could be mediated by a dose-response effect. Stratification by cancer histology revealed a higher risk for SQ (OR = 1.70 (1.24-2.33)) and SC (OR = 1.79 (1.24-2.59)) than for AD histology. Meta-analysis for the Kreyberg histological form I (five studies), in which the two histologies apparently more linked to smoking exposure are combined, i.e. SQ and SC, resulted in a meta-OR = 1.66 (1.29-2.12); the value was higher when estimates for heavy smokers were selected (OR=1.98 (1.41-2.78)), while the meta-OR for light smokers was not significantly elevated. All these studies used incident cases and population controls only and all were genotype-based.

LUNG CANCER: CASE-CASE STUDIES
Design

We identified three case-case studies investigating the prevalence of GSTM1null polymorphism in different subgroups of lung cancer; all of them were genotype-based and conducted on incident cases; smoking exposure was considered in two studies and occupational exposure to asbestos and mineral dusts in one; among covariates, ethnicity and cancer histology were considered in all studies and age and gender in one. Information on therapy was also reported in one study.

Results

The prevalence of GSTM1null polymorphism in lung cancer cases was investigated in three studies, two of which were performed on Caucasian populations and one on Asian subjects. In the latter, GSTM1null appeared to be associated with a worse prognosis, being significantly more frequent among non-operable patients in categories with worse performance status and with more advanced N-factor tumour grade and stage; the same study also found a significant interaction of GSTM1null with CYP1A1 MspI WM+MM genotypes in determining a lower survival time. The two studies on Caucasians failed to demonstrate significant associations of GSTM1 with cancer histology, tumour location or occupational exposure, even if a higher proportion of GSTM1null was found in cases exposed to asbestos compared to non-exposed cases; moreover, in one of the studies there was a significant excess of GSTM1+/MspI MM combined polymorphisms in cases with peripheral lung cancer.

BREAST CANCER: CASE-CONTROL STUDIES
Design

Only three case-control studies on the association between GSTM1 and breast cancer were found. Among these, only one used incident cases, two had a separate group of healthy controls, none reported response rates and all were based on genotyping; exposure to tobacco smoking was assessed in only one study; all the studies were restricted to only one ethnicity, but no other covariates were considered in two studies, while the third took age, education and family history of breast cancer into account; information about therapy was never reported; a statistical power greater than 80% (for an OR equal to or greater than 2 and $\alpha = 0.05$) was attained in two studies.

Results   (Annex Table 5)

All the studies reported ORs above 1.00.

In contrast to the older age groups, in the youngest one the risk for GSTM1null was significantly above unity. Stratification by smoking exposure in one study did not show a significant increase in risk among smokers.

In one study there was a non-significant interaction between GSTM1 and CYP1A1 Exon 7 polymorphisms.

Meta-analysis

Meta-analysis of the three studies resulted in an OR = 1.19 (0.92-1.54); the value was unchanged with restriction to Caucasian ethnicity.

BREAST CANCER: CASE-CASE STUDIES

In Caucasian breast cancer there was a significant excess of GSTM1null in patients who were younger, with a more advanced tumour grade and higher levels of cytosolic cathepsin D.

COLORECTAL CANCER: CASE-CONTROL STUDIES

Design

- We found eight case-control studies investigating the association between GSTM1 polymorphism and colorectal cancer.
- five studies used incident cases and three used prevalent cases;
- four studies had a group of healthy controls;
- three studies reported response rates ranging from 46% to 100%;
- seven studies were based on genotyping;
- exposure to tobacco smoking was assessed for cases and controls in three studies;
- the covariates most frequently considered were ethnicity in seven studies, and age, gender, cancer histology and tumour site in four studies;
- information about therapy was never reported;
- statistical power greater than 80% (for an OR equal to or greater than 2 and α = 0.05) was attained in three of seven studies, while in one it was impossible to calculate the power because of unavailability of the GSTM1null frequency in controls.

Results   (Annex Table 5)

Four of the eight studies on GSTM1 and colorectal cancer showed an overall risk above 1.00.

Stratification or restriction by tumour site revealed differences in risk, with an OR below 1.00 for the only study on anal cancer but excess risk in two of four studies on proximal colon cancer and

in three of four on distal colon cancer. For AD a risk above unity occurred in two of three studies; the only study on colorectal adenomas reported an OR below 1.00. One study reported a stratified OR below unity for smokers, while two others reported that significant excess risk was not found among smokers.

In a study on an Asian population the interaction with GSTT1 was tested; there was a non-significantly higher risk for GSTM1null/GSTT1null than for the GSTM1+/GSTT1+ genotype.

Meta-analysis

Meta-analysis of the ORs from the eight studies gave an OR = 1.01 (0.88-1.17) but the estimates were too heterogeneous to be pooled.

Meta-analysis restricted to Caucasians (five studies) gave an OR = 1.12 (0.94-1.33) but the single estimates lacked homogeneity. This problem persisted with genotype-based studies. Among these, restriction to estimates based on incident cases produced a meta-OR = 0.96 (0.79-1.20), computed on two studies. Stratification by cancer histology indicated for AD a meta-OR = 1.08 (0.72-1.62), whereas stratification by tumour site suggested a higher risk for cancers in the distal colon, with an OR = 1.40 (1.05-1.86), than for those in the proximal colon (OR =1.10 (0.84-1.44)), although the former estimate proved too heterogeneous. From the pooled analysis of the three studies on Asian subjects, all based on genotyping and incident cases, we obtained a meta-OR = 1.20 (0.77-1.86); on restriction to the two studies with healthy controls an increased value (OR = 1.54 (0.94-2.52)) was obtained but statistical significance was not reached.

GASTRIC CANCER: CASE-CONTROL STUDIES

Design

Five case-control studies were collected on GSTM1 polymorphism and gastric cancer; two used incident cases and healthy controls, four were genotype-based, and one reported the response rate (100%); smoking was considered in the analysis in one study, ethnicity in all studies, age, gender and cancer histology in three, tumour stage and tumour differentiation in two; therapy was never reported and only one study had a statistical power greater than 80% (for an OR equal to or greater than 2 and α = 0.05).

Results   (Annex Table 5)

Among the five studies, four found an OR above unity for GSTM1null carriers.

Only one study reported risk among smokers: there was a significantly elevated OR in light smokers, which decreased and lacked significance in heavy smokers.

Analysis by histology indicated a significantly higher risk for adenocarcinoma (AD) in two of three studies; stratification by gender was performed in one study, revealing a non-significant risk above unity in females but not in males.

Stratification by ethnicity showed an elevated risk in two of three studies on Asians and in one of two on Caucasians.

Interaction with GSTT1 was investigated in a study that found a non-significant risk above 1.00 for GSTM1null/GSTT1null compared to GSTM1+/GSTT1+.

Meta-analysis

Meta-analysis was performed on five studies, giving a meta-OR = 1.23 (0.95-1.58); however, this result was computed on estimates that were too heterogeneous.

The combined analysis of the two ORs relating to Caucasians gave a meta-OR = 1.04 (0.73-1.49), which also lacked homogeneity.

Meta-analysis restricted to the three studies on Asians, all genotype-based, gave a meta-OR = 1.44 (1.01-2.06); on combining the two estimates based on healthy controls the value increased to 1.87 (1.20-2.91).

Restriction to AD histology produced a significant meta-OR = 1.44 (1.00-2.07), although this was computed on risk estimates from three studies focusing on different ethnicities.

LIVER CANCER: CASE-CONTROL STUDIES
Design

We collected five case-control studies on GSTM1 and liver cancer; three used incident cases and healthy controls, all were genotype-based, two reported response rates (78.9-100%), and smoking exposure was considered in only one study; in one study, exposure to environmental aflatoxin was assessed on the basis of the AFB_1-albumin adduct level. With regard to covariates, age was considered in two studies,

gender in three, ethnicity and cancer histology in all studies, and HBV status in four; therapy was never reported and no study had a statistical power above 80% (for an OR equal to or greater than 2 and $\alpha = 0.05$).

Results   (Annex Table 5)

All five studies on GSTM1 and liver cancer concerned hepatocellular carcinoma (HCC) in Asian populations: three of them found a risk for GSTM1null above 1.00.

Stratification by smoking exposure, performed in one study, did not show a higher risk in smokers compared to non-smokers; in the study where exposure to aflatoxin was assessed on the basis of the AFB_1-adduct level an elevated but non-significant risk was demonstrated in categories of exposed subjects.

Meta-analysis

Meta-analysis of the risk estimates for HCC among Asians produced a pooled OR = 1.16 (0.82-1.65). Restriction to the three studies with incident cases gave a meta-OR = 0.85 (0.54-1.35), whereas restriction to the three based on healthy controls produced a meta-OR = 1.36 (0.86-2.14). It was impossible to estimate the effect produced by using both incident cases and healthy controls because only one study had such a design.

LARYNX CANCER: CASE-CONTROL STUDIES
Design

We found four case-control studies on GSTM1 polymorphism and larynx cancer; two used incident cases and four used healthy controls; three were based on genotyping; none reported response rates; two assessed smoking exposure, three considered ethnicity, two considered age and three considered cancer histology; therapy was never reported and only one had a statistical power above 80% (for an OR equal to or above 2 and $\alpha = 0.05$).

Results   (Annex Table 5)

The association with larynx cancer was evaluated in four studies but one of them reported only an overall risk for oral, pharyngeal and laryngeal squamous cell carcinoma (SQ); three studies found a risk above unity for GSTM1null.

Risk in smokers was analysed in two studies; the one performed on a Caucasian population reported a risk above 1.00, while that performed on an Asian population found an OR below 1.00 for all smokers pooled but a significantly elevated risk for smokers under 60 years of age.

The two studies that examined risk in Caucasians found risks above unity; in the study on Asians mentioned above the OR was below unity.

In three of four studies the histology considered was SQ, and in all three the reported risk for GSTM1null in this type of cancer exceeded 1.00.

Meta-analysis

Meta-analysis of the four studies, including the combined estimate for oral, pharyngeal and laryngeal SQ, yielded an OR = 1.42 (1.10-1.84); restriction to the three ORs for larynx cancer produced a value of 1.30 (0.99-1.72).

Pooled analysis for Caucasians produced a meta-OR = 1.41 (1.03-1.93), computed on risk estimates from two studies concerning only SQ histology.

On combining the two ORs reported for smokers we obtained a pooled OR = 1.49 (0.96-2.31); however, the estimates used, taken from two studies based on incident cases but relating to different ethnicities, were too heterogeneous.

SKIN CANCER: CASE-CONTROL STUDIES
Design

Six studies were identified, all performed on Caucasian subjects; three were conducted on incident cases, two had a group of healthy controls and five were genotype-based; the response rate was reported in one study (100%); smoking, age and gender were considered in two studies, cancer histology in all studies; information about therapy was reported in one study and five studies had a power greater than 80%, whereas for one study it was not possible to calculate the power because of the unavailability of the GSTM1null frequency in controls.

Results   (Annex Table 5)

For melanoma we found three studies, in two of which the risk was above unity and in one it was significant. Only one study reported stratification by gender, showing similar risks in male and female, while a study considering the number of melanomas found a non-significantly elevated OR in multiple melanomas.

Regarding basocellular carcinoma (BCC), we found two studies on the association with GSTM1null with risks around unity, while for multiple BCC a significantly higher risk was found in one of two studies. In another study, analysis concerning tumour site failed to find a higher risk in truncal BCC compared to BCC at other sites. Risk for squamous cell carcinoma was assessed in one study and that for nevoid basal cell carcinoma syndrome in another, both failing to find an increased risk for GSTM1null carriers.

SKIN CANCER: CASE-CASE STUDIES

A significant association was found among basal cell carcinoma (BCC) cases between GSTM1null and skin type in determining the number of tumours; there was an almost significant association of GSTM1null with the BCC appearance rate.

OTHER CANCERS: CASE-CONTROL STUDIES
(Annex Table 5)

The risk for GSTM1null carriers was found to be below unity in myelodisplastic syndrome (MDS), epithelial ovarian cancer and uterine cervical cancer. Such risk was not significantly above 1.00 in oesophageal cancer, astrocytoma and meningioma. Significantly elevated ORs were found for pituitary adenoma, endometrial cancer and acute lymphoblastic leukaemia (ALL), while in mesothelioma the higher risk approached significance. In ALL, stratification by ethnicity showed the risk to be higher for African-Americans than for Caucasians, with a significantly elevated risk for male African-Americans.

OTHER CANCERS: CASE-CASE STUDIES

A study concerning Caucasian cases of childhood lymphoblastic leukaemia found a significantly lower survival time in GSTM1+ carriers than in GSTM1null. A study on ovarian cancer cases did not show a significant association of GSTM1 polymorphism with any prognostic factor.

CROSS-SECTIONAL STUDIES

We identified 42 cross-sectional studies concerning the association between GSTM1 polymorphism and various markers of target dose and cytogenetic or genetic damage.

Regarding markers of target dose we found that DNA adduct levels were evaluated in 17 studies, in 14 of them as PAH-DNA adducts, in two as total DNA adducts and in one as benzidine-DNA adducts; protein adduct levels were evaluated in five studies, in two of them as PAH-albumin adducts, in two as aminobiphenyl-haemoglobin adducts and in one as aflatoxin B1-albumin adducts. Moreover in one study the association with the level of PAHs and their metabolites in urine was tested.

Association with markers of cytogenetic damage was investigated in 13 studies: sister chromatid exchange frequency was considered as an end point in ten studies, although in five of them the assay was performed in cultured lymphocytes treated *in vitro* with carcinogenic chemicals; the frequencies of micronuclei and chromosomal aberrations were evaluated in four studies.

Among markers of genetic damage we considered only p53 and Rb mutations, mutations in the hprt locus, loss of heterozygosity (LOH) and mutagenicity in urine, as indicated by the Ames test. Mutations in p53 gene were evaluated in nine studies, Rb mutations in one study, mutations in hprt locus in two studies, LOH in one study and mutagenicity in urine in five studies.

Design   *(Annex Table 2)*

The analysis of the design of the cross-sectional studies showed that:
- GSTM1 polymorphism was assessed by genotyping in 39 of 43 studies;
- exposure to smoking was assessed in 21 studies, occupational exposure in seven and alcohol exposure in two;
- the covariates most frequently considered were: age in 11 studies, gender in 16 and ethnicity in 34.

Results   *(Annex Table 6)*

Of the 14 studies investigating the association between GSTM1 polymorphism and PAH-DNA adduct levels, four found a significant association, two of them among smokers, while total DNA adducts were significantly elevated in GSTM1null carriers in one of two studies. Interactions between GSTM1 and other metabolic polymorphisms in determining PAH-DNA adduct levels were evaluated in five studies: in one with CYP1A1

MspI polymorphism, in two with CYP1A1 Exon 7 and in two with NAT2. Among these, significantly different PAH-DNA adduct levels were found in only one of the two studies testing for interaction with NAT2, while one study found an interaction with Exon 7 approaching significance.

PAH-albumin adduct levels were assessed in two studies, neither of which showed a significant association with GSTM1, while a significantly higher proportion of GSTM1null was found among subjects with higher levels of AFB_1-albumin adducts.

Regarding aminobiphenyl-haemoglobin adducts, one of two studies found significantly higher levels of 3-ABP-haemoglobin adducts in GSTM1null compared to GSTM1+ carriers. One study considering the interaction with NAT2 and CYP1A2 did not show significantly different ABP-haemoglobin adduct levels for different combinations of these polymorphisms.

SCE frequency was significantly higher for GSTM1null in four of nine studies, one of them in heavy smokers, although in two of the four studies SCEs were induced *in vitro* by carcinogenic substances. None of the four studies considering interaction with GSTT1 showed a significant increase in SCE frequency for combined GSTM1null/GSTT1null; one of these studies showed no significant interaction with NAT2 polymorphism.

None of the four studies evaluating the association with MN frequency found it to be significantly increased in GSTM1null carriers; two of four studies concerning CA showed a significantly higher CA frequency in GSTM1null, one of them in smokers, and an another study found an almost significant increase in smokers. Interactions with GSTT1 and NAT2 did not reveal significant differences in MN frequency, while one of two studies testing interaction with GSTT1 on CA frequency showed a significantly higher frequency for the combined GSTM1/GSTT1null polymorphism.

While Rb mutation frequency was not associated with GSTM1null in the only study focusing on it, p53 mutation frequency was found to be significantly higher in two of nine studies, and in another study the difference approached significance. In two other studies only p53 transversion mutations were significantly associated with GSTM1, one of them in heavy smokers; moreover, in one study a combined heterozygous + homozygous p53 mutation, but not the homozygous one, was significantly increased in GSTM1null. Nevertheless, the frequency of p53 mutations seems to be quite consistently elevated across the studies, especially among smokers. One study considering interactions with MspI and Exon 7 CYP1A1 polymorphisms found a highly significant increase in p53 mutation frequency for either GSTM1null/MspI MM or GSTM1null/Exon 7 MM polymorphism, while another study found a significant interaction with GSTT1 on p53 mutations.

Mutation frequency on the hprt locus was found to be significantly associated with GSTM1null polymorphism only in one study on a subgroup of garage workers.

Urinary mutagenicity was significantly associated with GSTM1 in two of four studies, one of them in smokers and one in non-smokers living in an area of high pollution; the other two studies showed non-significantly higher urinary mutagenicity in GSTM1null carriers. Interaction with other metabolic polymorphisms was tested in only one study on GSTM1 and NAT2, in which significantly higher urinary mutagenicity was found in smokers carrying GSTM1null/NAT2slow polymorphism.

GSTT1

The design of the case-control and case-case studies of GSTT1 is summarized in Annex Table 9. The corresponding results are presented in Annex Table 11.

BLADDER CANCER: CASE-CONTROL STUDIES
Design

We collected two case-control studies on GSTT1 and bladder cancer. Both of them were genotype-based; one used incident cases and one healthy controls; neither reported response rates; exposure to tobacco smoking was considered in one study for cases and controls and in one study for cases only (in this study there was no exposure to smoking in controls because they were newborn infants); among covariates, ethnicity, age, gender and cancer histology were taken into account in one study, while ethnicity was considered in both; information about therapy was never reported; one study had a statistical power greater than 80% (for an OR equal to or greater than 2 and α = 0.05).

Results

In contrast to all other sites of cancer, in bladder cancer the current hypothesis is that GSTT1+ carriers are at increased risk, and ORs have therefore been expressed for GSTT1+ compared to GSTT1null carriers.

In both studies there were small excess risks for GSTT1+; one study found a significant excess risk among non-smokers, while the other showed a significantly higher proportion of GSTT1+ among cases with past smoking exposure compared to cases who had never smoked. No significant interactions with GSTM1, NAT2, CYP2D6, CYP2E1 or CYP1A1 polymorphisms were found in one study.

Meta-analysis

Meta-analysis of estimates from the two studies, both concerning subjects of Caucasian ethnicity, yielded an OR = 1.18 (0.86-1.63).

LUNG CANCER: CASE-CONTROL STUDIES
Design

Two case-control studies on GSTT1 and lung cancer were found. Both of them were conducted on smokers and based on genotyping and incident cases, but only one included healthy controls; neither reported response rates; age, gender and cancer histology were taken into account in one study; information about therapy was reported in one study; neither had a statistical power greater than 80% (for an OR equal to or greater than 2 and α = 0.05)

Results

OR values above unity were obtained in both studies; one of the studies analysed the combined effect for carrying both the GSTT1null and GSTM1null genotypes, finding no significant interaction on lung cancer risk.

Meta-analysis

Meta-analysis of the two risk estimates for smokers produced an OR = 1.34 (0.74-2.43).

COLORECTAL CANCER: CASE-CONTROL STUDIES
Design

We collected three case-control studies on GSTT1 and colorectal cancer. All were genotype-based, two used incident cases and two had a group of healthy controls; one reported the response rate (100%); smoking was considered in one study; age, gender, ethnicity, cancer histology, tumour stage and tumour site were considered in two studies; information on therapy was never reported; one study had a statistical power above 80% (for an OR equal to or above 2 and $\alpha = 0.05$).

Results
Two of three studies found an overall risk above 1.00. Stratification by tumour site showed excess risk in one of two studies for the proximal colon, in two out of two for the distal colon and in the only study considering the rectal site. Restriction to AD histology showed a risk above unity in one of two studies. Stratification by smoking exposure was performed in one study, which did not find a higher risk for GSTT1null among smokers. Another study found a significantly higher proportion of GSTT1null among cases older than 70 years compared to younger ones. Interaction with GSTT1 was tested in two studies, one of which showed a non-significantly higher risk for GSTT1null/GSTM1null compared to GSTT1+/GSTM1+ subjects.

Meta-analysis
The combined estimate of the results from the three studies, all of which were genotype-based, produced a meta-OR = 1.46 (1.11-1.92). On restriction to Caucasians we obtained a pooled OR = 1.58 (1.14-2.19); among Caucasians, stratification by tumour site produced a meta-OR = 1.49 (0.97-2.30) for cancers in the distal colon (two studies); the two estimates for cancers in the proximal colon were too heterogeneous to be pooled.

GASTRIC CANCER: CASE-CONTROL STUDIES
Design
Two studies on GSTT1 and gastric cancer were collected; one was performed on a Caucasian population, the other on an Asian population. Both were based on genotyping and on incident cases; one had healthy controls; the response rate was reported in one study (100%) and smoking exposure was assessed in one; among the covariates, ethnicity, age and gender were considered in both studies and cancer histology was considered in one; therapy was never reported; one study had a statistical power above 80% (for an OR equal to or greater than 2 and $\alpha = 0.05$).

Results
One study found a small excess risk among GSTT1null carriers. Evaluation of the interaction with the GSTM1 polymorphism demonstrated a risk approaching significance, which was almost two times greater for the GSTT1null/GSTM1null genotype compared to the GSTT1+/GSTM1+ genotype.

Meta-analysis
Combined analysis of the two estimates yielded a meta-OR = 1.07 (0.75-1.52).

SKIN CANCER: CASE-CONTROL STUDIES
Design
Three case-control studies on GSTT1 and skin cancer were found, both genotype-based. One used incident cases, neither used healthy controls; one reported the response rate (100%); smoking exposure was taken into account in one study, age in two, and ethnicity, gender and cancer histology in all of the studies; information on therapy was reported in one study; two studies had a statistical power above 80% (for an OR equal to or greater than 2 and $\alpha = 0.05$), whereas it was impossible to calculate the power for the other because of the unavailability of information on GSTT1null frequency in controls.

Results
Two of the studies focused on basocellular carcinoma (BCC) and both found risks around unity. The third study, which included only truncal BCC cases and used cases with BCC at other sites as controls, found a significantly higher GSTT1 frequency among the former; there was a significant interaction in this study between GSTT1 and CYP1A1 Exon 7 polymorphism in the determination of the truncal site of BCC. Testing for interaction with other polymorphisms in the other two studies failed to give significant results.

SKIN CANCER: CASE-CASE STUDIES
We found one case-case study on GSTT1 and skin cancer which focused on BCC and showed a significantly higher BCC rate for carriers of GSTT1null. This study evaluated interactions with CYP1A1, CYP2D6 and GSTM1 polymorphisms without showing any significant result.

OTHER CANCERS: CASE-CONTROL STUDIES

The design and results of the studies on GSTT1 polymorphism and cancer at different sites are indicated in Table 9 and Table 11 respectively.

The association between GSTT1 polymorphism and liver cancer was examined in a study concerning hepatocellular carcinoma (HCC) in an Asian population; this study found a non-significantly lower risk for GSTT1null, although stratification for exposure to aflatoxin, assessed by means of the AFB_1 adduct level, produced an elevated but non-significant risk among exposed subjects.

The association with larynx cancer was evaluated in two studies, one of which reported only a non-significant overall risk for oral, pharyngeal and laryngeal squamous cell carcinoma (SQ), while the other found a significant association with GSTT1null polymorphism.

The risk for GSTT1null carriers was found to be significantly above unity in myelodisplastic syndrome (MDS), astrocytomas and meningiomas, while for endometrial cancer the excess was non-significant.

Stratification by smoking exposure showed a non-significant association between GSTT1null and epithelial ovarian cancer. There was a significant interaction with CYP2D6 in the determination of high-grade uterine cervical intraepithelial neoplasia (CIN) among smokers.

For acute lymphoblastic leukaemia (ALL), stratification by ethnicity found the risk to be above 1.00 only among African-Americans, and there was a significantly greater proportion of GSTT1null/GSTM1null in African-American cases compared to African-American controls.

CROSS-SECTIONAL STUDIES

We identified 11 cross-sectional studies concerning the association between GSTT1 polymorphism and various markers of target dose and cytogenetic or genetic damage. Their designs are summarized in Annex Table 10 and the results are given in Annex Table 12.

Design

The analysis of the design of the cross-sectional studies showed that:
- GSTT1 polymorphism was assessed by genotyping in 10 of 11 studies;

- exposure to smoking was assessed in three studies and occupational exposure in 3 studies;
- the covariates most frequently considered were age in four studies, gender in four, and ethnicity in eight.

Results

None of the cross-sectional studies investigated the association between GSTT1null and DNA or protein adduct levels.

SCE frequency was significantly higher for GSTT1null in five of nine studies, although in four of five studies SCEs were induced *in vitro* by carcinogenic substances. None of the four studies considering interaction with GSTM1 showed a significant increase in SCE frequency for the combined GSTT1null/GSTM1null, while one of these studies also showed no significant interaction with NAT2 polymorphism.

MN frequency was significantly associated with GSTT1 polymorphism in one of two studies, in particular in subjects exposed to butadiene, but not in unexposed ones; this study also found a significant association with CA frequency among workers exposed to butadiene, while two other studies on CA did not show significantly higher CA frequency in GSTT1null carriers.

The frequency of p53 mutations was almost significantly associated with GSTT1 in one of the two studies focusing on it; the same study found a significantly higher frequency of p53 mutations in GSTM1null/GSTT1null carriers.

GSTM3

The design of the case-control and case-case studies of GSTM3 is summarized in Annex Table 7. The corresponding results are presented in Annex Table 8.

CASE-CONTROL STUDIES

Design

Five case-control studies have been identified focusing on the association between GSTM3 polymorphism and the occurence of cancer in any site. The analysis of the study design showed that among these:
- two studies employed incident cases;
- one study used healthy controls;

- two studies reported response rates (100%);
- genotyping was performed in four studies;
- exposures to tobacco smoking and alcohol were assessed in one study;
- the covariates most frequently considered were age and gender in three studies, ethnicity in all studies and cancer histology in four studies;
- information about therapy was reported in two studies;
- a statistical power greater than 80% (for an OR equal to or greater than 2 and α = 0.05) was attained in one of three studies, while for one study it was impossible to calculate the power because of the unavailability of information on GSTM3 null frequency in the control group.

Results
LUNG CANCER
The only study on the association between GSTM3 polymorphism and lung cancer found a non-significant reduction in risk for subjects with low enzyme activity.

LARYNX CANCER
The association with larynx cancer was evaluated in one study. A significantly elevated risk was reported for laryngeal squamous cell carcinoma (SQ) in GSTM3 homozygous and homozygous + heterozygous for the A allele. Stratification by tumour site showed the risk to be particularly enhanced for glottic tumours.

SKIN CANCER
One study investigated the association between GSTM3 and the occurrence of single or multiple basocellular carcinoma (BCC), showing a risk around unity for A allele homozygosity and a non-significantly higher risk for homozygous + heterozygous A carriers. Another study concerning the association with truncal BCC failed to find either an association between GSTM3 and truncal BCC, or an interaction with CYP1A1, CYP2D6, GSTT1 and GSTM1 polymorphisms in determining the tumour site.

BRAIN TUMOURS
One study on the association with high-grade astrocytoma showed a risk around 1.00 for homozygous carriers of A allele and a non-significantly high-

er risk for homozygous + heterozygous A carriers; moreover a significant interaction on cancer risk was found with GSTT1 but not with GSTM1.

CASE-CASE STUDIES
Only one case-case study has been published on GSTM3, focusing on lung cancer. There was a significantly greater proportion of subjects with high enzyme expression among cases exposed to asbestos compared to non-exposed cases.

NAT2
The design of the case-control and case-case studies on NAT2 is summarized in Annex Table 17.

BLADDER CANCER: CASE-CONTROL STUDIES
Design
We identified 16 case-control studies concerning the association between NAT2 polymorphism and occurrence of bladder cancer. The designs of these studies had the following features:
- three studies had at least a group of incident cases, while 13 used prevalent cases only;
- eight studies used a separate healthy control group;
- no studies reported response rates;
- genotyping was performed in four studies;
- exposure to tobacco smoking was assessed in five studies for cases and controls and in five for cases only, occupational exposure to carcinogens in six studies for cases and controls and in six for cases only, and alcohol exposure in one study for cases and controls;
- the covariates most frequently considered were age in nine studies, gender in eight, ethnicity in all studies, cancer histology in eight studies, and tumour stage and tumour grade in five;
- information on therapy was reported in nine studies;
- a statistical power above 80% (for an OR equal to or greater than 2 and α = 0.05) was attained in three of 16 studies.

Results   (Annex Table 19)
The risk of developing bladder cancer for carriers of NAT2slow compared to NAT2rapid polymorphism was over 1.0 in 11 of 16 studies.
In three of four studies a higher risk was demonstrated among smokers, while stratifica-

tion by occupational exposure in three studies revealed a risk above unity in subjects exposed to bladder carcinogens in two of them, with significance in one study.

Seven studies reported results for transitional cell carcinoma, by far the commonest cancer histology, with an OR above 1.00 in three studies.

Restriction by ethnicity showed ORs over 1.00 for NAT2slow acetylators among Caucasians in 11 of 13 studies, while the risk linked to NAT2slow among Asians was under unity in the three studies performed on them.

With regard to interactions between metabolic polymorphisms in the determination of the risk of bladder cancer, one of two studies found a significantly higher risk for NAT2slow/GSTM1null carriers in comparison with NAT2rapid/GSTM1+ subjects, while another study revealed a significant increase in risk for NAT2slow/NAT1rapid. No significant interaction with CYP2D6 was found in two studies.

Meta-analysis   *(Graphs 6 and 7)*

Meta-analysis of overall ORs from the 16 studies produced an OR = 1.37 (1.20 - 1.57).

For Caucasians in 13 studies there was a meta-OR = 1.41 (1.23-1.61), which was much higher than the pooled estimate for Asian subjects (OR = 0.81 (0.44-1.51)) based on three studies.

Among Caucasians, meta-analysis did not show substantial differences between studies based on genotyping (three studies, meta-OR = 1.44 (1.18-1.75)) and phenotype-based studies (ten studies, meta-OR = 1.38 (1.14-1.67)), so in subsequent analyses we did not keep them separate. Restricting to estimates based on incident cases yielded a meta-OR = 1.41 (1.14-1.74), quite similar to that obtained combining all estimates on Caucasians; this was computed on three studies that all used hospital controls. Selecting only ORs based on healthy controls (six studies, all based on phenotyping and prevalent cases), meta-analysis gave a lower pooled estimate (meta-OR = 1.29 (0.98-1.71)), but individual estimates lacked homogeneity. No studies have been conducted both on incident cases and healthy controls. Restriction to TCC histology produced a meta-OR = 1.13 (0.83-1.95), computed on the results of five studies, all based on phenotyping and prevalent cases. Stratification by smoking

exposure showed for non-smokers (two studies) a meta-OR = 0.87 (0.47-1.62) and for smokers (three studies) a meta-OR = 1.58 (1.24-2.02), but the latter result was based on estimates that were too heterogeneous. Stratification by occupational exposure produced pooled estimates of 1.44 (1.10-1.87) for non-exposed subjects (four studies) and 1.98 (1.27-3.09) for subjects exposed to bladder carcinogens (two studies), all computed on estimates based on hospital controls.

Among Asians, restriction to TCC histology yielded a meta-OR = 0.97 (0.47-2.00); the two studies combined in this analysis were based on phenotyping and concerned prevalent cases. None of the studies conducted on Asians reported risks stratified by smoking exposure and only one related to stratification by occupational exposure.

BLADDER CANCER: CASE-CASE STUDIES

We found only one case-case study on NAT2 and bladder cancer, which more precisely concerned the association with urothelial cancer; this study showed a non-significantly higher NAT2slow frequency among cases who worked in the chemical or rubber industries, which approached significance on restriction to cases previously employed in the Bayer Company.

LUNG CANCER: CASE-CONTROL STUDIES
Design

Six case-control studies on NAT2 polymorphism and lung cancer have been published; three used incident cases and four used healthy controls; four were based on genotyping, one reported the response rate (98% for controls and 100% for cases), smoking exposure was assessed in two studies for cases and controls and in two for cases only, age in three studies (in one for cases and controls and in two for cases only), ethnicity and cancer histology in all studies; therapy was reported in two studies; three studies had a statistical power greater than 80% (for an OR equal to or greater than 2 and $\alpha = 0.05$).

Results   *(Annex Table 21)*

Three of six studies found an OR over unity for carriers of NAT2slow. In two studies a higher risk was also found for NAT2 homozygous rapid acetylators.

Neither of the two studies considering smoking exposure showed a risk above 1.00 for NAT2slow in smokers, while a significantly higher risk was found in one study for NAT2 homozygous rapid among subjects with a cumulative smoking exposure of 20-50 pack-years.

Stratification by cancer histology, performed in all studies, found risks around or below unity for NAT2slow in all histologies, except that in one study elevated risk was demonstrated in adenocarcinomas. In one study there was a higher risk among male subjects for NAT2 homozygous rapid acetylators in LC and mixed-cell histology.

With regard to interaction between metabolic polymorphisms in determining risk of lung cancer, a non-significant interaction between NAT2 and CYP2D6 polymorphisms in Caucasians was reported by one study.

Meta-analysis *(Graph 10)*

Because the study by Roots *et al.* (1988) is included in the one by Cascorbi *et al.* (1996) we considered the crude results of the latter but the estimates stratified by cancer histology of the former, which dealt with a greater number of subjects. Meta-analysis of the estimates for NAT2slow, computed for five studies, yielded an OR = 0.96 (0.82-1.12); this was virtually unchanged on restriction to the four estimates for Caucasians (meta-OR = 0.94 (0.80-1.10)).

Stratification by cancer histology produced, for all histologies, pooled estimates close to 1.00, in particular 1.08 (0.71-1.64) for AD (four studies), 0.98 (0.67-1.37) for SQ (four studies) and 0.78 (0.48-1.26) for SC (three studies).

BREAST CANCER: CASE-CONTROL STUDIES
Design

Eight case-control studies were found on NAT2 and female breast cancer. Among these, four were conducted on incident cases only, seven had a separate group of healthy controls and two were based on genotyping; one reported response rates; exposure to tobacco smoking was considered in two studies, age in three, ethnicity in five, menopausal status in three (in one for cases only) and cancer histology in one; information on therapy was reported in one study; a statistical power above 80% (for an OR equal to or greater than 2 and $\alpha = 0.05$) was attained in two studies.

Results *(Annex Table 22)*

Five of the eight studies reported ORs above unity for rapid versus slow acetylators.

Stratification by menopausal status, performed in two studies, failed to reveal significant differences in risk associated with NAT2rapid polymorphism; stratification by smoking exposure was reported in two studies, one of which showed a high risk among smokers. Only one study investigated the association between NAT2 and breast cancer among different histologies, finding a significantly higher risk for NAT2rapid only in lobular carcinoma.

Meta-analysis *(Graphs 11 and 12)*

Meta-analysis of the estimates from the eight studies produced an OR = 1.11 (0.93-1.32); this did not change on limiting the analysis to the seven studies covering Caucasians only, whose estimates however lacked homogeneity. Among Caucasians, meta-analysis of ORs based on phenotyping yielded a much higher pooled estimate (OR = 1.44 (1.04-2.00), five studies) than the one obtained from studies based on genotyping (OR = 0.90 (0.70-1.17), two studies). Restriction to studies based on phenotyping and healthy controls revealed a meta-OR = 1.80 (1.15-2.84), computed on three estimates, while a combined analysis of the two studies based on phenotyping and incident cases gave a meta-OR = 1.13 (0.68-1.88).

Meta-analysis of stratified results by menopausal status and smoking exposure, both reported in two studies, did not show increases in risk for any of these categories.

COLORECTAL CANCER: CASE-CONTROL STUDIES
Design

We found 12 case-control studies on NAT2 and colorectal cancer, with the following features:
- four studies used incident cases, five prevalent cases, one incident and prevalent cases together, and in two studies it was not possible to determine whether the cases were incident or prevalent;
- four studies had a group of healthy controls;
- three studies reported response rates, ranging from 82% to 100%;

- six studies were based on genotyping;
- exposure to tobacco smoking was assessed for cases and controls in two studies and occupation was considered in one;
- the covariates most frequently considered were ethnicity in eight studies, age in five studies, gender in four, and cancer histology and tumour site in three;
- information on therapy was reported in two studies;
- only one study had a statistical power greater than 80% (for an OR equal to or greater than 2 and $\alpha = 0.05$), while in two studies it was impossible to calculate the power because of the unavailability of information on GSTM1null frequency in controls.

Results   *(Annex Table 20)*

Eight of the 12 studies showed an overall risk above 1.00 for NAT2rapid acetylators.

For Caucasians the risk was over unity in all six studies concerned, while only one of three studies on Asians found an increased risk.

Stratification by tumour site showed no significant differences in risk for NAT2rapid, while analysis by histology showed a risk for AD above unity in one study; all three studies on colorectal adenoma reported ORs above 1.00. Stratification by smoking exposure was performed in two studies on colorectal adenoma; they failed to find a significantly higher risk for NAT2rapid among smokers.

Concerning interactions, one study showed a significant interaction of NAT2rapid with NAT1rapid on the risk of colorectal cancer and another found a significant interaction with CYP1A2rapid phenotype in increasing the risk of colorectal tumours.

Another study failed to demonstrate an interaction between NAT1 and NAT2 polymorphisms but found a significant interaction between NAT2rapid and GSTM1null genotypes on the risk of colorectal adenomas among Caucasian smokers.

Meta-analysis

Meta-analysis of the overall ORs in 12 studies yielded a meta-OR = 1.19 (1.02-1.39).

For Caucasians, stratification by ethnicity in six studies revealed a meta-OR = 1.31 (1.08-1.59); the pooled estimate for Asians was markedly different (0.89 (0.56-1.41)).

Among Caucasians the three studies based on phenotyping gave an OR = 1.48 (1.08-1.98), substantially higher than the value obtained by combining the estimates from the three genotype-based studies (meta-OR = 1.21 (0.94-1.56)). Among the latter, restriction to the two studies based on incident cases did not change the pooled estimate.

Only one study on Asians and one on Caucasians reported separate risks for cancer histology and for tumour site. Meta-analysis of the two reported ORs concerning adenomas produced a meta-OR = 1.24 (0.91-1.69), whereas the pooled analysis of the two estimates for only colon cancers gave a meta-OR = 1.19 (0.72-1.89).

OTHER CANCERS

In Annex Table 23 the results are reported on the association between NAT2 polymorphism and cancer in different sites.

One study found a significant excess of NAT2slow carriers among cases of familial adenomatous polyposis (FAP) compared to controls.

A significantly higher risk for NAT2slow was also found in cases of hepatocellular carcinoma (HCC), which increased when cases without viral markers were selected; moreover, this study showed a significant interaction between NAT2 and CYP2D6 polymorphisms in determining HCC cancer risk.

Another study revealed a significantly greater risk of mesothelioma for carriers of NAT2slow, a risk that was enhanced among subjects with high levels of cumulative exposure to asbestos. An interaction between NAT2 and GSTM1 polymorphism was also found, demonstrating a significantly higher risk for carriers of GSTM1null and NAT2slow compared to GSTM1+/NAT2rapid.

In one study a non-significantly higher risk of developing larynx cancer was found for NAT2rapid vs. NAT2slow. The risk for homozygous rapid acetylators was almost twice that for NAT2slow acetylators.

CROSS-SECTIONAL STUDIES

We identified 15 cross-sectional studies concerning the association between NAT2 polymorphism and various markers of target dose and cytogenetic or genetic damage. Their design is summarized in Annex Table 18 and the results appear in Annex Table 24.

Design

The analysis of the design of the cross-sectional studies showed that:

- NAT2 polymorphism was assessed by genotyping in 10 of the 15 studies;
- exposure to smoking was assessed in seven studies, occupational exposure in four and alcohol exposure in one;
- the covariates most frequently considered were age and gender in four studies and ethnicity in 11 studies.

Results

None of the five studies concerning NAT2 polymorphism and DNA adduct levels was able to find a significant association with NAT2slow, although a higher PAH-DNA adduct level approaching significance was shown by one study in garage workers; in this study a significant interaction between NAT2 and GSTM1 on the PAH-DNA adduct level was also demonstrated; this was not confirmed by another study. The interaction with NAT1 on the aromatic-DNA adduct level was tested in one study without showing significantly higher levels in carriers of NAT2slow/NAT1rapid polymorphism.

Regarding aminobiphenyl-haemoglobin adducts, two of three studies found significantly higher levels of 4-ABP-haemoglobin adducts in NAT2slow compared to NAT2rapid carriers; in one of these studies this occurred only in subjects without appreciable nicotine and cotinine levels in the urine; the third study found that only the level of 3-ABP-haemoglobin adducts was significantly elevated.

The only study investigating the association with SCE, MN and CA failed to find significant differences in their frequencies between NAT2slow and NAT2rapid acetylators; no significant interactions were demonstrated between NAT2 and GSTM1 or GSTT1 in the determination of their frequencies.

Neither mutations at the Rb or the hprt locus, both considered in one study, nor p53 mutation frequency, evaluated in three studies, were found to be significantly increased in carriers of NAT2slow. In another study, K-ras mutation frequency was significantly elevated in NAT2 homozygous rapid compared to other genotypes.

Among the three studies regarding urinary mutagenicity, one found it significantly increased only in NAT2slow acetylators occupationally exposed to arylamines, one reported the same only in smokers, and in the third study this approached significance only in non-smokers.

Interaction with other metabolic polymorphisms was tested in only one study on GSTM1 and NAT2, showing a significantly higher urinary mutagenicity in smokers who carry GSTM1null/NAT2slow polymorphism.

NAT1

CASE-CONTROL STUDIES

The design of the case-control studies on NAT1 is summarized in Annex Table 13. The corresponding results are presented in Annex Table 15.

Design

Three case-control studies have been found concerning the association between NAT1 polymorphism and the occurrence of cancer in any site. The analysis of the study design showed that among these:

- two studies had at least a group of incident cases, while it was not possible to attribute cases in the third;
- none of the studies used healthy controls;
- two studies reported response rates (ranging from 82 to 100%);
- genotyping was performed in all studies;
- exposure to tobacco smoking was assessed in two studies;
- the covariates most frequently considered were age and gender in two studies, ethnicity in all studies and cancer histology in two studies;
- information about therapy was never reported;
- a statistical power greater than 80% (for an OR equal to or greater than 2 and $\alpha = 0.05$) was attained in two of the studies.

Results
COLORECTAL CANCER

We considered one study on the association between NAT1 polymorphism and colorectal cancer, which showed a significant increase in risk for carriers of the NAT1rapid genotype and a significant interaction between this and NAT2rapid in the determination of cancer risk.

Another study, focusing on colorectal adenoma, found a significantly higher proportion of NAT1rapid among incident cases compared to controls, but not among prevalent ones; moreover, this study failed to demonstrate a significant interaction between NAT1 and NAT2 genotypes on the risk of developing adenomas.

BLADDER CANCER

The only study on NAT1 polymorphism and bladder cancer did not show significant differences in NAT1 genotype frequency on the whole or in smokers; moreover, a significantly higher frequency of NAT2slow/NAT1rapid was found in cases compared to controls, while no significant interaction was found between NAT1 and GSTM1 polymorphisms.

CROSS-SECTIONAL STUDIES

We identified two cross-sectional studies that investigated the association between NAT1 polymorphism and DNA adduct levels. Their design is summarized in Annex Table 14 and the results are presented in Annex Table 16.

Design

The analysis of the design of the cross-sectional studies showed that:
- NAT1 polymorphism was assessed also by genotyping in one of two studies;
- exposures were never assessed;
- the only covariate considered was NAT2 polymorphism in one study.

Results

Whereas one of the two studies failed to show that total-DNA adduct levels were significantly associated with NAT1 phenotype, the other found a significant correlation between NAT1 activity and aromatic-DNA adduct levels, revealing also a significant interaction between NAT1 and NAT2 polymorphisms on these levels.

CYP2D6

The design of the case-control and case-case studies on CYP2D6 is summarized in Annex Table 34.

BLADDER CANCER: CASE-CONTROL STUDIES
Design

We collected nine case-control studies on CYP2D6 polymorphism and bladder cancer. The design of these studies had the following features:

- only one study was conducted on incident cases and eight were conducted on prevalent cases only; for one study it was not possible to establish the ethnicity of the subjects;
- four studies had a separate group of healthy controls;
- none of them reported response rates;
- four studies were based on genotyping;
- exposure to tobacco smoking was assessed in four studies, occupational exposure was assessed in four studies for cases and controls and in two studies for cases only, and alcohol intake was considered in two studies;
- among covariates, age was considered in the analysis in four studies, gender in five, ethnicity in eight, cancer histology in five, and tumour stage and tumour grade in three;
- information about therapy was reported in four studies;
- none of the studies had a statistical power above 80% (for an OR equal to or greater than 2 and α = 0.05) to provide evidence for a difference in cancer risk for homozygous (EM) and heterozygous (IM) extensive metabolizers compared to homozygous poor metabolizers (PM). It was impossible to calculate the power of one study because of the lack of information on the frequency of CYP2D6 polymorphism in controls.

Results   *(Annex Table 37)*

Four of eight studies found risks above 1.00 for EM + IM compared to PM, while in one study it was impossible to calculate the overall OR.

Restriction to TCC histology showed excess risks in one of three studies; the only histological results reported were for TCC.

Stratification by tumour stage produced a significantly high risk for aggressive cancer (stage III) in one of three studies, whereas no significant differences in CYP2D6 frequency were found in three out of three studies between tumour grades.

Stratification by smoking exposure in two studies did not reveal significant differences in risk among smokers.

In two studies the frequency of EM + IM was significantly higher among cases occupationally exposed to bladder carcinogens compared to unexposed cases. In another study, stratification by occupational exposure did not show significant differences in CYP2D6 frequency.

ORs above 1.00 were found by two of four studies based on genotyping and by two of four based on phenotyping.

Stratification or restriction by ethnicity showed ORs above 1.00 for Caucasians in three of five studies, while for Asians the risk was below unity in two out of two studies.

With regard to interactions between metabolic polymorphisms in determining risk of bladder cancer, a significant interaction was reported between CYP2D6 and GSTM1, revealing a significantly higher risk for 2D6 EM/GSTM1null polymorphism compared to subjects PM for 2D6 and positive for GSTM1. No significant interactions with other metabolic polymorphisms were found in two other studies.

Meta-analysis   *(Graph 19)*

Meta-analysis of the overall ORs from the eight studies yielded a meta-OR = 1.12 (0.77-1.64).

This risk estimate was virtually unchanged after restriction to the five ORs concerning Caucasian populations (meta-OR = 1.14 (0.78-1.69)), whereas the two studies on Asians, because of the very low prevalence of PM polymorphism, gave an estimate with a very wide confidence interval: OR = 0.65 (0.09-4.61).

Among Caucasians, restriction to the estimates from the four genotype-based studies produced a meta-OR = 1.03 (0.68-1.56), which did not change after the exclusion from the meta-analysis of one OR based on hospital controls.

The three ORs reported for TCC histology gave a meta-OR = 1.82 (0.66-5.01), which, although the estimates were not too heterogeneous, was strongly influenced by the only estimate related to Caucasians because of the very low prevalence of PM polymorphism among Asians.

CASE-CASE STUDIES

We identified one case-case study on bladder cancer, which failed to demonstrate a significant association of CYP2D6 polymorphism with smoking history or tumour grade.

LUNG CANCER: CASE-CONTROL STUDIES

Design

We found 16 case-control studies on CYP2D6 polymorphism and lung cancer. Among these:

- nine studies used incident cases and seven used prevalent cases;
- nine used at least a group of healthy controls;
- three studies reported response rates ranging from 26% to 98%;
- genotyping was performed in seven studies;
- exposure to tobacco smoking was assessed for cases and controls in nine studies and for cases only in one study, occupational exposure to lung carcinogens was assessed in five studies, and alcohol exposure was assessed in one study;
- the covariates most frequently considered were age in seven studies, gender in six, ethnicity in all studies, and cancer histology in 14 studies;
- information about therapy was reported in eight studies;
- none of the studies had a statistical power greater than 80% (for an OR equal to or greater than 2 and $\alpha = 0.05$) to provide evidence of a difference in cancer risk for EM + IM compared to PM, but it was impossible to calculate the power of one study because of the lack of information on the frequency of CYP2D6 polymorphism among controls.

Results   *(Annex Table 36)*

Twelve of 16 studies on CYP2D6 and lung cancer reported ORs over 1.00 for extensive metabolizers (EM + IM).

Among genotype-based studies there was an excess risk for EM + IM in five of seven studies; in phenotype-based studies the same was true in seven of nine studies.

Among the six studies reporting smoking exposure, the OR for EM + IM among smokers was above 1.00 in three studies. Among the four studies considering at least two levels of smoking exposure, two studies reported excess risk estimates for heavy smokers, whereas the other two found risks above 1.00 for light smokers but below unity for heavy smokers.

Risks stratified by occupational exposure were reported in one study, showing a non-significantly higher risk among subjects exposed to PAHs compared to non-exposed subjects.

As regards cancer histology, ORs for EM + IM were above 1.00 in eight of ten studies among SQ cases, in six of nine among SC cases and in six of 12 studies among AD cases.

Restriction to Caucasian ethnicity showed that ten of 15 estimates were above unity, while the only study that reported risks for other ethnic groups found an excess risk among African-Americans.

With regard to interactions between metabolic polymorphisms in the determination of the risk of lung cancer, a non-significant interaction between NAT2 and CYP2D6 polymorphisms in Caucasians was reported by one study.

Because some of the studies focused also on the association between homozygous EM and lung cancer, we have also evaluated the risk linked to EM compared to IM + PM phenotype/genotype when such estimates were available or when it was possible to compute them.

In seven of ten studies, data on this association showed ORs above unity for EM; in three studies they were significant.

Among phenotype-based studies there was an excess risk in three of five studies and in two of them it was significantly increased, while four of five genotype-based studies found ORs above 1.00, which reached significance in one study.

Among Caucasians the risk linked to homozygous EM genotype/phenotype was in excess in seven of nine studies and in two of them it was significant, while among African-Americans the risk was significantly increased in two out of two studies.

Stratification by cancer histology revealed an increased risk in three out of three studies among SQ cases, significant in two of them, in three out of three studies among SC cases, significant in one, in two out of two studies among Kreyberg I cases and in three of four studies among AD histotype cases, reaching significance in two studies.

Stratification by smoking exposure showed ORs above unity in one of two studies: significantly higher risks for carrying homozygous EM were found in one study among light smokers and in the other one among heavy smokers.

Meta-analysis   *(Graphs 17 and 18)*

Meta-analysis of overall ORs for EM + IM compared to PM from the 16 studies produced a meta-OR = 1.26 (1.01-1.58) but the estimates lacked homogeneity. The pooled analysis of the risk estimates reported for Caucasians (15 studies), which

yielded a meta-OR = 1.21 (0.96-1.53), also lacked homogeneity. All the pooled estimates reported below concern Caucasians, because only two studies were conducted on mixed populations and one of them also reported results for Caucasians.

Heterogeneity of estimates related to Caucasians persisted following selection of the eight studies based on phenotyping (OR = 1.33 (0.98-1.80)), while meta-analysis of the ORs based on genotyping (seven studies) produced an OR = 1.10 (0.79-1.55) which did not change substantially on restriction to estimates based on healthy controls (meta-OR = 1.17 (0.78-1.75)).

Restriction to Caucasian smokers (eight studies) produced a meta-OR = 1.25 (0.87-1.79); the value for genotype-based studies (meta-OR = 0.86 (0.47-1.58), two studies) was much lower than that for phenotype-based studies (meta-OR = 1.53 (0.98-2.39), six studies), for which the estimates were, however, too heterogeneous. Stratification by level of smoking exposure, performed in four studies, produced an estimate of 0.75 (0.37-1.50) for light smokers and one of 1.13 (0.56-2.28) for heavy smokers.

Stratification by cancer histology produced pooled estimates below 1.00 for SC (meta-OR = 0.75 (0.45-1.27), eight studies) and significantly below unity for AD (meta-OR = 0.64 (0.43-0.95), 11 studies); combining separately the ORs for AD histology based on phenotyping and genotyping we still obtained a pooled estimate for the former significantly below unity (OR = 0.51 (0.27-0.95), four studies); for genotyping the value was higher and non-significant. Meta-analysis for SQ gave a non-significantly increased value (OR = 1.32 (0.86-2.04), nine studies). The latter estimate, however, decreased when the meta-analysis was restricted to ORs based on genotyping, incident cases and healthy controls (meta-OR = 1.13 (0.40-3.15), three studies).

Interaction between smoking and cancer histology revealed among smokers a meta-OR = 0.51 (0.26-1.00) for AD (three studies) and a pooled estimate of 1.52 (0.71-3.27) for Kreyberg I histology (SQ + SC), also computed for three studies, whereas it was not possible to evaluate the effect of interaction between smoking exposure and SQ histology, which was reported in only one study.

CASE-CASE STUDIES

One phenotype-based study on lung cancer, performed on a Caucasian population, did not show any significant difference in the frequency of CYP2D6 polymorphism between cancers with different histologies.

BREAST CANCER: CASE-CONTROL STUDIES
Design

Five case-control studies were found on breast cancer. Two used incident cases only, four had a separate group of healthy controls, none reported response rates and three were based on genotyping; exposure to tobacco smoking was not considered in any of the studies, ethnicity was considered in four, age and cancer histology in one, menopausal status in one for cases and controls and in one for cases only; information about therapy was reported in three studies; none of the studies had a statistical power greater than 80% (for an OR equal to or greater than 2 and $\alpha = 0.05$).

Results   (Annex Table 38)

Three of five studies reported ORs above 1.00 for PM in comparison with EM + IM; excess risk was found in two of three genotype-based studies and in one of two phenotype-based studies.

Stratification by age, menopausal status and cancer histology was performed in one study and failed to reveal significant differences in PM frequency between subgroups.

Meta-analysis   (Graph 20)

Meta-analysis of the ORs for PM compared to EM + IM polymorphism produced a meta-OR = 1.21 (0.83-1.75).

Restriction to the four estimates related to Caucasians yielded a pooled estimate of 1.32 (0.82-2.03); selection of the ORs from the three genotype-based studies (also based on healthy controls) gave a reduced value of 1.07 (0.63-1.80).

LARYNX CANCER: CASE-CONTROL STUDIES
Design

We found two case-control studies on CYP2D6 polymorphism and larynx cancer; one used incident cases and one healthy controls; one was based on genotyping; none reported response rates; smoking exposure was assessed in both studies, age and gender in one, ethnicity and can-

cer histology in both; therapy was reported in one study; one study did not have a statistical power greater than 80% (for an OR equal to or greater than 2 and $\alpha = 0.05$), while for the other it was impossible to compute the power because of the lack of information on the prevalence of CYP2D6 variants in controls.

Results   (Annex Table 39)

One study did not report a risk estimate but only that it did not find a significantly higher risk for carrying the extensive metabolizer (EM + IM) polymorphism. The other reported a risk slightly over 1.00 for this polymorphism which was increased in particular among subjects with a smoking exposure of 21-30 cigarettes a day but was non-significant. Both studies were restricted to SQ histology.

OTHER CANCERS: CASE-CONTROL STUDIES

Results on the association between CYP2D6 polymorphism and cancer in different sites are reported in Annex Table 39.

In two studies on BCC skin cancer, EM + IM polymorphism was not associated with cancer risk, whereas one of them found a significantly higher risk for EM compared to IM + PM among multiple BCC. In another study, analysis of tumour site failed to find a higher risk in truncal BCC compared to BCC in other sites.

Two studies on meningioma found an increased risk for PM which was significant in one study. One of them also found a significant association of PM genotype with astrocytoma.

A study on CYP2D6 and hepatocellular carcinoma (HCC) revealed a significantly higher risk for EM compared to IM + PM genotype, and also a significant interaction between NAT2slow and CYP2D6 EM polymorphisms.

Two studies on epithelial ovarian cancer did not find any significant association with the extensive metabolizer (EM + IM) genotype, but one of them showed a significantly higher risk for EM genotype compared to IM + PM in cases of cervical intraepithelial neoplasia.

OTHER CANCERS: CASE-CASE STUDIES

A study on basocellular skin carcinoma found a significant association between EM genotype and number of BCCs; there was also a significant interaction of CYP2D6 polymorphism with green-blue eye colour and male gender on BCC number.

CROSS-SECTIONAL STUDIES

We identified seven cross-sectional studies on the association between CYP2D6 polymorphism and various markers of target dose and cytogenetic or genetic damage. Their designs are summarized in Annex Table 35 and the results are presented in Annex Table 40.

Design

The analysis of the design of the cross-sectional studies showed that:

- CYP2D6 polymorphism was assessed by genotyping in five of seven studies;
- exposure to smoking was considered in three studies;
- the covariates most frequently considered were age in three studies, gender in two and ethnicity in five.

Results

The only study concerning the association between CYP2D6 polymorphism and DNA adducts found a significantly higher level of PAH-DNA adducts in EM + IM compared to PM, which was even higher among subjects with low levels of cotinine; only one study focused on aminobiphenyl-haemoglobin adducts, failing to demonstrate higher levels of 4-ABP-haemoglobin adducts in homozygous EM carriers.

The association with SCE was investigated by one study, which did not find significantly different SCE frequencies between different CYP2D6 genotypes. The frequency of mutations at the Rb locus was found to be significantly associated with CYP2D6 activity in one study, whereas p53 mutation frequency, evaluated by four studies, was never significantly different between different CYP2D6 polymorphisms, although in one study it approached significance.

CYP2E1

In the CYP2E1 gene, four different polymorphisms were found, apparently related to the occurrence of cancer: Pst I, Rsa I, Dra I and Taq I. The first two are located in the 5'-transcrip-

tion regulatory region and, because of the high correlation between them, they have often been considered a unique polymorphism under the denomination of 5'-flanking region polymorphism (5'-fr). For this reason we have treated together the data related to these two polymorphisms, and have kept separate the data concerning Dra I and Taq I.

Because the risk of cancer appears to be linked to a single polymorphism and not to the expression of the gene, only genotype-based studies, except for one cross-sectional study, have been performed on the association between CYP2E1 and cancer.

The designs of case-control and case-case studies on the different polymorphisms of CYP2E1 are presented in Annex Table 41 and the results are presented in Annex Tables 43 (lung cancer) and 44 (other cancers).

5-flanking region (Rsa I, Pst I)

BLADDER CANCER: CASE-CONTROL STUDIES

Design

Two case-control studies on 5'-fr polymorphism and bladder cancer were published; neither used incident cases; one used healthy controls; none reported response rates or information about therapy; restriction to Caucasian ethnicity was performed in both studies and one study considered smoking exposure, age, gender and cancer histology in the analysis; neither reached a statistical power greater than 80% (for an OR equal to or greater than 2 and $\alpha = 0.05$) to provide evidence of a difference in cancer risk for homozygous + heterozygous variants (WM + MM) compared to homozygous wild-type (WW).

Results

Both studies found risks below 1.00 for carriers of the WM + MM genotype. No significant interactions were found with other metabolic polymorphisms.

Meta-analysis

The pooled estimate of the two ORs was 0.53 (0.27-1.04), suggesting a possible association between WW genotype and bladder cancer.

LUNG CANCER: CASE-CONTROL STUDIES
Design
We collected seven case-control studies on 5'-fr polymorphism and lung cancer; five used incident cases and five used healthy controls; response rates were reported in one study (80.5% for cases and 99.1% for controls); smoking exposure was considered in six studies and occupational exposure to asbestos was considered in one study; among the covariates, ethnicity was considered in six studies, age in three, and gender and cancer histology in four; therapy was reported in two studies; two studies had a statistical power above 80% (for an OR equal to or above 2 and α = 0.05) to provide evidence of a difference in cancer risk between WM + MM and WW genotypes.

Results
Six of seven studies reported overall ORs below 1.00 for carriers of WM + MM compared to the WW genotype.

Of the risk estimates related to smokers reported in two studies, one was above unity and one was below unity.

Stratification by cancer histology revealed ORs for AD over 1.00 in two of three studies, whereas all three estimates for SQ were under 1.00. Only one OR for SC histology was reported: it too was below unity.

Meta-analysis   (Graph 21)
Meta-analysis of the seven overall ORs produced a meta-OR = 0.82 (0.67-1.01) for the WM + MM genotype, indicating a possible higher risk for the WW genotype. This value was not substantially altered by restriction to the five estimates based on healthy controls or by selection of only the three ORs based on incident cases and healthy controls.

Stratification by ethnicity did not reveal significant differences in cancer risk associated with the 5'-fr polymorphism among Caucasians, African-Americans and Asians.

Stratification by cancer histology, reported in three studies, showed a meta-OR = 1.10 (0.81-1.49) for AD, whereas the pooled estimate for SQ showed a non-significantly lower risk for WM + MM compared to the WW genotype (meta-OR = 0.73 (0.50-1.06).

OTHER CANCERS: CASE-CONTROL STUDIES
The results on the association between the CYP2E1 5'-fr polymorphism and cancer at different sites are indicated in Table 44.

Two studies on hepatocellular carcinoma found a risk below 1.00 for WM + MM; in one study this was significant and the risk appeared to be even lower among smokers.

The 5'-fr polymorphism was not significantly associated with breast cancer (one study), larynx cancer (one study), stomach cancer (two studies) or oesophageal cancer (two studies), whereas an association approaching significance was found in a study on an Asian population between the MM genotype and the occurrence of nasopharyngeal cancer, indicating a risk eight times greater for carriers of the MM genotype compared to WM + WW.

Dra I polymorphism

LUNG CANCER: CASE-CONTROL STUDIES
Design
Four case-control studies on Dra I polymorphism and lung cancer were found; two were conducted on incident cases and three on healthy controls; the response rate was never reported; smoking exposure was assessed in two studies for cases and controls and in one study for cases only, while occupational exposure to asbestos was considered in one study; age and gender were considered in one study, ethnicity in all studies and cancer histology in three studies; therapy was reported in one study; one study had a statistical power greater than 80% (for an OR equal to or greater than 2 and α = 0.05) to provide evidence of a difference in cancer risk between the WM + MM and WW genotypes.

Results
Two of four studies found overall ORs above 1.00 for carriers of WM + MM compared to WW.

Risk estimates related to smokers in two studies were both over unity; in one study a case-case analysis revealed a significant difference in WM + MM frequency between heavy and light smokers.

Stratification by cancer histology in three studies showed ORs above 1.00 for AD and SC histologies in two of them and for SQ in one study.

Meta-analysis

Meta-analysis of the four overall estimates yielded a meta-OR = 1.04 (0.73-1.47) for the WM + MM genotype; this was not modified on restriction of the pooled analysis to the three OR values for Caucasians: meta-OR = 0.95 (0.62-1.47).

Stratification by cancer histology produced no significant results; for SC histology the meta-OR (1.59 (0.73-3.45) (three studies)) was higher than that for AD and SQ.

Meta-analysis of the two estimates related to smokers obtained a non-significantly elevated risk for carriers of the WM + MM genotype (meta-OR = 1.96 (0.61-6.25)).

OTHER CANCERS: CASE-CONTROL STUDIES

Table 44 gives the results on Dra I and cancer in different sites. No significant associations were found between the WM + MM genotype and bladder cancer, breast cancer, hepatocellular carcinoma, and nasopharyngeal, oesophageal and upper aerodigestive tract cancers. Nevertheless the study on nasopharyngeal cancer found a non-significant risk almost five times greater for carriers of MM compared to the WM + WW genotypes.

Taq I polymorphism

Only two case-control studies on Taq I and cancer have been published. The first concerned lung cancer and was conducted on a Caucasian population: it found risks around unity for carrying the WM + MM genotype compared to WW.

The second study investigated the association between Taq I polymorphism and bladder cancer, finding a non-significantly higher risk for the WW genotype compared to WM + MM.

CROSS-SECTIONAL STUDIES

We identified four cross-sectional studies on CYP2E1 polymorphism and various markers of target dose or genetic damage. Their designs are summarized in Annex Table 42 and the results appear in Annex Table 45.

Design

The analysis of the design of the cross-sectional studies showed that:
- CYP2E1 polymorphism was assessed by genotyping in three of four studies;

- exposure to smoking was considered in one study and was assessed through the measurement of serum cotinine levels;
- the covariates most frequently considered were ethnicity in two studies and cancer histology in one study.

Results

One phenotype-based study on laryngeal cancer patients did not find any significant correlation between the total DNA adduct level and CYP2E1 activity, whereas a study on deceased cancer-free subjects showed a significant association between the DNA adduct level (methyl-dGMP) and the Dra I WM genotype compared to WW among subjects with low cotinine levels. Regarding p53 mutation frequency, in one study it was found to be significantly higher among carriers of the Rsa I MM genotype compared to WM + WW, whereas another study, investigating the association of p53 with Rsa I and Dra I polymorphism, did not show any significant association with these polymorphisms.

CYP1A1

Three different polymorphisms have been described in this gene which are apparently related to the occurence of cancer: Msp I, Exon 7 and AA polymorphism. While Msp I and Exon 7 appear to be present among subjects of every ethnicity, AA polymorphism has been found only in African and African-American populations.

Because these three polymorphisms show different associations with cancer in various sites they are treated separately.

Also treated separately are studies based on phenotyping, performed by measuring the activity of aryl hydrocarbon hydroxylase (AHH), the enzyme encoded by the CYP1A1 gene, because AHH activity reflects the presence of mutations in all three polymorphic sites (Msp I, Exon 7, AA).

The designs of case-control and case-case studies on the different polymorphisms of CYP1A1 are presented in Annex Table 25 and the results are given in Annex Tables 27 (lung cancer) and 28 (other cancers). Corresponding data for cross-sectional studies are reported in Annex Tables 26 (design) and 29 (results).

Msp I polymorphism

The prevalence of this polymorphism is very different as between Asian populations, among which the homozygous mutant (MM) and the heterozygous genotype (WM) are present respectively in about 10% and 40% of subjects, and other ethnicities, where the MM genotype is present in about 0.5-5% and WM in about 20% of subjects.

Among Asians the hypothesis mainly investigated related to a difference in cancer risk between the MM and WM + WW genotypes, while in other populations, because of the very low prevalence of the MM genotype, studies focused on differences in cancer risk between the MM + WM and the WW genotypes.

For this reason we treated studies related to Asian and non-Asian populations separately, either for matters concerning the analysis of the design or in the presentation of results and the meta-analysis of data.

Asian populations

LUNG CANCER: CASE-CONTROL STUDIES

Design

We collected five case-control studies conducted on Asians concerning the association between Msp I polymorphism and lung cancer. Their design had the following features: four studies were conducted on incident cases and all studies used healthy controls; none reported response rates; exposure to tobacco smoking was assessed in four studies and occupational exposure in one; among the covariates, gender was considered in one study and cancer histology in all studies; information about therapy was never reported; a statistical power greater than 80% (for an OR equal to or greater than 2 and $\alpha = 0.05$) to provide evidence of a difference in cancer risk between the homozygous mutant (MM) genotype compared to the heterozygous + homozygous wild-type (WM + WW) was attained in one study.

Results

Because the study by Nakachi *et al.* (1993) includes 45 SQ cases reported by Nakachi *et al.* (1991), and because the estimates reported in the two studies are quite similar, we excluded the former from the analysis of results and from the meta-analysis.

Three of four studies found significant overall ORs above 1.00 for MM carriers compared to theWM + WW genotype, whereas in the fourth study, restricted to male smokers, a risk below unity was determined.

Stratification by smoking exposure showed an excess risk among smokers in two of three studies; in studies considering two levels of smoking exposure the risk for the MM genotype was above 1.00 in two of three studies among both light smokers and heavy smokers.

Stratification by cancer histology, reported in all studies, revealed excess risk for SQ histology in three of four studies, for SC in two of four studies and for AD in three out of three studies.

With regard to interactions between metabolic polymorphisms in the determination of the risk of lung cancer, a significant interaction between GSTM1null and CYP1A1 Msp I MM polymorphisms in Asians was reported in one study only among light smokers, whereas in another no significant interaction was found.

Meta-analysis   (Graph 13)

All four studies on Asians were conducted in Japan and were based on healthy controls. Meta-analysis of the estimates from the four studies produced a meta-OR = 1.73 (1.30-2.31) for the MM genotype; restriction to the 3 ORs based on incident cases caused the value to change slightly to 1.64 (1.21-2.23).

Stratification by smoking exposure produced a meta-OR = 1.50 (1.00-2.49) for smokers (three studies); stratification by level of smoking in three studies revealed a much higher risk among light smokers (meta-OR = 2.41 (1.32-4.41)) compared to heavy smokers, for whom the pooled estimate was around unity; nevertheless, estimates related to light smokers lacked homogeneity.

Stratification by cancer histology yielded pooled estimates significantly above 1.00 for SQ (meta-OR = 2.08 (1.44-3.01), four studies) and SC (meta-OR = 1.82 (1.02-3.26), four studies), whereas a non-significantly lower risk was found for AD (three studies). Interaction between SQ histology and smoking exposure was explored in three studies, for which the combined results produced a meta-OR = 1.71 (1.08-2.71) for the MM genotype among smokers.

LUNG CANCER: CASE-CASE STUDIES

One case-case study on Asians focused on non-small-cell lung cancer, showing significant associations of Msp I WM+MM genotype with AD histology, shorter survival time, worse performance status and non-operability; it also found a significant interaction between the WM+MM and GSTM1null genotypes in determining a shorter survival time of cases.

OTHER CANCERS: CASE-CONTROL STUDIES

Table 28 gives the results concerning the association between Msp I polymorphism and cancer in different sites.

Among studies conducted on Asian populations, a significant association was found between the MM genotype and colon cancer *in situ*, whereas in another study no increase in risk was shown for pancreatic cancer.

Non-Asian populations

LUNG CANCER: CASE-CONTROL STUDIES
Design

Ten case-control studies on Msp I polymorphism and lung cancer have been conducted in non-Asian populations; nine of them were based on incident cases and six had a separate group of healthy controls; two reported response rates (ranging from 55.3% to 97.2%); exposure to tobacco smoking was assessed in four studies for cases and controls and in three for cases only, while occupational exposure was considered in three studies for cases and controls; among covariates, age was considered in four studies, gender in five, and ethnicity and cancer histology in all studies; information on therapy was reported in two studies; three studies had a statistical power over 80% (for an OR equal to or greater than 2 and $\alpha = 0.05$) to provide evidence of a difference in cancer risk between the WM + MM and WW genotypes.

Results

In four of ten studies the overall ORs were above 1.00 for carriers of the MM + WM genotype compared to WW.

Estimates related to smokers were above unity in two of four studies, while the risk among light smokers and heavy smokers was found to be in excess in one of three studies and in two of three studies respectively.

Stratification by cancer histology showed risks above unity for the MM + WM genotype in six of nine studies in SQ, in one of eight studies in SC and in two of nine studies in AD histology.

Four of ten risk estimates concerning Caucasians and two out of two ORs related to African-Americans were found above 1.00.

One study explored the interaction between GSTM1null and CYP1A1 MspI WM + MM polymorphisms, without finding a significant increase in risk.

Meta-analysis   *(Graph 14)*

Meta-analysis of the ten overall ORs yielded a meta-OR = 1.05 (0.87-1.28). Restriction to the ten estimates concerning Caucasians produced a meta-OR = 1.04 (0.85-1.27), which did not change substantially with restriction to studies employing only incident cases and healthy controls (meta-OR = 1.00 (0.77-1.31), four studies); among Caucasians, stratification by cancer histology showed that the risk for carrying WM + MM genotype was above unity only among SQ cases (meta-OR = 1.26 (0.95-1.66, seven studies), whereas combined estimates among either AD or SC histologies were non-significantly below 1.00; restriction to Caucasian smokers did not reveal any significant excess risk (meta-OR = 1.10 (0.51-2.38), two studies).

Meta-analysis of the two reported results for African-Americans gave a meta-OR = 1.10 (0.49-2.50).

Because only two estimates relating to Caucasian smokers were reported, and because meta-ORs for Caucasians and African-Americans were quite similar, we combined ORs relating to smokers even if they concerned populations of mixed ethnicities in order to better assess interaction between Msp I polymorphism and smoking exposure. Meta-analysis showed a meta-OR = 1.28 (0.82-2.01) for the WM + MM genotype among all smokers (four studies); a higher value was obtained for light smokers (OR = 1.51 (0.72-3.15), three studies) than for heavy smokers (OR = 1.19 (0.57-2.47), three studies), although statistical significance was not attained.

OTHER CANCERS: CASE-CONTROL STUDIES

Table 28 gives the results concerning the association between Msp I polymorphism and cancer in different sites.

In one study on Caucasians a significant association of the WM + MM genotype with endometrial cancer was found; other studies on Caucasian populations failed to demonstrate significant associations with oesophageal and upper digestive tract cancer, breast cancer, bladder cancer and BCC.

A significantly higher risk for carrying the WM + MM genotype was found among African-Americans in one study on breast cancer, and there was an even higher one for the MM genotype, compared to WM + WW.

CASE-CASE STUDIES

A case-case study on skin cancer found a significant association between the WW genotype and number of BCCs developed among cases, but it did not show a significant interaction between Msp I and CYP2D6 polymorphisms on the BCC rate.

CROSS-SECTIONAL STUDIES

We identified six cross-sectional studies on Msp I polymorphism and various markers of target dose and genetic or cytogenetic damage.

Design

The analysis of the design of the cross-sectional studies showed that:

- exposure to smoking was considered in four studies, occupational exposure to PAHs in one study and alcohol intake in one study;
- the covariates most frequently considered were: ethnicity in four studies, age in one study and gender in two studies.

Results

Three studies concerned the association between Msp I polymorphism and the level of PAH-DNA adducts: one of them found a significantly higher level of PAH-DNA adducts (p = 0.01) in subjects carrying the WW genotype compared to WM + MM, whereas none showed a significant association of the WM + MM genotype with the PAH-DNA adduct level.

No significant association of the WM + MM genotype was found with MN frequency in one study and with SCE frequency in another.

In one study the p53 mutation frequency in Asians was significantly higher in carriers of the MM genotype compared to WM + WW, whereas a study on Caucasians did not show any significant association between the WM + MM genotype and p53 mutations.

Exon 7 polymorphism

For Exon 7 polymorphism too the prevalences of the MM and WM genotypes show wide differences between Asians, where their frequencies are about 5% and 30-40% respectively, and other ethnicities, where the MM genotype is present in about 1% and WM in about 15% of subjects.

As mentioned above in connection with Msp I, for Exon 7 the hypothesis mainly investigated among Asians was that of a difference in cancer risk between the MM and WM+WW genotypes, while in other populations, because of the very low prevalence of the MM genotype, studies focused on differences in cancer risk between the MM+WM and WW genotypes. For Exon 7, therefore, studies relating to Asian and non-Asian populations were treated separately for either the analysis of design or the presentation of the results and the meta-analysis of data.

Asian populations

LUNG CANCER: CASE-CONTROL STUDIES

Design

We found three case-control studies concerning the association of Exon 7 and lung cancer among Asians; all studies were conducted on incident cases and all used healthy controls; none reported response rates; exposure to tobacco smoking was considered in two studies, occupational exposure in one study, gender in one, and ethnicity and cancer histology in all studies; information about therapy was never reported; none of the studies had a statistical power greater than 80% (for an OR equal to or greater than 2 and α = 0.05) to reveal a difference in cancer risk between the MM and WM + WW genotypes.

Results

Two of three studies found overall ORs above 1.00 for the MM genotype compared to the WM + WW genotype.

Among smokers, excess risk was found in one of two studies, whereas the only study considering two levels of smoking exposure found a statistically significant high risk limited to light smokers.

Stratification by cancer histology, reported in all studies, revealed excess risk in two of three studies for SQ and Kreyberg I histotypes, and in the one study for SC and AD histologies.

With regard to interactions between metabolic polymorphisms in the determination of the risk of lung cancer, a significant interaction between GSTM1null and CYP1A1 Exon7 MM polymorphisms was reported in one study, while in another the interaction was significant only among light smokers.

Meta-analysis   *(Graph 15)*

All three studies on Asians were conducted in Japan and were based on incident cases and healthy controls. Meta-analysis of the ORs yielded a meta-OR = 2.25 (1.37-3.69) for the MM genotype, a higher value than that for the pooled estimate related to smokers only (meta-OR = 1.85 (0.86-3.99), two studies).

Stratification by cancer histology produced combined estimates significantly in excess in SQ (meta-OR = 2.53 (1.36-4.70), three studies) and Kreyberg I histologies (meta-OR = 2.35 (1.38-3.99), three studies), but it was not possible to perform meta-analysis on other histologies because results for AD and SC were reported in only one study.

OTHER CANCERS: CASE-CONTROL STUDIES
Table 28 gives the results on the association between Exon 7 polymorphism and cancer in different sites.

In one study no significant association with the MM genotype was found for stomach, breast or colon cancer; similarly, no significant increase in risk was shown for colon cancer *in situ* (one study), oesophageal cancer (one study) and bladder cancer (one study).

Non-Asian populations

LUNG CANCER: CASE-CONTROL STUDIES
Design
In non-Asian populations the association between Msp I polymorphism and lung cancer was investigated in five case-control studies; all of them

were based on incident cases and two had a separate group of healthy controls; one study reported response rates (80.5% for cases and 99.1% for controls); exposure to tobacco smoking was assessed in two studies for cases and controls and in one for cases only, and occupational exposure was assessed in two studies for cases and controls; among the covariates, age was considered in three studies, gender and cancer histology in four, and ethnicity in all studies; information on therapy was reported in one study; none of the studies had a statistical power above 80% (for an OR equal to or greater than 2 and $\alpha = 0.05$) to provide evidence of a difference in cancer risk between the WM + MM and the WW genotypes.

Results
In one study a significant association between Exon 7 polymorphism and lung cancer was not found, but risk estimates were not reported.

Concerning the other four studies, two overall ORs were above 1.00 for carrying the MM + WM genotype, compared to WW.

The only reported OR related to smokers was below unity, whereas stratification by cancer histology revealed for the MM + WM genotype excess risks in one of two studies for AD and in two of three studies for SQ and SC histologies. Moreover, one study did not show a significantly different frequency of the WM+MM genotype in cases with past smoking exposure compared to cases who had never smoked.

Meta-analysis
Because only one risk estimate concerning ethnicities other than Caucasians was reported we performed a meta-analysis restricted to estimates related to Caucasians: a combined estimate of the four overall ORs gave a meta-OR = 1.30 (0.89-1.90).

Stratification by cancer histology failed to show a significant increase in risk for the MM + WM genotype in any histology, giving a meta-OR = 1.22 (0.55-2.72) for AD (two studies), a meta-OR = 1.28 (0.75-2.20) for SQ (three studies) and a pooled estimate around 1.00 for SC (three studies).

BREAST CANCER: CASE-CONTROL STUDIES
Design
Three case-control studies on Exon 7 and female breast cancer were found. All were con-

ducted on incident cases and healthy controls; one reported response rates (96.1% for cases, 94.8% for controls); exposure to tobacco smoking was considered in one study, age in one study and ethnicity in all studies; information about therapy was never reported; none of the studies had a statistical power greater than 80% (for an OR equal to or above 2 and $\alpha = 0.05$) to provide evidence of a difference in cancer risk between the WM + MM and WW genotypes.

Results

All three studies reported ORs above unity for the WM + MM genotype among Caucasians, while the only estimate concerning African-Americans was below 1.00.

Stratification by age in one study did not reveal differences in risk between younger and older subjects.

Only one study assessed cancer risk for the WM + MM genotype in smokers; there was a significant increase in risk among light smokers but a non-significant OR, below unity, among heavy smokers.

Meta-analysis

Meta-analysis of the three estimates for Caucasians yielded a meta-OR = 1.51 (0.95-2.43); all the studies were conducted in the USA on incident cases and healthy controls.

OTHER CANCERS: CASE-CONTROL STUDIES

Table 28 gives the results on the association between Exon 7 polymorphism and cancer in different sites.

The WM + MM genotype was significantly associated with endometrial cancer in one study.

A study on skin cancer indicated a significant association of WM + MM with BCC occurrence and a significant interaction between Exon 7 and GSTM3 polymorphisms in determining the number of BCCs.

Another study on BCC found a significantly higher frequency of the WW genotype in cases of truncal BCC compared to BCC in other sites, and there was a significant interaction between Exon 7 WW and GSTT1null in relation to the occurrence of truncal BCC.

There was no significant increase in risk for carriers of the WM + MM genotype in one study on bladder cancer.

OTHER CANCERS: CASE-CASE STUDIES

A case-case study on skin cancer did not show a significant association between the WW genotype and the BCC rate (p = 0.079); nor did this study find a significant interaction between Exon 7 and CYP2D6 polymorphisms in relation to BCC number.

CROSS-SECTIONAL STUDIES

Twelve cross-sectional studies were collected on the association between Exon 7 polymorphism and various markers of target dose and genetic or cytogenetic damage.

Design

The analysis of design was as follows:
- exposure to smoking was considered in eight studies, occupational exposure to PAHs in one and alcohol intake in one;
- the covariates most frequently considered were ethnicity in eight studies, age in three and gender in four.

Results

Seven studies focused on the association between Exon 7 polymorphism and the level of PAH-DNA adducts; only one of them found a significantly higher level of PAH-DNA adducts (p = 0.01) in smokers carrying the WM + MM genotype compared to WW, while another study showed an interaction approaching significance (p = 0.06) between GSTM1+ and Exon 7 WW in determining higher PAH-DNA adduct levels.

No significant association of the WM + MM genotype was found with MN frequency in one study and with SCE frequency in another study.

In one study on Asians, p53 mutation frequency was significantly increased in carriers of the MM genotype compared to WM + WW, while two other studies, one on Caucasians and the other on Asians, did not show any significant association between Exon 7 and p53 mutations.

AA polymorphism

This polymorphism was found only in African and African-American populations; because the prevalence of the homozygous mutant (MM) genotype seems to be very low (below 1%), studies investigating the association of this polymorphism with the occurrence of cancer focused on differences in cancer risk between the MM + WM and WW genotypes.

LUNG CANCER: CASE-CONTROL STUDIES
Design
We collected three case-control studies on AA polymorphism and lung cancer: all were conducted on incident cases and healthy controls; one reported response rates (86.2% for cases, 89.1% for controls); exposure to tobacco smoking was considered in all studies, occupational exposure in one study, age and gender in none, and cancer histology in all studies; information about therapy was reported in one study; none of the studies had a statistical power above 80% (for an OR equal to or greater than 2 and $\alpha = 0.05$) to provide evidence of a difference in cancer risk between the homozygous + heterozygous mutant (MM + WM) and the wild-type (WW) genotype.

Results
Two of three studies showed a risk above 1.00 for carriers of WM + MM compared to WW.

Among smokers, excess risk was found in two of three studies, while the risk for the MM + WM genotype was over 1.00 in two out of two studies for light smokers and in one of two studies for heavy smokers.

Stratification by cancer histology, reported in two studies, revealed excess risk in two studies for AD, in one for SQ and in none for SC.

Meta-analysis
All three studies were conducted on African-American subjects living in the USA and were based on incident cases and healthy controls. Meta-analysis of the overall ORs yielded a meta-OR = 1.01 (0.67-1.52) for the WM + MM genotype.

Stratification by smoking exposure in three studies showed a meta-OR = 1.58 (0.86-2.90) for the WM + MM genotype among smokers; stratification by level of smoking in two studies revealed a non-significantly higher risk in light smokers (meta-OR = 1.39 (0.69-2.83)) compared to heavy smokers, for whom the pooled estimate was around unity.

Stratification by cancer histology, reported in two studies, yielded a meta-OR = 1.91 (1.01-3.61) for AD, while the pooled estimate was around 1.00 for SC and slightly higher for SQ (meta-OR = 1.22 (0.55-2.70)).

OTHER CANCERS: CASE-CONTROL STUDIES
The only other study investigating the association between AA polymorphism and cancer concerned breast cancer and did not show a significant association of the WM + MM genotype with this cancer site.

AHH activity

LUNG CANCER: CASE-CONTROL STUDIES
Design
The association between AHH activity and lung cancer was explored in 17 case-control studies, ten of which were conducted on incident cases and seven on healthy controls only; none reported response rates; exposure to tobacco smoking was considered in seven studies, age in four, gender in one, ethnicity in ten and cancer histology in three; information about therapy was reported in eight studies.

Results
Eleven studies reported significant associations between high AHH activity or inducibility in PAM or lymphocytes and the occurrence of lung cancer.

Stratification by smoking exposure, reported in seven studies, showed a significant association among smokers in four of seven studies and among non-smokers in two out of two studies.

Stratification by cancer histology, reported in one study, did not reveal significant differences in AHH activity between AD and SQ cases.

LUNG CANCER: CASE-CASE STUDIES
One study performed in Finland on CYP1A1 phenotype and lung cancer found a significant association of CYP1A1 inducible phenotype with the peripheral location of the tumour but not with any histological type; this study also revealed a significant association between GSTM1 and tumour location among cases carrying CYP1A1 inducible polymorphism.

OTHER CANCERS: CASE-CONTROL STUDIES

Table 28 gives the results on the association between AHH activity and cancer in different sites.

One study on larynx cancer conducted in the USA did not find a significant difference in AHH activity between cases and controls, nor between cases of different age and family history of cancer. Nevertheless, another study found a highly significant association between AHH inducibility and larynx cancer; in the same study, AHH inducibility was also significantly associated with oral cancer, whereas no association was shown with urothelial cancer.

CROSS-SECTIONAL STUDIES

The association between AHH activity and the level of DNA adducts was examined in six cross-sectional studies.

Design
The analysis of design was as follows:
- exposure to smoking was taken into account in five studies and environmental exposure to PCB and PCDF in one;
- among covariates, only ethnicity was considered in four studies.

Results
Five of six studies found a significant association between AHH activity and the level of DNA adducts. AHH activity was significantly correlated with total DNA adducts in two of three studies and with BPDE-DNA and PAH-DNA adducts in three out of three studies, while one study on Taiwanese women did not find a significant association between the PCB/PCDF-DNA adduct level and AHH activity.

Among smokers a significant association between AHH activity and total- or aromatic-DNA adducts was demonstrated in three out of three studies.

CYP1A2

CASE-CONTROL STUDIES
The design and results of studies focusing on the association between CYP1A2 and cancer are reported in Annex Tables 30 and 32 respectively.

One study found a significant association of the CYP1A2 rapid phenotype with colorectal polyps but not with colorectal cancer; the same study showed a significant interaction between CYP1A2rapid and NAT2rapid phenotypes in increasing the risk of developing colorectal tumours. In another study, CYP1A2 activity was significantly higher in cases of familial adenomatous polyposis compared to controls.

A case-control study on bladder cancer found significantly higher CYP1A2 activity in cases compared to controls.

CROSS-SECTIONAL STUDIES
The only cross-sectional study on CYP1A2 investigated the association with Hb adducts, finding a significant association between the CYP1A2rapid phenotype and the level of Hb adducts among smokers but not among non-smokers (Annex Tables 31 and 33).

Publication bias
The relation between weight and natural logarithm of OR is displayed in Plots 1-21 (Annex) (the numbers correspond to the numbers of the graphs on meta-analysis).

Visual examination of these funnel plots suggested the presence of a publication bias concerning the following associations:

- GSTM1 and lung cancer
- GSTM1 and lung cancer - Caucasians
- GSTM1 and bladder cancer
- GSTM1 and bladder cancer - Caucasians
- NAT2 and breast cancer
- NAT2 and breast cancer - Caucasians
- CYP2D6 and lung cancer
- CYP2D6 and lung cancer - Caucasians

Linear regression confirmed a significant inverse association between the inverse of the variance (weight) and the natural logarithm of the ratio OR/meta-OR at a p-value <0.1 for:
- GSTM1 and bladder cancer - Caucasians (p = 0.041)
- CYP2D6 and lung cancer (p = 0.004)
- CYP2D6 and lung cancer - Caucasians (p = 0.008)

The constant of the linear regression did not include the origin of the SND at a p-value < 0.1 for the following associations:

- GSTM1 and bladder cancer (p = 0.088)
- GSTM1 and bladder cancer - Caucasians (p = 0.022)
- NAT2 and breast cancer (p = 0.053)
- NAT2 and breast cancer - Caucasians (p = 0.065)
- CYP2D6 and lung cancer (p = 0.001)
- CYP2D6 and lung cancer - Caucasians (p = 0.002)

Considering that the asymmetry of the two funnel plots concerning GSTM1 and lung cancer is quite slight, there is good agreement between the visual examination of funnel plots and the described test on the constant of the linear regression, while the significance of the linear regression is a less sensitive criterion for assessing publication bias, producing significant results only when the bias is more pronounced.

Consequently, the data support the presence of a publication bias concerning the associations listed above, for which we can expect the pooled estimates to be lower than those computed using ORs extracted from published papers.

Conclusions

GSTM1

Studies on bladder cancer suggest an association between GSTM1null polymorphism and risk of bladder cancer, because of the high consistency of the results and the statistical significance of pooled estimates, in spite of a lack of homogeneity of risk estimates related to Caucasians. Among Caucasians such heterogeneity disappears in estimates related to TCC histology and to smokers, for which there is a significant excess risk. Cancer risk seems comparable among different ethnicities, although not significant in African-Americans, indicating for carriers of GSTM1null a relative risk of bladder cancer probably around 1.5 compared to GSTM1+.

For lung cancer the risk seems to concern in particular SQ and SC histologies, which are known to be more linked to smoking exposure, although among Caucasians estimates for smokers are quite low and non-significant. Estimates for Asians show higher consistency and stronger association, confirming that the risk is concen-

trated among Kreyberg I histologies and demonstrating an interaction between GSTM1null and smoking exposure at high doses.

The association with breast cancer shows a high consistency among studies but the pooled estimate is low and non-significant. Nevertheless, results from a case-control and a case-case study support the presence of a significantly higher risk among younger women. Colorectal and liver cancer do not seem to be associated with GSTM1, showing low consistency among studies and low and non-significant cancer risk. Meta-analysis of results on colorectal cancer imply a significant risk for cancers located in the distal colon, but this suggestion is based on estimates lacking homogeneity.

For gastric cancer the risk for GSTM1null is very different between Caucasians, among whom it is around one, and Asians, who present a significantly higher risk that increases on restriction to studies with the best design, and there is good consistency among studies; the data suggest that the association concerns AD histology in particular, but this requires confirmation in future studies.

Studies on larynx cancer show good consistency but the pooled estimate is significant only on restriction to SQ histology.

For other cancer sites the data are insufficient to express an assessment of cancer risk for carriers of GTM1 null, although they suggest an association with pituitary adenoma, endometrial cancer and acute lymphoblastic leukaemia.

The excess risk of cancer linked to GSTM1null is consistent with the results from cross-sectional investigations, a substantial proportion of which show significantly higher levels of PAH-DNA and total-DNA adducts, and SCE, CA and p53 mutations among carriers of this polymorphism.

The results suggest the existence of an interaction of GSTM1 with CYP2D6 in relation to the risk of bladder cancer and with CYP1A1 polymorphisms, either MspI or Exon7, in relation to lung cancer risk.

GSTT1

The risk of bladder cancer, lung cancer and gastric cancer does not seem to be associated with GSTT1 polymorphism, although the data are too scarce to permit an evaluation of the results.

The risk of laryngeal cancer seems to indicate a consistent increase among GSTT1null carriers, but this association is based on too few studies.

With regard to colorectal cancer, although meta-analysis revealed a significantly higher risk for GSTT1null carriers, this result is unduly influenced by the only study that found a strong association with GSTT1null (Deakin *et al.*, 1996) and accounted for over half the subjects; the design of this study, based on hospital inpatient controls, could have biased the risk estimate.

For basocellular skin cancer the data suggest the possibility of associations only with the truncal site and with the rate of appearence of BCCs.

Among other cancer sites, results concerning HCC, endometrial cancer and epithelial ovarian cancer do not support an association with GSTT1, while the highly significant risks shown for astrocytoma, meningioma and myelodisplastic syndromes suggest the presence of a strong association with these cancers; this needs to be confirmed in future research.

GSTM3

Up to the present the studies that have been performed do not permit an evaluation of the risk of cancer linked to GSTM3, although one of them supports the possibility of an association between the A allele and laryngeal cancer; this needs further confirmation.

NAT2

The results on bladder cancer suggest an increased risk for carrying NAT2slow only among Caucasians, whose estimates are highly consistent and for whom meta-analysis is statistically significant. For Asians the risk is consistently below unity. The data indicate that in Caucasians there is a relative risk of approximately 1.4 for NAT2slow compared to NAT2rapid subjects; the risk seems to be higher among smokers and among subjects exposed to bladder carcinogens.

The risk of lung cancer does not seem to be associated with NAT2slow, because estimates are low and not consistent, while an increased risk for carrying NAT2 homozygous rapid polymorphism is suggested by the results of Cascorbi *et al.* (1996).

With regard to breast cancer, only studies based on phenotyping showed an increased risk for NAT2rapid carriers; a higher risk occurred on restriction to estimates from studies with the best design. The consistency of the results and the significance of the meta-analysis in phenotype-based studies indicate the likelihood of an association between NAT2rapid, as measured by phenotyping, and breast cancer. On the other hand, the discrepancy between genotype-based and phenotype-based estimates suggests the presence in this gene of mutations leading to slow phenotype which have not yet been identified.

In colorectal cancer, phenotype-based estimates suggest an association with NAT2rapid, given the high consistency of the results and the significance of the meta-analysis; however, this is not confirmed by genotype-based studies; these findings support the hypothesis that not all the mutations leading to slow phenotype have been discovered.

The data on other cancer sites, although insufficient to evaluate consistency among studies, suggest a possible association of NAT2slow with familial adenomatous polyposis, hepatocellular carcinoma and, among subjects strongly exposed to asbestos, mesothelioma.

The results suggest the existence of an interaction of NAT2slow with GSTM1null and NAT1rapid on the risk of bladder cancer, with GSTM1null on the risk of mesothelioma and with CYP2D6 on HCC risk, whereas NAT2rapid seems to interact with GSTM1null and NAT1rapid on colorectal cancer risk.

Data from cross-sectional studies support the association between NAT2 and bladder cancer, in that Hb adducts of 4-APB, a recognized risk factor for this cancer site, were consistently higher among NAT2slow carriers and statistically significant in two of three studies. The results for other biomarkers are controversial and do not help to elucidate the association of NAT2 with other cancer sites.

NAT1

The results on NAT1 are not sufficient to evaluate the association with cancer, although they support the existence of an increased risk of colorectal cancer and adenoma for NAT1rapid and of an interaction with NAT2rapid in relation to the risk of colorectal tumours. Data from one study would also suggest a possible interaction of NAT1rapid with NAT2slow on bladder cancer risk.

The interaction between NAT1 and NAT2 polymorphisms is consistent with the findings of one cross-sectional study.

CYP2D6

Data concerning bladder cancer do not indicate an association with CYP2D6 polymorphism because risk estimates are low and inconsistent.

Results on lung cancer show a difference between estimates from genotype-based and phenotype-based studies; the results from the latter are consistently higher; this finding suggests that for the CYP2D6 polymorphism, as with NAT2, some of the mutations leading to the extensive metabolizer phenotype have not yet been identified. The risk linked to EM + IM does not show variations between smokers and non-smokers and seems to concern only SQ histology, although the low strength of association and the lack of significance of the meta-OR do not support the hypothesis of an association between SQ histotype and CYP2D6 polymorphism. The risk of lung cancer linked to homozygous EM has not been evaluated through a formal meta-analysis, because estimates on it were not reported systematically; nevertheless, available data suggest an increased risk for EM compared to IM + PM, which is more consistant than that relating to EM + IM, but the subject needs further research.

Breast cancer, larynx cancer, basocellular carcinoma (BCC) and epithelial ovarian cancer do not appear to be associated with CYP2D6. Data regarding HCC and cervical intraepithelial neoplasia suggest for these neoplasms the existence of an association with homozygous extensive metabolizers (EM), but not with EM + IM, while for astrocytoma and meningioma the risk seems to be linked to the PM phenotype/genotype. These findings are based on very few studies and need further confirmation.

Results from cross-sectional studies are too scarce and controversial to permit an evaluation of the association of CYP2D6 with cancer, although the study by Kato *et al.* (1995) supports the existence of an interaction between EM and smoking on lung cancer risk.

The available data also suggest possible interactions between CYP2D6 EM + IM and GSTM1null on bladder cancer risk and between homozygous EM and NAT2slow on the risk of HCC.

CYP2E1
5'-flanking region polymorphism

Studies on bladder cancer suggest an association with the wild-type genotype (WW); further research is required because only two studies on this cancer site are available.

For lung cancer an association with the WW genotype is supported by the high consistency of the results, even though meta-analysis did not give a significant estimate; such increased risk seems to be confined to SQ and SC histologies.

Breast cancer, larynx cancer, stomach cancer and oesophageal cancer do not appear to be associated with the 5'-flanking region polymorphism. Results concerning HCC and nasopharyngeal cancer suggest associations with the WW genotype and the MM genotype respectively, but these findings need further confirmation.

Data from cross-sectional studies on 5'-fr are not consistent with the hypothesis of an increased risk of lung cancer for carriers of the WW genotype.

Dra I polymorphism

The Dra I polymorphism does not seem to be associated with lung cancer, because the consistency of the results and the pooled estimate are both low; nevertheless, the data suggest an interaction of the WM + MM genotype with SC histology and with smoking exposure; there is a need to explore this area in further studies.

Bladder cancer, breast cancer, HCC, oesophageal and upper aerodigestive tract cancers are apparently not associated with Dra I, while one study suggests the existence of an association between the MM genotype and nasopharyngeal cancer.

One study on DNA adducts supports a possible association of the WM + MM genotype with lung cancer.

Taq I polymorphism

Results on lung cancer and bladder cancer do not suggest an association with Taq I polymorphism.

CYP1A1
Msp I polymorphism - Asians

The data on lung cancer among Asians suggest the existence of an association with MM genotype, given the quality of the design of the studies and the significance of the meta-analysis; however, the results are not very consistent. There is a dose-response relationship with smoking exposure, the risk being more than doubled for light smokers and close to 1.00 for heavy smokers, and in particular appears to concern the SQ and SC histologies.

Sivaraman *et al.* (1994) found a strong association between the MM genotype and colon cancer *in situ*, suggesting a possible role of Msp I in the development of colon cancer; further research is required in this area.

The results of the only cross-sectional study on Asians support the association between MM and lung cancer, showing p53 mutations to be significantly more frequent among cases carrying this genotype.

Msp I polymorphism - non-Asians

Studies on non-Asian populations do not support the association between the WM + MM genotype and lung cancer, the pooled estimate being close to 1.00 and the consistency of the results quite low. The data suggest, however, that the risk could be limited to light smokers and SQ histology, but the weakness of these associations makes it impossible to assess their validity.

Bladder cancer, BCC, oesophageal cancer and upper digestive tract cancer do not appear to be associated with Msp I polymorphism, whereas studies on breast cancer and endometrial cancer suggest an association with WM + MM; the association with breast cancer seems to be higher in African-Americans, among whom the risk appears to be linked in particular to the MM genotype.

Data from cross-sectional studies are apparently consistent with the absence of an association between the WM + MM genotype and cancer.

Exon 7 - Asians

Studies on Asians suggest an association between the MM genotype and lung cancer because of the strong association found in two of them and the good design quality; however, only three studies were available and in one the risk was below 1.00. There are not enough data and further studies are needed on Exon 7 and lung cancer in order to evaluate the association fully.

For the other cancer sites examined the available data do not suggest any association with Exon 7 polymorphism.

The only cross-sectional study on Asians supports the hypothesis of an association between MM and lung cancer, showing p53 mutations to be significantly more frequent among cases carrying this genotype.

Exon 7 - non-Asians

Studies on non-Asian populations do not support the presence of an association between the WM + MM genotype and lung cancer because of the low consistency of the results, the weakness of the association and a lack of significance in the meta-analysis.

Breast cancer seems to be associated with the WM + MM genotype, given the quality of the design of the studies and the consistency of the results, with a risk of about 1.5, but a lack of significance in the meta-analysis indicates that further research is needed in order to confirm the association.

The data on other cancers suggest a possible association of the WM + MM genotype with endometrial cancer and BCC but not with bladder cancer.

Cross-sectional studies do not support the existence of an association between Exon 7 and cancer in non-Asian populations.

AA polymorphism - African-Americans

The results from studies on lung cancer are not sufficient to permit an evaluation of the association between the WM + MM genotype and this cancer site; whereas the overall pooled estimate is around one, the data suggest possible interactions with low-level smoking exposure and with AD histology, and this has to be confirmed in future studies.

A study on breast cancer did not indicate an association with the WM + MM genotype.

Aryl hydrocarbon hydroxylase activity

Studies on AHH activity and lung cancer suggest an association with the inducible phenotype, given the high consistency of the results and the statistical significance of the estimates.

The association of the inducible phenotype with larynx cancer is questionable because the strong association found in one study was not confirmed in another, this one instead showing a higher risk for the non-inducible phenotype.

Data from cross-sectional studies support an association with lung cancer, showing consistently and significantly higher levels of aromatic-DNA adducts in carriers of the inducible phenotype.

CYP1A2

Studies on CYP1A2 suggest possible associations of the rapid phenotype with colorectal polyps, familial adenomatous polyposis (FAP) and bladder cancer, which will have to be explored in additional studies in order to obtain confirmation.

The only cross-sectional study on CYP1A2 supports an association between the rapid phenotype and cancer, revealing significantly higher levels of Hb adducts in smokers who carry this phenotype.

References

Abe, S., Makimura, S., Ogura, S. & Nakajima, I. (1990) Pulmonary drug-metabolizing enzyme in alveolar macrophages in relation to cigarette smoking. *Jpn. J. Med.*, 29 (2), 164-167

Agundez, J.A.G., Ladero, J.M., Olivera, M., Abildua, R., Roman, J.M. & Benitez, J. (1995a) Genetic analysis of the arylamine N-acetyltransferase polymorphism in breast cancer patients. *Oncology*, 52, 7-11

Agundez, J.A.G., Ledesma, M.C., Benitez, J., Ladero, J.M., Rodriguez-Lescure, A., Diaz-Rubio, E. & Diaz-Rubio, M. (1995b) CYP2D6 genes and risk of liver cancer. *Lancet*, 345, 830-831

Agundez, J.A.G., Martinez, C., Ladero, J.M., Ledesma, M.C., Ramos, J.M., Martin, R., Rodriguez, A., Jara, C. & Benitez, J. (1994) Debrisoquine oxidation genotype and susceptibility to lung cancer. *Clin. Pharmacol. Ther.*, 55, 10-14

Agundez, J.A.G., Olivera, M., Ladero, J.M., Rodriguez-Lescure, A., Ledesma, M.C., Diaz-Rubio, M., Meyer, U.A. & Benitez, J. (1996). Increased risk for hepatocellular carcinoma in *NAT2*-slow acetylators and *CYP2D6*-rapid metabolizers. *Pharmacogenetics*, 6, 501-512

Alexandrie, A. K., Ingleman-Sundberg, M., Seidegard, J., Tornling, G. & Rannug, A. (1994) Genetic susceptibility to lung cancer with special emphasis on CYP1A1 and GSTM1: a study on host factors in relation to age at onset, gender and histological cancer types. *Carcinogenesis*, 15 (9), 1785-1790

Alexandrov, K., Rojas, M., Geneste, O., Castegnaro, M., Camus, A.M., Petruzzelli, S., Giuntini, C. & Bartsch, H. (1992). An improved fluorometric assay for dosimetry of benzo(a)pyrene diol-epoxide-DNA adducts in smokers' lung: comparisons with total bulky adducts and aryl hydroxylase activity. *Cancer Res.*, 52, 6248-6253

Ambrosone, C. B., Freudenheim, J.L., Graham, S., Marshall, J.R., Vena, J.E., Brasure, J.R., Laughlin, R., Nemoto, T., Michalek, A.M., Harrington, A., Ford, T.D. & Shields, P.G. (1995) Cytochrome P4501A1 and glutathione S-transferase (M1) genetic polymorphisms and postmenopausal breast cancer risk. *Cancer Res.*, 55, 3483-3485

Ambrosone, C.B., Freudenheim, J.L., Graham, S., Marshall, J.R., Vena, J.E., Brasure, J.R., Michalek, A.M., Laughlin, R., Nemoto, T., Gillenwater, K.A., Harrington, A.M. & Shields, P.G. (1996) Cigarette smoking, N-acetyltransferase 2 genetic polymorphisms, and breast cancer risk. *JAMA*, 276 (18), 1494-1501

Amos, C. I., Caporaso, N.E. & Weston, A. (1992) Host factors in lung cancer risk: a review of interdisciplinary studies. *Cancer Epidemiol. Biomarkers Prev.*, 1 (6), 505-13

Anttila, S., Hirvonen, A., Husgafvel-Pursiainen, K., Karjalainen, A., Nurminen, T. & Vainio, H. (1994) Combined effect of CYP1A1 inducibility and GSTM1 polymorphism on histological type of lung cancer. *Carcinogenesis*, 15, 1133-1135

Anttila, S., Luostarinen, L., Hirvonen, A., Elovaara, E., Karjalainen, A., Nurminen, T., Hayes, J.D., Vainio, H. & Ketterer, B. (1995) Pulmonary expression of glutathione S-transferase M3 in lung cancer patients: association with GSTM1 polymorphism, smoking, and asbestos exposure. *Cancer Res.*, 55, 3305-3309

Anwar, W.A., Abdel-Rahman, S.Z., El-Zein, R.A., Mostafa, H.M. & Au, W.W. (1996) Genetic polymorphism of GSTM1, CYP2E1 and CYP2D6 in Egyptian bladder cancer patients. *Carcinogenesis,* 17 (9), 1923-1929

Ayesh, R., Idle, J.R., Ritchie, J.C., Crothers, M. J. & Hetzel, M.R. (1984) Metabolic oxidation phenotypes as markers for susceptibility to lung cancer. *Nature,* 312, 169-170

Badawi, A.V., Hirvonen, A., Bell, D.A., Lang, N.P. & Kadlubar, F.F. (1995) Role of aromatic amine acetyltransferase, NAT1 and NAT2, in carcinogen-DNA adduct formation in the human urinary bladder. *Cancer Res.,* 55, 5230-5237

Baranov, V.S., Ivaschenko, T., Bakay, B., Aseev, M., Belotserkovskaya, R., Baranova, H., Malet, P., Perriot, J., Mouraire, P., Baskakov, V.N., Savitskyi, G.A., Gorbushin, S., Deyneka, S.I.., Michnin, E., Barchuk, A., Vakharlovsky, V., Pavlov, G., Shilko, V.I., Guembitzkaya, T. & Kovaleva, L. (1996) Proportion of the GSTM1 0/0 genotype in some Slavic populations and its correlation with cystic fibrosis and some multi-factorial diseases. *Hum. Genet.,* 97, 516-520

Bartsch, H., Castegnaro, M., Rojas, M., Camus, A.M., Alexandrov, K. & Lang, M. (1992a) Expression of pulmonary cytochrome P4501A1 and carcinogen DNA adduct formation in high-risk subjects for tobacco-related lung cancer. *Toxicol. Lett.,* 64/65, 477-483

Bartsch, H., Petruzzelli, S., De Flora, S., Hietanen, E., Camus, A.M., Castegnaro, M., Alexandrov, K., Rojas, M., Saracci, R. & Giuntini, C. (1992b) Carcinogen metabolism in human lung tissues and the effect of tobacco smoking: results from a case-control multicenter study on lung cancer patients. *Environ. Health Perspect.,* 98, 119-124

Bartsch, H., Rojas, M., Alexandrov, K., Camus, A.M., Castegnaro, M., Malaveille, C., Anttila, S., Hirvonen, K., Husgafvel-Pursiainen, K., Hietanen, E. & Vainio, H. (1995) Metabolic polymorphism affecting DNA binding and excretion of carcinogens in humans. *Pharmacogenetics,* 5, S84-S90

Bell, D.A., Stephens, E.A., Castranio, T., Umbach, D.M., Watson, M., Deakin, M., Elder, J., Hendrickse, C., Duncan, H. & Strange, R.C. (1995) Polyadenylation polymorphism in the acetyltransferase 1 gene (*NAT1*) increases risk of colorectal cancer. *Cancer Res.,* 55, 3537-3542

Bell, D.A., Taylor, J.A., Paulson, D.F., Robertson, C.N., Mohler, J.L. & Lucier, G.W. (1993) Genetic risk and carcinogen exposure: a common inherited defect of the carcinogen-metabolism gene glutathione S-transferase M1 (GSTM1) that increases susceptibility to bladder cancer. *J. Natl. Cancer Inst.,* 85 (14), 1159-1164

Benhamou, S., Bouchardy, C., Paoletti, C. & Dayer, P. (1996) Effects of CYP2D6 activity and tobacco on larynx cancer risk. *Cancer Epidemiol. Biomarkers Prev.,* 5, 683-686

Benitez, J., Ladero, J.M., Fernandez-Gundin, M.J., Llerena, A., Cobaleda, J., Martinez, C., Munoz, J.J., Vargas, E., Prados, J., Gonzales-Rozas, F., Rodriguez-Molina, J. & Uson, A.C. (1990) Polymorphic oxidation of debrisoquine in bladder cancer. *Ann. Med.,* 22, 157-160

Benitez, J., Ladero, J.M., Jara, C., Carrillo, J.A., Cobaleda, J., Llerena, A., Vargas, E. & Munoz, J.J. (1991) Polymorphic oxidation of debrisoquine in lung cancer patients. *Eur. J. Cancer,* 27 (2), 158-161

Bernardini, S., Pelin, K., Peltonen, K., Jarventaus, H., Hirvonen, A., Neagu, C., Sorsa, M. & Norppa, H. (1996) Induction of sister chromatid exchange by 3,4-epoxybutane-1,2-diol in cultured human lymphocytes of different *GSTT1* and *GSTM1* genotypes. *Mutat. Res.,* 361, 121-127

Binkova, B., Lewtas, J., Miskova, I., Rossner, P., Cerna, M., Mrackova, G., Peterkova, K., Mumford, J., Meyer, S. & Sram, R. (1996) Biomarker studies in Northern Bohemia. *Environ. Health Perspect.,* 104, 591-597

Board, P., Coggan, M., Johnston, P., Ross, V. & Suzuki, T.G.W. (1990) Genetic heterogeneity of the human glutathione transferase: a complex of gene families. *Pharmacol. Ther.,* 48, 357-369

Bouchardy, C., Benhamou, S. & Dayer, P. (1996) The effect of tobacco on lung cancer risk depends on CYP2D6 activity. *Cancer Res.*, 56, 251-253

Bouchardy, C., Wikman, H., Benhamou, S., Hirvonen, A., Dayer, P. & Husgafvel-Pursiainen, K. (1997) CYP1A1 genetic polymorphism, tobacco smoking and lung cancer risk in a French Caucasian population. *Biomarkers*, 2, 131-134

Brockmöller, J., Cascorbi, I., Kerb, R. & Roots, I. (1996a) Combined analysis of inherited polymorphisms in arylamine N-acetyltransferase 2, glutathione S-transferases M1 and T1, microsomal epoxide hydrolase, and cytochrome P450 enzymes as modulators of bladder cancer risk. *Cancer Res.*, 56, 3915-3925

Brockmöller, J., Kaiser, R., Kerb, R., Cascorbi, I., Jaeger, V. & Roots, I. (1996b) Polymorphic enzymes of xenobiotic metabolism as modulators of acquired P53 mutations in bladder cancer. *Pharmacogenetics*, 6, 535-545

Brockmöller, J., Kerb, R., Drakoulis, N., Nitz, M. & Roots, I. (1993) Genotype and phenotype of glutathione S-transferase class mu isoenzymes mu and psi in lung cancer patients and controls. *Cancer Res.*, 53, 1004-1011

Brockmöller, J., Kerb, R., Drakoulis, N., Staffeldt, B. & Roots, I. (1994) Glutathione S-transferase M1 and its variants A and B as host factors of bladder cancer susceptibility: a case-control study. *Cancer Res.*, 54, 4103-4111

Brosen, K., Gram, L.F., Haghfelt, T. & Bertilsson, L. (1987) Extensive metabolizers of debrisoquine become poor metabolizers during quinidine treatment. *Pharmacol. Toxicol.*, 60, 312-314

Buchert, E.T., Woosley, R.L., Swain, S.M., Oliver, S.J., Coughlin, S.S., Pickle, L., Trock, B. & Riegel, A.T. (1993) Relationship of CYP2D6 (debrisoquine hydroxylase) genotype to breast cancer susceptibility. *Pharmacogenetics*, 3, 322-327

Bulovskaya, L.N., Krupkin, R.G., Bochina, T.A., Shipkova, A.A. & Pavlova, M.V. (1978) Acetylator phenotype in patients with breast cancer. *Oncology*, 35, 185-188

Burgess, E.J. & Trafford, J.A.P. (1985) Acetylator phenotype in patients with lung carcinoma - a negative report. *Eur. J. Respir. Dis.*, 67, 17-19

Caporaso, N., Hayes, R.B., Dosemeci, M., Hoover, R., Ayesh, R., Hetzel, M. & Idle, J. (1989) Lung cancer risk, occupational exposure, and debrisoquine metabolic phenotype. *Cancer Res.*, 49, 3675-3679

Caporaso, N., Tucker, M.A., Hoover, R.N., Hayes, R.B., Pickle, L.W., Issaq, H.J., Muschik, G.M., Green-Gallo, L., Buivys, D., Aisner, S., Resau, J.H., Trump, B.F., Tollerud, D., Weston, A. & Harris, C.C. (1990) Lung cancer and debrisoquine metabolic phenotype. *J. Natl. Cancer Inst.*, 82, 1264-1272

Caporaso, N.E., Shields, P.G., Landi, M.T., Shaw, G.L., Tucker, M.A., Hoover, R., Sugimura, H., Weston, A. & Harris, C.C. (1992) The debrisoquine metabolic phenotype and DNA-based assays: implications of misclassification for the associations of lung cancer and debrisoquine metabolic phenotype. *Environ. Health Perspect.*, 98, 101-105

Cartwright, R.A., Philip, P.A., Rogers, H.J. & Glashan, R.W. (1984) Genetically determined debrisoquine oxidation capacity in bladder cancer. *Carcinogenesis*, 5, 1191-1192

Cartwright, R.A., Rogers, H.J., Barham-Hall, D., Glashan, R.W., Ahmad, R.A., Higgins, E. and Kahn, M.A. (1982). Role of N-acetyltransferase phenotypes in bladder carcinogenesis: a pharmacogenetic epidemiological approach to bladder cancer. *Lancet*, 2, 842-845

Cascorbi. I., Brockmöller, J., Mrozikiewicz, P.M., Bauer, S., Loddenkemper, R. & Roots, I. (1996) Homozygous rapid arylamine N-acetyltransferase (NAT2) genotype as a susceptibility factor for lung cancer. *Cancer Res.*, 56, 3961-3966

Chen, C., Madeleine, M.M., Lubinski, C., Weiss, N.S., Tickman, E.W. & Daling, J.R. (1996) Glutathione S-transferase *M1* genotypes and the risk of anal cancer: a population-based case-control study. *Cancer Epidemiol. Biomarkers Prev.*, 5, 985-991

Chen, C.J., Yu, M.W., Liaw, Y.F., Wang, L.W., Chiamprasert, S., Matin, F., Hirvonen, A., Bell, D.A. & Santella, R.M. (1996) Chronic hepatitis B carriers with null genotype of glutathione S-transferase M1 and T1 polymorphisms who are exposed to aflatoxin are at increased risk of hepatocellular carcinoma. *Am. J. Hum. Genet.*, 59, 128-134

Chen, C.L., Liu, Q., Pui, C.H., Rivera, G.K., Sandlund, J.T., Ribeiro, R., Evans, W.E. & Relling, M.V. (1997) Higher frequency of glutathione S-transferase deletions in black children with acute lymphoblastic leukemia. *Blood*, 89 (5), 1701-1707

Chen, H., Sandler, D.P., Taylor, J.A., Shore, D.L., Liu, E., Bloomfield, C.D. & Bell, D.A. (1996) Increased risk for myelodisplastic syndromes in individuals with glutathione transferase theta 1 (GSTT1) gene defect. *Lancet*, 347, 295-297

Chenevix-Trench, G., Young, J., Coggan, M. & Board, P. (1995) Glutathione S-transferase M1 and T1 polymorphisms: susceptibility to colon cancer and age of onset. *Carcinogenesis*, 16 (7), 1655-1657

Cheng, T.J., Christiani, D.C., Xu, X., Wain J.C., Wiencke, J.K. & Kelsey, K.T. (1995a) Glutathione S-transferase mu genotype, diet, and smoking as determinants of sister chromatid exchange frequency in lymphocytes. *Cancer Epidemiol. Biomarkers Prev.*, 4, 535-542

Cheng, T.J., Christiani, D.C., Liber, H.L., Wain, J.C., Xu, X., Wiencke, J.K. & Kelsey, K.T. (1995b) Mutant frequency at the hrprt locus in human lymphocytes in a case-control study of lung cancer. *Mutat. Res.*, 332, 109-118

Cheng, T.J., Christiani, D.C., Wiencke, J.K., Wain, J.C., Xu, X. & Kelsey, K.T., (1995c) Comparison of sister chromatid exchange frequency in peripheral lymphocytes in lung cancer cases and controls. *Mutat. Res.*, 348, 75-82

Chinegwundoh, F.I. & Kaisary, A.V. (1996) Polymorphism and smoking in bladder carcinogenesis. *Br. J. Urol.*, 77, 672-675

Cosma, G.N., Crofts, F., Currie, D., Wirgin, I., Toniolo, P. & Garte, S.J. (1993). Racial differences in restriction fragment length polymorphisms and messenger RNA inducibility of the human CYP1A1 gene. *Cancer Epidemiol. Biomarkers Prev.*, 2 (1), 53-57

Crespi, C.L., Penman, B.W., Gelboin, H.V. & Gonzalez, F.J. (1991) A tobacco-smoke derived nitrosamine, 4-(methylnitrosamino)-1-(3-pyridyl)-1-butanone, is activated by multiple human P-450s including the polymorphic cytocrome P-4502D6. *Carcinogenesis*, 12, 1197-1201

Crofts, F., Cosma, G., Currie, D., Taioli, E., Toniolo, P. & Garte, S.J. (1993) A novel CYP1A1 gene polymorphism in African-Americans. [Erratum published in *Carcinogenesis*, 1993, 14 (12): 2652] *Carcinogenesis*, 14 (9), 1729-1731

Crofts, F., Taioli, E., Trachman, J., Cosma, G.N., Currie, D., Toniolo, P., & Garte, S.J. (1994) Functional significance of different human CYP1A1 genotypes. *Carcinogenesis*, 15 (12), 2961-2963

Daly, A.K., Thomas, D.J., Cooper, J., Pearson, W.R., Neal, D.E. & Idle, J.R. (1993) Homozygous deletion of gene for glutathione S-transferase M1 in bladder cancer. *Br. Med. J.*, 307, 481-482

Deakin, M., Elder, J., Hendrickse, C., Peckham, D., Baldwin, D., Pantin, C., Wild, N., Leopard, P., Bell, D.A., Jones, P., Duncan, H., Branningan, K., Alldersea, J., Fryer, A.A. & Strange, R.C. (1996) Glutathione S-transferase GSTT1 genotypes and susceptibility to cancer: studies of interactions with GSTM1 in lung, oral, gastric and colorectal cancers. *Carcinogenesis*, 17 (4), 881-884

Degawa, M., Stern, S.J., Martin, M.V., Guengerich, F.P., Fu, P.P., Ilett, K. F., Kaderlik, R. K. & Kadlubar, F. F. (1994) Metabolic activation and carcinogen-DNA adduct detection in human larynx. *Cancer Res.*, 54, 4915-4919

DerSimonian, R. & Laird, N. (1986) Meta-analysis in clinical trials. *Controlled Clin. Trials*, 7(3), 177-188

Dolzan, V., Rudolf, Z. & Breskvar, K.. (1995) Human CYP2D6 gene polymorphism in Slovene cancer patients and healthy controls. *Carcinogenesis*, 16 (11), 2675-2678

Drakoulis, N., Cascorbi, I., Brockmöller, J., Gross, C.R. & Roots, I. (1994) Polymorphisms in the human *CYP1A1* gene as susceptibility factors for lung cancer: exon-7 mutation (4889 *A* to *G*), and a *T* to *C* mutation in the 3'-flanking region. *Clin. Investigator*, 72, 240-248

Duche, J.C., Joanne, C., Barre, J., De Cremoux, H., Dalphin, J.C., Depierre, A., Brochard, P., Tillement, J.P. & Bechtel, P. (1991) Lack of a relationship between the polymorphism of debrisoquine oxidation and lung cancer. *Br. J. Clin. Pharmacol.*, 31, 533-536

Egger, M., Smith G., D., Schneider, M. & Minder, C. (1997) Bias in meta-analysis detected by a simple, graphical test. *Br. Med. J.*, 315, 629-634

Elexpuru-Camiruaga, J., Buxton, N., Kandula, V., Dias, P.S., Campbell, D., McIntosh, J., Broome, J., Jones, P., Inskip, A., Alldersea, J., Fryer, A.A. & Strange, R.C. (1995) Susceptibility to astrocytoma and meningioma: influence of allelism at glutathione S-transferase (GSTT1 and GSTM1) and cytochrome P-450 (CYP2D6) loci. *Cancer Res.*, 55, 4237-4239

El-Zein, R.A., Zwishenberger, J.B., Abdel-Rahman, S.Z., Sankar, A.B. & Au, W.W. (1997) Polymorphism of metabolizing genes and lung cancer histology: prevalence of CYP2E1 in adenocarcinoma. *Cancer Letters*, 112, 71-78

Emery, A.E., Anand, R., Danford, N., Duncan, W. & Paton, L. (1978) Aryl-hydrocarbon-hydroxylase inducibility in patients with cancer. *Lancet*, 1, 470-472

Esteller, M., Garcia, A., Martinez-Palones, J.M., Xercavins, J. & Reventos, J. (1997) Susceptibility to endometrial cancer: influence of allelism at

p53, glutathione S-transferase (GSTM1 and GSTT1) and cytochrome P-450 (CYP1A1) loci. *Br. J. Cancer*, 75 (9), 1385-1388

Evans, D.A.P. (1989) N-acetyltransferase. *Pharmacol. Ther.*, 42, 157-234

Evans, D.A.P. & White, T.A. (1964) Human acetylation polymorphism. *J. Lab. Clin. Med.*, 63, 394-403

Evans, D.A.P., Eze, L.C. & Whibley, E.J. (1983) The association of the slow acetylator phenotype with bladder cancer. *J. Med. Genet.*, 20, 330-333

Evans, D.A.P., Manley, K.A. & McKusick, V.A. (1960) Genetic control of isoniazid metabolism in man. *Br. Med. J.*, 2, 485-491

Fleiss, J.L. & Gross, A.J. (1991) Meta-analysis in epidemiology, with special reference to studies of the association between exposure to environmental tobacco smoke and lung cancer: a critique. *J. Clin. Epidemiol.*, 44(2), 127-139

Fleiss, J.L., Tytun, A. & Ury, H.K. (1980) A simple approximation for calculating sample sizes for comparing independent proportions. *Biometrics*, 36, 343-346

Fontana, X., Peyrotte, I., Valente, E., Rossi, C., Ettore, F., Namer, M. & Bussiere, F. (1997) Glutathione S-transferase mu 1 (*GSTM1*): gène de susceptibilité du cancer du sein. *Bull. Cancer*, 84 (1), 35-40

Fryer, A.A., Zhao, L., Alldersea J., Boggild, M.D., Perrett, C.W., Clayton, R.N., Jones, P.W. & Strange, R.C. (1993) The glutathione S-transferases: polymerase chain reaction studies on the frequency of the GSTM1 0 genotype in patients with pituitary adenomas. *Carcinogenesis*, 14 (4), 563-566

Gabbani, G., Hou, S.M., Nardini, B., Marchioro, M., Lambert, B. & Clonfero, E. (1996) *GSTM1* and *NAT2* genotypes and urinary mutagens in coke oven workers. *Carcinogenesis*, 17 (8), 1677-1681

Gahmberg, C.G., Sekki, A., Kosunen, T.U., Holsti, L.R. & Makela, O. (1979) Induction of aryl hydrocarbon hydroxylase activity and pulmonary carcinoma. *Int. J. Cancer*, 23 (3), 302-305

Gallagher, J.E., Everson, R.B., Lewtas J., George, M. & Lucier, G.W. (1994) Comparison of DNA adduct levels in human placenta from polychlorinated biphenyl exposed women and smokers in which CYP1A1 levels are similarly elevated. *Teratogenesis Carcinog. Mutagen.*, 14, 183-192

Ge, H., Lam, W.K., Lee, J., Wong, M.P., Yew, W.W. & Lung, M. L. (1996) Analysis of *L-myc* and *GSTM1* genotypes in Chinese non-small-cell lung carcinoma patients. *Lung Cancer*, 15, 355-366

Geneste, O., Camus., A.M., Castegnaro, M., Petruzzelli, S., Macchiarini, P., Angeletti, C.A., Giuntini, C. & Bartsch, H. (1991) Comparison of pulmonary DNA adduct levels, measured by ^{32}P-postlabelling and aryl hydrocarbon hydroxylase activity in lung parenchyma of smokers and ex-smokers. *Carcinogenesis*, 12 (7), 1301-1305

Golka, K., Prior, V., Blaszkewicz, M., Cascorbi, I., Schops, W., Kierfeld, G., Roots, I. & Bolt, H.M. (1996) Occupational history and genetic N-acetyltransferase polymorphism in urothelial cancer patients of Leverkusen, Germany. *Scand. J. Work Environ. Health*, 22, 332-338

Goto, I., Yoneda, S., Yamamoto, M. & Kawajiri, K. (1996) Prognostic significance of germ line polymorphisms of the *CYP1A1* and glutathione S-transferase genes in patients with non-small-cell lung cancer. *Cancer Res.*, 56, 3725-3730

Grant, D.M. (1993) Molecular genetics of the N-acetyltransferase. *Pharmacogenetics*, 3, 45-50

Greenland, S. (1987) Quantitative methods in the review of epidemiologic literature. *Epidemiol. Rev.*, 9, 1-30

Grinberg-Funes, R.A., Singh, V.N., Perera, F.P., Bell, D.A., Young, T.L., Dickey, C., Wang, L.W. & Santella, R.M. (1994) Polycyclic aromatic hydrocarbon-DNA adducts in smokers and their relationship to micronutrient levels and the glutathione-S-transferase M1 genotype. *Carcinogenesis*, 15 (11), 2449-2454

Guirgis, H.A., Lynch, H.T., Mate, T., Harris, R.E., Wells, I., Caha, L., Anderson, J., Maloney, K. & Rankin, L. (1976) Aryl-hydrocarbon hydroxylase activity in lymphocytes from lung cancer patients and normal controls. *Oncology*, 33 (3), 105-109

Guo, J., Wan, D., Zeng, R & Zhang, Q. (1996) The polymorphism of GSTM1, mutagen sensitivity in colon cancer and healthy control. *Mutat. Res.*, 372, 17-22

Hall, A.G., Autzen, P., Cattan, A.R., Malcolm, A.J., Cole, M., Kernahan, J. & Reid, M.M. (1994) Expression of μ-class glutathione *S*-transferase correlates with event-free survival in childhood acute lymphoblastic leukaemia. *Cancer Res.*, 54, 5251-5254

Hamada, G.S., Sugimura, H., Suzuki, J., Nagura, K., Kiyokawa, E., Iwase, T., Tanaka, M., Takahashi, T., Watanabe, S., Kino, I. & Tsugane, S. (1995) The haem-binding region polymorphism of cytochrome P4501A1 (CYP1A1), rather than the RsaI polymorphism of P450IIE1 (CYPIIE1), is associated with lung cancer in Rio de Janeiro. *Cancer Epidemiol. Biomarkers Prev.*, 4 (1), 63-67

Hand, P.A., Inskip, A., Gilford, J., Alldersea, J., Elexpuru-Camiruaga, J., Hayes, J.D., Jones, P.W., Strange, R.C. & Fryer, A.A. (1996) Allelism at the glutathione S-transferase GSTM3 locus: interactions with GSTM1 and GSTT1 as risk factors for astrocytoma. *Carcinogenesis*, 17 (9), 1919-1922

Hanke, J. & Krajewska, B. (1990) Acetylation phenotypes and bladder cancer. *J. Occup. Med.*, 32, 917-918

Hanssen, H.P., Agarwal, D.P., Goedde, H.W., Bucher, H., Huland, H., Brachmann, W. & Ovenback, R. (1985) Association of N-acetyltransferase polymorphism and environmental factors with bladder carcinogenesis. Study in a North German population. *Eur. Urol.*, 11, 263-266

Harada, S., Misawa, S., Nakamura, T., Tanaka, N., Ueno, E. & Mutzumi, N. (1992) Detection of GST1 gene deletion by polymerase chain reaction and its possible correlation with stomach cancer in Japanese. *Hum. Genet.*, 90, 62-64

Hayashi, S., Watanabe, J. & Kawajiri, K. (1992) High susceptibility to lung cancer analysed in terms of combined genotypes of P450IA1 and mu-class glutathione S-transferase genes. *Jpn. J. Cancer Res.*, 83, 866-870

Hayes, R.B., Bi, W., Rothman, N., Broly, F., Caporaso, N., Feng, P., You, X., Yin, S., Woosley, R.L. & Meyer, U.A. (1993) N-acetylation phenotype and genotype and risk of bladder cancer in benzidine-exposed workers. *Carcinogenesis*, 14 (4), 675-678

Heagerty, A.H.M., Smith, A., English, J., Lear, J., Perkins, W., Bowers, B., Jones, P., Gilford, J., Alldersea, J., Fryer, A.A. & Strange, R.C. (1996) Susceptibility to multiple cutaneous basal cell carcinomas: significant interactions between glutathione S-transferase GSTM1 genotypes, skin type and male gender. *Br. J. Cancer*, 73, 44-48

Heagerty, A.H.M., Fitzgerald, D., Smith, A., Bowers, B., Jones, P., Fryer, A.A., Zhao, L., Alldersea, J. & Strange, R.C. (1994) Glutathione S-transferase GSTM1 phenotypes and protection against cutaneous tumours. *Lancet*, 343, 266-268

Hearse, D.J. & Weber, W.W. (1973) Multiple N-acetyltransferase and drug metabolism. *Biochem. J.*, 132, 519-526

Heckbert, S.R., Weiss, N.S., Hornung, S.K., Eaton, D.L. & Motulsky, A.G. (1992) Glutathione S-transferase and epoxide hydrolase activity in human leukocytes in relation to risk of lung cancer and other smoking-related cancers. *J. Natl. Cancer Inst.*, 84, 414-422

Heim, M.H. & Mayer, U.A. (1991) Genetyc polymorphism of debrisoquine oxidation: restriction fragment analysis and allele-specific amplification of mutant alleles of CYP2D6. *Methods Enzymol.*, 206, 173-183

Hemminki, K., Dickey, C., Karlsson, S., Bell, D., Hsu, Y., Tsai, W., Mooney, L.A., Savela, K. & Perera, F.P. (1997) Aromatic DNA adducts in foundry workers in relation to exposure, lifestyle and CYP1A1 and glutathione transferase M1 genotype. *Carcinogenesis*, 18 (2), 345-350

Henning, S., Cascorbi, I., Jahnke, V. & Roots, I. (1996) The *rapid* arylamine N-acetyltransferase (*NAT2*) genotype: a hereditary susceptibility factor for laryngeal cancer. *Head Neck Cancer*, 465-468

Hildesheim, A., Chen, C., Caporaso, N.E., Cheng, Y., Hoover, R.N., Hsu, M., Levine, P.H., Chen, I., Chen, J., Yang, C., Daly, A.K. & Idle, J.R. (1995) Cytochrome P4502E1 genetic polymorphisms and risk of nasopharyngeal carcinoma: results from a case-control study conducted in Taiwan. *Cancer Epidemiol. Biomarkers Prev.*, 4, 607-610

Hirvonen, A., Husgafvel-Pursiainen, K., Karjalainen, A., Anttila, S. & Vainio, H. (1992a) Point-mutational MspI and Ile-Val polymorphisms closely linked in the CYP1A1 gene: lack of association with susceptibility to lung cancer in a Finnish study population. *Cancer Epidemiol. Biomarkers Prev.*, 1 (6), 485-489

Hirvonen, A., Husgafvel-Pursiainen, K., Anttila, S., Karjalainen, A., Sorsa, M. & Vainio, H. (1992b) Metabolic cytochrome P450 genotypes and assessment of individual susceptibility to lung cancer. *Pharmacogenetics*, 2, 259-263

Hirvonen, A., Husgafvel-Pursiainen, K., Anttila, S. & Vainio, H. (1993a) The GSTM1 null genotype as a potential risk modifier for squamous cell carcinoma of the lung. *Carcinogenesis*, 14 (7), 1479-1481

Hirvonen, A., Husgafvel-Pursiainen, K., Anttila, S., Karjalainen, A., Pelkonen, O. & Vainio, H. (1993b) PCR-based CYP2D6 genotyping for Finnish lung cancer patients. *Pharmacogenetics*, 3, 19-27

Hirvonen, A., Husgafvel-Pursiainen, K., Anttila, S., Karjalainen, A. & Vainio, H. (1993c) Polymorphism in CYP1A1 and CYP2D6 genes: possible association with susceptibility to lung cancer. *Environ. Health Perspect.*, 3, 101, suppl. 109-112

Hirvonen, A., Husgafvel-Pursiainen, K., Anttila, S., Karjalainen, A. & Vainio, H. (1993d) The human CYP2E1 and lung cancer: DraI and RsaI restriction fragment length polymorphisms in a Finnish study population. *Carcinogenesis*, 14 (1), 85-88

Hirvonen, A., Nylund, L., Kociba, P., Husgafvel-Pursiainen, K. & Vainio, H. (1994) Modulation of urinary mutagenicity by genetically determined carcinogen metabolism in smokers. *Carcinogenesis*, 15 (5), 813-815

Hirvonen, A., Pelin, K., Tammilehto, L., Karjalainen, A., Mattson, K. & Linnainmaa, K. (1995) Inherited *GSTM1* and *NAT2* defects as concurrent risk modifiers in asbestos-related human malignant mesothelioma. *Cancer Res.*, 55, 2981-2983

Horai, Y., Fujita, K. & Ishizaki, T. (1989) Genetically determined N-acetylation and oxidation capacities in Japanese patients with non-occupational urinary bladder cancer. *Eur. J. Clin. Pharmacol.*, 37, 581-587

Horsmans, Y., Desager, J.P. & Harvengt, C. (1991) Is there a link between debrisoquine oxidation phenotype and lung cancer susceptibility? *Biomed. Pharmacother.*, 45, 359-362

Hou, S., Lambert, B. & Hemminki, K. (1995) Relationship between hrpt mutant frequency, aromatic DNA adducts and genotypes for *GSTM1* and *NAT2* in bus maintenance workers. *Carcinogenesis*, 16 (8), 1913-1917

Hsieh, L., Huang, R., Yu, M., Chen, C. & Liaw, Y. (1996) L-*myc* GST M1 genetic polymorphism and hepatocellular carcinoma risk among chronic hepatitis B carriers. *Cancer Lett.*, 103, 171-176

Ichiba, M., Hagmar, L., Rannug, A., Hogstedt, B., Alexandrie, A., Carstensen, U. & Hemminki, K. (1994) Aromatic DNA adducts, micronuclei and genetic polymorphism for *CYP1A1* and *GST1* in chimney sweeps. *Carcinogenesis*, 15 (7), 1347-1352

Idle, J.R., Mahgoub, A., Lancaster, R. & Smith, R.L. (1978) Hypotensive response to debrisoquine and hydroxylation phenotype. *Life Sci.*, 22, 979-984

Idle, J.R., Mahgoub, A., Sloan, T.P., Smith, R.L., Mbanefo, C.O. & Babubunmi, E.A. (1981) Some observations on the phenotype status of Nigerian patients presenting with cancer. *Cancer Lett.*, 11, 331-338

Ilett, K.F., David, B.M., Detchon, P., Castleden, W.M. & Kwa, R. (1987) Acetylator phenotype in colorectal carcinoma. *Cancer Res.*, 47, 1466-1469

Ilett, K.F., Detchon, P., Ingram, D. M. & Castleden, W.M. (1990) Acetylator phenotype is not associated with breast cancer. *Cancer Res.*, 50, 6649-6651

Jacquet, M., Lambert, V., Baudoux, E., Muller, M., Kremers, P. & Gielen, J. (1996) Correlation between P450 CYP1A1 inducibility, MspI genotype and lung cancer incidence. *Eur. J. Cancer*, 32A (10), 1701-1706

Jahnke, V., Matthias, C., Fryer, A. & Strange, R. (1996) Glutathione S-transferase and cytochrome-P-450 polymorphism as risk factors for squamous cell carcinoma of the larynx. *Am. J. Surg.*, 172, 671-673

Jaiswal, A.K., Gonzales, F.J. & Nebert, D.W. (1985) Human P1-450 gene sequence and correlation of mRNA with genetic differences in benzo[a]pyrene metabolism. *Nucleic Acids Res.*, 13 (12), 4503-4520

Jennings, M., Sweetland, H., Smith, C.A.D., Wolf, C.R., Lennard, M.S., Tucker, G.T., Woods, H.F. & Rogers, K. (1996) Lack of relationship between the debrisoquine (CYP2D6) and mephenytoin (CYP2C19) oxidation polymorphisms and susceptibility to breast cancer. *Breast*, 5, 254-258

Kadlubar, F.F., Butler, M.A., Kaderlik, K.R., Chou, H.C. & Lang, N.P. (1992) Polymorphisms for aromatic amine metabolism in humans: relevance for human carcinogenesis. *Environ. Health Perspect.*, 98, 69-74

Kaisary, A., Smith, P., Jaczq, E., McAllister, C.B., Wilkinson, G.R., Ray, W.A. & Branch, R.A. (1987) Genetic predisposition to bladder cancer: ability to hydroxylate debrisoquine and mephenytoin as risk factors. *Cancer Res.*, 47, 5488-5493

Karakaya, A.E., Cok, I., Sardas, S., Gogus, O. & Sardas, O.S. (1986) N-acetyltransferase phenotype of patients with bladder cancer. *Hum. Toxicol.*, 5, 333-335

Karki, N.T., Pokela, R., Nuutinen, L. & Pelkonen, O. (1987) Aryl hydrocarbon hydroxylase in lymphocytes and lung tissue from lung cancer patients and controls. *Int. J. Cancer*, 39, 565-570

Kato, S., Shields, P.G., Caporaso, N.E., Hoover, R.N., Trump, B.F., Sugimura, H., Weston, A. & Harris, C.C. (1992) Cytochrome P450IIE1 genetic polymorphisms, racial variation, and lung cancer risk. *Cancer Res.*, 52, 6712-6715

Kato, S., Shields, P.G., Caporaso, N.E., Sugimura,H., Trivers, G.E., Tucker, M.A., Trump, B.F., Weston, A. & Harris, C.C. (1994) Analysis of cytochrome P450 2E1 genetic polymorphisms in relation to human lung cancer. *Cancer Epidemiol. Biomarkers Prev.*, 3, 515-518

Kato, S., Bowman, E.D., Harrington, A.M., Blömeke, B. & Shields, P.G. (1995a) Human lung carcinogen-DNA adduct levels mediated by genetic polymorphisms *in vivo*. *J. Natl. Cancer Inst.*, 87 (12), 902-907

Kato, S., Onda, M., Matsukura, N., Tokunaga, A., Tajiri, T., Kim, D.Y., Tsuruta, H., Matsuda, N., Yamashita, K. & Shields, P.G. (1995b) Cytochrome P4502E1 (CYP2E1) genetic polymorphism in a case-control study of gastric cancer and liver disease. *Pharmacogenetics*, 5, S141-S144

Kato, S., Onda, M., Matsukura, N., Tokunaga, A., Matsuda, N., Yamashita, K. & Shields, P.G. (1996) Genetic polymorphisms of the cancer-related gene and *Helicobacter pylori* infection in Japanese gastric cancer patients. *Cancer*, 77, 8 Suppl. 1654-1661

Katoh, T., Inatomi, H., Nagaoka, A. & Sugita, A. (1995) Citochrome P4501A1 gene polymorphism and homozygous deletion of the glutathione S-transferase M1 gene in urothelial cancer patients. *Carcinogenesis*, 16 (3), 655-657

Katoh, T., Nagata, N., Kuroda, Y., Itoh, H., Kawahara, A., Kuroki, N., Ookuma, R. & Bell, D.A. (1996) Glutathione S-transferase M1 (GSTM1) and T1 (GSTT1) genetic polymorphism and susceptibility to gastric and colorectal adenocarcinoma. *Carcinogenesis*, 17 (9), 1855-1859

Kawajiri, K., Nakachi, K., Imai, K., Yoshii, A., Shinoda, N. & Watanabe, J. (1990) Identification of genetically high-risk individuals to lung cancer by DNA polymorphisms of the cytochrome P450IA1 gene. *FEBS Lett.*, 263 (1), 131-133

Kawajiri, K. & Fujii-Kuriyama, Y. (1991) P450 and human cancer. *Jpn. J. Cancer Res.*, 82 (12), 1325-1335

Kawajiri, K., Eguchi, H., Nakachi, K., Sekiya, T. & Yamamoto, M. (1996) Association of CYP1A1 germ line polymorphisms with mutations of the p53 gene in lung cancer. *Cancer Res.*, 56, 72-76

Kellermann, G., Shaw, C.R. & Luyten-Kellermann, M. (1973) Aryl hydrocarbon hydroxylase inducibility and bronchogenic carcinoma. *New Engl. J. Med.*, 289 (18), 934-937

Kelsey, K.T., Wiencke, J.K. & Spitz, M.R. (1994) A race-specific genetic polymorphism in the CYP1A1 gene is not associated with lung cancer in African-Americans. *Carcinogenesis*, 15 (6), 1121-1124

Kempkes, M., Golka, K., Reich, S., Reckwitz, T. & Bolt, H.M. (1996) Glutathione S-transferase GSTM1 and GSTT1 null genotypes as potential risk factors for urothelial cancer of the bladder. *Arch. Toxicol.*, 71, 123-126

Ketterer, B., Harris, J.M., Talaska, G., Meyer, D.J., Pemble, S.E., Taylor, J.B., Lang, N.P. & Kadlubar, F.K. (1992) The human glutathione S-transferase supergene family, its polymorphism, and its effects on susceptibility to lung cancer. *Environ. Health Perspect.*, 98, 87-94

Kihara, M., Kihara, M. & Noda, K. (1994) Lung cancer risk of GSTM1 null genotype is dependent on the extent of tobacco smoke exposure. *Carcinogenesis*, 15 (2), 415-418

Kihara, M., Kihara, M. & Noda, K. (1995a) Distribution of *GSTM1* null genotype in relation to gender, age and smoking status in Japanese lung cancer patients. *Pharmacogenetics*, 5, S74-S79

Kihara, M., Noda, K. & Kihara, M. (1995b) Risk of smoking for squamous and small cell carcinomas of the lung modulated by combinations of CYP1A1 and GSTM1 gene polymorphisms in a Japanese population. *Carcinogenesis*, 16 (10), 2331-2336

Kihara, M., Kihara, M., Kubota, A., Furukawa, M. & Kimura, H. (1997) *GSTM1* gene polymorphism as a possible marker for susceptibility to head and neck cancers among Japanese smokers. *Cancer Lett.*, 112, 257-262

Kirlin, W.G., Ogolla, F., Andrews, A.F., Trinidad, A., Ferguson, R.J., Yerokun, T., Mpezo, M. & Hein, D.W. (1991) Acetylator genotype-dependent expression of arylamine N-acetyltransferase in human colon cytosol from non-cancer and colorectal cancer patients. *Cancer Res.*, 51, 549-555

Korsgaard, R., Trell, E., Simonsson, B.G., Stiksa, G., Janzon, L., Hood, B. & Oldbring, J. (1984) Aryl hydrocarbon hydroxylase induction levels in patients with malignant tumors associated with smoking. *J. Cancer Res. Clin. Oncol.*, 108, 286-289

Kouri, R.E., McKinney, C.E., Slomiany, D.J., Snodgrass, D.R., Wray, N.P. & McLemore, T.L. (1982) Positive correlation between high aryl hydrocarbon hydroxylase activity and primary lung cancer as analysed in cryopreserved lymphocytes. *Cancer Res.*, 42 (12), 5030-5037

Ladero, J.M., Kwok, C.K., Jara, C., Fernandez, L., Silmi, A.M., Tapia, D. & Uson, A.C. (1985) Hepatic acetylator phenotype in bladder cancer patients. *Ann. Clin. Res.*, 17, 96-99

Ladero, J.M., Fernandez, M.J., Palmeiro, R., Munoz, J.J., Jara, C., Lazaro, C. & Perez-Manga, G. (1987) Hepatic acetylator polymorphism in breast cancer patients. *Oncology*, 44, 341-344

Ladero, J.M., Gonzalez, J.F., Benitez, J., Vargas, E., Fernandez, M.J., Baki, W. & Diaz-Rubio, M. (1991a) Acetylator polymorphism in human colorectal carcinoma. *Cancer Res.*, 51, 2098-2100

Ladero, J.M., Benitez, J., Jara, C., Llerena, A., Valdivielso, M.J., Munoz, J.J. & Vargas, E. (1991b) Polymorphic oxidation of debrisoquine in women with breast cancer. *Oncology*, 48, 107-110

Ladona, M., Abildua, R.E., Ladero, J.M., Roman, J.M., Plaza, M.A., Agundez, J.A.G., Munoz, J.J. & Benitez, J. (1996) CYP2D6 genotypes in Spanish women with breast cancer. *Cancer Lett.*, 99, 23-28

Lafuente, A., Pujol, F., Carretero, P., Perez Villa, J. & Cuchi, A. (1993) Human glutathione S-transferase μ (GSTμ) deficiency as a marker for susceptibility to bladder and larynx cancer among smokers. *Cancer Lett.*, 68, 49-54

Lafuente, A., Molina, R., Palou, J., Castel, T., Moral, A., Trias, M. & the MMM Group (1995) Phenotype of glutathione S-transferase Mu (GSTM1) and susceptibility to malignant melanoma. *Br. J. Cancer*, 72, 324-326

Landi, M.T., Zocchetti, C., Bernucci, I., Kadlubar, F.F., Tannenbaum, S., Skipper, P., Bartsch, H., Malaveille, C., Shields, P., Caporaso, N.E. & Vineis, P. (1996a) Cytochrome P4501A2: enzyme induction and genetic control in determining 4-aminobiphenyl-haemoglobin adduct levels. *Cancer Epidemiol. Biomarkers Prev.*, 5, 693-698

Landi, S., Ponzanelli, I., Hirvonen, A., Norppa, H. & Barale, R. (1996b) Repeated analysis of sister chromatid exchange induction by diepoxybutane in cultured human lymphocytes: effect of glutathione S-transferase T1 and M1 genotype. *Mutat. Res.*, 351, 79-85

Lang, N.P., Chu, D.Z.J., Hunter, C.F., Kendall, D.C., Flammang, T.J. & Kadlubar, F.F. (1986) Role of aromatic amine acetyltransferase in human colorectal cancer. *Arch. Surg.*, 121, 1259-1261

Lang, N.P., Butler, M.A., Massengill, J., Lawson, M., Stotts, R.C., Hauer-Jensen, M. & Kadlubar, F.F. (1994) Rapid metabolic phenotypes for acetyltransferase and cytochrome P4501A2 and putative exposure to food-borne heterocyclic amines increase the risk for colorectal cancer or polyps. *Cancer Epidemiol. Biomarkers Prev.*, 3, 675-682

Law, M.R., Hetzel, M.R. & Idle, J.R. (1989) Debrisoquine metabolism and genetic predisposition to lung cancer. *Br. J. Cancer*, 59, 686-687

Lear, J.T., Heagerty, A.H.M., Smith, A., Bowers, B., Payne, C.R., Dale Smith, C.A., Jones, P.W., Gilford, J., Yengi, L., Alldersea, J., Fryer, A.A. & Strange, R.C. (1996) Multiple cutaneous basal cell carcinomas: glutathione *S*-transferase (GSTM1, GSTT1) and cytochrome P450 (CYP2D6, CYP1A1) polymorphisms influence tumour numbers and accrual. *Carcinogenesis*, 17 (9), 1891-1896

Lear, J.T., Smith, A.G., Bowers, B., Heagearty, A.H.M., Jones, P.W., Gilford, J., Alldersea, J., Strange, C. & Fryer, A.A. (1997) Truncal tumour site is associated with high risk of multiple basal cell carcinoma and is influenced by glutathione *S*-transferase, GSTT1, and cytochrome P450, CYP1A1 genotypes, and their interaction. *J. Invest. Dermatol.*, 108 (4), 519-522

Lee, S.W., Jang, I., Shin, S., Lee, K., Yim, D., Kim, S., Oh, S. & Lee, S. (1994) CYP1A2 activity as a risk factor for bladder cancer. *J. Korean Med. Sci.*, 9, (6), 482-489

Legrand, M., Stucker, I., Marez, D., Sabbagh, N., Lo-Giudice, J.M. & Broly, F. (1996) Influence of a mutation reducing the catalytic activity of cytochrome P450 CYP2D6 on lung cancer susceptibility. *Carcinogenesis*, 17 (9), 2267-2269

Lin, H.J., Han, C.Y., Bernstein, D.A., Hsiao, W., Lin, B.K. & Hardy, S. (1994) Ethnic distribution of the glutathione transferase M1-1 (GSTM1) null genotype in 1473 individuals and application to bladder cancer susceptibility. *Carcinogenesis*, 15 (5), 1077-1081

Lin, H.J., Probst-Hensch, NM., Ingles, S.A., Han, C.Y., Lin, B.K., Lee, D.B., Frankl, H.D., Lee, E.R., Longnecker, M.P. & Haile, R.W. (1995) Glutathione transferase (GSTM1) null genotype, smoking, and prevalence of colorectal adenomas. *Cancer Res.*, 55, 1224-1226

Liu, L. & Wang, L.H. (1988) Correlation between lung cancer prevalence and activities of aryl hydrocarbon hydroxylase and glutathione S-transferase in human lung tissues. *Biomed. Environ. Sci.*, 1, 277-282

London, S.J., Daly, A.K., Cooper, J., Navidi, W.C., Carpenter, C.L. & Idle, J.R. (1995a) Polymorphism of glutathione *S*-transferase M1 and lung cancer risk among African-Americans and Caucasians in Los Angeles County, California. *J. Natl. Cancer Inst.*, 87 (16), 1246-1253

London, S.J., Daly, A.K., Fairbrother, K.S., Holmes, C., Carpenter, C.L., Navidi, W.C. & Idle, J.R. (1995b) Lung cancer risk in African-Americans in relation to a race-specific CYP1A1 polymorphism. *Cancer Res.*, 55, 6035-6037

London, S.J., Daly, A.K., Leathart, J.B., Navidi, W.C., Carpenter, C.C. & Idle, J.R. (1997) Genetic polymorphism of CYP2D6 and lung cancer risk in African-Americans and Caucasians in Los Angeles County. *Carcinogenesis*, 18 (6), 1203-1214

Lower, G.M., Nilsson, T., Nelson, C.E., Wolf, H., Gamsky, T.E. & Bryan, G.T. (1979) N-acetyltransferase phenotype and risk in urinary bladder cancer: approaches in molecular epidemiology. Preliminary results in Sweden and Denmark. *Environ. Health Perspect.*, 29, 71-79

Lucas, D., Menez, C., Floch, F., Gourlaouen, Y., Sparfel, O., Joannet, I., Bodenez, P., Jezequel, J., Gouerou, H., Berthou, F., Bardou, L.G. & Menez, J.F. (1996) Cytochromes P4502E1 and P4501A1 genotypes and susceptibility to cirrhosis or upper aerodigestive tract cancer in alcoholic Caucasians. *Alcoholism: Clin. Experiment. Res.*, 20 (6), 1033-1037

Mahgoub, A., Idle, J.R., Dring, L.G., Lancaster, R. & Smith, R.L. (1977) Polymorphic hydroxylation of debrisoquine in man. *Lancet*, 2, 584-586

Manchester, D. K., Bowman, E. D., Parker, N. B., Caporaso, N. E. & Weston, A. (1992) Determinants of polycyclic aromatic hydrocarbon-DNA adducts in human placenta. *Cancer Res.*, 52, 1499-1503

Mannervik, B. (1985).The isozymes of glutathione S-transferase. *Adv. Enzymol.*, 57, 357-417

Martinez, C., Agundez, J.A.G., Olivera, M., Martin, R., Ladero, J.M. & Benitez, J. (1995) Lung cancer and mutations at the polymorphic NAT2 gene locus. *Pharmacogenetics*, 5, 207-214

McGlynn, K.A., Rosvold, E.A., Lustbader, E.D., Hu, Y., Clapper, M.L., Zhou, T., Wild, C.P., Xia, X.L., Baffoe-Bonnie, A., Ofori-Adjei, D., Chen, G.C., London, W.T., Shen, F.M. & Buetow, K.H. (1995) Susceptibility to hepatocellular carcinoma is associated with genetic variation in the enzymatic detoxification of aflatoxin B_1. *Proc. Natl. Acad. Sci. USA*, 92, 2384-2387

McLemore, T.L., Martin, R.R., Busbee, D.L., Ritchie, R.C., Springer, R.R., Toppell, K.L. & Cantrell, E.T. (1977) Aryl hydrocarbon hydroxylase activity in pulmonary macrophages and lymphocytes from lung cancer and noncancer patients. *Cancer Res.*, 37 (4), 1175-1181

McLemore, T.L., Martin, R.R., Wray, N.P., Cantrell, E.T. & Busbee, D.L. (1978) Dissociation between aryl hydrocarbon hydroxylase activity in cultured pulmonary macrophages and blood lymphocytes from lung cancer patients. *Cancer Res.*, 38 (11), 3805-11

McLemore, T.L., Martin, R.R., Springer, R.R., Wray, N., Cantrell, E.T. & Busbee, D.L. (1979) Aryl hydrocarbon hydroxylase activity in pulmonary alveolar macrophages and lymphocytes from lung cancer and noncancer patients: a correlation with family histories of cancer. *Biochem. Genet.*, 17 (9-10), 795-806

Meyer, C.F., Zanger, U.M., Grant, D. & Blume, M. (1990) Genetic polymorphism of drug metabolism. *Adv. Drug Res.*, 19, 198

Miller, M.E. & Cosgriff, J.M. (1983) Acetylator phenotype in human bladder cancer. *J. Urol.*, 130, 65-66

Mommsen, S., Barfod, N.M. & Aagaard, J. (1985) N-acetyltransferase phenotypes in the urinary bladder carcinogenesis of a low-risk population. *Carcinogenesis*, 6 (2), 199-201

Mooney, L. A., Bell, D.A., Santella, R.M., Van Bennekum, A.M., Ottman, R., Paik, M., Blaner, W.S., Lucier, G.W., Covey, L., Young, T., Cooper, T.B., Glassman, A.H. & Perera, F.P. (1997) Contribution of genetic and nutritional factors to DNA damage in heavy smokers. *Carcinogenesis*, 18 (3), 503-509

Moreira, A., Martins, G., Monteiro, M.J., Alves, M., Dias, J., Duro da Costa, J., Melo, M.J., Matias, D., Costa, A., Cristovao, M., Rueff, J. & Monteiro, C. (1996) Glutathione S-transferase mu polymorphism and susceptibility to lung cancer in the Portuguese population. *Teratogenesis Carcinog. Mutagen.*, 16, 269-274

Morita, S., Yano, M., Shiozaki, H., Tsujinaka, T., Ebisui, C., Morimoto, T., Kishibuti, M., Fujita, J., Ogawa, A., Taniguchi, M., Inoue, M., Tamura, S., Yamazaki, K., Kikkawa, N., Mizunoya, S. & Monden, M. (1997) CYP1A1, CYP2E1 and GSTM1 polymorphisms are not associated with susceptibility to squamous-cell carcinomas of the esophagus. *Int. J. Cancer*, 71, 192-195

Nakachi, K., Imai, K., Hayashi, S., Watanabe, J. & Kawajiri, K. (1991) Genetic susceptibility to squamous cell carcinoma of the lung in relation to cigarette smoking dose. *Cancer Res.*, 51 (19), 5177-80

Nakachi, K., Imai, K., Hayashi, S. & Kawajiri, K. (1993) Polymorphisms of the CYP1A1 and glutathione S-transferase genes associated with susceptibility to lung cancer in relation to cigarette dose in a Japanese population. *Cancer Res.*, 53, 2994-2999

Nakajima, T., Elovaara, E., Anttila, S., Hirvonen, A., Camus, A.M., Hayes, J.D., Ketterer, B. & Vainio, H. (1995) Expression and polymorphism of glutathione S-transferase in human lungs: risk factors in smoking-related cancer. *Carcinogenesis*, 16 (4), 707-711

Nazar-Stewart, V., Motulsky, A.G., Eaton, D.L., White, E., Hornung, S.K., Leng, Z.T., Stapleton, P. & Weiss, N.S. (1993) The glutathione S-transferase μ polymorphism as a marker for susceptibility to lung carcinoma. *Cancer Res.*, 53, 2313-2318

Nebert, D.W. & Gonzalez, F.J. (1987). P450 genes: structure, evolution and regulation. *Annu. Rev. Biochem.*, 56, 945-993

Nielsen, P.S., De Pater, N., Okkels, H. & Autrup, H. (1996a) Enviromental air pollution and DNA adducts in Copenhagen bus drivers - Effect of GSTM1 and NAT2 genotypes on adduct levels. *Carcinogenesis*, 17 (5), 1021-1027

Nielsen, P., Okkels, H., Sigsgaard, T., Kyrtopoulos, S. & Autrup, H. (1996b) Exposure to urban and rural air pollution: DNA and protein adducts and effect of glutathione *S*-transferase genotype on adduct levels. *Int. Arch. Occup. Environ. Health*, 68, 170-176

Norppa, H., Hirvonen, A., Jarventaus, H., Uuskula, M., Tasa, G., Ojajarvi, A. & Sorsa, M. (1995) Role of GSTT1 and GSTM1 genotypes in determining individual sensitivity to sister chromatid exchange induction by diepoxybutane in cultured human lymphocytes. *Carcinogenesis*, 16 (6), 1261-1264

Oda, Y., Tanaka, M. & Nakanishi, I. (1994) Relation between the occurrence of K-ras gene point mutations and genotypes of polymorphic N-acetyltransferase in human colorectal carcinomas. *Carcinogenesis*, 15 (7), 1365-1369

Ohshima, S. & Xu, Y. (1997) p53 gene mutation, and CYP1A1 and GSTM1 genotypes in pulmonary squamous cell carcinomas. *J. Clin. Pathol. Mol. Pathol.*, 50, 108-110

Okada, T., Kawashima, K., Fukushi, S., Minakuchi, T. & Nishimura, S. (1994) Association between a cytochrome *P450 CYP1A1* and incidence of lung cancer. *Pharmacogenetics*, 4, 333-340

Okkels, H., Sigsgaard, T., Wolf, H. & Autrup, H. (1996) Glutathione S-transferase μ as a risk factor in bladder tumors. *Pharmacogenetics*, 6, 251-256

Okkels, H., Sigsgaard, T., Wolf, H. & Autrup, H. (1997) Arylamine N-acetyltransferase 1 (NAT1) and 2 (NAT2) polymorphisms in susceptibility to bladder cancer: the influence of smoking. *Cancer Epidemiol. Biomarkers Prev.*, 6, 225-231

Oyama, T., Kawamoto, T., Mizoue, T., Sugio, K., Kodama, Y., Mitsudomi, T. & Yasumoto, K. (1997a) Cytochrome P450 2E1 polymorphism as a risk factor for lung cancer in relation to p53 gene mutation. *Anticancer Res.*, 17, 583-588

Oyama, T., Kawamoto, T., Mizoue, T., Yasumoto, K., Kodama, Y. & Mitsudomi, T. (1997b) N-acetylation polymorphism in patients with lung cancer and its association with p53 gene mutation. *Anticancer Res.*, 17, 577-582

Paigen, B., Gurtoo, H.L., Minowada, J., Houten, L., Vincent, R., Paigen, K., Parker, N.B., Ward, E. & Hayner, N.T. (1977) Questionable relation of aryl hydrocarbon hydroxylase to lung-cancer risk. *New Engl. J. Med.*, 297, 346-350

Pelin, K., Hirvonen, A. & Norppa, H. (1996) Influence of erythrocyte glutathione *S*-transferase T1 on sister chromatid exchanges induced by diepoxybutane in cultured human lymphocytes. *Mutagenesis*, 11 (2), 213-215

Perrett, C.W., Clayton, R.N., Pistorello, M., Boscaro, M., Scanarini, M., Bates, A.S., Buckley, N., Jones, P., Fryer, A.A., Gilford, J., Alldersea, J. & Strange, R.C. (1995) *GSTM1* and *CYP2D6* genotype frequencies in patients with pituitary tumours: effects on *P53*, *ras* and *gsp*. *Carcinogenesis*, 16 (7), 1643-1645

Persson, I., Johansson, I., Bergling, H., Dahl, M., Seidegard, J., Rylander, R., Rannug, A., Hogberg, J. & Ingelman Sundberg, M. (1993) Genetic polymorphism of cytochrome P4502E1 in a Swedish population. Relationship to incidence of lung cancer. *FEBS Lett.*, 319 (3), 207-211

Petruzzelli, S., Camus, A.M., Carrozzi, L., Ghelarducci, L., Rindi, M., Menconi, G., Angeletti, C.A., Ahotupa, M., Hietanen, E., Aitio, A., Saracci, R., Bartsch, H. & Giuntini, C. (1988) Long-lasting effects of tobacco smoking on pulmonary drug-metabolizing enzyme: a case-control study on lung cancer patients. *Cancer Res.*, 48, 4695-4700

Philip, P.A., Rogers, H.J., Millis, R.R., Rubens, R.D. & Cartwright, R.A. (1987) Acetylator status and its relationship to breast cancer and other diseases of the breast. *European Journal of Cancer and Clinical Oncology*, 23 (11), 1701-1706

Philip, P.A., Fitzgerald, D.L., Cartwright, R.A., Peake, M.D. & Rogers, H.J. (1988) Polymorphic N-acetylation capacity in lung cancer. *Carcinogenesis*, 9 (3), 491-493

Probst-Hensch, N.M., Haile, R.W., Ingles, S.A., Longnecker, M.P., Han, C.Y., Lin, B.K., Lee, D.B., Sakamoto, G.T., Frankl, H.D., Lee, E.R. & Lin, H.J. (1995) Acetylation polymorphism and prevalence of colorectal adenomas. *Cancer Res.*, 55, 2017-2020

Probst-Hensch, N.M., Haile, R.W., Li, D.S., Sakamoto, G.T., Louie, A.D., Lin, B.K., Frankl, H.D., Lee, E.R. & Lin, H.J. (1996) Lack of association between the polyadenylation polymorphism in the *NAT1* (acetyltransferase 1) gene and colorectal adenomas. *Carcinogenesis*, 17 (10), 2125-2129

Rebbeck, T.R., Godwin, A.K. & Buetow, K.H. (1996) Variability in loss of constitutional heterozygosity across loci and among individuals: association with candidate genes in ductal breast carcinoma. *Mol. Carcinogenesis*, 17, 117-125

Rebbeck, T.R., Rosvold, E.A., Duggan, D.J., Zhang, J. & Buetow, K.H. (1994) Genetics of CYP1A1: coamplification of specific alleles by polymerase chain reaction and association with breast cancer. *Cancer Epidemiol. Biomarkers Prev.*, 3 (6), 511-514

Risch, A., Wallace, D.M.A., Bathers, S. & Sim, E. (1995) Slow N-acetylation genotype is a susceptibility factor in occupational and smoking-related bladder cancer. *Hum. Mol. Genet.*, 4 (2), 231-236

Roberts-Thomson, I.C., Ryan, P., Khoo, K.K., Hart, W.J., McMichael, A.J. & Butler, R.N. (1996) Diet, acetylator phenotype, and risk of colorectal neoplasia. *Lancet*, 347, 1372-1374

Rodriguez, J.W., Kirlin, W.G., Ferguson, R.J., Doll, M.A., Gray, K., Rustan, T.D., Lee, M.E., Kemp, K., Urso, P. & Hein, D.W. (1993) Human acetylator genotype: relationship to colorectal cancer incidence and arylamine N-acetyltransferase expression in colon cytosol. *Arch. Toxicol.*, 67, 445-452

Romkes, M., Chern, H., Lesnick T.G., Becich, M.J., Persad, R., Smith, P. & Branch, R.A. (1996) Association of low CYP3A activity with *p53* mutation and CYP2D6 activity with *Rb* mutation in human bladder cancer. *Carcinogenesis*, 17 (5), 1057-1062

Roots, I., Drakoulis, N., Ploch, M., Heinemeyer, G., Loddenkemper, R., Minks, T., Nitz, M., Otte, F. & Koch, M. (1988) Debrisoquine hydroxylation phenotype, acetylation phenotype, and AB0 blood groups as genetic host factors of lung cancer risk. *Klin. Wochenschr.*, 66, suppl. XI, 87-97

Rothman, K.J. (1986) *Modern Epidemiology*, Boston; Little, Brown & Co.; 358 pp

Rothman, N., Hayes, R.B., Zenser, T.V., Demarini, D.M., Bi, W., Hirvonen, A., Talaska, G., Bhatnagar, V.K., Caporaso, N.E., Brooks, L.R., Lakshmi, V.M., Feng, P., Kashyap, S.K., You, X., Eischen, B.T., Kashyap, R., Shelton, M.L., Hsu, F.F., Jaeger, M., Parikh, D.J., Davis, B.B., Yin, S. & Bell, D.A. (1996) The glutathione S-transferase M1 (*GSTM1*) null genotype and benzidine-associated bladder cancer, urine mutagenicity, and exfoliated urothelial cell DNA adducts. *Cancer Epidemiol. Biomarkers Prev.*, 5, 979-983

Rothman, N., Stewart, W.F., Caporaso, N.E. & Hayes, R.B. (1993) Misclassification of genetic susceptibility biomarkers: implications for case-control studies and cross-population comparison. *Cancer Epidemiol. Biomarkers Prev.*, 2, 299-303

Rothman, N., Shields, P.G., Poirier, M.C., Harrington, A.M., Ford, D.P. & Strickland, P.T. (1995) The impact of glutathione S-transferase M1 and cytochrome P450 1A1 genotypes on white-blood-cell polycyclic aromatic hydrocarbon-DNA adduct levels in humans. *Mol. Carcinogen.*, 14, 63-68

Ryberg, D., Hewer, A., Phillips, D.H. & Haugen, A. (1994a) Different susceptibility to smoking-induced DNA damage among male and female lung cancer patients. *Cancer Res.*, 54, 5801-5803

Ryberg, D., Kure, E., Lystad, S., Skaug, V., Stangeland, L., Mercy, I., Borresen, A. & Haugen, A. (1994b) p53 mutations in lung tumours: relationship to putative susceptibility markers for cancer. *Cancer Res.*, 54, 1551-1555

Sardas, S., Cok, I., Sardas, O.S., Ilhan, O. & Karakaya, A.E. (1990) Polymorphic N-acetylation capacity in breast cancer patients. *Int. J. Cancer*, 46 (6), 1138-1139

Sarhanis, P., Redman, C., Perrett, C., Brannigan, K., Clayton, R.N., Hand, P., Musgrove, C., Suarez, V., Jones, P., Fryer, A.A., Farrell, W.E. & Strange, R.C. (1996) Epithelial ovarian cancer: influence of polymorphism at the glutathione S-transferase GSTM1 and GSTT1 loci on p53 expression. *Br. J. Cancer*, 74, 1757-1761

Sato, K. (1989) Glutathione transferases as markers of preoplasia and neoplasia. *Adv. Cancer Res.*, 52, 205-255

Scarpato, R., Migliore, L., Hirvonen, A., Falck, G. & Norppa, H. (1996) Cytogenetic monitoring of occupational exposure to pesticides: characterization of *GSTM1*, *GSTT1*, and *NAT2* genotypes. *Environ. Mol. Mutagen.*, 27, 263-269

Scarpato, R., Hirvonen, A., Migliore, L., Falck, G. & Norppa, H. (1997) Influence of *GSTM*1 and *GSTT1* polymorphisms on the frequency of chromosome aberrations in lymphocytes of smokers and pesticide-exposed greenhouse workers. *Mutat. Res.*, 389, 227-235

Schroder, K.R., Wiebel, F.A., Reich, S., Dannappel, D., Bolt, H.M. & Hallier, E. (1995) Glutathione-S-transferase (GST) theta polymorphism influences background SCE rate. *Arch. Toxicol.*, 69, 505-507

Seidegard, J., De Pierre, J., Birberg, W., Pilotti, A. & Pero, R.W. (1984) Characterization of soluble glutathione transferase activity in resting mononuclear leukocytes from human blood. *Biochem. Pharmacol.*, 33, 3053-3058

Seidegard, J. & Pero, R.W. (1985) The hereditary trasmission of high glutathione transferase activity towards trans-stilbene oxide in human mononuclear leukocytes. *Hum. Genet.*, 69, 66-68

Seidegard, J., Pero, R.W., Miller, D.G. & Beattie, E.J. (1986) A glutathione transferase in human leukocytes as a marker for the susceptibility to lung cancer. *Carcinogenesis*, 7 (5), 751-753

Seidegard, J., Vorachek, W.R., Pero, R.W. & Pearson, W.R. (1988) Hereditary differences in the expression of human glutathione transferase activity on trans-stilbene oxide are due to a gene deletion. *Proc. Natl. Acad. Sci. USA*, 85, 7293-7297

Seidegard, J., Pero, R.W., Markovitz, M.M., Roush, G., Miller, D.G. & Beattie, E.J. (1990) Isoenzyme(s) of glutathione transferase (class Mu) as a marker for the susceptibility to lung cancer: a follow up study. *Carcinogenesis*, 11 (1), 33-36

Shanley, S.M., Chevenix-Trench, G., Palmer, J. & Hayward, N. (1995) Glutathione S-transferase *GSTM1* null genotype is not overrepresented in Australian patients with nevoid basal cell carcinoma syndrome or sporadic melanoma. *Carcinogenesis*, 16 (8), 2003-2004

Shaw, G.L., Falk, R.T., Deslauriers, J., Frame, J.N., Nesbitt, J.C., Pass, H.I., Issaq, H.J., Hoover, R.N. & Tucker, M.A. (1995) Debrisoquine metabolism and lung cancer risk. *Cancer Epidemiol. Biomarkers Prev.*, 4, 41-48

Shibuta, K., Nakashima, T., Abe, M., Mashimo, M., Mori, M., Ueo, H., Akiyoshi, T., Sugimachi, K. & Suzuki, T. (1994) Molecular genotyping for N-acetylation polymorphism in Japanese patients with colorectal cancer. *Cancer*, 74 (12), 3108-3112

Shields, P.G., Ambrosone, C.B., Graham, S., Bowman, E.D., Harrington, A.M., Gillenwater, K.A., Marshall, J.R., Vena, J.E., Laughlin, R., Nemoto, T. & Freudenheim, J.L. (1996) A cytochrome P4502E1 genetic polymorphism and tobacco smoking in breast cancer. *Mol. Carcinogen.*, 17, 144-150

Shields, P.G., Bowman, E.D., Harrington, A.M., Doan, V.T. & Weston, A. (1993a) Polycyclic aromatic hydrocarbon-DNA adducts in human lung and cancer susceptibility genes. *Cancer Res.*, 53, 3486-3492

Shields, P.G., Caporaso, N.E., Falk, R.T., Sugimura, H., Trivers, G.E., Trump, B.F., Hoover, R.N., Weston, A. & Harris, C.C. (1993b) Lung cancer, race, and a CYP1A1 genetic polymorphism. *Cancer Epidemiol. Biomarkers Prev.*, 2 (5), 481-485

Sinues, B., Perez, J., Bernal, M.L., Saenz, M.A., Lanuza, J. & Bartolome, M. (1992) Urinary mutagenicity and N-acetylation phenotype in textile industry workers exposed to arylamines. *Cancer Research*, 52, 4885-4889

Sivaraman, L., Leatham, M.P., Yee, J., Wilkens, L.R., Lau, A.F. & Le Marchand, L. (1994) CYP1A1 genetic polymorphisms and *in situ* colorectal cancer. *Cancer Res.*, 54 (14), 3692-3695

Sorsa, M., Osterman-Golkar, S., Peltonen, K., Saarikoski, S.T. & Sram, R. (1996) Assessment of exposure to butadiene in the process industry. *Toxicology*, 113, 77-83

Speirs, C.J., Murray, S., Davies, D.S., Biola Mabadeje, A.F. & Boobis, A.R. (1990) Debrisoquine oxidation phenotype and susceptibility to lung cancer. *Br. J. Clin. Pharmacol.*, 29, 101-109

Spigelman, A.D., Farmer, K.C.R., Oliver, S., Nugent, K.P., Bennett, P.N., Notarianni, L.J., Dobrocky, P. & Phillips, R.K.S. (1995) Caffeine phenotyping of cytochrome P4501A2, N-acetyltransferase, and xanthine oxidase in patients with familial adenomatous polyposis. *Gut*, 36, 251-254

Spurr, N.K., Gough, A.C., Chinegwundoh, F.I. & Dale Smith, C.A. (1995) Polymorphisms in drug-metabolizing enzymes as modifiers of cancer risk. *Clin Chem.*, 41 (12), 1864-1869

Strange, R.C., Matharoo, B., Faulder, G.C., Jones, P., Cotton, W., Elder, J.B. & Deakin, M. (1991) The human glutathione S-transferase: a case-control study of the incidence of the GST1 0 phenotype in patients with adenocarcinoma. *Carcinogenesis*, 12 (1), 25-28

Stücker, I., Cosme, J., Laurent, P., Cenee, S., Beaune, P., Bignon, J., Depierre, A., Milleron, B. & Hemon, D. (1995) CYP2D6 genotype and lung cancer risk according to histologic type and tobacco exposure. *Carcinogenesis*, 16 (11), 2759-2764

Sugimura, H., Caporaso, N.E., Shaw, G.L., Modali, R.V., Gonzalez, F.J., Hoover, R.N., Resau, J.H., Trump, B.F., Weston, A. & Harris, C.C. (1990) Human debrisoquine hydroxylase gene polymorphism in cancer patients and controls. *Carcinogenesis*, 11 (9), 1527-1530

Sugimura, H., Suzuki, I., Hamada, G.S., Iwase, T., Takahashi, T., Nagura, K., Iwata H., Watanabe S., Kino I. & Tsugane, S. (1994) Cytochrome P-450 1A1 genotype in lung cancer patients and controls in Rio de Janeiro, Brazil. *Cancer Epidemiol. Biomarkers Prev.*, 3 (2), 145-148

Taioli, E., Crofts, F., Trachman, J., Demopoulos, R., Toniolo, P. & Garte, S.J. (1995a) A specific African-American CYP1A1 polymorphism is associated with adenocarcinoma of the lung. *Cancer Res.*, 55 (3), 472-473

Taioli, E., Trachman, J., Chen, X., Toniolo, P. & Garte, S.J. (1995b) A CYP1A1 restriction fragment length polymorphism is associated with breast cancer in African-American women. *Cancer Res.*, 55, 3757-3758

Tefre, T., Daly, A.K., Armstrong, M., Leathart, J.B.S., Idle, J.R., Brogger, A. & Borresen, A.L. (1994) Genotyping of the CYP2D6 gene in Norwegian lung cancer patients and controls. *Pharmacogenetics*, 4, 47-57

Tefre, T., Ryberg, D., Haugen, A., Nebert, D.W., Skaug, V., Brogger, A. & Borresen, A.L. (1991) Human CYP1A1 (cytochrome P_1450) gene: lack of association between the Msp I restriction fragment length polymorphism and incidence of lung cancer in a Norwegian population. *Pharmacogenetics*, 1 (1), 20-25

To-Figueras, J., Gene, M., Gomez-Catalan, J., Galan, C., Firvida, J., Fuentes, M., Rodamilans, M., Huguet, E., Estape, J. & Corbella, J. (1996) Glutathione S-transferase M1 and codon 72 p53 polymorphisms in a northwestern Mediterranean population and their relation to lung cancer susceptibility. *Cancer Epidemiol. Biomarkers Prev.*, 5, 337-342

Topinka, J., Binkova, B., Mrackova, G., Stavkova, Z., Benes, I., Dejmek, J., Lenicek, J. & Sram, R.J. (1997) DNA adducts in human placenta as related to air pollution and to GSTM1 genotype. *Mutat. Res.*, 390, 59-68

Trell, E., Korsgaard, R., Hood, B., Kitzing, P., Norden, G. & Simonsson, B.G. (1976) Aryl hydrocarbon hydroxylase inducibility and laryngeal carcinomas. *The Lancet*, 2, 140

Trizna, Z., Clayman, G.L., Spitz, M.R., Briggs, K.L. & Goepfert, H. (1995) Glutathione S-transferase genotypes as risk factors for head and neck cancer. *Am. J. Surg.*, 170, 499-501

Uematsu, F., Ikawa, S., Kikuchi, H., Sagami, I., Kanamaru, R., Abe,T., Satoh, K., Motomiya, M. & Watanabe, M. (1994) Restriction fragment length polymorphism of the human CYP2E1 (cytochrome P450IIE1) gene and susceptibility to lung cancer: possible relevance to low smoking exposure. *Pharmacogenetics*, 4, 58-63

Uuskula, M., Jarventaus, H., Hirvonen, A., Sorsa, M. & Norppa, H. (1995) Influence of GSTM1 genotype on sister chromatid exchange induction by styrene-7,8-oxide and 1,2-epoxy-3-butene in cultured human lymphocytes. *Carcinogenesis*, 16 (4), 947-950

Van Poppel, G., De Vogel, N., Van Balderen, P.J. & Kok, F.J. (1992) Increased cytogenetic damage in smokers deficient in glutathione S-transferase isozyme μ. *Carcinogenesis*, 13 (2), 303-305

Van Poppel, G., Verhagen, H., Van't Veer, P. & Van Bladeren, P.J. (1993) Markers for cytogenetic damage in smokers: associations with plasma antioxidants and glutathione S-transferase μ. *Cancer Epidemiol. Biomarkers Prev.*, 2, 441-447

Vatsis, K.P. & Weber, W.W. (1993) Structural heterogeneity of Caucasian N-acetyltransferase at the NAT1 gene locus. *Arch. Biochem. Biophys*, 301, 71-76

Vineis, P., Bartsch, H., Caporaso, N., Harrington, A.M., Kadlubar, F.F., Landi, M.T., Malaveille, C., Shields, P.G., Skipper, P., Talaska, G. & Tannenbaum, S.R. (1994) Genetically based N-acetyltransferase metabolic polymorphism and low-level enviromental exposure to carcinogens. *Nature*, 369, 154-156

Vineis, P., Caporaso, N., Tannenbaum, S.R., Skipper, P.L., Glogowski, J., Bartsch, H., Coda, M., Talaska, G. & Kadlubar, F. (1990) Acetylation phenotype, carcinogen-hemoglobin adducts, and cigarette smoking. *Cancer Res.*, 50, 3002-3004

Wang, Y., Ichiba, M., Oishi, H., Iyadomi, M., Shono, N. & Tomokuni, K. (1997) Relationship between plasma concentrations of β-carotene and α-tocopherol and lifestyle factors and levels of DNA adducts in lymphocytes. *Nutr. Cancer*, 27 (1), 69-73

Ward, E., Paigen, B., Steenland, K., Vincent, R., Minowada, J., Gurtoo, H.L., Sartori, P. & Havens, M.B. (1978) Aryl hydrocarbon hydroxylase in persons with lung or laryngeal cancer. *Int. J. Cancer*, 22, 384-389

Warholm, M., Guthenberg, C., Mannervik, B. & von Bahr, C. (1981) Purification of a new glutathione S-transferase (transferase μ) from human liver having high activity with benzo(a)pyrene-4,5-oxide. *Biochem. Biophys. Res. Commun.*, 98, 512-519

Warwick, A.P., Redman, C.W.E., Jones, P.W., Fryer, A.A., Gilford, J., Alldersea, J. & Strange, R.C. (1994a) Progression of cervical intraepithelial neoplasia to cervical cancer: interactions of cytochrome P450 CYP2D6 EM and glutathione S-transferase GSTM1 null genotypes and cigarette smoking. *Br. J. Cancer*, 70, 704-708

Warwick, A.P., Sarhanis, P., Redman, C., Pemble, S., Taylor, J.B., Ketterer, B., Jones, P., Alldersea, J., Gilford, J., Yengi, L., Fryer, A.A. & Strange, R.C. (1994b) Theta class glutathione S-transferase GSTT1 genotypes and susceptibility to cervical neoplasia: interactions with GSTM1, CYP2D6 and smoking. *Carcinogenesis*, 15 (12), 2841-2845

Watanabe, J., Yang, J., Eguchi, H., Hayashi, S., Imai, K., Nakachi, K. & Kawajiri, K. (1995) An Rsa I polymorphism in the CYP2E1 gene does not affect lung cancer risk in a Japanese population. *Jpn. J. Cancer Res.*, 86, 245-248

Webster, D.J.T., Flook, D., Jenkins, J., Hutchings, A. & Routledge, P.A. (1989) Drug acetylation in breast cancer. *Br. J. Cancer*, 60, 236-237

Weston, A., Caporaso, N.E., Taghizadeh, K., Hoover, R.N., Tannenbaum, S.R., Skipper, P..L., Resau, J.H., Trump, B.F. & Harris, C.C. (1991) Measurement of 4-aminobiphenyl-haemoglobin adducts in lung cancer cases and controls. *Cancer Res.*, 51, 5219-5223

Wiencke, J.K., Kelsey, K.T., Lamela, R.A. & Toscano, W.A. (1990) Human glutathione S-transferase deficiency as a marker of susceptibility to epoxide-induced cytogenetic damage. *Cancer Res.*, 50, 1585-1590

Wiencke, J.K., Pemble, S., Ketterer, B. & Kelsey, K.T. (1995) Gene deletion of glutathione S-transferase θ: correlation with induced genetic damage and potential role in endogenous mutagenesis. *Cancer Epidemiol. Biomarkers Prev.*, 4, 253-259

Wohlleb, J.C., Hunter, C.F., Blass, B., Kadlubar, F.F., Chu, D.Z.J. & Lang, N.P. (1990) Aromatic amines acetyltransferase as a marker for colorectal cancer: environmental and demographic associations. *Int. J. Cancer*, 46, 22-30

Wolf, C.R. (1986) Cytocrome P450s: a multigene family involved in carcinogen metabolism. *Trend Genet.*, 2, 209-214

Wolf, C.R., Dale Smith, C.A., Gough, A.C., Moss, J.E., Vallis, K.A., Howard, G., Carey, F.J., Mills, K., McNee, W., Carmichael, J. & Spurr, N.K. (1992) Relationship between the debrisoquine hydroxylase polymorphism and cancer susceptibility. *Carcinogenesis*, 13 (6) 1035-1038

Woodhouse, K.W., Adams, P.C., Clothier, A., Mucklow, J.C. & Rawlins, M.D. (1982) N-acetylation phenotype in bladder cancer. *Hum. Toxicol.*, 1, 443-445

Wrigley, E.C., McGown, A.T., Buckley, H., Hall, A. & Crowther, D. (1996) Glutathione S-transferase activity and isoenzyme levels measured by two methods in ovarian cancer, and their value as markers of disease outcome. *Br. J. Cancer*, 73, 763-769

Wu, X., Shi, H., Kemp, B., Jang, H., Kemp, B., Hong, W.K., Delclos, G.L. & Spitz, M.R. (1997) Associations between cytochrome P4502E1 genotype, mutagen sensitivity, cigarette smoking and susceptibility to lung cancer. *Carcinogenesis*, 18 (5), 967-973

Wundrack, I., Meese, E., Mullenbach, R. & Blin, N. (1994) Debrisoquine hydroxylase gene polymorphism in meningioma. *Acta Neuropathol.*, 88, 472-474

Xu, X., Kelsey, K.T., Wiencke, J.K., Wain, J.C. & Christiani, D.C. (1996) Cytochrome P450 CYP1A1 MspI polymorphism and lung cancer susceptibility. *Cancer Epidemiol. Biomarkers Prev.*, 5, 687-692

Yengi, L., Inskip, A., Gilford, J., Alldersea, J., Bailey, L., Smith, A., Lear, J.T., Heagerty, A.H., Bowers, B., Hand, P., Hayes, J.D., Jones, P.W., Strange, R.C. & Fryer, A.A. (1996) Polymorphism at the glutathione S-transferase locus GSTM3: interactions with cytochrome P450 and glutathione S-transferase genotypes as risk factors for multiple cutaneous basal cell carcinoma. *Cancer Res.*, 56, 1974-1977

Yoshikawa, M., Arashidani, K., Kawamoto, T. & Kodama, Y. (1994) Aryl hydrocarbon hydroxylase activity in human lung tissue: in relation to cigarette smoking and lung cancer. *Environ. Res.*, 65 (1), 1-11

Yu, M.C., Ross, R.K., Chan, K.K., Henderson, B.E., Skipper, P.L., Tannenbaum, S.R. & Coetzee, G.A. (1995a) Glutathione S-transferase M1 genotype affects aminobiphenyl-haemoglobin adduct levels in white, black, and Asian smokers and non-smokers. *Cancer Epidemiol. Biomarkers Prev.*, 4 (8), 861-864

Yu, M.W., Gladek-Yarborough, A., Chiamprasert, S, Santella, R.M., Liaw, Y.F. & Chen, C.J. (1995b) Cytochrome P450 2E1 and glutathione S-transferase M1 polymorphisms and susceptibility to hepatocellular carcinoma. *Gastroenterol.*, 109, 1266-1273

Yu, M.C., Skipper, P.L., Taghizadeh, K., Tannenbaum, S.R., Chan, K.K., Henderson, B.E. & Ross, R.K. (1991) Acetylator phenotype, amino-biphenyl-haemoglobin adduct levels, and bladder cancer risk in white, black, and Asian men in Los Angeles, California. *J. Natl. Cancer Inst.*, 86 (9), 712-716

Zhong, S., Howie, A.F., Ketterer, B., Taylor, J., Hayes, J.D., Beckett, G.J., Wathen, C.G., Wolf, C.R. & Spurr, N.K. (1991) Glutathione transferase mu locus: use of genotyping and phenotyping assays to assess association with lung cancer susceptibility. *Carcinogenesis*, 12 (9), 1533-1537

Zhong, S., Wyllie, A.H., Barnes, D., Wolf, C.R. & Spurr, N.K. (1993) Relationship between the GSTM1 genetic polymorphism and susceptibility to bladder, breast and colon cancer. *Carcinogenesis*, 14 (9), 1821-1824

Corresponding author
Angelo d'Errico
Regional Environmental Protection Agency,
Turin, Italy

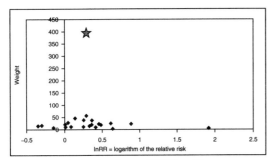

Plot 1. Funnel plot of studies on GSTM1 and lung cancer

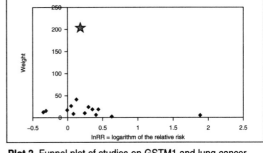

Plot 2. Funnel plot of studies on GSTM1 and lung cancer – Caucasians

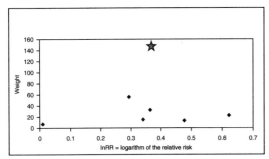

Plot 3. Funnel plot of studies on GSTM1 and lung cancer – Asians

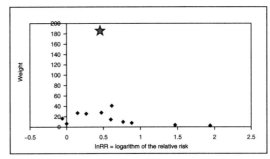

Plot 4. Funnel plot of studies on GSTM1 and bladder cancer

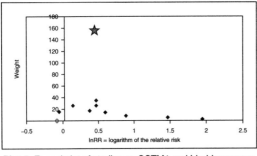

Plot 5. Funnel plot of studies on GSTM1 and bladder cancer – Caucasians

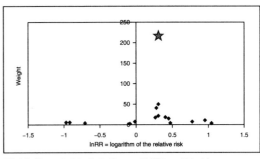

Plot 6. Funnel plot of studies on NAT2 and bladder cancer

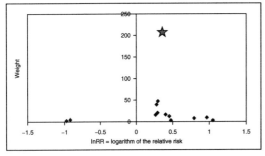

Plot 7. Funnel plot of studies on NAT2 and bladder cancer – Caucasians

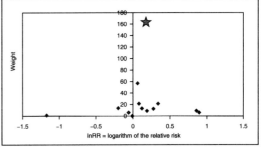

Plot 8. Funnel plot of studies on NAT2 and colorectal cancer

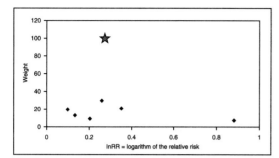

Plot 9. Funnel plot of studies on NAT2 and colorectal cancer – Caucasians

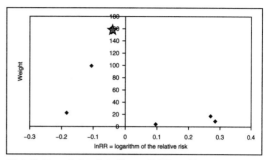

Plot 10. Funnel plot of studies on NAT2 and lung cancer

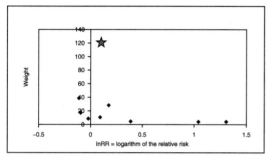

Plot 11. Funnel plot of studies on NAT2 and breast cancer

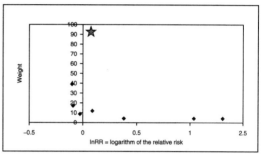

Plot 12. Funnel plot of studies on NAT2 and breast cancer – Caucasians

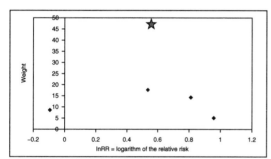

Plot 13. Funnel plot of studies on CYP1A1 MspI and lung cancer – Asians

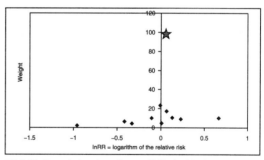

Plot 14. Funnel plot of studies on CYP1A1 MspI and lung cancer – Caucasians

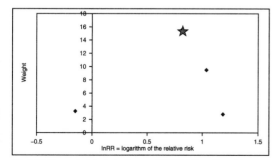

Plot 15. Funnel plot of studies on CYP1A1 Exon7 and lung cancer – Asians

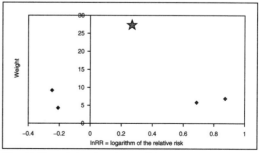

Plot 16. Funnel plot of studies on CYP1A1 Exon7 and lung cancer – Caucasians

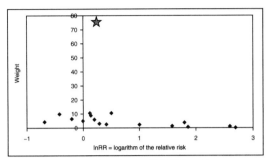

Plot 17. Funnel plot of studies on CYP2D6 and lung cancer

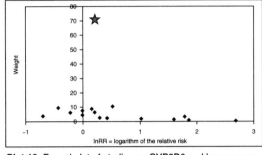

Plot 18. Funnel plot of studies on CYP2D6 and lung cancer – Caucasians

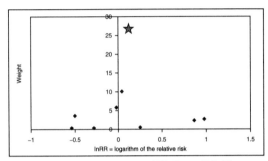

Plot 19. Funnel plot of studies on CYP2D6 and bladder cancer

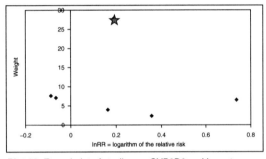

Plot 20. Funnel plot of studies on CYP2D6 and breast cancer

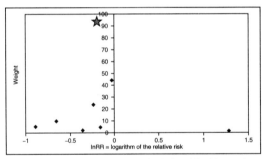

Plot 21. Funnel plot of studies on CYP2E1 5'-flanking region and lung cancer

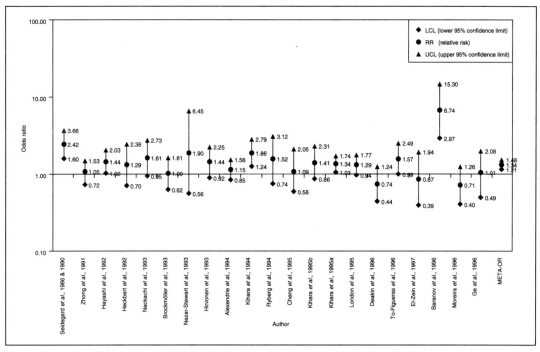

Graph 1. Meta-analysis of studies on GSTM1 polymorphism and lung cancer

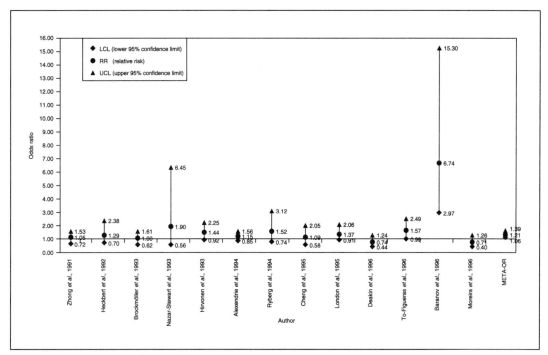

Graph 2. Meta-analysis of studies on GSTM1 polymorphism and lung cancer – Caucasians

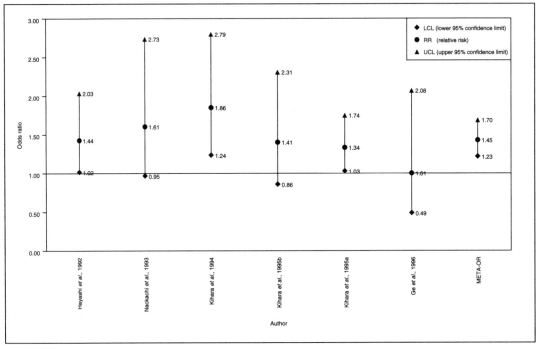

Graph 3. Meta-analysis of studies on GSTM1 polymorphism and lung cancer – Asians

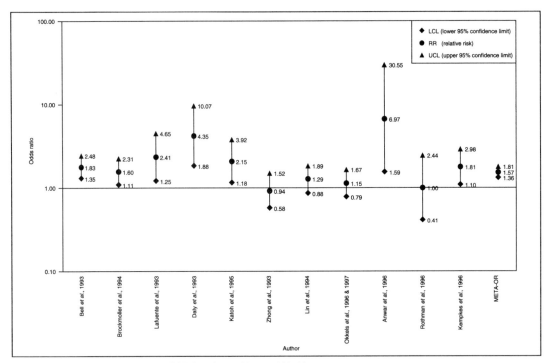

Graph 4. Meta-analysis of studies on GSTM1 polymorphism and bladder cancer

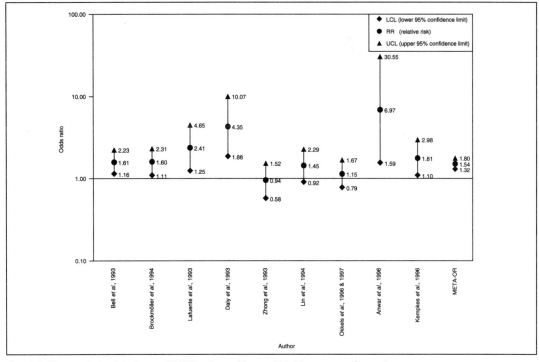

Graph 5. Meta-analysis of studies on GSTM1 polymorphism and bladder cancer – Caucasians

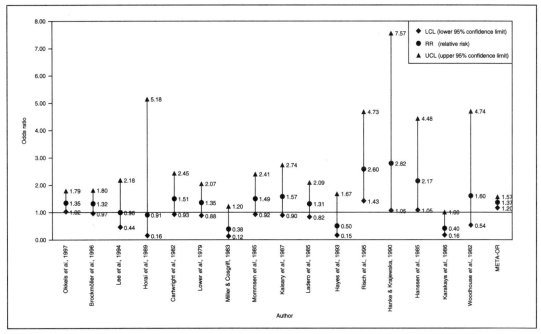

Graph 6. Meta-analysis of studies on NAT2 polymorphism and bladder cancer

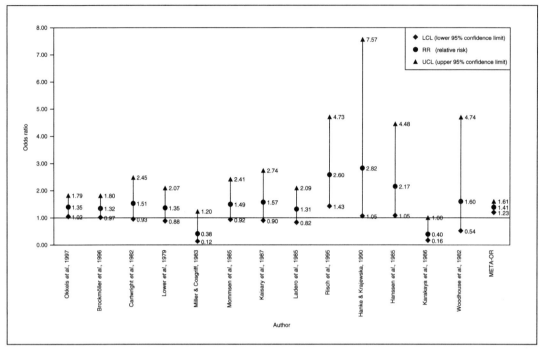

Graph 7. Meta-analysis of studies on NAT2 polymorphism and bladder cancer – Caucasians

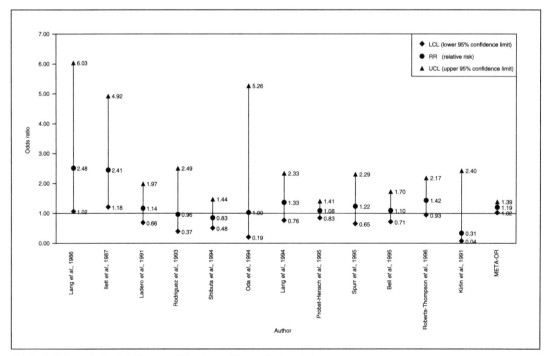

Graph 8. Meta-analysis of studies on NAT2 polymorphism and colorectal cancer

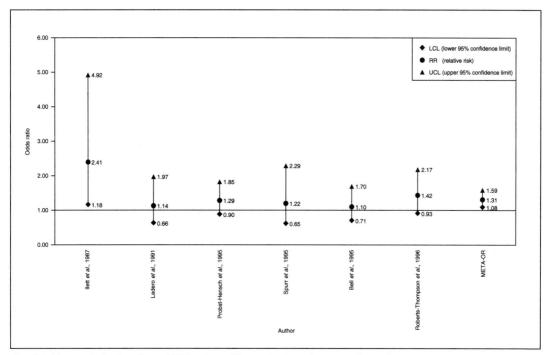

Graph 9. Meta-analysis of studies on NAT2 polymorphism and colorectal cancer – Caucasians

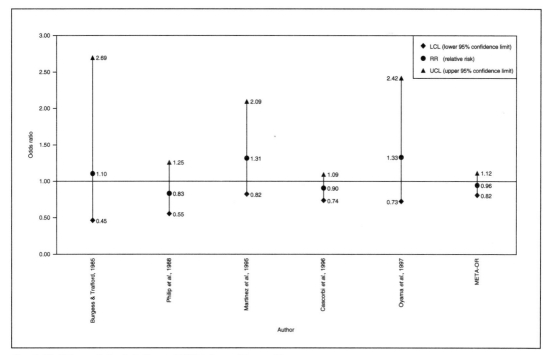

Graph 10. Meta-analysis of studies on NAT2 polymorphism and lung cancer

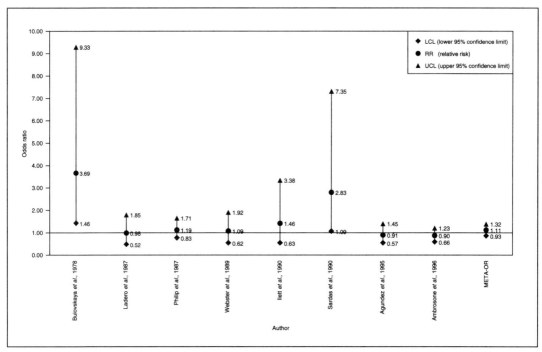

Graph 11. Meta-analysis of studies on NAT2 polymorphism and breast cancer

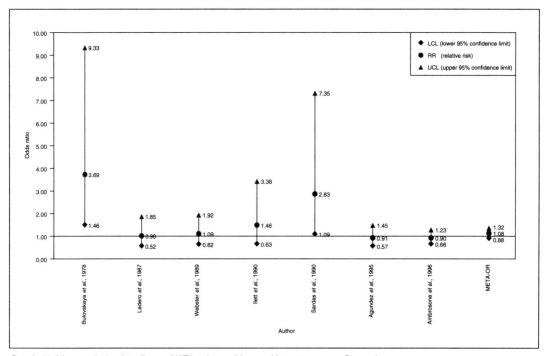

Graph 12. Meta-analysis of studies on NAT2 polymorphism and breast cancer – Caucasians

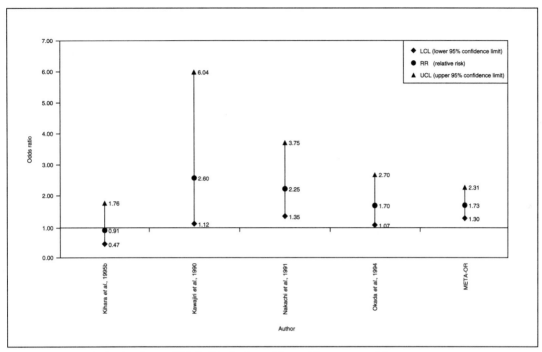

Graph 13. Meta-analysis of studies on CYP1A1 Msp I polymorphism and lung cancer – Asians

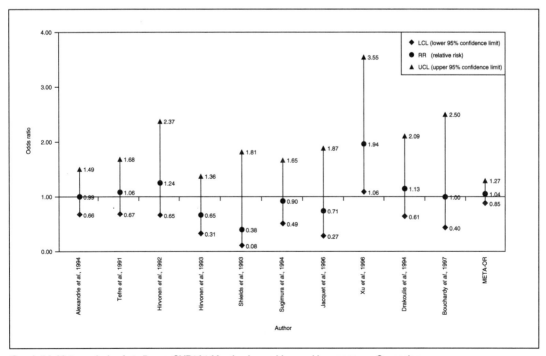

Graph 14. Meta-analysis of studies on CYP1A1 Msp I polymorphism and lung cancer – Caucasians

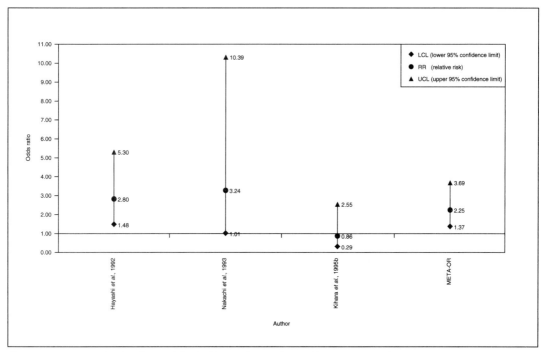

Graph 15. Meta-analysis of studies on CYP1A1 Exon7 polymorphism and lung cancer – Asians

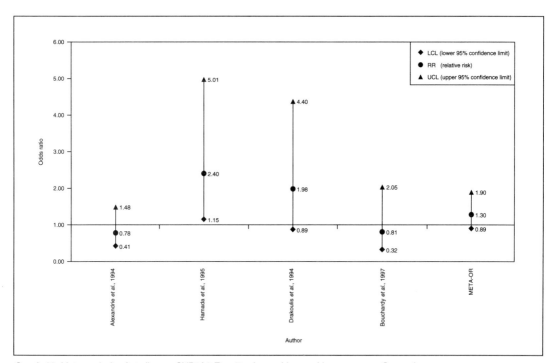

Graph 16. Meta-analysis of studies on CYP1A1 Exon7 polymorphism and lung cancer – Caucasians

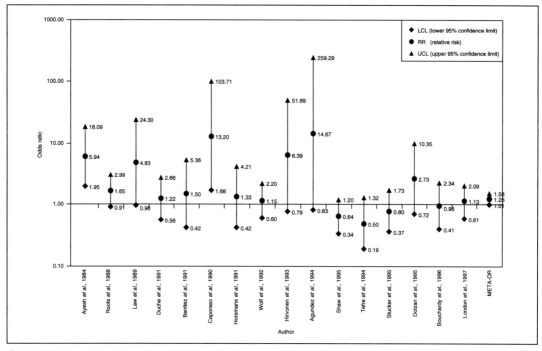

Graph 17. Meta-analysis of studies on CYP2D6 polymorphism and lung cancer

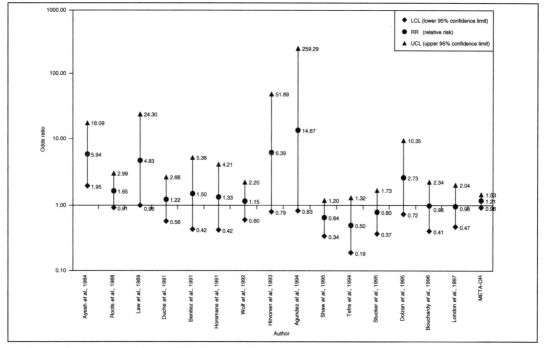

Graph 18. Meta-analysis of studies on CYP2D6 polymorphism and lung cancer – Caucasians

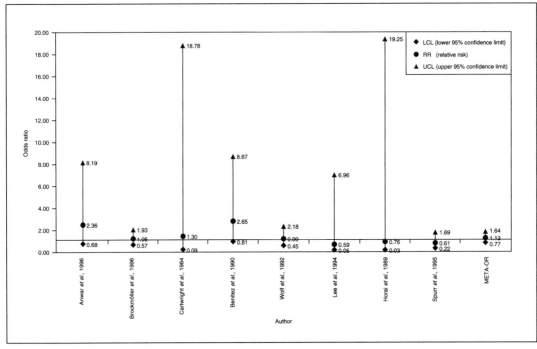

Graph 19. Meta-analysis of studies on CYP2D6 polymorphism and bladder cancer

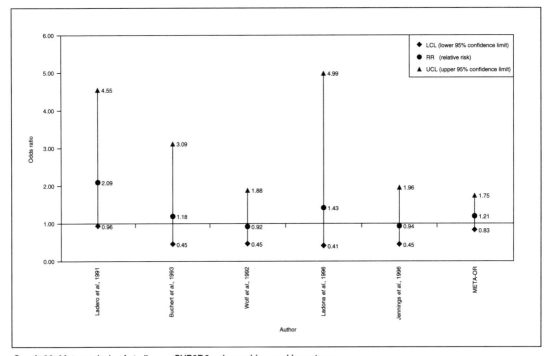

Graph 20. Meta-analysis of studies on CYP2D6 polymorphism and breast cancer

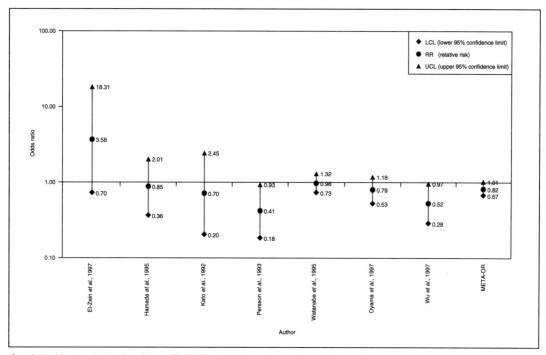

Graph 21. Meta-analysis of studies on CYP2E1 5'-flanking region polymorphism and lung cancer

Metabolic Polymorphisms and Susceptibility to Cancer
W. Ryder
IARC Scientific Publications No. 148
International Agency for Research on Cancer, Lyon, 1999

Chapter 24. Genetic analysis of metabolic polymorphisms in molecular epidemiological studies: social and ethical implications

Pierre Hainaut and Kirsi Vähäkangas

The use of genetic biomarkers in epidemiological studies raises specific social and ethical issues related to the selection of molecular markers and methods of analysis, obtaining participation, the storage of biological samples and their linkage with individual data, the disclosure of information and the publication of results. Several of these issues are similar to those associated with the use of any type of biomarker in epidemiology. Other problems are specifically related to the use of genetic material and the perception that genetic information raises special concerns regarding privacy, risk of abuse and psychosocial impact. In this Chapter we define how genetic studies performed in the context of molecular epidemiological studies (genetic analysis) differ from genetic screening or genetic testing conducted in a clinical or public health context. We then examine the ethical implications of this distinction and describe how general ethical principles may apply to genetic analysis in the area of molecular epidemiology. In particular we discuss specific questions such as those of obtaining participation, working with archival samples and communicating results. We advocate an approach whereby ethical issues are tackled as an intrinsic part of study design; this requires broad discussion with all the parties involved.

Molecular epidemiological research involves the collection, storage and use of individual biological samples and of data on individuals and communities on a large scale. In this context, ethical conflicts often arise between the potential benefits of research and the risks it entails for individuals and communities. The International Ethical Guidelines for Biomedical Research Involving Human Subjects state that three ethical principles are essential, namely respect for persons, beneficence and justice. How these ethical principles should be upheld in biomedical research involving human subjects is described in the World Medical Association Declaration of Helsinki (CIOMS, 1993).

The identification of ethical conflicts is not always easy and requires increased awareness within society as well as among scientists (Goodman & Prineas, 1996). We describe below some of the social and ethical issues that may arise in the course of molecular epidemiological studies involving genetic analysis of metabolic

polymorphisms, and we discuss their practical implications. These issues relate to the specific status of genetic analysis in epidemiology, the design of studies, the stringency and reliability of methods for genetic analysis, the need to inform all parties involved in studies, obtaining consent from individual subjects, the use of archival tissue specimens, the communication of results and the respect of privacy and confidentiality. Many of these questions have been considered by Schulte (1992), Smith & Suk (1994), Pereira & Whyatt (1994), Vineis & Schulte (1995), Clayton et al. (1995) and Schulte et al. (1997).

Specificity of genetic analysis in molecular epidemiology

Molecular epidemiology is based on the use of molecular methods for assessing internal exposure, individual susceptibility and early disease (Harris, 1996). The analysis of metabolic polymorphisms and other genetic biomarkers in molecular epidemiology requires individual biologi-

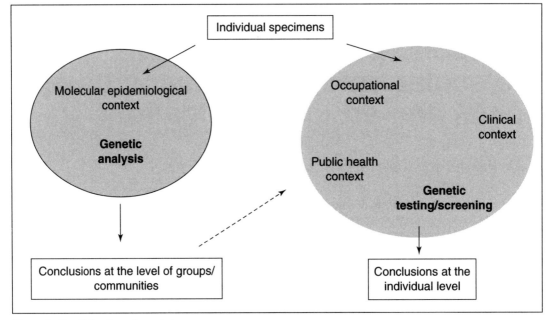

Figure 1. Specificity of genetic analysis.

Genetic analysis is carried out in the context of molecular epidemiological studies. Individual samples are used but the conclusions are drawn at the level of groups and populations. In this respect, genetic analysis differs from genetic screening and testing. The latter are conducted in clinical, occupational and public health contexts and are aimed at drawing conclusions at the individual level. However, the conclusions from molecular epidemiological studies involving genetic analysis can lead to genetic testing or screening in appropriate contexts. Ethical requirements for these two types of genetic assessment are different (see text).

cal samples for the extraction and analysis of genetic material. The use of genetic material in studies involving any kind of genetic screening or testing generates concerns in the public mind with regard to privacy, risk of abuse and psychosocial impact (Wald, 1996). These concerns are legitimate, although they may be reinforced by the misconception that genetic information has more value than information from other sources such as questionnaires or biological monitoring.

The degree of risk and the significance of the type of genetic analysis which is carried out in molecular epidemiological studies need to be clearly identified (Fig. 1). Firstly, it has to be realized that most molecular epidemiological approaches are still at a developmental stage and that their significance and relevance remain ambiguous. More epidemiological and mechanistic research is necessary in order to reduce this ambiguity. Secondly, although they are based on individual data, molecular epidemiological stud-

ies are aimed at drawing conclusions at the level of groups or communities. In many cases the results of molecular epidemiological analysis do not carry a clear and unambiguous significance at the individual level. In studies of individual susceptibility, genetic factors such as metabolic polymorphisms may at best represent only one of the many factors that influence susceptibility. Other factors, such as exposure, lifestyle and medical condition, can minimize or maximize the degree of risk.

A distinction can be made between genetic assessment within the context of molecular epidemiology and genetic screening and testing, which are carried out in clinical or occupational settings and may carry much greater significance for the individual tested. To clarify this matter we recommend the use of the term "genetic analysis" (rather than genetic screening or genetic testing) to describe the type of genetic assessment conducted in the context of molecular epidemiology.

This underlines that genetic analysis raises ethical issues that are distinct from those of genetic screening or genetic testing, but does not imply that lower ethical standards should apply to genetic analysis. Indeed, genetic analysis may raise ethical issues that are not essential in genetic screening or testing. For example, the results of genetic analysis may affect not only individuals but also the groups and communities to which the study subjects belong (see, for example, Goldgar & Reilly, 1995). Studies investigating ethnic, cultural or social groups may be perceived as exposing these groups to kinds of harm and injustice such as stigmatization, blame or discrimination. In addition, it has to be kept in mind that molecular epidemiological studies may lead to the development of interventions involving genetic testing or screening in a clinical, occupational or public health context.

Ethical questions in genetic analysis
Study design
The first ethical question that arises when planning a study involving genetic analysis is whether and how genetic markers should be included. A single polymorphic gene is seldom significant and multiple polymorphisms often have to be analysed. The resources, manpower and time required for such analysis should be carefully considered. For example, the cost of analysing one tissue specimen for a genetic polymorphism by a methodology based on PCR and restriction digestion may be US$ 100-200 (including manpower, equipment and consumables for all steps of the procedure). Commercial companies commonly charge US$ 50-80 for sequence analysis of a single purified DNA fragment. The emergence of new technologies (such as microchip-based assays) is expected to significantly decrease the cost of such analyses. However, failure to realize the material implications of the study may lead to unethical situations, such as the collection and storage of tissue specimens that may never be analysed because of excessive demands on manpower and resources.

The analysis of multiple genes often requires the cooperation of several laboratories. This raises additional problems in relation to the storage and processing of specimens as well as to the confidentiality of individual data. The setting up of integrated, multidisciplinary consortiums may help to facilitate cooperation and exchange between research teams, to coordinate the efforts of individual groups and to limit the number of tissue specimens needed for a particular study.

Stringency and reliability of methods
Most methods for genetic analysis are still at a preliminary stage of development. A methodology that works in the laboratory may not have sufficient power and reliability in a molecular epidemiological study. Mistakes or inconsistencies at this level may result in important samples being lost or wasted.

Many common methods for genetic analysis are based on the polymerase chain reaction (PCR). In this method, multiple copies of a DNA fragment are enzymatically generated *in vitro*. When performed under appropriate conditions, PCR is powerful and specific but it is at best semiquantitative and is prone to errors through contamination by foreign DNA or polymerase errors. The risk of contamination is particularly high in laboratories where large numbers of samples are analysed for the same region of DNA, as it is the case in molecular epidemiological studies. It is therefore essential that extraction of DNA from tissue specimens, assembly of the PCR reaction, and running the PCR reaction should be carried out in physically separated locations, and that controls should be run in each set of PCR reactions. In addition, it is absolutely necessary to confirm results by repeating analyses with independent PCR reactions.

Talking to everyone involved
Studies in molecular epidemiology often involve multidisciplinary research groups, only a few members of which have contact with the study subjects. Nevertheless, all the personnel involved, including laboratory scientists, technicians and statisticians, are ethically responsible. Before starting a study the main investigator has the responsibility of ensuring that all staff members are aware of the objectives and the potential risks and benefits for all participants.

In molecular epidemiology, individuals are studied as members of communities or groups (e.g. social, cultural or ethnic communities, or groups of individuals defined by specific dietary habits or lifestyles). Investigators have to take care that the study respects the cultural values and social codes of conduct of the communities or groups they investigate. The potential impact of the study on these groups and communities should be taken into account. Before starting a study it is important to consider the need to inform the groups and communities involved and the possibility that the results may create harm for other members of these groups and communities (e.g. groups of workers and their representatives in a study involving occupational risk factors). This requires contact with the communities and their representatives in order to explain and answer questions before starting the study, as well as dialogue throughout the study. The interests of the groups and communities should also be considered with regard to the disclosure of results (Schulte & Singall, 1996).

Obtaining participation

How individuals are recruited and involved as study subjects has serious ethical and social implications (Schulte *et al.*, 1997). The central problem relates to how the individual is informed and what is his or her degree of awareness of the implications of agreeing to participate. There is now overall agreement that informed consent is required for all genetic research using linkable samples (that is, samples that can be traced back to one particular individual), unless some strict conditions for limitation or "waiver" are met.

The nature of informed consent and how specific it should be is still a grey area. Obtaining consent is a complex process that is initiated when contacts are made with prospective subjects and continued by the communication of specific, individual information, by repetition and explanation, and by answering the subjects' questions (CIOMS, 1993). The establishment of the actual document of informed consent is a critical step in this process. The form and language of this document should be adapted to each particular situation. It is the responsibility of the investigator to ensure that the prospective subject has adequately understood all the implications of consent.

In practice this implies that both written information and discussion sessions are arranged, the latter providing opportunities for prospective participants to ask questions. Signing the informed consent should be done separately from this process and should not happen during the initial contacts. A few basic rules apply to informed consent (CIOMS, 1993). First, the aim of the study has to be defined and stated with as much precision as possible, and the information given should be understood by prospective participants. It should be concise and accurate, and unnecessary technical details should be avoided. A single consent may be requested in respect of the analysis of several distinct genes (such as several different polymorphic metabolic genes). However, asking for a generic consent (e.g. to "provide tissue for research") that would allow the same biological samples to be used for other, unrelated genetic studies, should be considered with extreme caution. Second, the potential risks and benefits should be explained in detail, particularly the physical risks associated with sample collection. Third, the policy for communicating the results of the test and/or study should be clearly described, and possible implications for the participant should be fully explained. It is essential that the individual should not be directly or indirectly coerced to participate. Giving false expectations on the outcome of the analysis has to be seen as a form of coercion. It is not ethically acceptable for refusal to participate to have adverse consequences on the medical care or the employment of the individuals concerned. Finally, giving informed consent is not a final and definitive agreement, and participants should be free to withdraw at any stage, irrespective of the consequences for the research programme.

There is no agreement on the conditions under which the requirement to obtain informed consent can be waived. Informed consent may not be required in the case of anonymous tissue specimens (Clayton *et al.*, 1995). This means that samples should be unidentifiable by investigators and anyone else, and this implies the irreversible destruction of individual identifiers. However, it has to be stressed that destroying links may also be seen as unethical, since this may result in the loss of potentially important information.

Working with archival biological samples

Obtaining consent can be particularly complicated in studies using archival samples. The individual who is the source of the sample may be very difficult to trace or may have died, and obtaining consent may be physically impossible. Archival samples (such as, for example, pathology collections) are a well-characterized source of biological material that is relatively simple to use. However, it is important to note that the use of archival samples raises a number of ethical issues concerning, for instance, the right of ownership of the tissues, the criteria for storage, and the right of access to the samples (Clayton *et al.*, 1995; Marshall *et al.*, 1996).

A distinction can be made between specimens that have already been collected for other purposes and specimens that are to be collected in the future. The first case includes specimens from pathology collections which can be particularly useful in many studies, as they have already been characterized for a number of biological end points and may therefore yield informative results with no additional risk of collection for the source individuals. In such cases, asking retrospective consent is often very difficult.

We believe that it is ethical to use such specimens for genetic analysis of metabolic polymorphisms, provided that a number of conditions are met. First, the design of the study has to be reviewed by institutional ethical review committees, and the decision to grant a "waiver" on the requirement for informed consent has to be taken by these committees on a case-by-case basis (Levine, 1996). Second, strict rules of confidentiality should be applied. For example, it is not ethical to provide all investigators with copies of pathology protocols carrying names or identifiers, such as social security numbers; this information should be kept strictly confidential. Third, the study design should include a clear description of whether and how results of the analysis would be communicated, especially in the case of individuals whose results are at the extreme of the distribution of the test in question.

In the case of samples to be collected in the future, the strictest rules for obtaining informed consent should apply. Tissue specimens should not be kept for analyses other than those described in the informed consent. Unless consent has been specifically given the specimens should not be kept after completion of the study. Specimens should be either destroyed or made anonymous by irreversibly removing all individual identifiers.

Communication of results

The release of results has several ethical implications (Schulte & Singall, 1996). In communicating results, investigators performing molecular epidemiology work should consider themselves as health professionals. As such, they have an ethical obligation to release information that is in the public interest (CIOMS, 1993).

First of all, communication of the results may affect the individuals who are involved as subjects of study. The strategy for communication with these persons should be carefully planned and discussed with them prior to the study. In many instances, individuals may wish to be regarded as collaborators rather than subjects and may wish to be informed of their individual results (Clayton *et al.*, 1995). However, particularly in translational studies it may be considered as ethical not to disclose this information as it seldom carries any significance at the individual level. The study design should also clearly state how individuals whose results are at the extreme of the distribution of the analysis are to be managed, since in such cases it may be necessary to repeat the analysis, tissue sampling or clinical evaluation of the subject (Schulte *et al.*, 1997). Although it is not possible to establish any definitive guidelines on these matters, an essential principle should be that obtaining a tissue specimen entails a responsibility of the researcher towards the individual who is the source of the specimen. As a part of this responsibility, scientists have to provide information as well as material and/or psychosocial assistance to help the individual to cope with the implications of the analysis.

The need to inform the communities and groups to which the subjects belong should also be considered, especially in studies where the results have the potential to stimulate changes in individual or social behaviour, occupational practice, lifestyle or dietary habits. Investigators have an ethical duty to anticipate these changes and to present their results so as to avoid misrepresentation or misinterpretation of the data.

Finally, the publication and communication of the results in the scientific community also have ethical implications. Authors should keep in mind that the way they report their results will affect the design of further studies and that the information they release in the scientific community should meet the highest possible standards. The IARC database of p53 mutations in human cancers is particularly significant in this respect. Mutations in p53 may be interpreted as "fingerprints" of carcinogens and thus represent an important source of information on carcinogenic exposure. The database rests exclusively on material reported in the peer-reviewed literature (Hainaut et al., 1997). It consistently happens that about 20% of the published reports contain mistakes, ranging from simple misprints to gross errors relating, for instance, to non-existent codons or errors in the selection of the reading frame. Many publications also have to be left out of the database as they contain incomplete or ambiguous reports. As a result, important data are misinterpreted. It is an ethical responsibility of authors, reviewers and editors to ensure that published data on molecular epidemiology meet the highest standards.

Confidentiality and privacy

During and after any study involving genetic analysis it is essential that all individual data are kept strictly confidential and that the study does not threaten privacy (Gold, 1996). This requires the adoption of safe coding systems for all information collected and in particular for tissue specimens. It is common practice to store such information in computers, yet they cannot be considered as safe places for keeping linkable individual information. We recommend that the key to each code should be kept in a physically closed area under the responsibility of the principal investigator, who is also required to keep this information confidential even after the completion of the study and publication of the results. This may be particularly difficult if the principal investigator is moving to another position and has to leave behind files containing linkable individual information. In some cases, ethical review boards may recommend that this information be destroyed after the completion of a study. In all circumstances the study design should clearly indicate who is responsible for keeping the individual records and how long these should be retained.

There is a risk that results from genetic analysis may be requested by third parties and used as a basis for discrimination against susceptible individuals, for example in connection with access to

work or insurance (Masood, 1996; Vineis et al., 1995). We believe it unethical to use the results of genetic analysis in molecular epidemiology in any other context than that of scientific research. By definition, the results of such genetic analysis represent an assessment of an individual's character as a member of a group or community and thus carry little significance at the individual level (Fig.1). Using this information for discrimination or "adverse selection" should be legally prohibited. For example, participation in a molecular epidemiological study should not be classified as "genetic testing" with respect to registration with insurance companies or applications for jobs.

Conclusions and perspectives

Ethical conflicts arise against a background of profound scientific and societal change, and there is great uncertainty as to how they should be resolved. The solutions are not exclusively a matter for legislation and regulation, and will always involve making difficult individual and collective choices.

We have tried to show that solving ethical problems has very practical, material implications, and is not only a question of principles. Some of the implications are directly relevant to good scientific practice. We believe it important to fight the misconception that concern for ethics may restrict scientific autonomy and freedom: ethical research is good quality research. In this respect, resolving ethical conflicts is also a matter of methodology. An ethical approach to conflict resolution involves broad discussion with all the parties involved, awareness of the ideas and attitudes of others, systematic analysis of the sources of conflict, and adoption of specific solutions adapted to each particular situation. However, such an ethical approach is time-consuming and entails additional costs, in particular for the information and recruitment of prospective study subjects and for the organization of proper procedures for the storage of specimens. We think that these costs should be clearly identified when a study is being planned and that they should be identified in grant applications. This would help to increase awareness of these issues among both scientists and scientific policy-makers.

The lack of public awareness for scientific issues has a dramatic influence on many ethical issues.

Scientific education and the dissemination of information among the general public on scientific matters is now becoming a major ethical challenge. There is an urgent need for a new "contract" between the scientific community and the public, based on a commitment to inform in simple but accurate terms, to demonstrate respect for persons and communities, to promote justice and to protect those who are most vulnerable. Several recent widely publicized events have reinforced the public perception of the scientific community as being secretive and insensitive. This is a major source of misunderstanding that could greatly hinder the achievement of the goals of biomedical research.

Acknowledgements

This paper is partly based on the final discussion and conclusions of the International Meeting on Molecular Epidemiology and Ethics held in Oulu, Finland, on 10-12 December 1995.

References

CIOMS (Council for International Organizations of Medical Sciences). (1993) World Declaration of Helsinki (as amended by the 41st World Medical Assembly, Hong Kong, September, 1989). Reprinted as Annex I in: Council for International Organizations of Medical Sciences, International Ethical Guidelines for Biomedical Research Involving Human Subjets. Geneva, CIOMS

Clayton, E.W., Steinberg, K.K, Khoury, M.J., Thomson, E., Andrews, L., Kahn, M.J.E., Kopelman, L.M. & Weiss, J.O. (1995) Informed consent for genetic research on stored tissue samples. *JAMA*, 274, 1786-1792

Gold, E. (1996) Confidentiality and privacy protection in epidemiologic research. In: Coughlin, S.S. & Beauchamp, T.L., eds, *Ethics and Epidemiology.* New York and Oxford; Oxford University Press; pp. 129-141

Goldgar, D.E. & Reilly, P.R. (1995) A common BRCA1 mutation in the Ashkenazim. *Nature Genet.*, 11, 113-114

Goodman, K.W. (1996) Codes of ethics in occupational and environmental health. *J. Occup. Environ. Med.*, 38, 882-883

Goodman, K.W. & Prineas, R.J. (1996) Towards an ethics curriculum in epidemiology. In: Coughlin, S.S. & Beauchamp, T.L., eds, *Ethics and Epidemiology.* New York and Oxford; Oxford University Press; pp. 290-303

Hainaut, P., Soussi, T., Shomer, B., Hollstein, M., Greenblatt, M., Hovig, E., Harris, C.C. & Montesano, R. (1997) Database of p53 gene somatic mutations in human tumours and cell lines: updated compilation and future prospects. *Nucleic Acids Res.*, 25, 151-157

Harris, C.C. (1996) The 1995 Walter Hubert Lecture - molecular epidemiology of human cancer: insights from the mutational analysis of the p53 tumour-suppressor gene. *Br. J. Cancer*, 73, 261-269

Levine, R.J. (1996) The institutional review board. In: Coughlin, S.S. & Beauchamp, T.L., eds, *Ethics and Epidemiology*. New York and Oxford; Oxford University Press; pp. 257-273

Marshall, E. (1996) Policy on DNA research troubles tissue bankers. *Science*, 271, 440

Masood, E. (1996) Gene tests: who benefits from risk? *Nature*, 379, 389-392

Perera, F.P. & Whyatt, R.M. (1994) Biomarkers and molecular epidemiology in mutation/cancer research. *Mutat. Res.*, 313, 117-129

Schulte, P.A. (1992) Biomarkers in epidemiology: scientific issues and ethical implications. *Environ. Health Perspect.*, 98, 143-147

Schulte, P.A., Hunter, D. & Rothman, N. (1997) Ethical and social issues in the use of biomarkers in epidemiologic research. *IARC Sci. Publ.*, 142, 313-318

Schulte, P.A. & Singall, M. (1996) Ethical issues in the relation with subjects and disclosure of the results. In: Coughlin, S.S. & Beauchamp, T.L., eds, *Ethics and Epidemiology.* New York and Oxford; Oxford University Press; pp.178-196

Smith, M.T. & Suk, W.A. (1994) Application of molecular biomarkers in epidemiology. *Environ. Health Perspect.*, 102, 229-235

Vineis, P. & Schulte, P.A. (1995) Scientific and ethical aspects of genetic screening of workers for cancer risk: the case of the N-acetyltransferase phenotype. *J. Clin. Epidemiol.*, 48,1 89-197

Wald, N.J. (1996) What is genetic screening anyway? *J. Med. Screening*, 3, 57

Corresponding author
Pierre Hainaut
Unit of Mechanisms of Carcinogenesis,
International Agency for Research on Cancer,
150 cours Albert Thomas, F-69372,
Lyon cedex 08, France

Metabolic Polymorphisms and Susceptibility to Cancer
W. Ryder
IARC Scientific Publications No. 148
International Agency for Research on Cancer, Lyon, 1999

Chapter 25. Overall evaluation and research perspectives

Paolo Vineis, Angelo d'Errico, Núria Malats and Paolo Boffetta

Methodological considerations

In addition to important conceptual aspects, the present volume has raised several methodological issues that deserve consideration by specialists involved in studies on the interaction between carcinogenic exposures and metabolic polymorphisms, by those who interpret the scientific merits of research, and by public health professionals who are expected to apply well-established epidemiological knowledge. Methodological issues are relevant both to the assessment of cause-effect relationships and to practical applications.

An issue relevant to all epidemiological investigations aimed at interactions between exposures and genetic traits (gene-environment interactions) is that of statistical power (sample size). Statistical power is usually inadequate in most studies on this subject (see Chapter 23). Appropriate *a priori* calculations of the size required to detect an interaction are needed (see Chapter 11). A related issue is that of subgroup analysis: statistically significant associations may arise by chance when multiple comparisons are made within a single study. As Cuzick points out in Chapter 11, this is not just a statistical problem, i.e. one that can be solved with mathematical tools. Rather, the role of sound *a priori* scientific hypotheses (when a study is undertaken) is crucial to avoid false positive results due to multiple comparisons. A further, strictly related, issue is known as "publication bias". Because of small sample size and multiple comparisons, a number of chance findings arise. This phenomenon would probably be insignificant if all findings had the same probability of becoming accessible to the scientific community. However, researchers and journal editors have little interest in publishing "negative" findings, unless they clearly falsify a previously held hypothesis. "False positive" results have much greater chances of appearing in

the literature than both "false" and genuine negative findings. In the literature, therefore, the ratio of false to true positive results is inflated because of publication bias. It is not easy to estimate the extent of such bias but an attempt is made to do so in Chapter 23.

The best way to avoid the pitfalls associated with subgroup analysis, multiple comparisons and publication bias is to define sound scientific hypotheses *a priori*. This can be accomplished only by ensuring strong cooperation among all the persons involved, i.e. geneticists, biochemists, molecular biologists, epidemiologists and biostatisticians. A sound *a priori* hypothesis implies (a) that evidence has been provided that a genetic polymorphism is implicated in the metabolism of a given carcinogen; (b) that the polymorphism can be measured with a reasonably small degree of misclassification; (c) that epidemiological tools allow the researcher to identify the exposed subjects with sufficient accuracy (i.e. exposure assessment is sound). On this basis, sample size is computed to test for the interaction between exposure and the polymorphism (both assessed with a known or expected degree of misclassification). Associations observed *a posteriori* may be taken into consideration only if they are interpreted with great caution.

Establishment of causality

The assessment of cause-effect relationships based on *a posteriori* evaluation of evidence derived from published studies is a difficult task that is best accomplished by consensus in groups of experts from different disciplines. Although in the case of the metabolic polymorphisms considered in this volume we have not formally attempted to establish causality, the systematic review in Chapter 23 leads us to certain conclusions. These, as Rebbeck (1997) suggested, are based on the guidelines developed by Hill (1965) for the evaluation of cause-effect relationships in observational studies:

Strength of association: weak associations are more likely to be explained by bias, including publication bias, or confounding. Although most of the direct associations (polymorphism-disease) are weak, the effects of interaction between a polymorphism and an exposure on a specific disease are larger (Rebbeck, 1997).

Dose-response relationship: a criterion that applies to both genotyping, when two mutations are more effective that one, and to phenotyping, when the association with cancer risk is proportional to enzyme activity. Genotype-environmental and genotype-genotype interactions could also be considered as dose-dependent interactions with an environmental factor (smoking) or with high-risk genotypes (GSTM1-0 and CYP1A1 Val/Val) (Nakachi *et al.*, 1993).

Reproducibility of association: in studies conducted in different populations with different designs. There is no evidence of consistency of associations involving enzyme polymorphisms in different populations except for GSTM1 enzyme, for which most of the studies find a slight excess risk of lung cancer for GSTM1 null subjects.

Internal coherence: for example, the association is observed in both genders unless there is a strong biological background to justify gender differences.

Biological plausibility: see above re the need for sound biological hypotheses; a particularly important issue is knowledge of the compounds (xeno- and endobiotics) metabolized by the polymorphic enzyme involved in carcinogenesis. This condition is not clearly fulfilled for all polymorphic enzymes (i.e. CYP2D6).

Specificity of association: for example, the N-acetyltransferase polymorphism is associated with bladder cancer, a target site for arylamines.

Animal models: these are expected to become more frequently available for studies on metabolic polymorphisms with the development of the "transgenic mice" technology.

Time sequence: although the genotype does not change with time, and its measurement within a cross-sectional design is meaningful, there are subtle problems of interpretation. For example, there is evidence that some polymorphisms influence the survival of cancer patients; therefore the

measurement of the genotype within a cross-sectional design may simply imply the observation of a survival effect.

Summary of results

We summarize below the main results derived from the review of studies on metabolic polymorphisms and cancer. Table 1 provides an overview of our conclusions. We only present here the results on polymorphisms studied in greatest detail. Readers can refer to other parts of this volume in order to obtain more information about the biological and epidemiological evidence of the roles of the enzymes in carcinogenesis.

CYP1A1
Msp I polymorphism
Data on lung cancer among Asians suggest the existence of an association with the mutated genotype, despite a lack of consistency in the results of the individual studies. The risk is modified by smoking, being more than double among light smokers and close to 1.00 among heavy smokers, and concerns squamous and small-cell carcinomas in particular. Studies in non-Asian populations do not support the association between mutated genotype and lung cancer, although there is a suggestion of a small increase in risk among light smokers and for squamous cell carcinoma.

Bladder, oesophageal and upper digestive cancers and basal cell carcinoma of the skin do not appear to be associated with Msp I polymorphism, whereas studies on breast cancer and endometrial cancer would suggest an association with the mutated genotype; the association with breast cancer seems to be higher in African-Americans, among whom the risk appears to be linked in particular to the mutated genotype. Data from cross-sectional studies are apparently consistent with the absence of an association between the WM + MM genotype and cancer.

Exon 7 polymorphism
The available studies do not consistently support the presence of an association between mutated genotype and lung cancer: Two out of three studies conducted among Asians, however, found a strong association.

Table 1. Evaluation of the available evidence on the associations between selected metabolic polymorphisms and human cancers

	CYP1A1	CYP1A1	CYP1A1	CYP1A2	CYP2D6	CYP2E1	CYP2E1	GSTM1	GSTT1	NAT1	NAT2
Polymorphism	Msp I	Exon 7	AHH ind	Rapid	EM	5'FR	Dra I	Null	Null	Slow	Slow
Lung	+ A	(+) A	+	NA	+ P	(-)	(=)	+	(-)	NA	=
	(=) C	(=) C			= G						
Bladder	(=)	(=)	NA	(+)	=	NA	(=)	(+)	(-)	NA	= A
											+ C
Breast	(+)	(+)	NA	NA	(=)	(=)	(=)	(+)	NA	NA	(-) P
											(=) G
Colorectum	(+)	NA	NA	(+)	NA	NA	NA	(+) D	(+)	(-)	(+) P
								(=) O			(=) G
Larynx	(=)	NA	(=)	NA	(=)	(=)	(=)	(+)	(+)	NA	NA
Stomach	NA	NA	NA	NA	NA	(=)	NA	NA	(-)	NA	NA
Liver	NA	NA	NA	NA	(+)	(-)	(=)	NA	NA	NA	(+)
Endometrium	(+)	(+)	NA	NA	NA	NA	NA	(+)	NA	NA	NA
BCC	(=)	(+)	NA	NA	(=)	NA	NA	NA	(+)	NA	NA
Brain	NA	NA	NA	NA	(-)	NA	NA	NA	(+)	NA	NA

+	Increased risk	(+)	Suggested increased risk
		(-)	Suggested reduced risk
=	No effect	(=)	Suggested no effect
NA	Available data do not allow any conclusion	BCC	Basal cell carcinoma of the skin
A	Asians	C	Caucasians
D	Distal colon	O	Other parts of colon
P	Phenotype-based studies	G	Genotype-based studies

Breast cancer seems to be associated with mutated genotype, there being a non-significant overall relative risk of about 1.5. Data on other cancers suggest a possible association of mutated genotype with endometrial cancer and basal cell skin cancer, but not with bladder cancer.

African-American polymorphism

Results from studies on lung cancer are not sufficient to permit an evaluation of the association with the mutated genotype; whereas the pooled relative risk estimate is close to one, the data suggest a possible interaction with low-level smoking. One study on breast cancer does not indicate an association with mutated genotype.

Aryl hydrocarbon hydroxylase (AHH) activity

Studies on AHH activity and lung cancer suggest an association with the inducible phenotype, given the high consistency of the results and the statistical significance of the estimates. The association of the inducible phenotype with larynx cancer is controversial, because the strong association found in one study was not confirmed in another that instead showed a higher risk for the non-inducible phenotype.

CYP1A2

A few studies on CYP1A2 polymorphism suggest possible associations of the rapid metabolizing phenotype with colorectal polyps, familial adenomatous polyposis and bladder cancer.

CYP2D6

Phenotype-based studies of lung cancer consistently show an increased risk, while no association is reported in genotype-based studies, suggesting that some of the mutations leading to the extensive metabolizer (EM) phenotype have not yet been identified. Risk linked to the EM phenotype is not modified by smoking. The risk of lung cancer linked to homozygous EM has not been evaluated through a formal meta-analysis, because estimates on it were not reported sistematically: nevertheless, available data suggest an increased risk for EM compared to IM + PM, which is more consistent than relating to EM + IM, but the subject needs further research.

Data on bladder cancer do not indicate an association with CYP2D6 polymorphism. Similarly, breast cancer, larynx cancer, basal cell carcinoma of the skin and ovarian cancer do not appear to be associated with CYP2D6 polymorphism. Data on liver cancer and cervical intraepithelial neoplasms, based on only a few studies, suggest an association with the homozygous EM genotype but not with the heterozygous genotype, while for brain cancer the risk seems to be linked to the poor metabolizing phenotype or genotype.

CYP2E1

5'-flanking region polymorphism

An association with the wild genotype is suggested for lung cancer and in particular for squamous cell and small-cell carcinomas: meta-analysis, however, did not indicate a statistically significant increased risk.

Two studies on bladder cancer suggest an association with wild-type genotype, while breast, laryngeal, stomach and oesophageal cancers do not appear to be associated with 5'-flanking region polymorphism. Results concerning liver and nasopharyngeal cancers suggest associations with the wild and the mutated genotypes respectively, but these findings need confirmation.

Dra I polymorphism

Dra I polymorphism does not seem to be associated with lung cancer: the consistency of the results and the pooled risk estimate are low. Similarly, bladder, breast, liver, oesophageal and upper aerodigestive tract cancers do not appear to be associated with Dra I polymorphism, while one study suggests an association between the mutated genotype and nasopharyngeal cancer.

Taq I polymorphism

Results on lung cancer and bladder cancer do not suggest the presence of an association with Taq I polymorphism.

GSTM1

Studies on lung cancer suggest an association with GSTM1 null genotype. The risk seems to be higher for squamous and small-cell carcinomas. Risk estimates among Caucasians tend to be low and non-significant, while results for Asians show a higher consistency, a stronger association and an interaction with heavy smoking.

Studies on bladder cancer suggest an association with GSTM1 null genotype (overall relative risk of the order of 1.5) in all ethnic groups. There is some heterogeneity of risk estimates in Caucasians, which is reduced when only results for transitional cell carcinomas and smokers are taken into consideration.

The pooled estimate of breast cancer risk among GSTM1 null carriers is low and non-significant. Nevertheless, results from a few studies support the presence of a significantly higher risk among younger women. Colorectal and liver cancers do not seem to be consistently associated with GSTM1 polymorphism, with the exception of cancers of the distal colon, for which an increased risk, based on heterogeneous risk estimates, is suggested. For gastric cancer the risk for GSTM1 null carriers differs between Caucasians, for whom it is about one, and Asians, who present a significant association, especially in the best-designed studies and those dealing with adenocarcinoma. Studies of laryngeal cancer consistently suggest an increased risk linked to the GSTM1 null genotype, but the pooled estimate is significant only for squamous cell carcinoma.

The available data are insufficient to assess the risk for other cancers, although they suggest an association of the GSTM1 null genotype with pituitary adenoma, endometrial cancer and acute lymphoblastic leukaemia.

GSTM3

The available studies do not permit an evaluation of the risk of cancer linked to GSTM3 polymorphism, although one study reported an association between A allele and laryngeal cancer.

GSTT1

The risk of lung, bladder and gastric cancers does not seem to be associated with GSTT1 polymorphism, although the data are insufficient to rule out a weak association. A few studies on laryngeal cancer suggest an increase among GSTT1 null carriers. Regarding colorectal cancer, meta-analysis revealed a significantly higher risk for GSTT1 null carriers: this result, however, is strongly influenced by a single large hospital-based study. Other suggested associations for the GSTT1 null genotype, based on a few studies, include basocellular skin cancer of the trunk and myelodisplastic syndrome, as well as cancers of the brain and cervix.

NAT1

The results on NAT1 polymorphism are not sufficient for conclusions to be drawn regarding the presence or absence of an association with any cancer, although they support the existence of an increased risk of colorectal cancer and adenoma among NAT1 rapid carriers.

NAT2

The risk of lung cancer does not seem to be associated with NAT2 polymorphism. The results on bladder cancer show an increased risk among Caucasians carrying the NAT2 slow genotype, while for Asians the risk estimates are consistently below unity. The relative risk in Caucasians is around 1.4 and seems to be higher among smokers and among subjects exposed to occupational carcinogens.

Regarding breast cancer, phenotype-based studies but not genotype-based studies consistently showed an increased risk among NAT2 rapid carriers; this was also true when consideration was restricted to the best-designed studies. The discrepancy between the two types of study suggests the presence of mutations leading to the slow phenotype which have not been yet identified. For colorectal cancer, phenotype-based estimates suggested an association with NAT2 slow phenotype, while no such association was confirmed in genotype-based studies.

Data on other cancer sites, although insufficient to evaluate consistency among studies, suggest a possible association of NAT2 slow polymorphism with familial adenomatous polyposis, liver cancer and, among subjects heavily exposed to asbestos, mesothelioma.

Interactions between metabolic polymorphisms

In a few studies the risk of cancer associated with the combined genotype or phenotype of more than one metabolic enzyme has been estimated. Great caution should be applied to the interpretation of these data, since the general limitations of studies on metabolic polymorphisms outlined above (limited statistical power, multiple comparisons and selective reporting) are particularly important when more than one gene is considered. The available evidence suggests (i) an increased risk of lung cancer for carriers of the GSTM1 null genotype and either the CYP1A1 Msp I or the CYP1A1 exon 7 high-risk alleles; (ii) an increased risk of bladder cancer and a decreased risk of colorectal cancer among carriers of the GSTM1 null and the NAT2 slow genotypes; (iii) a decreased risk of bladder cancer among carriers of NAT1 rapid and NAT2 slow genotypes; and (iv) an increased risk of liver cancer among NAT2 slow acetylators and CYP2D6 extensive metabolizers.

Public health applications

Chapter 24 deals with ethical issues related to the potential application of metabolic polymorphisms in a public health context. Such issues go far beyond obtaining informed consent. The use of metabolic polymorphisms to identify highly susceptible individuals has several implications that should be discussed thoroughly before any field application is approved: (i) the distribution of polymorphisms is uneven according to ethnic groups; this means that any job-related selection - on the basis of genetic susceptibility - would imply ethnic discrimination; (ii) the role of insurance companies must be clarified, if personal information on genetic susceptibility to cancer is released; and (iii) metabolic susceptibility to cancer is such a complex issue that it can hardly be used to select susceptible individuals for any meaningful purpose.

Recommendations for future studies

A few recommendations can be made for future studies on cancer and metabolic polymorphisms in humans:

(i) Attention should be paid to important aspects of study design for investigations on metabolic polymorphism and cancer, including the definition of the study base, the choice of controls, the avoidance of misclassification, the performance of state-of-the-art assays, the control of known confounding factors and the performance of appropriate statistical analysis.

(ii) Studies should have adequate statistical power for the detection of expected differences in the prevalence of polymorphisms. This applies in particular to analyses aimed at assessing the interaction between polymorphisms and environmental factors. Multicentric studies are encouraged.

(iii) Results should be reported for all analyses performed; it is important to avoid selective reporting of positive or significant results.

(iv) Efforts aimed at pooling the results of comparable studies, using appropriate statistical methods, should be encouraged.

References

Hill, A.B. (1965) The environment and disease: association or causation? *Proc. R.. Soc. Med.*, 58, 295-300

Nakachi, K., Imai, K., Hayashi, S. & Kawajiri, K. (1993) Polymorphisms of the CYP1A1 and glutathione S-transferase genes associated with susceptibility to lung cancer in relation to cigarette dose in a Japanese population. *Cancer Res.*, 53, 2994-2999

Rebbeck, T.R. (1997) Molecular epidemiology of the human glutathione S-transferase genotypes GSTM1 and GSTT1 in cancer susceptibility. *Cancer Epidemiol. Biomarkers Prev.*, 6, 733-743

Corresponding author
Paolo Vineis
Unit of Cancer Epidemiology,
S. Giovanni Battista Hospital and University of Turin,
Italy

Metabolic Polymorphisms and Susceptibility to Cancer
W. Ryder
IARC Scientific Publications No. 148
International Agency for Research on Cancer, Lyon, 1999

Annex

Table 1. Study design: GSTM1 and cancer (case–case studies shaded grey)

Author	# of cases	# of controls	Response	Phenotyping/ genotyping	Exposures	Covariates	Therapy	GSTM1null in controls	Power (α=0.05, OR>2)
Alexandrie et al., 1994 (Sweden)	296 incid. lung cancer histolog. confirmed (Caucas.)	329 healthy controls from laboratory personnel, chimney sweeps and welders <65 yrs; 79 COPD patients (Caucas.)		TSO conjugation in leukocytes; PCR		age (<65, >65 yrs), gender, cancer histology, CYP1A1 polym., race		52.2% all, 52.9% healthy, 45.7% hosp. <65 yrs, 52.3% hosp >65 yrs	99.1% vs. all contr., 98.4% vs. healthy contr., 73.4% vs. hosp. contr.
Ambrosone et al., 1995 (USA)	439 incid. post-menopausal breast cancer histolog. confirmed (Caucas.)	494 healthy controls frequency matched by age and county residence (Caucas.)		PCR	smoking (non-smokers, smokers <29 PY, >29 PY)	CYP1A1 polym., age (at diagnos., menarche, first pregnancy and menopause), education, BMI, family history of breast cancer, race		50.2% all, 41% <58 yrs, 58% 58-63 yrs, 45% 64-69 yrs, 55% >69 yrs	91.1%
Anttila et al., 1994 (Finland)	54 incid. lung cancer histolog. confirmed undergoing surgery, smokers (Caucas.)			PCR		cancer histology, CYP1A1 polym., tumour location			
Anttila et al., 1995 (Finland)	100 incid. lung cancer histolog. confirmed undergoing surgery, current+ former smokers (Caucas.)			PCR	smoking (current smokers, recent and long-term former smokers), occupation (exp. to asbestos and mineral dusts)	cancer histology, GSTM3 polym.			
Anwar et al., 1996 (Egypt)	22 prev. bladder cancer histolog. confirmed (Caucas.)	21 healthy controls matched by age and smoking (Caucas.)		PCR		race, CYP2E1 and CYP2D6 polym.		47.6%	12.2%
Baranov et al., 1996 (Russia)	58 prev. lung cancer, 37 prev. digestive cancer (stomach + colon) histolog. confirmed (Caucas.)	67 healthy controls (Caucas.)		PCR		race		38.8%	40.9% (lung cancer), 31.2% (digestive cancer)
Bell et al., 1993 (USA)	229 incid.+ prev. bladder transitional cell carcinoma histolog. confirmed (mixed)	211 urology clinic patients matched by race, gender, age; 466 healthy controls (mixed)		PCR	smoking (non-smokers, 1-50, >50 PY) for cases and hosp. controls	race, tumour grade, cancer histology		49% (Caucas.), 35% (Afric.-Americ.)	93.7%, 92.1% Caucas. 6.7% Afric.-Americ.
Brockmöller et al., 1993 (Germany)	117 incid. Lung cancer histolog. confirmed <85 yrs (Caucas.)	155 hosp. controls, mainly pulmonary; 200 hosp. controls from an intensive care unit (Caucas.)		TSO conjugation in leukocytes; ELISA; PCR	smoking for cases and 155 controls (non-smokers, 1-20, >20 PY)	age (<70, >70 yrs), gender, cancer histology, race	no chemotherapy or radiotherapy before phenotyping/ genotyping	52.9% all, 53.7% <70 yrs, 51.1% >70 yrs, 49.4% male, 56.9% female	86.4%

Table 1 (Contd). Study design: GSTM1 and cancer (case-case studies shaded grey)

Author	# of cases	# of controls	Response	Phenotyping/ genotyping	Exposures	Covariates	Therapy	GSTM1null in controls	Power (α=0.05, OR>2)
Brockmöller et al., 1994 (Germany) (part of Brockmöller et al., 1996a)	296 prev. bladder cancer histolog. confirmed (Caucas.)	400 cancer-free hosp. controls (Caucas.)		TSO conjugation and ELISA in serum; PCR	smoking (non smokers, 1-20, 20-50, >50 PY), occupation (exp. to bladder carcinog.) for cases and 296 controls	age (<55, 55-65, 65-75, >75 yrs), gender, tumour grade and stage, cancer histology, race		50.7% all, 59.2% <55 yrs, 49.6% 55-65 yrs, 54.3% 65-75 yrs, 36.4% >75 yrs, 48.8% male, 54.0% female	99.2%
Brockmöller et al., 1996a (Germany)	374 incid. + prev. bladder cancer histolog. confirmed (Caucas.)	373 hosp. cancer-free controls (Caucas.)		PCR	smoking, occupation (>1 year in jobs at high risk for bladder cancer)	age, gender, race, cancer histology, tumour stage and grade, NAT2, GSTT1, CYP2D6, CYP2E1 and CYP1A1 polym.		51.1%	99.6%
Chen et al., 1996 (Taiwan)	32 incid. HCC histolog. confirmed from a cohort of HBsAg carriers, male (Asians)	73 healthy controls from a cohort of HBsAg carriers, male, matched by age, clinic and date of specimen collection (Asians)		PCR	smoking, alcohol, aflatoxin (AFB, - albumin adducts: high, low, undetectable)	race, age, gender, HBV status, cancer histology		58.9%	23.4%
Chen et al., 1996 (USA)	92 incid. myelodisplastic syndrome (Caucasian, Afric.-Americ.)	201 urology clinic patients (Caucasian, Afric.-Americ.)		PCR		age (<60, >60 yrs), gender, cancer histology	no therapy before genotyping	48.0%	73.1%
Chen et al., 1996 (USA)	71 incid. anal cancer histolog. confirmed, (mixed)	360 healthy controls selected random-digit dialing frequency matched by age (5 yrs), gender and year of diagnosis (mixed)	46% male cases, 73.3% female cases; 52.7% male controls, 61.8% female controls	PCR	smoking (never, former, current)	gender, age (<50, >50 yrs)		56.7% all, 53.4% male, 57.7% female, 56.5% <50 yrs, 56.9% >50 yrs	65.2%
Chen et al., 1997 (USA)	197 prev. childhood acute lymphoblastic leukaemia histolog. confirmed (mixed)	416 healthy blood donors (mixed)		PCR		race, gender, GSTT1 polym.		53.5% all, 49.5% male, 57.8% female (Caucas.); 27.6 all, 22.3% male, 33.0% female (Afric.-Americ.)	97.5%, 87.4% (Caucas.), 38.4% (Afric.-Americ.)
Chenevix-Trench et al., 1995 (Australia)	132 prev. colorectal adenocarcinoma histolog. confirmed (Caucas.)	100 healthy controls, 100 cancer-free geriatric patients (Caucas.)		PCR		age (<70, >70 yrs), race, gender, cancer histology, tumour stage and differentiation		50.5%	82.7%
Cheng et al., 1995c (USA)	78 incid. lung cancer (95% Caucas.)	78 healthy controls (95% Caucas.)		PCR	smoking (current, former, never smokers)			56.0%	47.0%

Reference	Cases	Controls	Method		Smoking	Matching/confounding factors	Treatment before genotyping	%	%
Daly et al., 1993 (UK)	53 prev. bladder transitional cell carcinoma (Caucas.?)	52 urology clinic patients with negative cytoscopy; 58 healthy volunteers (Caucas.?)	PCR			cancer histology		57.4%	41.8%
Deakin et al., 1996 (UK)	108 incid. lung cancer smokers, 40 incid. SQ oral cancer, 136 incid. gastric cancer, 252 incid. colorectal cancer (Caucas.)	129 COPD smokers controls, 577 hosp. controls with non-malignant diseases (Caucas.)	PCR		smoking (never, former, current smokers); for lung cancer cases and COPD controls	GSTT1 polym.; age (<65, >65 yrs), gender, race, tumour site, t. stage, t. differentiation (for colorectal cases)		54.8%	66.5% (lung), 43.4% (oral), 92.4% (gastric), 99.2% (colorectal)
Elexpuru-Camiruaga et al., 1995 (UK)	109 incid. astrocytoma, 49 incid. meningioma histolog. confirmed (Caucas.)	577 hosp. cancer-free controls (Caucas.)	PCR	100% cases		gender, age, race, cancer histology, CYP2D6 and GSTT1 polym.	no radiotherapy or chemotherapy before genotyping	54.6%	86.6% (astrocytoma), 52.6% (meningioma)
El-Zein et al., 1997 (USA)	52 incid. lung cancer histolog. confirmed, smokers (Caucas.?)	48 healthy controls matched by smoking habit, age and gender (Caucas. ?)	PCR		smoking	cancer histology	no radiotherapy or chemotherapy before genotyping	46%	32%
Esteller et al., 1997 (Spain)	80 incid. endometrial cancer histolog. confirmed undergoing surgery (Caucas.)	60 healthy controls from the same area (Caucas.)	PCR			race	no radiotherapy or treatment with hormones before genotyping	46.6%	44.8%
Fontana et al., 1997 (France)	373 incid. breast cancer histolog. confirmed (Caucas.)		PCR			age (<55, >55 yrs), cancer histology, tumour size, grade and stage, preogesterone and estrogen receptor status			
Fryer et al., 1993 (UK)	113 pituitary adenomas histolog. confirmed (Caucas.)	89 healthy controls (Caucas.)	PCR			race, cancer histology		44.0%	72.8%
Ge et al., 1996 (Hong Kong)	89 incid. non-SC lung cancer histolog. confirmed (Asians)	25 healthy and 28 hosp. controls (Asians)	PCR			race	no chemotherapy or radiotherapy before genotyping	67%	35.9%
Goto et al., 1996 (Japan)	232 incid. non-SC lung cancer histolog. confirmed (Asians)		PCR		smoking (non-smokers, smokers)	age (<65, 65+ yrs), gender, cancer histology, tumour stage and grade, CYP1A1 polym., survival time, operability	no radio-chemotherapy or surgery before genotyping		
Guo et al., 1996 (China)	19 incid. colon cancer histolog. confirmed (Asians)	23 healthy controls frequency matched by place of birth, age (2 yrs) and gender (Asians)	PCR			race		26.1%	10.7%

Table 1 (Contd). Study design: GSTM1 and cancer (case–case studies shaded grey)

Author	# of cases	# of controls	Response	Phenotyping/genotyping	Exposures	Covariates	Therapy	GSTM1 null in controls	Power (α=0.05, OR>2)
Hall et al., 1994 (UK)	71 incid. childhood acute lymphoblastic leukaemia histolog. confirmed (Caucas.)		100%	immunohis-toche-mistry in bone marrow blasts		gender, age and WBC at diagnosis, year of diagnosis, treatment protocol			
Harada et al., 1992 (Japan)	19 prev. stomach cancer, 32 prev. HCC, 65 prev. breast cancer (Asians)	84 healthy blood donors (Asians)		PCR		race		47.6%	27.8% (stomach), 47.1% (breast), 28.9% (HCC)
Hayashi et al., 1992 (Japan)	212 inc. lung cancer histolog. confirmed (Asians)	358 healthy controls, chosen randomly from a cohort study (Asians)		PCR		cancer histology, CYP1A1 polym., race		46.6%	97%
Heagerty et al., 1994 (UK)	629 incid. cutaneous tumours (435 BCC, 64 melanoma, 85 SQ, 45 multiple cutaneous cancer, 33 BCC+SQ) histolog. confirmed (Caucas.)	153 healthy controls (Caucas.)		PCR		cancer histology, race		52%	93.9% BCC, 54.8% melanoma, 64.6% SQ, 42.6% multiple cancers, 32.6% multiple BCC+SQ
Heagerty et al., 1996 (UK)	699 incid. BCC (454 single, 245 multiple) histolog. confirmed (Caucas.)	561 hosp. controls (Caucas.)		PCR	smoking (never, former, current)	gender, skin type, hair and eye colour, race, cancer histology, GSTT1 and CYP2D6 polym.		54.5%	99.9%
Heckbert et al., 1992 (USA)	66 incid. lung cancer (Caucas.)	120 healthy controls selected random-digit dialing and randomly from Social Security lists (Caucas.)	cases: 59%; controls: 80% (random dialing); 87% (Soc. Sec.)	TSO conjugation in leukocytes	smoking (<20, >20 PY), occupation (exp. to lung carcinog.), alcohol (never, ex-, current drinkers)	gender, race	no change after chemotherapy, radiation therapy, surgery	58%	48.8%
Hirvonen et al., 1993a (Finland)	138 incid. lung cancer histolog. confirmed (Caucas.)	142 healthy controls, 36 hosp. controls having a benign lung tumour (Caucas.)		PCR	smoking (non-smokers, smokers <40, >40 PY) for cases and 36 controls	cancer histology, race		43.7%	83.2% vs. all contr., 78.8% vs. healthy contr.; 38.3% vs. hosp. contr.
Hirvonen et al., 1995 (Finland)	44 incid. mesothelioma histolog. confirmed (Caucas.)	270 healthy blood donors (Caucas.)		PCR	occupation (exp. to asbestos: high, moderate, low), smoking (never, former, current smokers)	NAT2 polym., age, race, cancer histology		46.0%	48.8%

Reference	Cases	Controls	Genotyping	Method	Exposure	Matching/adjustment variables	%	%
Hsieh et al., 1996 (Taiwan)	46 incid. HCC undergoing surgery, male HBsAg carriers (Asians)	88 healthy male HBsAg carriers frequency matched by age (Asians)	100% for cases	PCR		race, gender, cancer histology, HBV status	53.4%	36.5%
Jahnke et al., 1996 (UK)	269 prev. laryngeal SQ carcinoma histolog. confirmed undergoing surgery (Caucas.)	216 healthy controls (Caucas.)		PCR		race, cancer histology, tumour location (glottic, supraglottic), grade and stage	52.0%	95.0%
Kato et al., 1996 (Japan)	82 prev. gastric AD histolog. confirmed who did not undergo gastrectomy (Asians)	151 controls affected by benign gastric diseases matched by age and gender (Asians)		PCR		gender, race, age, cancer histology, pepsinogen I levels, pepsinogen I/II ratios, H. pylori IgG, L-myc and CYP2E1 genotypes	51%	63.6%
Katoh et al., 1995 (Japan)	83 prev. transitional cell carcinoma histolog. confirmed (65 of the bladder, 12 renal pelvis, 6 ureter) (Asians)	101 healthy controls from a community (Asians)		PCR		race, cancer histology	42.6%	58.3%
Katoh et al., 1996 (Japan, USA)	139 incid. gastric AD, 103 incid. colorectal AD histolog. confirmed (Asians)	126 healthy controls undergoing a general health check-up (Asians)	100% for cases and controls	PCR	smoking (non-smokers, smokers <40, >40 PY)	age, gender, race, cancer histology, tumour location (only for colorectal cancer), tumour differentiation, GSTT1 polym.	43.6%	76.3% (gastric cancer), 68.9% (colorectal cancer)
Kempkes et al., 1996 (Germany)	113 prev. bladder cancer histolog. confirmed (Caucas.)	170 newborns controls (Caucas.)		PCR	smoking (for cases only)		54%	74.3%
Kihara et al., 1994 (Japan)	178 incid. lung cancer histolog. confirmed, <69 yrs, smokers (Asians)	201 healthy controls, <69 yrs, smokers, from a general health ceck-up (Asians)		PCR	smoking (<800, 800-1200, >1200 cig. x day x yrs), occupation (no exp. to lung carcinog.)	gender, cancer histology, race	45.3% all, 45.0% male, 45.9% female	89.9%
Kihara et al., 1995a (Japan)	447 incid. lung cancer histolog. confirmed (Asians)	469 healthy controls >50 yrs undergoing a general health check-up (Asians)		PCR	smoking (non-smokers, ex-smokers, current smokers <800, >800, >1200 cig. per day x yrs)	gender, age, race	48.7% all, 45.2% female, 50.5% male, 48.1% <70 yrs, 54.1% >70 yrs	99.9%
Kihara et al., 1995b (Japan)	118 incid. lung cancer histolog. confirmed (71 SQ, 47 SC) <70 yrs (Asians)	331 healthy controls <70 yrs (Asians)		PCR	smoking (non-smokers, ex-smokers, current smokers <800, >800, >1200 cig. per day x yrs), occupation (no exp. to lung carcinog.)	cancer histology, gender, CYP1A1 polym., race	50.7% male	86.1%
Kihara et al., 1997 (Japan)	150 incid. head and neck cancer histolog. confirmed >50 yrs (Asians)	474 healthy controls >50 yrs (Asians)		PCR	smoking (non-smokers, smokers)	age (<60, >60 yrs), race	48.7% all, 50.7% male, 45.2% female	95.3% (all cancers), 59.8% (larynx cancer), 74.7% (non-larynx cancer)

Table 1 (Contd). Study design: GSTM1 and cancer (case–case studies shaded grey)

Author	# of cases	# of controls	Response	Phenotyping/ genotyping	Exposures	Covariates	Therapy	GSTM1null in controls	Power (α=0.05, OR=2)
Lafuente et al., 1993 (Spain)	75 incid. bladder transitional cell carcinoma, 78 incid. SQ larynx cancer histolog. confirmed; smokers (Caucas.)	127 healthy controls, smokers, matched by age and smoking history (Caucas.)		ELISA in leukocytes	smoking (non-smokers, smokers; light, heavy smokers for cases only)	age, tumour grade and tumour penetration, race, cancer histology	no chemotherapy or radiotherapy before phenotyping	44.9%	57.8%
Lafuente et al., 1995 (Spain)	183 incid. malignant melanoma histolog. confirmed (Caucas.)	147 hosp. cancer-free controls from a surgery department (Caucas.)		ELISA in leukocytes	smoking	gender, race, age at onset, skin photo-type, cancer histology, tumour depth	no chemotherapy or radiotherapy before phenotyping	40.9% all, 45.2% male, 35.4% female	85.1%
Lear et al., 1996 (UK)	827 incid BCC histolog. confirmed (Caucas.)			PCR		gender, cancer histology, skin type, eye colour, number of BCC, BCC rate, CYP1A1, GSTT1 and CYP2D6 polym.			
Lear et al., 1997 (UK)	74 prev. BCC histolog. confirmed with at least one truncal tumour (Caucas.)	263 prev. BCC controls without truncal tumours (Caucas.)	100%	PCR		age, gender, race, cancer histology, BCC number, tumour site, CYP1A1, GSTT1, GSTM3 and CYP2D6 polym.			
Lin et al., 1994 (USA)	114 incid. bladder cancer histolog. confirmed (mixed)	1104 healthy controls (mixed)		PCR		race		49% Caucas., 45% Afric.-Americ., 48% Asians	92.2% Caucas., 80.7% Caucas., 11.7% Afric.-Americ.
Lin et al., 1995 (USA)	446 incid. colorectal adenomas histolog. confirmed (mixed)	488 controls undergoing sigmoidoscopy (mixed)	84% cases, 82% controls	PCR	smoking (non-smokers, ex, current smokers)	race, tumour size, cancer histology		N.D.	N.D.
London et al., 1995a (USA)	342 incid. lung cancer histolog. confirmed, collected from 35 hospitals (167 Afric.-Americ., 189 Caucas.)	716 healthy controls (251 Afric.-Americ., 465 Caucas.)	41.4% cases, 68.8% controls	PCR	smoking (never, former, current smokers, <40 PY, >40 PY), occupation (none, possible, probable exposure to asbestos)	race, age, gender, diet (vit. C, E and b-carotene intake)		44.0%, 27.1% Afric.- Americ., 52.5% Caucas., 44.4% female, 43.2% male	99.9%, 87.9% Afric.-Americ., 96.6% caucas.
McGlynn et al., 1995 (USA, China)	52 prev. HCC histolog. confirmed (Asians)	116 healthy controls (Asians)		PCR		HBV status, race, cancer histology		41.0%	47.5%
Moreira et al., 1996 (Portugal)	98 prev. lung cancer histolog. confirmed (Caucas.)	84 healthy controls (Caucas.)		PCR		cancer histology, race		52.4%	54.9%
Morita et al., 1997 (Japan)	53 incid. oesophageal SQ histolog. confirmed undergoing surgery (Asians)	132 healthy controls (Asians)		PCR	smoking (non-smokers, smokers), alcohol (non-drinkers, drinkers)	cancer histology, race, CYP1A1 and CYP2E1 polym.		41.7%	49.7%

Reference	Study population	Method	Exposure stratification	Adjustment / matching	Note		
Nakachi et al., 1993 (Japan)	85 incid. SQ of the lung histolog. confirmed (Asians); 170 healthy controls randomly from a cohort study, >40 yrs, matched by gender and age (Asians)	PCR	smoking (<44 PY, >44 PY)	CYP1A1 polym., race, cancer histology		49.4%	67.4%
Nazar-Stewart et al., 1993 (USA)	35 incid. deceased or operat. lung cancer histolog. confirmed; >30 yrs; >100 cig. in lifetime (mixed: 2 non-white cases); 43 controls deceased or operated for causes unrelated with smoking; 30-80 yrs; >100 cig. in lifetime (mixed: 3 non-white controls)	TSO conjugation in leukocytes; immunological assay with GST-μ antibodies; RFLP	smoking (<54, >54 PY)	age (<64, >64 yrs), gender, race, cancer histology		48.3% (mixed)	23.8%
Okkels et al., 1996 & 1997 (Denmark)	95 incid. and 159 prev. bladder cancer histolog. confirmed (Caucas.); 242 controls affected by noncancerous urinary tract diseases (Caucas.)	PCR	smoking (smokers 1-20, 21-50, >50 PY; non-smokers; ex-smokers for 2-9, 10-19, >19 yrs), occupation (exp. to bladder carcinogens)	gender, age, race, cancer histology, tumour grade, NAT1 and NAT2 polym.		50%	95.9%
Rothman et al., 1996 (China, USA)	38 prev. bladder cancer histolog. confirmed, exp. to benzidine (Asians); 43 controls with negative cytology exp. to benzidine, frequency matched by age (Asians)	PCR	smoking (none, <20, >20 cig/day); occupation (benzidine exposure estimated: low, medium, high)	gender, age (50-59, 60-69, >69 yrs), residence, weight, NAT2 polym., race		60.0%	21.6%
Ryberg et al., 1994a (Norway, UK)	63 incid. non-SC lung cancer undergoing surgery (Caucas.); 177 healthy controls (Caucas.)	PCR	total DNA-adducts (low, high) for cases only	race	no treatment before genotyping	50.3%	38.7%
Sarhanis et al., 1996 (UK)	84 incid. epithelial ovarian cancer histolog. confirmed, (Caucas.); 312 hosp. controls undergoing hysterectomy (Caucas.)	PCR		race	no treatment before genotyping	61.5%	67.0%
Seidegard et al., 1986 (USA, Sweden)	66 incid. lung cancer histolog. confirmed >45 yrs; smokers >20 cig/day (Caucas.?); 78 incid. lung cancer randomly from a cohort study, matched by age and smoking; >45 yrs; smokers >20 cig/day (Caucas.?)	TSO conjugation in leukocytes	smoking (heavy, light smokers)	age (>65, <65 yrs), gender, cancer histology		41.6% all, 52.3% <65 yrs, 33.0% <65 yrs, 44.9% male, 35.4% female	90.6%
Seidegard et al., 1990 (USA)	125 incid. lung cancer histolog. confirmed; smokers >20 PY (Caucas.?); 114 healthy controls from a cohort study, matched by age and smoking; smokers >20 PY (Caucas.?)	TSO conjugation in leukocytes	smoking	age (<65, >65 yrs), gender, cancer histology		41.6% all, 52.3% >65 yrs, 33.0% <65 yrs, 44.9% male, 35.4% female	90.6%
Shanley et al., 1995 (Australia)	124 prev. malignant melanoma, 62 prev. NBCCS histolog. confirmed (Caucas.); 100 healthy controls, 100 cancer-free geriatric patients (Caucas.)	PCR		age at onset, race, cancer histology		50.5%	81.1% (melanoma), 57.8% (NBCCS), 20.6% (multiple melanoma)

Table 1 (Contd). Study design: GSTM1 and cancer (case-case studies shaded grey)

Author	# of cases	# of controls	Response	Phenotyping/ genotyping	Exposures	Covariates	Therapy	GSTM1null in controls	Power (α=0.05, OR>2)
Strange et al., 1991 (UK)	26 prev. operated colon AD. and 19 stomach AD histolog. confirmed (Caucas.)	49 controls deceased for cardiovasc. diseases (Caucas.)		starch gel electrophoresis on liver tissue		race, tumour stage, cancer histology		40.8%	21.3% (colon), 16.7% (stomach)
To-Figueras et al., 1996 (Spain)	139 incid. histolog. confirmed lung cancer (Caucas.)	147 healthy controls (Caucas.)		PCR	smoking (<50 PY, >50 PY)	age (<59, >59 yrs), cancer histology, race	no therapy before genotyping	45.6%	79.4%
Trizna et al., 1995 (USA)	186 SQ of mouth, pharynx or larynx histolog. confirmed (mixed)	42 healthy controls matched by age, gender and race (mixed)		PCR		cancer histology		48.0%	45.9%
Warwick et al., 1994a (UK)	175 prev. CIN (cervical intraepithelial neoplasia), 77 SQ (Caucas.)	180 cancer-free controls affected by menorrhagia (Caucas.)		PCR	smoking (non-smokers, smokers: >10 cig./day for at least 5 yrs)	CYP2D6 polym., race, cancer histology		58.4%	59.5% (SQ), 84.1% (CIN)
Wrigley et al., 1996 (UK)	97 prev. ovarian cancer histolog. confirmed			Western blot in tumour tissue (immunoelectrophoresis)		age, tumour grade and stage, cancer histology, post-operative status, response to treatment			
Yengi et al., 1996 (UK)	286 prev. basal cell carcinoma (92 single BCC, 194 multiple BCC) histolog. confirmed (Caucas.)	300 cancer-free hosp. controls (Caucas.)		PCR		age, gender, skin type, CYP1A1, CYP2D6, GSTM3, GSTT1 polym., race, cancer histology		57.3%	92.5% (all BCC), 69.2% (single BCC), 84.3% (multiple BCC)
Yu et al., 1995b (Taiwan, USA)	30 incid. HCC histolog. confirmed, males (Asians)	150 healthy controls, males, matched by age (Asians)	78.9% cases, 98.7% controls	PCR		race, gender, cancer histology, HBV status, CYP2E1 polym.		63.3%	29.3%
Zhong et al., 1991 (UK)	228 prev. lung cancer histolog. confirmed, smokers (Caucas.)	225 controls chosen randomly from 2 hospitals and a group of volunteers (Caucas.)		RIA in leukocytes; RFLP	smoking (non-smokers, smokers 1-17.4 PY, 17.5-29.2 PY, >29.2 PY)	cancer histology, race		41.8%	94.7%
Zhong et al., 1993 (UK)	97 prev. bladder cancer, 197 prev. breast cancer, 196 prev. colon cancer (Caucas.)	225 randomly from 2 hospitals and a group of volunteers (Caucas.)		PCR		race, tumour site (proximal, distal) for colon cancer		41.8%	77.6% (bladder), 93.1% (breast), 93% (colon)

Table 2. Study design: GSTM1 and outcomes other than cancer

Author	Subjects	Analysis	Phenotyping/ genotyping	Exposures	Covariates	GSTM1 null (%)
Bartsch et al., 1995 (Finland)	230 patients with or without malignant lung disease (Caucas.)	^{32}P-postlabelling assay of PAH-DNA and BPDE-DNA adducts in parenchymal lung tissue	PCR	smoking (smokers, non-smokers, ex-smokers)	race	
Bernardini et al., 1996 (Finland)	22 healthy volunteers non-smokers (Caucas.)	SCE induction with 3,4-epoxybutane-1,2-diol (EBD) in cultured lymphocytes	PCR		race, GSTT1 polym	45.0%
Binkova et al., 1996 (Czech Republic)	51 women working outdoors about 30% of their daily time from 2 areas with different air pollution levels (Caucas.)	SCE and CA in lymphocytes; PAHs and their metabolites in urines by HPLC and GC; PAH-DNA adducts in WBC by ^{32}P-postlabelling; PAH-albumin adducts in WBC by ELISA; Ames assay on urines in Salmonella typhimurium YG10241 and TA98 strains	PCR	smoking	age, gender, race, diet, residence	50.0%
Brockmöller et al., 1996b (Germany)	69 bladder cancer histolog. confirmed (Caucas.)	p53 mutations by PCR	PCR		race	
Cheng et al., 1995a (USA)	78 healthy controls (95% Caucas.)	SCE in lymphocytes	PCR	smoking (current, former, never smokers), alcohol	age, gender, diet (vit. A, C, E, folate	56.0%
Cheng et al., 1995b (USA)	40 lung cancer and 66 healthy controls (mixed)	mutant frequency at hprt locus in lymphocytes	PCR		cloning efficency	59.0%
Gabbani et al., 1996 (Italy)	46 coke oven workers exp. to PAH (Caucas.)	Ames assay on urines in Salmonella typhimurium TA98 strain (number of revertant colonies per mmol creatinine)	PCR	smoking	race, NAT2 polym.	60.9%
Grinberg-Funes et al., 1994 (USA)	63 male volunteers cigarette smokers (Caucas.?)	PAH-DNA adducts in lymphocytes and monocytes by ELISA	PCR	smoking (cig. smoked/day)	gender, serum levels of vitamins A, C, E and b-carotene	51.0%
Hemminki et al., 1997 (Finland, USA)	100 foundry workers (Caucas.)	^{32}P-postlabelling assay of PAH-DNA adducts in lymphocytes	PCR	smoking, occupation (exposure to PAH), diet (charcoal broiled food)	race	38.8%
Hirvonen et al., 1994 (Finland)	healthy males exp. to asbestos: 10 smokers, 29 non-smokers; patients with malignant lung cancer or non-malignant lesions: 7 smokers, 6 non-smokers (Caucas.)	Ames assay in Salmonella typhimurium YG1024 and TA98 strains (number of revertant colonies per 100 ml urine)	PCR	smoking, occupation (asbestos)	race, gender	46%
Hou et al., 1995 (Sweden)	47 healthy non-smokers bus maintainance workers; 22 healthy non-smokers controls (Caucas.)	^{32}P-postlabelling assay of PAH-DNA adducts in lymphocytes; mutant frequency in hprt gene	PCR	occupation (garage workers, mechanics, others)	NAT2 polym., race, age (for mutant frequency only)	49.3%
Ichiba et al., 1994 (Sweden)	69 male chimney sweeps, 35 male healthy controls lacking a definite PAH exposure (Caucas.)	^{32}P-postlabelling assay of PAH-DNA adducts in total white blood cells; micronuclei in B- and T-lymphocytes	PCR	smoking, occupation (exp. to PAH)	race, gender	50%

Table 2 (Contd). Study design: GSTM1 and outcomes other than cancer

Author	Subjects	Analysis	Phenotyping/ genotyping	Exposures	Covariates	GSTM1 null (%)
Kato et al., 1995a (USA)	90 cancer-free autopsy donors (mixed)	32P-postlabelling assay of PAH-DNA adducts (PAH-dGMP) in parenchymal lung tissue	PCR	smoking (serum cotinine levels)		52.0%
Kawajiri et al., 1996 (Japan)	187 non-SC lung cancers: 75 SQ, 112 AD (Asians)	p53 mutations by PCR	PCR	smoking (current or former smokers, never smokers)	race, CYP1A1 polym.	53.4%
Ketterer et al., 1992 (UK)	12 lung cancer smokers (Caucas.?)	32P-postlabelling assay of PAH-DNA adducts in parenchymal lung tissue	immunoassay (western blotting)			
Landi M.T et al., 1996 (Italy, USA)	45 healthy male blood donors 45-64 yrs old (Caucas.)	4-aminobiphenyl-haemoglobin adducts level	PCR	smoking (smokers, non-smokers, cotinine and nicotine in urine)	race, NAT2 and CYP1A2 polym.	55.8%
Landi S. et al., 1996 (Italy)	7 healthy non-smokers (Caucas.)	SCE induction with DEB 2 or 4 M in cultured lymphocytes	PCR		race, GSTT1 polym.	
McGlynn et al., 1995 (Ghana, China)	49 healthy males (Africans), 52 prev. HCC histolog. confirmed, 116 healthy controls (Asians)	serum aflatoxin B1-albumin adducts by ELISA (Africans); p53 mutations in codon 249 by restriction endonuclease assay (Asians)	PCR		gender, race, HBV status	38.8% (Africans), 41% (Asians)
Mooney et al., 1997 (USA)	159 heavy smokers enrolled in a smoking cessation programme (mixed, 90% Caucas.)	PAH-DNA adducts in WBC by ELISA	PCR	smoking (>20 cig./day for >1 year)	Msp I and Exon 7 CYP1A1 polym., serum levels of retinol, α-tocopherol, and β-carotene	47.2%
Nielsen et al., 1996a (Denmark)	90 healthy non-smoking bus drivers, 60 healthy subjects from a rural area (Caucas.)	32P-postlabelling assay of PAH-DNA adducts in lymphocytes	PCR	smoking (smokers, non-smokers) for rural controls	race, NAT2 polym., driving area (centre, suburban, dormitory) for bus drivers	40.0%
Nielsen et al., 1996b (Denmark)	120 non-smoking healthy males: 91 from a urban area, 29 from a rural area (Caucas.)	32P-postlabelling assay of total-DNA adducts in lymphocytes; PAH-albumin adducts by ELISA	PCR		gender, race, residence (urban, rural)	47.0%
Norppa et al., 1995 (Finland)	20 healthy volunteers current non-smokers (Caucas.)	SCE induction by DEB in cultured lymphocytes	PCR	diepoxybutane (DEB)	gender, race, age, replication index, GSTT1 polym.	
Ohshima et al., 1997 (Japan)	35 SQ lung cancer histolog. confirmed (Asians)	p53 mutations by PCR	PCR		race, cancer histology, family history of cancer	54.3%
Perrett et al., 1995 (UK)	136 pituitary tumours histolog. confirmed (Caucas.)	p53 mutations by immunohistochemical analysis	PCR		race	54.0%
Rebbeck et al., 1996 (USA)	28 prev. ductal breast cancer histolog. confirmed (Caucas.?)	loss of heterozygosity (LOH) in tumour tissue	PCR		gender	46.0%

Reference	Subjects	Assay	Technique	Exposure	Confounders	%
Romkes et al., 1996 (UK)	93 transitional cell bladder carcinoma histolog. confirmed (Caucas.?)	p53 and Rb mutations in tumour tissue by immunohistochemistry	PCR		cancer histology, tumour grade	60.9%
Rothman et al., 1996 (India)	30 workers exp. to benzidine (15 benzidine dye workers and 15 benzidine production workers), 15 unexp. subjects (Caucas.)	Ames assay in Salmonella typhimurium YG1024 strain (number of revertant colonies per 100 ml urine); 32P-postlabelling assay of benzidine-DNA adducts in exfoliated urothelial cells	PCR	occupation (exp. to benzidine)	race	
Rothman et al., 1995 (USA)	47 nonsmoking fire-fighters (mixed)	PAH-DNA adducts in WBC by ELISA	PCR	alcohol (drinks per week)	race, age, gender, season of blood collection, CYP1A1 polym.	59.6%
Ryberg et al., 1994a (Norway, UK)	63 primary non-SC lung cancer patients (Caucas.)	32P-postlabelling assay of PAH-DNA adducts in normal lung tissue	PCR		gender, race	50%
Ryberg et al., 1994b (Norway)	108 previously untreated non-SC lung cancers (Caucas.)	p53 mutations by PCR	PCR	smoking (non-smokers, light and heavy smokers)	race	51.0%
Sarhanis et al., 1996 (UK)	64 epithelial ovarian cancer histolog. confirmed, 20 hosp. controls (Caucas.)	p53 mutations by immunohistochemical analysis (monoclonal antibody DO-7)	PCR		race, cancer histology, stage and grade, gender, GSTT1 and CYP2D6 polym.	61.5%
Scarpato et al., 1996 (Italy)	23 floriculturists occup. exp. to pesticides; 22 bank clerks matched by gender, age and smoking (Caucas.)	SCE, CA and MN in lymphocytes	PCR	smoking, occupation	GSTT1 and NAT2 polym., race, age, gender	
Scarpato et al., 1997 (Italy, Finland)	30 floriculturists occup. exp. to pesticides; 32 bank clerks matched by gender, age and smoking (Caucas.)	CA in lymphocytes	PCR	smoking, occupation (exposure to pesticides)	GSTT1 polym., age, race, gender	58.1%
Shields et al., 1993a (USA)	38 cancer-free autopsy donors (12 Afro-Amer., 26 Caucas.)	32P-postlabelling assay of PAH-DNA adducts in parenchymal lung tissue	PCR	smoking (serum cotinine levels) for 30 cases	age, gender, race	47% (mixed)
Sorsa et al., 1996 (Finland, Portugal, Czech Republic)	53 workers exp. to butadiene, 46 unexp. subjects (Caucas.)	SCE, MN and CA in lymphocytes	PCR	occupation (exp. to butadiene)	race	57.6%
To-Figueras et al., 1996 (Spain)	139 histolog. confirmed lung cancers (Caucas.)	p53 Pro/Arg mutation in codon 72 by PCR	PCR	smoking (<50 PY, >50 PY)	race, age (<59, >59 yrs), cancer histology	45.6%
Topinka et al., 1997 (Czech Republic)	98 non-smoking pregnant women (Caucas.)	32P-postlabelling assay of total-DNA adducts in placental tissue	PCR		race, gender, sampling season, residence (low, high air pollution area)	48.0%
Uuskula et al., 1995 (Finland)	12 healthy volunteers current non-smokers (Caucas.)	SCE induction by SO and MEB in cultured lymphocytes	PCR	styrene-7,8-oxide (SO); 1,2-epoxy-3-butene (MEB)	race, gender, replication rate	45.5%
van Poppel et al., 1993 (Netherlands)	healthy male volunteers: 154 smokers > 15 cig./day for > 2 yrs, 38 non-smokers (Caucas.)	MN in smokers' sputum epithelial cells (count in 3000 cells);	immunoassay (ELISA)	smoking (light, heavy smokers, non-smokers; cig./day, yrs of smoking; plasma cotinine levels)	age, race, gender, BMI, culturing day, observer variation)	45%

Table 2 (Contd). Study design: GSTM1 and outcomes other than cancer

Author	Subjects	Analysis	Phenotyping/ genotyping	Exposures	Covariates	GSTM1null (%)
van Poppel et. al., 1992 (Netherlands)	healthy male volunteers: 155 smokers > 15 cig./day for > 2 yrs, 66 non-smokers (Caucas.)	SCE in lymphocytes	immunoassay (ELISA)	smoking (light, heavy smokers, non-smokers; plasma cotinine levels)	age, race, gender, BMI	45%
Wang et al., 1997 (Japan)	104 healthy male workers employed in a food products factory (Asians)	32P-postlabelling assay of PAH-DNA adducts in lymphocytes	PCR	smoking (smokers, non-smokers)	race, gender, serum levels of β-carotene and α-tocopherol	
Wiencke et al., 1990 (USA)	45 healthy volunteers (Caucas.?)	SCE in cultured lymphocytes untreated or treated with TSO	TSO conjugation in lymphocytes			47.0%
Yu et. al., 1995a (USA)	151 male healthy volunteers (mixed)	aminobiphenyl-haemoglobin adduct levels	PCR	smoking (smokers, non-smokers)	race, gender	57% (Caucas.) 23% (Afric.-Americ.) 32% (Asians)

Table 3. Results: GSTM1 and lung cancer (case-case studies shaded grey)

Author	OR - lung cancer (GSTM1null/non-null)	OR - stratified by ethnicity (GSTM1null/non-null)	OR - stratified by smoking (GSTM1null/non-null)	OR - stratified by cancer histology (GSTM1null/non-null)	OR - (interactions between polym.)	Other comments
Seidegard et al., 1986 and 1990 (USA)			2.42 (1.60-3.65), 3.52 (2.0-6.22) <65 yrs, 1.57 (0.85-2.87) >65 yrs, 2.14 (1.30-3.54) males, 3.10 (1.50-6.39) females (smokers)	1.81 (1.02-3.24) SQ, 4.2 (1.00-24.70) SC, 3.25 (1.92-5.51) AD		
Zhong et al., 1991 (UK)	1.05 (0.72-1.53)			1.51 (0.94-2.42) SQ, 0.56 (0.29-1.05) AD, 1.00 (0.58-1.7) others		
Hayashi et al., 1992 (Japan)	1.44 (1.02-2.02)			2.19 (1.27-3.77) SQ, 1.05 (0.67-1.65) AD, 1.87 (1.22-2.87) Kreyberg I	5.83 (2.38-14.28); 9.07 (2.95-27.93) SQ; 3.45 (1.04-11.49) AD; 7.94 (2.99-21.08) Kreyberg I (GSTM1null/Exon7 MM vs. GSTM1+/Exon7 WW)	
Heckbert et al., 1992 (USA)	1.29 (0.7-2.4)		1.98 (0.96-4.11) >20 PY			
Nakachi et al., 1993 (Japan)			1.77 (0.99-3.16) smokers, 1.31 (0.59-2.92) <44 PY, 2.48 (1.06-5.81) >44 PY	1.61 (0.95-2.74) SQ	23.20 (5.15-104.85) <44 PY, 1.82 (0.30-11.02) >44 PY (GSTM1null/MspI MM vs. GSTM1+/MspI WW+WM), 20.67 (3.60-118.50) <44 PY, 1.83 (0.15-21.64) >44 PY (GSTM1null/Exon7 MM vs. GSTM1+/Exon7 WW+WM)	
Brockmöller et al., 1993 (Germany)	1.00 (0.62-1.62), 1.1 (0.6-1.99) male, 1.01 (0.42-2.44) female, 0.96 (0.53-1.74) < 70 yrs, 1.10 (0.48-2.52) > 70 yrs		0.75 (0.11-5.11) non-smokers, 0.98 (0.59-1.65) smokers, 0.51 (0.16-1.62) 1-20 PY, 1.16 (0.65-2.06) >20 PY	1.19 (0.39-3.58) SC, 1.26 (0.63-2.52) SQ, 0.89 (0.42-1.91) AD		
Nazar-Stewart et al., 1993 (USA)			3.32 (1.26-8.73)			
Hirvonen et al., 1993a (Finland)	1.44 (0.92-2.25) vs. all controls, 1.45 (0.90-2.32) vs. healthy controls, 1.40 (0.67-2.94) vs. hosp. controls		1.38 (0.58-3.32) smokers, 0.83 (0.28-2.46) <40 PY, 3.96 (0.74-21.3) >40 PY	2.10 (1.17-3.77) SQ, 0.77 (0.40-1.48) AD, 2.15 (0.66-7.57) others (vs. healthy controls); 2.04 (0.90-4.60) SQ, 0.74 (0.31-1.77) AD, 2.08 (0.62-6.96) others (vs. hosp. controls)		

Table 3 (Contd). Results: GSTM1 and lung cancer (case–case studies shaded grey)

Author	OR - lung cancer (GSTM1null/non-null)	OR - stratified by ethnicity (GSTM1null/non-null)	OR - stratified by smoking (GSTM1null/non-null)	OR - stratified by cancer histology (GSTM1null/non-null)	OR - (interactions between polym.)	Other comments
Alexandrie et al., 1994 (Sweden)	1.15 (0.85-1.56), 1.12 (0.82-1.54) vs. healthy controls, 1.29 (0.79-2.12) vs. hosp. controls			0.80 (0.40-1.59) SQ, 2.3 (1.01-5.43) SC, 1.52 (0.80-2.87) AD (vs. healthy controls)	1.23 (0.69-2.19); 1.14 (0.54-2.41) SQ; 1.55 (0.56-4.25) SC; 1.20 (0.48-3.04)AD (GSTM1null/Mspl MM+WM vs. GSTM1+/Mspl WW)	
Kihara et al., 1994 (Japan)			1.86 (1.24-2.81), 1.16 (0.57-2.35) S.I.<800, 1.86 (0.82-4.18) S.I.800-1200, 2.10 (0.73-6.04) S.I.>1200 (cig./day x yrs of smoking); 1.69 (1.06-2.67) males, 5.01 (1.38-22.44) females	2.13 (1.17-3.89)SQ, 2.07 (1.01-4.24) SC, 1.44 (0.83-2.48) AD; 3.32 (1.31-8.39) Kreyberg I, males, smokers S.I.>1200 (cig./day x yrs of smoking)		
Ryberg et al., 1994a (Norway, UK)	1.52 (0.74-3.10) non-SC					no significant difference of GSTM1null frequency in high vs. low DNA-adducts group (p=0.10)
Anttila et al., 1994 (Finland)	non-significant association between GSTM1 polym. and cancer histology (p=0.26) or tumour location (p=0.34) (WM+MM/WW)				almost significant association between GSTM1 polym. and cancer histology among CYP1A1 inducible polym. (p=0.064); significant association between GSTM1 positive polym. and peripheral tumour location among CYP1A1 inducible polym. (p=0.037)	
Cheng et al., 1995c (USA)	1.09 (0.58-2.08)		4.38 (0.53-53.23) never smokers, 0.74 (0.28-1.91) former smokers, 0.79 (0.16-3.77) current smokers, 0.76 (0.37-1.58) current + former smokers			
Kihara et al., 1995a (Japan)	1.34 (1.03-1.74); 1.21 (0.89-1.65) males; 1.68 (1.03-2.72) females; 1.51 (1.12-2.02) <70 yrs; 0.85 (0.41-1.77) >70 yrs		1.00 (0.63-1.60) non-smokers; 1.45 (0.97-2.16) smokers; 1.45 (0.81-2.59) S.I. <800; 1.78 (0.89-3.59) 800 < S.I. <1200; 1.80 (0.80-4.07) S.I. >1200; 1.96 (1.16-3.31) S.I.>800, 2.17 (0.89-5.27) SQ + SC smokers, 1.82 (1.02-3.24) SQ + SC, S.I. >800	1.41 (0.96-2.06) SQ, 1.81 (1.06-3.08) SC, 1.22 (0.88-1.69) AD, 1.52 (1.09-2.12) SQ + SC, 7.28 (1.53-68.34) SQ, female, 9.71 (1.24-435.33) SC, female, 8.09 (2.25-43.71) SC + SQ, female		

Reference					
London et al., 1995a (USA)	1.29 (0.94-1.77), 0.94 (0.56-1.56) female, 1.55 (1.04-2.32) male, 1.03 (0.68-1.55) no exp. to asbestos, 1.89 (1.03-3.46) possible exp. to asbestos, 1.51 (0.55-4.15) probable exp. to asbestos (adjusted for age, ethnicity, gender and smoking history)	1.20 (0.72-2.00) Afric-Americ., 1.37 (0.91-2.06) Caucas. (adjusted for age, gender and smoking history)	1.23 (0.40-3.73) never smokers, 1.46 (0.89-2.38) former smokers, 1.12 (0.71-1.76) current smokers, 1.77 (1.11-2.82) <40 PY, 0.90 (0.56-1.44) >40 PY (adjusted for age, ethnicity and gender)	4.06 (1.77-9.31) SQ <40 PY, 0.59 (0.27-1.27) SQ >40 PY, 1.33 (0.45-3.87) SC <40 PY, 0.90 (0.36-2.23) SC >40 PY, 1.33 (0.67-2.65) AD <40 PY, 1.28 (0.67-2.44) AD >40 PY (adjusted for age, ethnicity and gender)	no significant association of GSTM1 polym. with β-carotene, vit. C or vit. E intake;
Kihara et al., 1995b (Japan)		1.41 (0.86-2.32) male smokers	1.36 (0.76-2.43) SQ smokers, 1.51 (0.73-3.11) SC smokers (male)	1.95 (0.82-4.61) (GSTM1 null/Mspl MM vs. GSTM1+/Mspl WM+WW)	
Antilla et al., 1995 (Finland)	almost significant excess of GSTM1null in cases with definite/probable or possible exp. to asbestos vs. cases with unlikely exp. (p=0.095)			significantly higher GSTM3 expression in GSTM1+ vs. GSTM1null in all cases (p<0.001), in smokers (p<0.001) and in recent ex-smokers (p=0.004)	
Deakin et al., 1996 (UK)		0.74 (0.44-1.24)		no significant interaction between GSTM1 and GSTT1 polym.	
To-Figueras et al., 1996 (Spain)	1.57 (0.99-2.51), 1.33 (0.76-2.35) <59 yrs, 1.88 (1.04-3.39) >59 yrs	1.56 (1.04-2.35) smokers, 1.77 (1.01-3.10) <50 PY, 1.36 (0.75-2.46) >50 PY	1.55 (0.80-3.03) SQ, 1.93 (0.90-4.14) AD, 1.89 (0.97-3.65) SC, 2.84 (1.17-6.89) SC <50 PY, 1.19 (0.49-2.93) SC >50 PY, 1.55 (0.64-3.76) SC <59 yrs, 2.26 (0.94-5.39) SC >59 yrs		
Baranov et al., 1996 (Russia)	6.74 (2.97-15.30)				
Moreira et al., 1996 (Portugal)	0.71 (0.40-1.28)		0.55 (0.27-1.11) SQ, 1.06 (0.44-2.56) AD, 0.82 (0.30-2.22) SC		significantly lower frequency of GSTM1 B in controls vs. cases (p=0.038)

Table 3 (Contd). Results: GSTM1 and lung cancer (case-case studies shaded grey)

Author	OR - lung cancer (GSTM1null/non-null)	OR - stratified by ethnicity (GSTM1null/non-null)	OR - stratified by smoking (GSTM1null/non-null)	OR - stratified by cancer histology (GSTM1null/non-null)	OR - (interactions between polym.)	Other comments
Ge et al, 1996 (Hong Kong)	1.01 (0.49-2.07) vs. all controls, 1.11 (0.44-2.80) vs. healthy controls, 0.93 (0.38-2.31) vs. hosp. controls					no significant association of GSTM1 polym. with age, gender, lymph node metastasis, smoking history, cancer histology and tumour size; significant higher survival rate in GSTM1null vs. non-null cases at 16-24 months post-operation (p<0.05)
Goto et al, 1996 (Japan)	significantly higher proportion of GSTM1 null polym. in cases characterized by non operability (p=0.037), worse performance status (p=0.025), high categories of N-factor (p=0.024) and tumor stage (p=0.032)				significantly lower survival time in GSTM null / MspI WM+MM vs. GSTM1+ / MspI WW (p=0.017)	
El-Zein et al. 1997 (USA)			0.87 (0.39-1.91) smokers	0.82 (0.29-2.27) SQ smokers, 0.74 (0.28-1.95) AD smokers		

424

Table 4. Results: GSTM1 and bladder cancer

Author	OR - bladder cancer (GSTM1null/non-null)	OR - stratified by ethnicity (GSTM1null/non-null)	OR - stratified by smoking (GSTM1null/non-null)	OR - stratified by cancer histology (GSTM1null/non-null)	OR - (interactions between polym.)	Other comments
Bell et al., 1993 (USA)		1.61 (1.16-2.23) all cases, 2.40 (1.08-5.34) incid. cases, 1.56 (1.10-2.20) prev. cases (Caucas.); 1.86 (0.67-5.19) Afric.-Americ. (vs. all controls)	1.85 (1.15-2.96) smokers, 1.27 (0.58-2.74) non-smokers (Caucas.)	1.83 (1.35-2.48) vs. all controls, 1.7 (1.2-2.5) vs. all controls (adjusted for ethnicity), 1.68 (1.15-2.46) vs. hosp. controls, 1.88 (1.36-2.59) vs. healthy controls (TCC)		no significant association between GSTM1 polym. and tumour grade (p=0.11)
Lafuente et al., 1993 (Spain)			2.41 (1.25-4.67) TCC			no significant difference of GSTM1null frequency in heavy vs. light smokers (p=0.30) cases, early vs. late age at diagnosis (p=0.66), tumour penetration (p=0.60) and grade (p=0.18)
Daly et al., 1993 (UK)				4.35 (1.88-10.10) vs all controls, 3.81 (1.50-9.70) vs. hosp. controls, 4.90 (1.97-12.20) vs. healthy controls (TCC)		
Zhong et al., 1993 (UK)	0.94 (0.58-1.52)					
Brockmöller et al., 1994 (Germany)	1.4 (1.04-1.90) crude, 1.54 (1.12-2.13) adjusted for age and gender, 2.43 (1.26-4.71) 55-65 yrs, 1.96 (1.17-3.26) >65 yrs, 1.30 (0.87-1.94) males, 1.50 (1.03-2.19) males, 1.26 (0.74-2.12) females, 1.44 (0.77-2.77) occup. exp. to bladder carcino., 1.39 (0.95-2.06) occup. not exp.		1.96 (0.96-3.99) non-smokers, 1.30 (0.92-1.85) smokers, 1.10 (0.69-1.74) >20 PY, 1.35 (0.70-2.59) <20 PY	1.38 (1.02-1.88) TCC, 1.78 (0.65-4.90) other histologies		no significant association of GSTM1null frequency with tumour aggressivity (p=0.65), tumour grade (p=0.32) and stage (p=0.10)
Lin et al., 1994 (USA)	1.29 (0.88-1.91)	1.45 (0.92-2.29) Caucas., 1.11 (0.31-4.01) Afric.-Americ. 4.75 (0.52-225.89) Asians				
Katoh et al., 1995 (Japan)				2.15 (1.19-3.89) TCC		

Table 4 (Contd). Results: GSTM1 and bladder cancer

Author	OR - bladder cancer (GSTM1null/non-null)	OR - stratified by ethnicity (GSTM1null/non-null)	OR - stratified by smoking (GSTM1null/non-null)	OR - stratified by cancer histology (GSTM1null/non-null)	OR - (interactions between polym.)	Other comments
Anwar et al., 1996 (Egypt)	6.97 (1.34-45.69)				no significant interaction between GSTM1 and CYP2E1 polym.; 8.4 (1.26-56.03) (2D6WW+WM/GSTM1null vs. 2D6MM/GSTM1+)	
Rothman et al., 1996a (China, USA)	1.00 (0.41-2.45) all, 0.67 (0.15-3.05) low exp., 1.04 (0.13-8.61) medium exp., 3.33 (0.16-61.70) high exp. to benzidine				no significant interaction with NAT2 polym. in determining bladder cancer risk	the effects of smoking and residence have been evaluated as confounders, not as effect modifiers
Brockmöller et al., 1996a (Germany)	1.29 (0.97-1.72); 1.6 (1.1-2.3) adjusted for age, gender, smoking and occupation		lack of increasing risk linked to GSTM1null with increasing exposure to tobacco smoking		significant interaction with NAT2 polym. (p=0.007); no significant interaction with GSTT1, CYP2E1, CYP1A1 or CYP2D6 polym.	1.9 (1.2-3.2) in cases lacking A allele compared to controls (adjusted for age, gender, smoking and occupation); no significant association of GSTM1 polym. with cancer histology, stage and grade
Kempkes et al., 1996 (Germany)	1.81 (1.10-2.98)					no significant difference of GSTM1null frequency in smokers (current + former) vs. non-smokers (p=0.40) cases
Okkels et al., 1996 & 1997 (Denmark)	1.15 (0.79-1.69) all cases, 0.82 (0.50-1.37) incid. cases, 1.44 (0.93-2.23) prev. cases (adjusted for age, gender and smoking)		non-significant association of GSTM1null with cancer risk among smokers		1.51 (0.89-2.55) NAT2slow/GSTM1null vs. NAT2rapid/GSTM1+	

Table 5. Results: GSTM1 and other cancers (case-case studies shaded grey).

Author	OR - breast cancer (GSTM1null/non-null)	OR - stratified by ethnicity	OR - stratified by smoking	OR - (interactions between polym.)	Other comments
Harada et al., 1992 (Japan)	1.21 (0.63-2.31)				
Zhong et al., 1993 (UK)	1.27 (0.87-1.87)				
Ambrosone et al., 1995 (USA)	1.10 (0.73-1.64), 2.53 (1.10-5.84) <58 yrs, 1.43 (0.82-2.48) <64 yrs, 1.06 (0.61-1.84) >64 yrs		1.09 (0.61-1.98) non-smokers, 0.82 (0.31-2.16) smokers <29 PY, 1.08 (0.43-2.72) smokers >29 PY (adjusted for age, education, BMI, family history of breast cancer)	1.69 (0.82-3.48) (Exon7 WM+MM/GSTM1null vs. Exon7 WW/GSTM1+)	
Fontana et al., 1997 (France)	significant association of GSTM1null with age <55 yrs (p=0.01), with tumour grade III (p=0.02) and with levels of cytosolic cathepsin >40 pmol/mg (p=0.03)				

Author	OR - digestive cancer (GSTM1null/non-null)	OR - stratified by ethnicity	OR - stratified by smoking	OR - (interactions between polym.)	Other comments
Strange et al., 1991 (UK)	2.32 (0.88-6.14) colon AD, 4.06 (1.13-16.45) stomach AD, 2.90 (1.25-6.73) colon-stomach AD				no significant association between GSTM1 polym. and tumour stage
Harada et al., 1992 (Japan)	3.08 (0.92-10.86) stomach, 1.61 (0.70-3.67) HCC				
Zhong et al., 1993 (UK)	1.78 (1.21-2.62) colon, 1.66 (1.04-2.66) distal colon, 3.38 (1.91-6.00) proximal colon				
McGlynn et al., 1995 (USA, China)	1.9 (0.94-3.63) HCC			1.86 (0.38-9.10) (GSTM1null/2E1 WW vs. GSTM1+/2E1 WM+MM)	no significant association of GSTM1 polym. with age at diagnosis (p=0.31), gender, tumour stage and differentiation (p>0.10); significant association with L-myc genotype among cases (p=0.015)
Chenevix-Trench et al., 1995 (Australia)	0.92 (0.59-1.43) colorectal, 0.87 (0.42-1.80) proximal tumours, 0.94 (0.58-1.53) distal tumours				
Yu et al., 1995b (Taiwan, USA)	0.7 (0.3-1.5) HCC		0.8 (0.3-2.3) non-smokers, 0.5 (0.2-1.8) smokers		
Lin et al., 1995 (USA)	0.85 (0.65-1.10) colon	0.98 (0.69-1.40) Caucas., 0.84 (0.43-1.66) Hispanics, 0.61 (0.26-1.44) Afric.-Americ., 0.43 (0.16-1.14) Asians			no significant association of GSTM1 polym. with smoking (p=0.27) and tumour size

Table 5 (Contd). Results: GSTM1 and other cancers (case-case studies shaded grey)

Author	OR - digestive cancer (GSTM1null/non-null)	OR - stratified by ethnicity	OR - stratified by smoking	OR - (interactions between polym.)	Other comments
Deakin et al., 1996 (UK)	1.6 (0.53-1.92) oral SQ, 0.93 (0.64-1.35) gastric, 0.95 (0.71-1.28) colorectal, 1.16 (0.75-1.81) rectal, 0.90 (0.62-1.29) proximal colon				
Kato et al., 1996 (Japan)	0.88 (0.48-1.62) stomach AD, 0.55 (0.25-1.19) males, 1.77 (0.63-5.00) females; 1.26 (0.55-2.90) adjusted for age, gender, pepsinogen I levels, pepsinogen I/II ratios, H. pylori IgG, L-myc and CYP2E1 polym.				
Baranov et al., 1996 (Russia)	2.91 (1.26-6.71) stomach + colon				
Katoh et al., 1996 (Japan, USA)	1.70 (1.05-2.76) stomach AD, 1.53 (0.91-2.60) colorectal, 1.19 (0.61-2.31) proximal tumours, 2.03 (1.06-3.89) distal tumours		1.90 (0.88-4.09) non-smokers, 5.76 (1.18-28.3) smokers <40 PY, 1.24 (0.59-2.61) smokers >40 PY stomach AD, no significant higher frequency of GSTM1null in colorectal cases vs. controls, stratified by smoking history	1.89 (0.95-3.77) stomach AD, 1.74 (0.86-3.55) colorectal cancer (GSTM1null/GSTT1null vs. GSTM1+/GSTT1+)	no significantly higher frequency of GSTM1null in gastric cases <50 yrs than older cases (p=0.22); no significant association with tumour differentiation
Chen et al., 1996 (USA)	0.5 (0.3-0.9) anal cancer, 0.4 (0.1-1.1) male, 0.6 (0.3-1.1) female, 0.7 (0.3-1.6) <50 yrs, 0.4 (0.2-0.9) >50 yrs (adjusted for age and gender)		1.6 (0.3-3.3) non-smokers, 0.4 (0.2-1.2) former smokers, 0.5 (0.2-1.1) current smokers (adjusted for age and gender)		
Chen et al., 1996 (Taiwan)	0.79 (0.34-1.82) HCC, 0.35 (0.10-1.22) undetectable AFB1-adducts, 1.43 (0.34-6.08) low AFB1-adducts, 3.00 (0.16-63.73) high AFB1-adducts				the effects of smoking and alcohol drinking have been evaluated as confounders, not as effect modifiers
Hsieh et al., 1996 (Taiwan)	1.04 (0.51-2.12) HCC				
Guo et al., 1996 (China)	1.65 (0.36-7.60) colon cancer				
Morita et al., 1997 (Japan)	1.6 (0.6-2.0) oesophageal cancer, 1.4 (0.6-3.1) male drinkers		1.6 (0.6-3.9) males smokers	significant interactions between Exon7, CYP2E1 and GSTM1 polym.	

Author	OR - other cancers (GSTM1null/non-null)	OR - stratified by ethnicity	OR - stratified by smoking	OR - (interactions between polym.)	Other comments
Fryer et al., 1993 (UK)	1.77 (1.07-2.93) all adenomas, 2.56 (1.27-5.18) prolactinoma, 2.03 (0.88-4.68) corticotrophinoma, 1.46 (0.72-2.96) somatotrophinoma, 1.41 (0.74-2.70) non-functional adenoma				
Latuente et al., 1993 (Spain)			2.46 (1.28-4.70) larynx cancer		no significant difference of GSTM1null frequency in heavy vs. light smokers (p=0.11) cases, early vs. late age at diagnosis (p=0.42) and grade (p=0.06); significant difference in tumour penetration (p=0.01)
Heagerty et al., 1994 (UK) (all BCC are included also in Heagerty et al., 1996)	1.06 (0.73-1.53) all BCC, 1.08 (0.63-1.83) multiple BCC, 1.00 (0.56-1.79) melanoma, 0.76 (0.44-1.29) SQ, 2.31 (1.12-4.73) multiple cancers with any histology, 2.15 (0.90-5.23) multiple BCC-SQ				
Warwick et al., 1994a (UK)	0.77 (0.45-1.32) SQ, 0.79 (0.52-1.20) CIN, 0.60 (0.36-0.99) low-grade CIN, 1.05 (0.62-1.77) high-grade CIN			1.60 (0.43-6.78) low-gr. CIN, 0.44 (0.07-2.87) high-gr. CIN, 0.34 (0.10-1.13) SQ (non-smokers); 2.22 (0.69-7.94) low-gr. CIN, 1.92 (0.71-5.37) high-gr. CIN, 2.17 (0.61-8.97) SQ (smokers) (2D6 WW / GSTM1null vs. 2D6 MM+WM / GSTM1+)	
Hall et al., 1994 (UK)	ALL (acute lymphoblastic leukaemia); significantly lower survival in GSTM1+ vs. GSTM1null (p=0.01)				
Latuente et al., 1995 (Spain)	1.99 (1.56-2.41) malignant melanoma, 1.96 (1.35-2.56) male, 2.1 (1.45-2.74) female				no significant association of GSTM1 polym. with skin type, age at diagnosis or smoking among cases
Shanley et al., 1995 (Australia)	1.05 (0.67-1.64) malignant melanoma, 1.82 (0.70-4.75) multiple melanoma, 1.05 (0.59-1.85) NBCCS				no significant association of GSTM1 polym. with age at onset for NBCCS (p=1.0) or melanoma (p=0.31)
Trizna et al., 1995 (USA)	2.37 (1.20-4.67) oral, pharyngeal and laryngeal SQ				
Elexpuru-Camiruaga et al., 1995 (UK)	1.23 (0.81-1.86) astrocytoma, 1.24 (0.79-1.93) low-grade astrocyt., 1.19 (0.45-3.16) high-grade astrocyt., 1.02 (0.57-1.83) meningioma			no significant interaction between GSTM1 and GSTT1 or CYP2D6 polym.	

Table 5 (Contd). Results: GSTM1 and other cancers (case-case studies shaded grey)

Author	OR - other cancers (GSTM1null/non-null)	OR - stratified by ethnicity	OR - stratified by smoking	OR - (interactions between polym.)	Other comments
Hirvonen et al., 1995 (Finland)	1.84 (0.96-3.54) all, 1.42 (0.57-3.53) low/moderate exp. to asbestos, 2.32 (0.96-5.60) high exp. to asbestos (mesothelioma)			3.59 (1.35-9.58) all, 1.70 (0.46-6.31) low/moderate exp. to asbestos, 7.37 (1.60-33.98) high exp. to asbestos (GSTM1null/NAT2slow vs. GSTM1+/NAT2rapid)	no significant difference in GSTM1null frequency in cases compared to controls in different age groups and smoking categories
Chen et al., 1996 (USA)	0.8 (0.5-1.3) all MDS, 0.5 (0.2-1.5) non-aggressive MDS (RA/RAS), 1.0 (0.5-1.7) aggressive MDS (RAEB/RAEB-t)				
Yengi et al., 1996 (UK)	0.99 (0.68-1.44) all BCC, 0.97 (0.59-1.59) single BCC, 1.01 (0.66-153) multiple BCC, 1.44 (1.14-1.80) multiple BCC (adjusted for age, gender and skin type)			significant interaction between GSTM1 and GSTM3 polym. on the number of tumours (p<0.001)	
Jahnke et al., 1996 (Germany)	1.19 (0.83-1.70) laryngeal SQ				
Heagerty et al., 1996 (UK)	0.97 (0.78-121), 0.76 (0.51-1.14) male, 1.03 (0.67-157) female (all BCC); 0.90 (0.70-1.16), 0.63 (0.41-0.98) male, 1.07 (0.68-1.68) female (single BCC); 1.11 (0.82-1.50), 1.02 (0.63-1.65) male, 0.94 (0.55-1.62) female (multiple BCC)		no significant association between GSTM1null and BCC in smokers	no significant interaction with GSTT1 and CYP2D6 polym.	significantly lower frequency of GSTM1 AB in cases vs. controls (p=0.02); no significant association of GSTM1null with tumour stage, grade or location
Sarhanis et al., 1996 (UK)	0.79 (0.35-1.80) epithelial ovarian cancer				significantly lower frequency of AB genotype in multiple BCC compared to controls (p=0.048)

Reference			
Lear et al., 1996 (UK)	significant interaction between GSTM1 polym. and skin type 1 in determining an increased number of BCC: p<0.001, (adjusted by age); almost significant association of GSTM1null and BCC rate (p=0.067)		no significant interactions between GSTM1 and other polym. in determining an increased number of BCC and BCC rate
Wrigley et al., 1996 (UK)	no significant correlation of GSTM1 activity with response to treatment, progression-free, survival or clinico-patholog. parameters		
Kihara et al., 1997 (Japan)	1.29 (0.90-1.86) head and neck cancer	1.39 (0.90-2.15) smokers, 1.32 (0.84-2.08) male smokers, 2.50 (0.52-11.93) female smokers, 0.97 (0.45-2.10) non-smokers (head and neck cancer); 0.98 (0.54-1.79) smokers, 3.89 (1.06-14.32) smokers <60 yrs, 0.62 (0.31-1.26) smokers >60 yrs (laryngeal cancer); 1.78 (1.05-3.04) smokers, 1.91 (0.85-4.32) smokers <60 yrs, 1.71 (0.90-3.25) smokers >60 yrs (non-laryngeal cancer)	
Esteller et al., 1997 (Spain)	2.01 (1.02-3.97) endometrial cancer		
Chen et al., 1997 (USA)	2.18 (1.57-3.02) ALL (acute lymphoblastic leukaemia)	1.07 (0.71-1.61) all, 1.04 (0.59-1.83) males, 1.10 (0.61-2.01) females (Caucas.); 1.84 (0.87-3.89) all, 2.90 (1.11-7.56) males, 1.02 (0.28-3.62) females (Afric.-Americ.)	significantly higher proportion of GSTM1null/GSTT1null in ALL cases vs. controls among Afric.-Americ. (p=0.0005), but not among Caucas. (p=0.68)
Lear et al., 1997 (UK)	no significant association between GSTM1 polym. and presence of truncal BCC	no significant interactions with CYP1A1, CYP2D6, GSTT1 or GSTM3 polym.	no significant association of GSTM1 or combined GSTM1/GSTT1 polym. with survival

Table 6. Results: GSTM1 and outcomes other than cancer

Author	SCE (GSTM1null/non-null)	MN and CA (GSTM1null/non-null)	Mutagenicity (GSTM1null/non-null)	DNA adducts (GSTM1null/non-null)	Hb and albumin adducts (GSTM1null/non-null)	OR - (interactions between polym.)	Other comments
Wiencke et al., 1990 (USA)	non-significantly higher SCE frequency in untreated cells (p=0.69); significantly higher SCE frequency in cells treated with TSO (p<0.001)						
van Poppel et al., 1992 (Netherlands)	4.67/4.65, p=0.79 (non-smokers); 5.24/4.97, p=0.09 (smokers); 5.50/4.97, p=0.01 (heavy smokers: > 315 ng/ml cotinine in blood); 5.47/4.99, p=0.02 (heavy smokers; adjusted for age, BMI, smoking, cotinine levels) (SCE/cell)						
Ketterer et al., 1992 (UK)				significant inverse correlation between PAH-DNA adducts level and GSTM1 activity (rs −0.58, p=0.04)			
van Poppel et al., 1993 (Netherlands)		non-significantly lower MN frequency					
Shields et al., 1993a (USA)				significantly higher proportion of subjects with detectable PAH-DNA adducts in GSTM1null vs. GSTM1+ (p=0.038)			
Hinvonen et al., 1994 (Finland)			2527/766 in YG1024 strain, p<0.001 (smokers); 336/123 in TA98 strain, p<0.001 (smokers); 249/274 in YG1024 strain, p=0.48 (non-smokers); 37/50 in TA98 strain, p=0.27 (non-smokers) (revertants/100ml urine)				
Ichiba et al., 1994 (Sweden)		MN: (per 3000 cells) 5.5/5.4 in B-lymphocytes (p=0.40); 5.0/5.0 in T-lymphocytes (p>0.50)		0.66/0.65, p>0.50 (all); 0.77/0.77, p>0.50 (smokers); 0.54/0.62, p>0.50 (non-smokers); (per 10^8 nucleotides)			
Carstensen et al., 1993							significant correlation between DNA adducts and MN levels in T-lymphocytes (r=0.30, p=0.04)

Reference			
Ryberg et al., 1994a (Norway)		non-significantly higher level of PAH-DNA adducts in male GSTM1null vs. GSTM1+ (p=0.29)	
Grinberg-Funes et al., 1994 (USA)		non-significant difference in PAH-DNA adduct level: 4.75/4.01, p=0.50 (per 10^8 nucleotides)	
Ryberg et al., 1994b (Norway)		OR=1.73 (0.75-4.02); OR=11.33 (1.29-99.3) in heavy smokers, including only transversion mutations at the G:C base pairs (p53 mutations)	
Yu et al., 1995a (USA)	significantly higher levels of 4-ABP Hb adducts (p=0.04); almost significantly higher levels of 3-ABP Hb adducts (p=0.07)		
Uuskula et al., 1995 (Finland)			significantly higher SCE levels in lymphocytes treated with MEB 250 mM (p=0.02)
Hou et al., 1995 (Sweden)		non-significantly higher mutant frequency in hprt gene (p=0.20); significantly higher mutant frequency in hprt gene in garage workers (p=0.049)	
Perrett et al., 1995 (UK)		non-significantly lower frequency of GSTM1 null in p53 positive tumours (p=0.16)	
Kato et al., 1995a (USA)		significantly higher proportion of GSTM1 null carriers among subjects with detectable PAH-DNA adducts: OR=8.62 (1.03-100)	
Cheng et al., 1995a (USA)			significantly higher SCE frequency, p=0.05 (adjusted for age, gender, smoking and vitamin A intake)

significantly higher PAH-DNA adduct level in GSTM1null/NAT2slow vs. GSTM1+/NAT2rapid (p=0.03)

significant correlation between levels of DNA adducts and frequencies of hprt mutations (p=0.008)

Table 6. (Contd). Results: GSTM1 and outcomes other than cancer

Author	SCE (GSTM1 null/non-null)	MN and CA (GSTM1 null/non-null)	Mutagenicity (GSTM1 null/non-null)	DNA adducts (GSTM1 null/non-null)	Hb and albumin adducts (GSTM1 null/non-null)	OR - (interactions between polym.)	Other comments
McGlynn et al., 1995 (Ghana, China)			almost significantly higher frequency of p53 mutations in codon 249 (p=0.08)		significantly higher proportion of GSTM1 null carriers among subjects with AFB$_1$-albumin adducts >5 pg/mg vs. <5pg/mg; OR=3.74 (1.11-12.67)		
Bartsch et al., 1995 (Finland)			significantly greater urinary mutagenicity among smokers	non-significantly higher PAH-DNA adduct level in smokers and non-smokers, but significantly higher in ex-smokers (p<0.01)			
Rothman et al., 1995 (USA)				no significantly different PAH-DNA adduct level (p=0.45)		almost significantly higher PAH-DNA adduct level in GSTM1+/Exon7 WW vs. GSTM1 null/ Exon7 WM+MM (p=0.06)	
Cheng et al., 1995b (USA)			non-significant association between mutant frequency at hprt locus and GSTM1 polym.				
Norppa et al., 1995 (Finland)	non-significantly different SCE levels in lymphocytes treated with DEB 2 or 5 mM					no significant interaction with GSTT1 polym. in determining SCE levels	
Kawajiri et al., 1996 (Japan)			OR=1.61 (0.82-3.17) in current or ex-smokers (p53 mutations)			OR=9.24 (2.38-35.93) (MspI MM/GSTM1null vs. MspI WW/GSTM1+); OR=8.17 (1.74-38.47) (Exon7 MM/GSTM1null vs. Exon7 WW/GSTM1+) (p53 mutations)	
To-Figueras et al., 1996 (Spain)			non-significantly higher frequency of MM p53 mutation in codon 72 (p=0.63); significantly higher frequency of WM+MM: OR=1.97 (1.03-3.73)				
Nielsen et al., 1996a (Denmark)				non-significantly higher PAH-DNA adduct level (p=0.17)		no significant interaction with NAT2 polym. in determining PAH-DNA adduct level	

Reference	SCE	MN / CA	Mutations / adducts		
Sorsa et al., 1996 (Finland, Portugal, Czech Republic)	non-significant difference in SCE frequency	non-significant difference in MN frequency; significant higher CA frequency in unexp. subjects (p<0.05), but not in subjects exp. to butadiene			no significant association with tumour grade
Romkes et al., 1996 (UK)			OR=1.56 (0.65-3.74) (p53 mutations); OR=0.62 (0.22-1.76) (Rb mutations)		
Brockmöller et al., 1996b (Germany)			non-significantly different p53 mutations frequency (p=0.41); almost significant association of GSTM1 null with tranversions vs. transitions mutations (p=0.06)		
Landi S. et al., 1996 (Italy)					non-significant interaction between GSTM1 and GSTT1 polym. in determining SCE frequency
Scarpato et al., 1996 (Italy)	no correlation between SCE sensitivity to DEB and GSTM1null	non-significant difference in MN frequency (p=0.58), almost significant differences in CA frequency (p=0.058) (smokers)			non-significant interaction between GSTM1, GSTT1 and NAT2 polym. in determining SCE, MN or CA frequency
Sarhanis et al., 1996 (UK)			significant association between p53 mutations frequency and GSTM1null polym. (p=0.002)		significant association between p53 mutations frequency and GSTM1null/GSTT1null polym. (p=0.049)
Gabbani et al., 1996 (Italy)			non-significantly higher urinary mutagenicity in smokers (p=0.32)		significantly higher urinary mutagenicity in smokers GSTM1null/NAT2slow vs. GSTM1+/NAT2rapid (p<0.05)
Binkova et al., 1996 (Czech Republic)	non-significantly higher SCE frequency (p=0.24)	non-significant difference in CA frequency	significantly higher urinary levels of PAHs and their metabolites in non-smokers from a high-pollution area (p=0.037); significantly higher urinary mutagenicity in YG1041 strain in non-smokers (p=0.033)	almost significantly higher PAH-DNA adduct level (p=0.09) (adjusted by age, diet, PAH exposure and sampling period)	non-significant difference in PAH-albumin adduct level
Nielsen et al., 1996b (Denmark)			non-significant association between total-DNA adducts and GSTM1null (p=0.96)		non-significant association between PAH-albumin adducts and GSTM1null (p=0.83)

Table 6. (Contd). Results: GSTM1 and outcomes other than cancer

Author	SCE (GSTM1null/non-null)	MN and CA (GSTM1null/non-null)	Mutagenicity (GSTM1null/non-null)	DNA adducts (GSTM1null/non-null)	Hb and albumin adducts (GSTM1null/non-null)	OR - (interactions between polym.)	Other comments
Rothman et al., 1996 (India)			non-significantly higher urinary mutagenicity in benzidine dye workers (p=0.69) and benzidine production workers (p=0.28)	non-significantly higher benzidine-DNA adducts in benzidine dye workers (p=0.27) and benzidine production workers (p=0.38)			
Landi M.T. et al., 1996 (Italy)					non-significant difference in ABP-Hb adduct level (p=0.46)	non-significant interaction between GSTM1, NAT2 and CYP1A2 in determining ABP-Hb adduct level	
Rebbeck et al., 1996 (USA)			non-significantly higher LOH frequency (p=0.14)				
Bernardini et al., 1996 (Finland)	non-significantly different SCE frequency in untreated or EBD-treated lymphocytes					non-significantly different SCE frequency in untreated or EBD-treated lymphocytes between GSTM1null/GSTT1null and GSTM1+/GSTT1+ polym.	
Mooney et al., 1997 (USA)				non-significant difference in PAH-DNA adduct level (p=0.74)		no significant interaction of GSTM1 with CYP1A1 Exon7 or MspI polym. on PAH-DNA adducts level	
Hemminki et al., 1997 (Finland)				no significantly different PAH-DNA adduct level (p=0.95)			
Scarpato et al., 1997 (Italy, Finland)		non-significantly different CA frequency (p=0.13); significantly higher CA frequency in smokers (p=0.026)					
Ohshima et al., 1997 (Japan)			non-significant difference in p53 mutations frequency (p=0.15)			significantly higher CA frequency in carriers of GSTM1null/GSTT1null vs. GSTM1+/GSTT1null polym. (p=0.012)	
Topinka et al., 1997 (Czech Republic)				significantly higher total-DNA adduct level in subjects from the high pollution area (p=0.047), but not in those from the low pollution area (p=0.092)			significant inverse correlation between β-carotene plasma levels and PAH-DNA adducts (p=0.05) in subjects with GSTM1null genotype
Wang et al., 1997 (Japan)				no significant difference in PAH-DNA adduct level			

Table 7. Study design: GSTM3 (case–case study shaded grey)

Author	# of cases	# of controls	Response	Genotyping/phenotyping	Exposures	Covariates	Therapy	GSTM3 variants in controls	Power (α=0.05, OR≥2)
Anttila et al., 1995 (Finland)	100 incid. lung cancer histolog. confirmed undergoing surgery (Caucas.)			immunohisto-chemistry in lung tissue	smoking (smokers, recent and long-term ex-smokers), occupation (exp. to asbestos and mineral dusts)	GSTM1 polym., cancer histology			
Hand et al., 1996 (UK)	89 incid. high-grade astrocytoma histolog. confirmed (Caucas.)	300 hospital controls (Caucas.)	100% for cases	PCR		age, gender, cancer histology, GSTM1 and GSTT1 polym.	no radiotherapy or chemotherapy before genotyping	73.7% AA, 21.3% AB, 5.0% BB	51.2% (AA/AB+BB), 6.5% (AA+AB/BB)
Jahnke et al., 1996 (UK)	269 prev. laryngeal SQ carcinoma histolog. confirmed undergoing surgery (Caucas.)	216 healthy controls (Caucas.)		PCR	smoking (never, light, moderate, heavy); alcohol (never, light, moderate, heavy)	tumour location (glottic, supraglottic), grading, staging		66.5% AA, 27.0% AB, 6.5% BB polym.	89.7% (AA/AB+BB), 29.4% (AA+AB/BB)
Lear et al., 1997 (UK)	74 prev. BCC histolog. confirmed with at least one truncal tumour (Caucas.)	263 prev. BCC controls without truncal tumours (Caucas.)	100%	PCR		age, sex, BCC number, GSTT1, GSTM1, CYP1A1 and CYP2D6 polym.			
Nakajima et al., 1995 (Finland)	27 incid. lung cancer histolog. confirmed (Caucas.)	11 non-lung cancer controls (Caucas.)		immunoblot analysis, enzyme assay			no chemotherapy or radiotherapy before phenotyping	73% (low activity enzyme)	6.8%
Yengi et al., 1996 (UK)	286 prev. basal cell carcinoma (92 single BCC, 194 multiple BCC) histologic. confirmed (Caucas.)	300 cancer-free hospital controls (Caucas.)		PCR		age, gender, skin type, CYP1A1, CYP2D6, GSTM1 and GSTT1 polym.		73.7% AA, 21.3% AB, 5.0% BB polym.	78.1% (AA/AB+BB), 18.2% (AA+AB/BB)

Table 8. Results: GSTM3 and cancer (case-case study shaded grey)

Author	OR - cancer	OR - interactions between polymorphisms	Other comments
Nakajima et al., 1995 (Finland)	0.89 (0.05-1.52) lung cancer (low vs. high enzyme activity)		
Anttila et al., 1995 (Finland)	significantly higher GSTM3 expression in cases with definite/probable or possible vs. cases with unlikely exp. to asbestos (p = 0.04)		significantly higher GSTM3 expression in GSTM1+ vs. GSTM1null in all cases (p<0.001), in smokers (p<0.001) and in recent ex-smokers (p = 0.04)
Jahnke et al., 1996 (UK)	1.48 (1.00-2.19) larynx cancer (AA/AB+BB); 4.59 (1.49-14.16) larynx cancer, 6.90 (1.55-30.74) glottic, 2.29 (0.51-10.33) supraglottic (AA+AB/BB)		
Yengi et al., 1996 (UK)	0.95 (0.66-1.37) all BCC, 0.93 (0.62-1.39) multiple BCC (AA/AB+BB); 1.20 (0.55-2.61) all BCC, 1.99 (0.71-5.57) multiple BCC (AA+AB/BB)	significant interaction of GSTM3 AA with GSTM1 (p<0.001) and CYP1A1 Hspl polym. (PC 0.001) on the number of tumours. no significant interaction with GSTT1 or CYP2D6 polym. (adjusted for age and gender)	significant interaction of GSTM3 AA with skin type 1 on the number of tumours (p<0.001) (adjusted for age and gender)
Hand et al., 1996 (UK)	2.29 (0.51-10.21) high-grade astrocytoma (AA+AB/BB); 0.97 (0.57-1.65) (AA/AB+BB)	significantly higher risk for GSTM3 AA / GSTT1null vs. GSTM3 AB+BB/ GSTT1+ (p = 0.023); no significant interaction with GSTM1	
Lear et al., 1997 (UK)	no significant association between GSTM3 polymorph. and presence of truncal BCC	no significant interaction with CYP1A1, CYP2D6, GSTT1, GSTM1 polym.	

Table 9. Study design: GSTT1 and cancer (case–case study shaded grey)

Author	# of cases	# of controls	Response rates	Genotyping/ phenotyping	Exposures	Covariates	Therapy	GSTT1 null in controls	Power (α=0.05, OR>2)
Brockmöller et al., 1996a (Germany)	374 incid. bladder cancer histolog. confirmed (Caucas.)	373 hospital cancer-free controls (Caucas.)		PCR	smoking, occupation	age, gender, race, cancer histology, tumour stage, tumour grade, NAT2, GSTM1, CYP2D6, CYP2E1 and CYP1A1 polym.		20.8%	90.5%
Chen C.J. et al., 1996 (Taiwan)	32 incid. HCC histolog. confirmed from a cohort of HBsAg carriers (Asians)	73 healthy controls from a cohort of HBsAg carriers, matched by age, recruitment clinic and date of specimen collection (Asians)		PCR	aflatoxin (AFB1-albumin adducts level: high, low, undetectable)	smoking, alcohol, race, HBV status		51.4%	23.4%
Chen C.L. et al., 1997 (USA)	197 incid. childhood acute lymphoblastic leukaemia (ALL) histolog. confirmed (mixed)	416 healthy blood donors (mixed)		PCR		race, gender, GSTM1 polym.		15.0% (Caucas.), 24.1% (African-Americans)	92.5% all, 71.7% (Caucas.), 37.0% (African-Americans)
Chen H. et al., 1996 (USA)	92 incid. myelodisplastic syndrome (Caucas., African-Americans)	190 urology clinic patients (Caucas., African-Americans)		PCR		age (<60, >60 yrs), gender, MDS aggressivity	no therapy before genotyping	16.0%	56.4%
Chenevix-Trench et al., 1995 (Australia)	125 prev. colorectal AD histolog. confirmed (Caucas.)	94 healthy controls, 54 cancer-free geriatric patients (Caucas.)		PCR		age (<70, >70 yrs), race, gender, cancer histology, tumour stage and differentiation, L-myc, K-ras		19% (healthy controls), 9% (geriatric controls)	58.7%
Deakin et al., 1996 (UK)	108 incid. lung cancer smokers, 40 incid. SQ oral cancer, 136 incid. gastric cancer, 252 incid. colorectal cancer (Caucas.)	129 COPD smokers controls, 577 hospital controls with non-malignant diseases (Caucas.)	100% cases	PCR	smoking (smokers) for lung cancer cases and COPD controls	age (<65, >65 yrs), race, gender, GSTM1 polym.; tumour site, stage and grade for colorectal cases		14.0%	47.8% (lung), 37.7% (oral), 80.1% (gastric), 94.3% (colorectal)
Elexpuru-Camiruaga et al., 1995 (UK)	109 incid. astrocytoma, 49 incid. meningioma histologic. confirmed (Caucas.)	577 hospital cancer-free controls (Caucas.)		PCR		gender, age, race, CYP2D6 and GSTM1 polym.	no radio- or chemotherapy before genotyping	18.4%	78.2% (astrocytoma), 48.1% (meningioma)
El-Zein et al., 1997 (USA)	52 incid. lung cancer histologic. confirmed, smokers (Caucas.?)	48 healthy controls matched by smoking habit, age (5 yrs) and gender (Caucas.?)		PCR	smoking (smokers)	cancer histology	no radio- or chemotherapy before genotyping	12.5%	16.8%

Table 9 (Contd). Study design: GSTT1 and cancer (case–case study shaded grey)

Author	# of cases	# of controls	Response	Phenotyping/genotyping	Exposures	Covariates	Therapy	GSTT1 null in controls	Power (α=0.05, OR>2)
Esteller et al., 1997 (Spain)	80 incid. endometrial cancer histolog. confirmed undergoing surgery (Caucas.)	60 healthy controls from the same area (Caucas.)		PCR		race	no treatment before genotyping	20%	33.8%
Heagerty et al., 1996 (UK)	584 incid. BCC (384 single, 200 multiple) histologic. confirmed (Caucas.)	484 hospital controls (Caucas.)		PCR	smoking (never, former, current)	gender, race, skin colour, cancer histology, GSTM1 and CYP2D6 polym.		18.6%	99.7%
Jahnke et al., 1996 (UK)	269 prev. laryngeal SQ carcinoma histolog. confirmed undergoing surgery (Caucas.)	216 healthy controls (Caucas.)	100% for cases and controls	PCR		race, tumour location (glottic, supraglottic), grade and stage		12.9%	77.5%
Katoh et al., 1996 (Japan)	139 incid. gastric AD, 103 incid. colorectal AD histolog. confirmed (Asians)	126 healthy controls undergoing a general health check-up (Asians)		PCR	smoking	age, gender, race, tumor location (only for colorectal cancer), tumour grade and GSTM1 polym.		44.4%	76.2% (gastric cancer), 68.8% (colorectal cancer)
Kempkes et al., 1996 (Germany)	113 prev. bladder cancer histolog. confirmed (Caucas.)	170 newborns controls (Caucas.)		PCR	smoking (for cases only)			18%	39.7%
Lear et al., 1996 (UK)	827 incid. BCC histolog. confirmed (Caucas.)			PCR		sex, skin type, eye colour, number of BCC, BCC rate, CYP1A1, GSTM1 and CYP2D6 polym.			
Lear et al., 1997 (UK)	74 prev. BCC histolog. confirmed with at least one truncal tumour (Caucas.)	263 prev. BCC controls without truncal tumours (Caucas.)	100%	PCR		age, gender, race, cancer histology, BCC number, CYP1A1, GSTM1, GSTM3 and CYP2D6 polym.			
Sarhanis et al., 1996 (UK)	81 incid. epithelial ovarian cancer histologic. confirmed, (Caucas.)	325 hospital controls (Caucas.)		PCR		cancer histology, stage and grade, gender, CYP2D6 and GSTM1 polym.	no treatment before genotyping	18.8%	64.6%
Trizna et al., 1995 (USA)	127 SQ carcinoma of mouth, pharynx or larynx histolog. confirmed (mixed)	42 healthy controls matched by age, gender and race (mixed)		PCR				36.0%	40.5%
Warwick et al., 1994b (UK)	160 prev. cervical intraepithelial neoplasia and 68 prev. SCC histolog. confirmed (Caucas.)	167 hospital controls (Caucas.)		PCR	smoking	race, gender, CIN grade (low, high), GSTM1 and CYP2D6 polym.		16.1%	47.2% (SQ), 67.7% (CIN)

| Yengi et al., 1996 (UK) | 286 prev. basal cell carcinoma (92 single BCC, 194 multiple BCC) histologic. confirmed (Caucas.) | 300 cancer-free hospital controls (Caucas.) | PCR | | age, gender, race, skin type, CYP1A1, CYP2D6, GSTM3 and GSTM1 polym. | 19.7% | 92.7% (all BCC), 68.4% (single BCC), 85.1% (multiple BCC) |

Table 10. Study design: GSTT1 and outcomes other than cancer

Author	Subjects	Analysis	Phenotyping/ genotyping	Exposures	Covariates	GSTT1null (%)
Bernardini et al., 1996 (Finland)	22 healthy volunteers non-smokers (Caucas.)	SCE induction with EBD in cultured lymphocytes	PCR		race, GSTM1 polym.	25.0%
Brockmöller et al., 1996b (Germany)	69 bladder cancer histologic. confirmed (Caucas.)	p53 mutations by PCR	PCR		race	
Landi S. et al., 1996 (Italy)	7 healthy non-smoking volunteers (Caucas.)	SCE induction with DEB 2 mM or 5 mM in whole-blood lymphocyte cultures	PCR		race, GSTM1 polym.	
Norppa et al., 1995 (Finland)	20 healthy volunteers current non-smokers (Caucas.)	SCE in whole-blood lymphocyte cultures untreated or treated with DEB 2 μM or 5 μM	PCR	diepoxybutane (DEB)	gender, age, race, replication index, GSTM1 polym.	40.0%
Pelin et al., 1996 (Finland)	8 healthy non-smoking volunteers (Caucas.)	SCE in whole-blood and isolated lymphocyte cultures untreated or treated with DEB 2 μM or 5 μM	PCR			
Sarhanis et al., 1996 (UK)	64 epithelial ovarian cancer histolog. confirmed, 20 hospital controls (Caucas.)	p53 mutations by immunohistochemical analysis (monoclonal antibody DO-7)	PCR		race, cancer histology, tumour stage and grade, GSTM1 and CYP2D6 polym.	18.8%
Scarpato et al., 1996 (Italy, Finland)	23 floriculturists occupationally exposed to pesticides; 22 bank clerks matched by gender, age and smoking (Caucas.)	SCE, CA and MN in lymphocytes	PCR	smoking, occupation	GSTM1 polym., NAT2 polym., race, age, gender	
Scarpato et al., 1997 (Italy, Finland)	30 floriculturists occupationally exposed to pesticides; 32 bank clerks matched by gender, age and smoking (Caucas.)	CA in lymphocytes	PCR	smoking, occupation (exp. to pesticides)	GSTM1 polym., age, gender, race	14.5%
Schroeder et al., 1995 (Germany)	30 healthy volunteers (Caucas.?)	SCE in untreated lymphocytes	GSTT1 activity in RBCs	smoking		50.0%
Sorsa et al., 1996 (Finland, Portugal, Czech Republic)	53 workers exposed to butadiene, 46 unexposed subjects (Caucas.)	SCE, MN and CA in lymphocytes	PCR	occupation (exp. to butadiene)	race	17.2%
Wiencke et al., 1995 (USA)	78 healthy subjects (Caucas.?)	SCE in whole-blood lymphocyte cultures untreated or treated with DEB (diepoxybutane)	PCR	diepoxybutane (DEB)	age, gender, residence	15.4%

Table 11. – Results: GSTT1 and cancer (case–case study shaded grey)

Author	OR - other cancers (GSTT1null/non-null)	OR - interactions between polymorphisms	Other comments
Chenevix-Trench et al., 1995 (Australia)	0.86 (0.43-1.68) colorectal AD, 0.66 (0.32-1.37) vs. healthy contr., 1.54 (0.54-4.42) vs geriatric contr., 0.37 (0.08-1.68) proximal colon, 1.03 (0.51-2.10) distal colon		no significant association with gender, L-myc genotype, K-ras mutations, tumour stage and differentiation; significantly higher proportion of GSTT1null among cases >70 yrs compared to cases <70 yrs (p=0.028)
Deakin et al., 1996 (UK)	1.88 (1.30-2.72) colorectal cancer, 1.50 (0.84-2.68) right colon, 2.33 (1.28-4.24) left colon, 1.84 (1.18-2.86) colon, 1.87 (1.08-3.23) rectum, 0.59 (0.15-1.73) mouth cancer, 1.00 (0.59-1.68) gastric cancer	no significant interaction between GSTT1 and GSTM1 genotypes	
Katoh et al., 1996 (Japan, USA)	1.13 (0.70-1.83) gastric AD, 1.18 (0.70-1.99) colorectal AD	1.89 (0.95-3.77) gastric AD, 1.74 (0.86-3.55) colorectal AD (GSTM1-/GSTT1- vs. GSTM1+/GSTT1+)	non-significant increase of cancer risk in GSTT1null smoker
Chen C.J. et al., 1996 (Taiwan)	0.71 (0.29-1.71) all HCC, 0.51 (0.11-2.44) low AFB1-adducts, 3.33 (0.11-235.24) high AFB1-adducts		

Author	OR - lung cancer (GSTT1null/non-null)	OR - interactions between polymorphisms	Other comments
Deakin et al., 1996 (UK)	1.15 (0.56-2.36) smokers	no significant interaction between GSTT1 and GSTM1 genotypes	
El-Zein et al., 1997 (USA)	1.88 (0.64-5.55) 2.06 (0.55-7.66) SQ, 1.67 (0.46-6.10) AD (smokers)		

Author	OR - bladder cancer (GSTT1null/non-null)	OR - interactions between polymorphisms	Other comments
Brockmöller et al., 1996a (Germany)	1.24 (0.85-1.79), 2.6 (1.1-6.0) non-smokers	no significant interactions with GSTM1, NAT2, CYP2D6, CYP2E1 or CYP1A1 polym.	
Kempkes et al., 1996 (Germany)	1.04 (0.56-1.93)		significantly higher proportion of GSTT1non-null in smokers (current + former) vs. non-smokers cases (p=0.005)

Author	OR - other cancers (GSTT1null/non-null)	OR - interactions between polymorphisms	Other comments
Warwick et al., 1994a,b (UK)	0.76 (0.36-1.61), 1.94 (0.72-5.17) smokers (low-grade CIN); 0.88 (0.41-1.89), 1.18 (0.47-2.99) smokers (high-grade CIN); 0.77 (0.34-1.74), 1.45 (0.50-4.20) smokers(SQ)	1.35 (0.43-4.27) CIN low-grade, 2.13 (0.80-5.67) CIN high-grade, 3.31 (1.10-9.94) CIN high-grade smokers, 0.94 (0.28-3.21) SQ (GSTT1null/CYP2D6 WM+WW vs. GSTT1+/CYP2D6 MM); no significant interaction between GSTT1 and GSTM1 polym.	

Reference	OR (95% CI) / cancer type	Interactions	Conclusions
Trizna et al., 1995 (USA)	1.47 (0.71-3.02) oral, pharyngeal and laryngeal SQ		
Elexpuru-Camiruaga et al., 1995 (UK)	2.09 (1.32-3.32) astrocytoma, 2.36 (1.41-3.94) high-grade astrocytoma, 0.95 (0.27-3.37) low-grade astrocytoma, 3.58 (1.93-6.64) meningioma		
Jahnke et al., 1996 (UK)	1.77 (1.08-2.89) laryngeal SQ		no significant association of GSTM1null with tumour stage, grade or location
Sarhanis et al., 1996 (UK)	0.83 (0.28-2.49) epithelial ovarian cancer		no significant difference in risk after adjusting for age and gender
Chen H. et al., 1996 (USA)	4.3 (2.5-7.4) all myelodisplastic syndromes (MDS), 6.4 (2.6-16.0) non-aggressive MDS (RA or RAS), 4.6 (2.5-8.6) aggressive MDS (RAEB or RAEB-t)		
Heagerty et al., 1996 (UK)	0.87 (0.64-1.20) all BCC; 0.76 (0.53-1.10) single BCC; 1.09 (0.72-1.76) multiple BCC; no significant association between GSTT1null and BCC in smokers	no significant interaction with GSTM1 and CYP2D6 polym.	
Yengi et al., 1996 (UK)	1.05 (0.69-1.59) all BCC, 0.99 (0.55-1.79) single BCC, 1.08 (0.67-1.73) multiple BCC	no significant interactions with GSTM1, GSTM3, CYP2D6 or CYP1A1 polym.	
Lear et al., 1996 (UK)	non-significant association of GSTT1 polymorph. with number of BCC (adjusted by age), but significant association with BCC rate (p<0.001)	no significant interactions between GSTT1 and other polym. in determining an increased number of BCC and BCC rate	
Esteller et al., 1997 (Spain)	1.25 (0.55-2.82) endometrial cancer		
Chen C.L. et al., 1997 (USA)	0.89 (0.58-1.39) acute lymphoblastic leukemia (ALL); 0.93 (0.52-1.66), 1.09 (0.50-2.36) male, 0.76 (0.31-1.83) female (Caucas.); 1.71 (0.79-3.71), 1.53 (0.58-4.04) male, 1.88 (0.52-6.83) female (African-Americans)	significantly higher proportion of GSTM1null/GSTT1null in African-American ALL vs. African-American controls (p=0.0005); no significant association of combined GSTM1/GSTT1 poly-morph. with survival	no significant association of GSTT1 with survival
Lear et al., 1997 (UK)	1.44 (1.24-1.66) truncal BCC (adjusted for age, gender and BCC number)	3.56 (1.52-8.34) adjusted for age, gender and BCC number (Exon7 WW/GSTT1null vs. Exon7 WM+MM/GSTT1+); no significant interactions with GSTM1, GSTM3 or CYP2D6 polym.	

443

Table 12. Results: GSTT1 and outcomes other than cancer

Author	SCE (GSTT1null/non null)	MN and CA (GSTT1null/non-null)	Mutagenicity (GSTT1null/non-null)	DNA adducts (GSTT1null/non-null)	Hb and albumin adducts (GSTT1null/non-null)	OR - (interactions between polymorphisms)	Other comments
Norppa et al., 1995 (Finland)	significantly higher SCE background frequency (p=0.09), significantly higher SCE frequency in lymphocytes treated with DEB 2μM (p<0.000001) and 5 μM (p<0.000001)					no significant interaction with GSTM1 polymorphism in determining SCE levels	
Schroeder et al., 1995 (Germany)	significantly higher SCE frequency (p=0.0037) in all group and in non-smokers (p=0.046); almost significantly higher SCE frequency in smokers (p=0.086)						
Wiencke et al., 1995 (USA)	significantly higher SCE background frequency (p<0.001); significantly higher SCE frequency in lymphocytes treated with DEB (p<0.001)						
Bernardini et al., 1996 (Finland)	non-significantly different SCE frequency in untreated or EBD-treated lymphocytes					non-significantly different SCE frequency in untreated or EBD-treated lymphocytes between GSTM1-/GSTT1- and GSTM1+/GSTT1+	
Brockmöller et al., 1996b (Germany)			no significant association between p53 mutations and GSTT1 polymorph. (p=0.34)				
Landi S. et al., 1996 (Italy)	100% concordance between SCE sensitivity to DEB and GSTT1 null					non-significant interaction between GSTM1 and GSTT1 polymorphisms in determining SCE frequency	
Pelin et al., 1996 (Finland)	significantly higher DEB-induced SCE frequency (p<0.001)						
Sarhanis et al., 1996 (UK)			almost significant association between p53 mutation frequency and GSTT1null (p=0.057)			significant association between p53 mutation frequency and GSTM1null/GSTT1null (p=0.049)	

Scarpato et al., 1996 (Italy, Finland)	SCE frequency almost significantly lower in GSTT1 null vs. non-null (p=0.058)	no significant differences in MN levels (p=0.75) and CA levels (p=0.81) in GSTT1 null vs. non-null	non-significant interaction between GSTM1, GSTT1 and NAT2 polymorph. in determining SCE, MN or CA frequency
Sorsa et al., 1996 (Finland, Portugal, Czech Republic)	non-significant difference in SCE frequency	significantly higher MN and CA frequency in subjects exposed to butadiene (p<0.05), but not in unexposed subjects	
Scarpato et al., 1997 (Italy, Finland)	non-significantly different CA frequency (p=0.54, all subjects; p=0.77 smokers)	significantly higher CA frequency in carriers of GSTM1-/GSTT1- vs. GSTM1+/GSTT1- (p=0.012)	

Table 13. Study design: NAT1 and cancer

Author	# of cases	# of controls	Response	Phenotyping/ genotyping	Exposures	Covariates	Therapy	Rapid acetyl. in controls	Power (α=0.05, OR>2)
Bell et al., 1995 (USA)	202 incid. colorectal AD histolog. confirmed (Caucas.)	112 hospital cancer-free controls (Caucas.)	100% cases, 97% controls	PCR		race, cancer histology, tumour stage, NAT2 polym.		29.0%	76.4%
Okkels et al., 1997 (Denmark)	95 incid. and 159 prev. bladder cancer histolog. confirmed (Caucas.)	242 controls affected by noncancerous urinary tract diseases (Caucas.)		PCR	smoking (smokers 1-20, 21-50, >50 PY; ex-smokers for 2-9, 10-19, >19 yrs; non-smokers)	sex, age, race, cancer histology, tumour grade, GSTM1 and NAT2 polym.		44.0%	96.3%
Probst-Hensch et al., 1996 (USA)	441 incid.+ prev. colorectal adenoma histolog. confirmed undergoing sigmoidoscopy (mixed)	484 controls without current or past polyps undergoing sigmoidoscopy, matched by age, gender, clinic and date of sigmoidoscopy (mixed)	84% cases, 82% controls	PCR	smoking (never, former, current smokers)	age (5-yrs), gender, race, date of sigmoidoscopy (6-month intervals), clinic, tumour size, NAT2 polym.		20.9% (Caucas.), 50.0% (Asians), 42.6% (African-Americans), 30.5% (Hispanics)	99.9%

Table 14. Study design: NAT1 and outcomes other than cancer

Author	Subjects	Analysis	Phenotyping/ genotyping	Exposures	Covariates	Rapid acetylator (%)
Badawi et al., 1995 (USA)	26 healthy subjects (Caucas.?)	32P-postlabelling assay of aromatic -DNA adducts in normal bladder mucosa	bladder cytosol treated with PABA 0.5 μM in vitro, analysis performed by HPLC; PCR		NAT2 polym.	
Degawa et al., 1994 (USA)	25 laryngeal cancer patients (Caucas.?)	32P-postlabelling assay of total DNA adducts in normal laryngeal mucosa	laryngeal cytosol treated with PABA 0.5 μM in vitro; analysis performed by HPLC			

Table 15. Results: NAT1 and cancer

Author	OR - colorectal cancer (rapid vs. slow acetylators)	OR - stratified by smoking	OR - (interactions between polymorphisms)	Other comments
Bell et al., 1995 (UK)	1.92 (1.2-3.1). 2.5 (1.3-4.7) among cases in Duke's C tumour stage,		2.8 (1.4-5.7) NAT1rapid/NAT2rapid vs. NAT1slow/NAT2rapid; 2.0 (1.1-3.8) NAT1rapid/NAT2rapid vs. NAT1slow/NAT2slow	
Probst-Hensen et al., 1996 (USA)	1.04 (0.79-1.36) all adenomas, 1.81 (1.12-2.92) incid. cases, 2.29 (1.23-4.24) incid. cases with negative sigmoidoscopy in last 5 yrs, 1.02 (0.75-1.39) small adenomas, 1.04 (0.69-1.56) large adenomas (adjusted for age, gender, race, clinic and date of sigmoidoscopy)		1.11 (0.79-1.56) all adenomas, 1.50 (0.73-3.10) incid. cases (NAT1rapid/NAT2rapid vs. NAT1slow/NAT2slow) (adjusted for age, gender, race, clinic and date of sigmoidoscopy)	

Author	OR - bladder cancer (rapid vs. slow acetylators)	OR - stratified by smoking	OR - (interactions between polymorphisms)	Other comments
Okkels et al., 1997 (Denmark)	0.99 (0.98-1.01)	non-significant association among smokers	non-significant interaction between NAT1 and GSTM1 polym.; 3.76 (1.07-13.31) adjusted for sex, age and smoking (NAT2slow/NAT1rapid vs. NAT2rapid/NAT1slow)	

Table 16. Results: NAT1 and outcomes other than cancer

Author	DNA adducts	Interactions between polymorphisms	Other comments
Degawa et al., 1994 (USA)	non-significant correlation between total DNA adducts and NAT1 activity		
Badawi et al., 1995 (USA)	significant correlation between DNA adducts and NAT1 activity (r=0.52, p<0.01)	significant increase of DNA adduct level in NAT1rapid/NAT2slow vs. NAT1slow/NAT2slow (p=0.009)	significant correlation between NAT1 activity and NAT1 heterozygous genotype (p=0.026)

Table 17. Study design: NAT2 and cancer (case–case study shaded grey)

Author	# of cases	# of controls	Response rates	Phenotyping/ genotyping	Exposures	Covariates	Therapy	NAT2 slow in controls	Power (α=0.05, OR>2)
Agundez et al.,1995a (Spain)	160 incid. breast cancer histolog. confirmed (Caucas.)	132 healthy controls (Caucas.)		PCR		race, cancer histology, menopausal status (pre- or post-)		50.8%	79.3%
Agundez et al., 1996 (Spain)	100 incid. HCC histolog. confirmed (Caucas.)	258 healthy volunteers (Caucas.)	100% cases, 98% controls	PCR		race, cancer histology, CYP2D6 polym., HBV-HCV markers		53.9%	76.9%
Ambrosone et al., 1996 (USA)	304 incid. breast cancer histolog. confirmed (Caucas.)	327 healthy controls <65 years frequency matched by age and county of residence (Caucas.)	66% cases, 62% controls (pre-menopausal); 54% cases, 44% controls (post-menopausal)	PCR	smoking (non-smokers, smokers <16, 16-20, >20 cig/day, 20 yrs before the study)	race, age (at diagnosis, at menarche, at first pregnancy and at menopause), education, BMI, family history of breast cancer		54.4% all, 57% (pre-menop., 53% (post-menop.)	98.9% all, 70.3% pre-menop., 91.2% post-menop.
Bell et al., 1995 (UK)	202 incid. colorectal AD histolog. confirmed (Caucas.)	112 hospital cancer-free controls (Caucas.)	100% cases, 97% controls	PCR		race, NAT1 polym., tumour stage, cancer histology		55.0%	80.1%
Brockmöller et al., 1996a(Germany)	374 incid. bladder cancer histolog. confirmed (Caucas.)	373 hospital cancer-free controls (Caucas.)		PCR	smoking, occupation	age, gender, race, cancer histology, tumour grade, tumour stage, GSTM1, GSTT1, CYP2D6, CYP2E1 and CYP1A1 polym.		57.6%	99.3%
Bulovskaya et al., 1978 (USSR)	41 prev. breast cancer (Caucas.)	38 healthy controls matched for age (Caucas.)		sulfamethazine: <51 kg-500 mg, 51-83 kg-750 mg, >83 kg -1000 mg; blood and urine collected after 6 hours; analysis performed by spectrophotometry		race		63.0%	24.8%

Table 17 (Contd). Study design: NAT2 and cancer (case–case study study shaded grey)

Author	# of cases	# of controls	Response rates	Phenotyping/ genotyping	Exposures	Covariates	Therapy	NAT2 slow in controls	Power (α=0.05, OR>2)
Burgess & Trafford, 1985 (UK)	53 incid. lung cancer histolog. confirmed (Caucas.)	31 hospital controls (Caucas.)		sulfamethazine 40 mg/kg orally; blood collected after 6 hours		race, cancer histology		58.0%	23.2%
Cartwright et al., 1982 (UK)	111 prev. bladder cancer histolog. confirmed (Caucas.)	95 hospital, 112 healthy controls (Caucas.)		dapsone 50 mg orally; blood collected after 2-6 hours; MR=0.3 (MADDS/DDS); analysis performed by HP thin-layer chromatography	smoking for cases (>5 yrs, 5 yrs before diagnosis); occupation for cases (engineers, clerical, dye workers)	gender, age, race, tumour stage	no radio- or chemotherapy before phenotyping, nor therapy with: sulphonamides, isoniazid, procainamide, hydralazine	57.0%	75.4%
Cascorbi et al., 1996 (Germany)	544 prev. lung cancer histolog. confirmed (Caucas.)	967 hospital controls and 278 healthy volunteers (Caucas.)		PCR (155 cases and 588 controls); caffeine (1 cup) orally, urine coll. after 5 hours; analysis performed by HPLC (389 cases and 657 controls)	smoking (1-20, 20-50, >50 PY)	gender, race, cancer histology		53.0%	99.9% (slow/rapid), 38.1% (homozyg. rapid vs. heterozyg. rapid + slow)
Golka et al., 1996 (Germany)	196 prev. urothelial cancer histolog. confirmed (Caucas.)			PCR for 54 cases; caffeine 1-2 cups orally, urine coll. after 2-3 hours; analysis performed by HPLC; MR =1.0 (AFMU/1MX)	smoking, occupation (exp. to aromatic amines)	age, tumour grade			
Hanke & Krajewska, 1990 (Poland)	67 prev. bladder cancer (Caucas.)	22 healthy controls, 90 workers exposed to benzidine Caucas.)		isoniazid	occupation for cases (exposed or not to aromatic amines)	race		45.4% healthy contr., 67% workers exp. to benzidine	21.2% vs. healthy contr., 12.4% vs. workers exp. to benzidine
Hanssen et al., 1985 (Germany)	105 prev. bladder cancer histolog. confirmed (Caucas.)	42 healthy controls (Caucas.)		sulfamethazine, MR = 0.3	smoking and occupation for cases (exp. to bladder carcinog.)	race, drug abuse (analgetics, artif. sweeteners); tumour grade, tumour stage	no chemotherapy before phenotyping	42.9%	39.8%
Hayes et al., 1993 (China)	38 prev. bladder cancer histolog. confirmed, exposed to benzidine (Asians)	43 controls with negative cytology exposed to benzidine (Asians)		PCR; dapsone 100 mg orally; blood collected after 3 hours; MR = 0.3; analysis performed by HPLC	occupation (benzidine exposure estimated: low, medium, high)	gender, age (50-59, 60-69, >69 yrs), race, residence, weight, smoking		23.2%	21.5%

Study	Cases	Controls	Phenotyping/genotyping	Exposure	Confounders/matching	Notes		
Henning et al., 1996 (Germany)	179 incid. larynx cancer (Caucas.)	358 controls matched by age and gender (Caucas.)	PCR		race		58.4%	95.8%
Hirvonen et al., 1995 (Finland)	44 mesothelioma histolog. confirmed (Caucas.)	270 healthy blood donors (Caucas.)	PCR	occupation (exp. to asbestos: high, moderate, low), smoking	race, GSTM1 polym., age		51.0%	46.5%
Horai et al., 1989 (Japan)	51 prev. transitional cell bladder cancer histolog. confirmed (Asians)	23 healthy controls (Asians)	dapsone 100 mg orally, blood collected after 3 hours; MR~0.3 (MADDS/DDS); analysis performed by HPLC	smoking (none, <20, >20 cig/day); occupation for cases (no exposure to β-naphthylamine, benzidine, 4-aminobiphenyl)	race, gender, age, tumour grade, cancer histology	no drugs known to influence the phenotyping	6.4%	22.4%
Ilet et al., 1987 (Australia)	49 incid. colorectal cancer histolog. confirmed (Caucas.)	41 old hospital controls or volunteers matched for age, gender, smoking; 45 young healthy volunt. (Caucas.)	sulfamethazine 15 mg/kg orally, blood coll. after 5, 6, 7, 8, 9 hours, urine coll. after 5-6 and 7-8 hours; MR = 0.6; analysis performed by HPLC	occupation (no exposure to known carcinog.)	race	no chemotherapy before phenotyping	66.3%	40.7%
Ilet et al., 1990 (Australia)	45 incid. breast cancer histolog. confirmed (Caucas.)	28 healthy and 20 hospital controls (Caucas.)	sulfamethazine 500 mg orally, blood collected after 6 hours; MR = 0.6; analysis performed by HPLC	smoking	race, age (5-yrs), tumour stage, sex hormones receptor status (for cases)		64.6%	29.6%
Kaisary et al., 1987 (USA, UK)	98 prev. transitional cell bladder cancer histolog. confirmed (Caucas.)	110 urolog. patients (Caucas.)	dapsone 100 mg orally, blood collected after 8 hours; MR~0.4 (MADDS/DDS); analysis performed by HPLC	smoking, alcohol, occupation (no exposure to known bladder carcinog.)	gender, age, race, tumour stage, cancer histology	no drugs known to influence the dapsone metabolism before phenotyping	49.0%	63.4%
Karakaya et al., 1986 (Turkey)	23 prev. transitional cell bladder cancer histolog. confirmed (Caucas.)	109 healthy volunteers (Caucas.)	sulfamethazine 40 mg/kg orally; blood collected after 6 hours; analysis performed by spectrophotometry		race, cancer histology	no chemotherapy before phenotyping	61.5%	17.1%
Kirlin et al., 1991 (USA)	25 colorectal cancer (mixed)	12 hospital controls (mixed)	NAT enzyme activity in colon tissue				75%	6.4%
Ladero et al., 1985 (Spain)	130 prev. transitional cell bladder cancer histolog. confirmed (Caucas.)	157 healthy controls (Caucas.)	sulfamethazine 10 mg/kg orally; blood and urine collected after 6 hours; analysis performed by spectrophotometry	smoking and occupation for cases (exp. to bladder carcinog.)	age, race, tumour grade, cancer histology		57.4%	74.8%

449

Table 17 (Contd). Study design: NAT2 and cancer (case–case study shaded grey)

Author	# of cases	# of controls	Response	Phenotyping/genotyping	Exposures	Covariates	Therapy	NAT2 slow in controls	Power (α=0.05, OR>2)
Ladero et al., 1987 (Spain)	81 incid. breast cancer histolog. confirmed (Caucas.)	75 healthy or suffering for diseases not related to the acetylator phenotype (Caucas.)		sulfamethazine 10 mg/kg orally, blood and urine coll. after 6 hours; analysis performed by spectrophotometry		race, menopausal status	no hormonal, radio- or chemotherapy before phenotyping, nor drugs known to influence the sulfamethazine metabolism	60%	50.8%
Ladero et al., 1991a (Spain)	61 prev. colon cancer and 48 prev. rectal cancer histolog. confirmed (Caucas.)	96 healthy controls (Caucas.)		sulfamethazine 10 mg/kg orally, blood and urine coll. after 6 hours; analysis performed by spectrophotometry		age, gender, race, surgery treatment, tumour site (colon, rectum)	no drugs known to influence the sulfamethazine metabolism before phenotyping; surgery treatment for 74 cases	58.3%	63.9%
Lang et al., 1986 (USA)	43 prev. colorectal cancer, male, 45-75 yrs old (mixed)	41 hospital controls, male, 45-75 yrs old (mixed)		sulfamethazine 10 mg/kg orally, blood and urine coll. after 4.5 hours; analysis performed by HPLC		gender		68.3% (mixed)	25.6%
Lang et al., 1994 (USA)	41 incid. colorectal polyp and 34 colorect. cancer histolog. confirmed (mixed)	205 healthy controls randomly digit dialing selected (mixed)		caffeine 100 mg orally, urine coll. after 5 hours; analysis performed by HPLC; MR=0.6 (AFMU/1MX)	smoking (smokers, non-mokers)	age (<35, >35 yrs, <60, >60 yrs), CYP1A2 polym.		44.9%, 43% (Caucas.), 56% (African-Americans)	67.2% for combined cases; 37.9% for colon cancer, 44.5% for colon polyps
Lee et al., 1994 (Korea)	100 prev. transitional cell bladder cancer histolog. confirmed (Asians)	84 outpatients from the same department matched by age and gender (Asians)		isoniazid 400 mg orally, urine coll. after 8 hours; MR = 0.99 (acetyl-isoniazid/ isoniazid); analysis performed by fluorophotometry	occupation (no exposure to bladder carcinogens)	age, gender, race, smoking, cancer histology, tumour stage (I, II, III)	no drugs known to influence NAT2 metabolism	16.7%	40.8%
Lower et al., 1979 (Sweden, Denmark)	186 prev. bladder cancer histolog. confirmed (Caucas.)	192 hospital and healthy controls (Caucas.)		sulfamethazine 10 mg/kg orally, blood and urine coll. after 4.5 hours; analysis performed by spectrophotometry	smoking for cases (light smokers <1 pack/day; heavy smok. >1pack/day)	residence (rural, urban), race		51.4% (urban), 66.9% (rural)	89.0%
Martinez et al., 1995 (Spain)	108 incid. lung cancer histolog. confirmed (Caucas.)	243 healthy controls (Caucas.)	100% cases, 98% controls	PCR	smoking (for cases only)	age, gender, race, cancer histology		58.4%	76.0%

Reference	Cases	Controls	Participation	Method	Factors considered	Other factors	Conditions	%	%
Miller & Cosgriff, 1983 (USA)	26 prev. transitional cell bladder cancer histolog. confirmed (Caucas.)	26 healthy controls (Caucas.)		sulfamethazine: <51 kg-500 mg, 51-83 kg-750 mg, >83 kg - 1000 mg; blood and urine collected after 6 hours; analysis performed by spectrophotometry	smoking for cases (non-smokers, smokers>1 pack/ day for>5 yrs, 15 yrs before diagnosis); occupation for cases (exp. to bladder carcinog.)	race, cancer histology	no chemotherapy before phenotyping	69.0%	10.8%
Mommsen et al., 1985 (Denmark)	228 incid. bladder cancer histolog. confirmed from a rural area (Caucas.)	100 cancer-free urolog. patients matched for age from a rural area (Caucas.)		sulfamethazine 1 g orally, blood and urine collected after 4.5 hours; analysis performed by spectrophotometry		residence (rural), race	no chemotherapy before phenotyping, nor therapy with: sulphonamides, isoniazid, hydralazine	54.0%	76.5%
Oda et al., 1994 (Japan)	36 colorectal cancer histolog. confirmed (Asians)	36 autopsied controls matched for age (Asians)		RFLP		race		8.3%	10.2%
Okkels et al., 1997 (Denmark)	95 incid. and 159 prev. bladder cancer (benign + malignant) histolog. confirmed (Caucas.)	242 hospital controls affected by non-cancerous urinary tract diseases (Caucas.)		PCR	smoking (non-smokers, smokers 1-20, 21-50, >50 PY; ex-smokers for 2-9, 10-19, >19 yrs)	gender, age, race, tumour grade, GSTM1 and NAT1 polym.		55.8%	94.9%
Oyama et al., 1997 (Japan)	124 incid. lung cancer histolog. confirmed undergoing surgery (Asians)	376 healthy factory workers (Asians)		PCR	smoking (for cases)	race, cancer histology, tumour stage, gender, age for cases only (<65, >65 yrs)		11.0%	64.1%, 47.8% (AD), 37.7% (SQ)
Philip et al., 1987 (UK)	181 incid. breast cancer and 136 incid. benign breast disease histolog. confirmed (mixed)	337 healthy controls of both genders (Caucas.)		dapsone 50 mg orally, blood collected after 2-6 hours; MR=0.3 (MADDS/DDS); analysis performed by HPLC		age, tumour stage, sex hormones receptor status		55.2%	95.4% for breast cancer, 90.8% for benigne disease
Philip et al., 1988 (UK)	126 prev. lung cancer histolog. confirmed (Caucas.)	82 hospital controls, 191 hospital controls > 65 yrs old (Caucas.)		dapsone 100 mg orally, blood collected after 1.5-4 hours; MR=0.3 (MADDS/DDS); analysis performed by HPLC	smoking for cases and for 82 controls	race, cancer histology	no therapy before phenotyping	50.5%	86.8%
Probst-Hensch et al., 1995 & 1996 (USA)	447 incid. colorectal adenoma histolog. confirmed undergoing sigmoidoscopy (mixed)	487 controls without current or past polyps by sigmoidoscopy, matched by age, gender, clinic and date of sigmoidoscopy (mixed)	84% cases, 82% controls	PCR	smoking (never, former, current smokers)	age (5-yrs), gender, race, date of sigmoidoscopy (6-months intervals), cancer histology, clinic, tumour size, GSTM1 polym.			
Risch et al., 1995 (UK)	189 prev. bladder cancer (Caucas.)	59 urolog. controls matched for age (Caucas.)		RFLP	smoking for 186 cases and 43 controls, occupation for all cases and 43 controls	age, gender, race		44.1%	58.2%

451

Table 17 (Contd). Study design: NAT2 and cancer (case-case study shaded grey)

Author	# of cases	# of controls	Response rates	Phenotyping/ genotyping	Exposures	Covariates	Therapy	NAT2 slow in controls	Power (α=0.05, OR>2)
Roberts-Thompson et al., 1996 (Australia)	61 incid. + prev. colorectal cancer and 89 incid. colorectal adenoma histolog. confirmed (Caucas.)	110 hospital controls (Caucas.)	83,0%	sulfamethazine 20 mg/kg orally; blood coll. after 1 and 4 hours; analysis performed by HPLC		age, gender, race, diet, tumour site and cancer histology			
Rodriguez et al., 1993 (USA)	44 prev. colorectal cancer (mixed)	28 hospital cancer-free controls (mixed)		PCR				53.6%	21.5%
Roots et al., 1988 (Germany)	220 prev. lung cancer histolog. confirmed <80 yrs (Caucas.)	245 hospital controls <80 yrs (Caucas.)		caffeine 300 mg orally, urine coll. after 2-6 hours; analysis performed by HPLC; MR=0,48 (AFMU/1MX)		race, age (<50, >50 yrs) for cases, cancer histology, CYP2D6 polym.	no therapy before phenotyping	53.5%	94.0%
Sardas et al., 1990 (Turkey)	28 prev. breast cancer (Caucas.)	51 healthy volunteers (Caucas.)		sulfamethazine 25 mg/kg orally; blood collected after 6 hours; analysis performed by spectrophotometry		race		35.3%	22.9%
Shibuta et al., 1994 (Japan)	234 prev. colorectal cancer histolog. confirmed (Asians)	329 healthy volunteers (Asians)		PCR		age (<60, >60 yrs), race, tumour site (colon, rectum), tumour stage (well, moderately, poor differentiated)		9.6%	44.9%
Spigelman et al., 1994 (UK)	29 prev. familial adenomatous polyposis (Caucas.)	54 healthy volunteers matched by age and gender (Caucas.)		caffeine 300 mg orally, urine coll. after 2-6 hours; analysis performed by HPLC; MR=0,48(AAMU/AAMU+1MU+1MX)		race, cancer histology	no significant difference in NAT2 status before and after colectomy	63.6%	17.4%
Spurr et al., 1995 (UK)	103 prev. colon cancer (Caucas.)	96 outpatients controls (Caucas.)		PCR		race		64.6%	52.0%
Webster et al., 1989 (UK)	100 incid. + prev. breast cancer histolog. confirmed (Caucas.)	32 breast lumps and 68 healthy controls (Caucas.)		isoniazid 200 mg orally, blood collected after 3 hours; analysis performed by HPLC		race		59%	62.9%
Woodhouse et al., 1982 (UK)	30 prev. transitional cell bladder cancer histolog. confirmed (all smokers, except 2) (Caucas.)	27 hospital controls (Caucas.)		isoniazid 10 mg/kg orally, blood collected after 1.5-6 hours; analysis performed by spectrophotometry	occupation (no exp. to bladder carcinogens)	race, cancer histology	no drugs known to influence the isoniazid metabolism before phenotyping	59,0%	15.2%

Table 18. Study design: NAT2 and outcomes other than cancer

Author	Subjects	Analysis	Phenotyping/ genotyping	Exposures	Covariates	NAT2 slow %
Badawi et al., 1995 (USA)	26 healthy subjects (Caucas.?)	32P-postlabelling assay of aromatic amines-DNA adducts in normal bladder mucosa	PCR		NAT1 polym.	57.7%
Brockmöller et al., 1996b (Germany)	69 bladder cancer histolog. confirmed (Caucas.)	p53 mutations by PCR	PCR			62.3%
Degawa et al., 1994 (USA)	25 laryngeal cancer patients (Caucas.?)	32P-postlabelling assay of total DNA adducts in normal laryngeal mucosa	laryngeal cytosol treated with sulfamethazine 0.5 µM in vitro; analysis performed by HPLC			
Gabbani et al., 1996 (Italy, Sweden)	46 coke oven workers exposed to PAHs (Caucas.)	Ames assay in Salmonella typhimurium TA98 strain (number of revertant colonies per mmol creatinine)	PCR	smoking	race, GSTM1 polym.	73.3%
Hirvonen et al., 1994 (Finland)	healthy male exposed to asbestos: 10 smokers, 29 non-smokers; patients with malignant lung cancer or non-malignant lesions: 7 smokers, 6 non-smokers (Caucas.)	Ames assay in Salmonella typhimurium YG1024 and TA98 strains (number of revertant colonies per 100 ml urine)	PCR	smoking, occupation (asbestos exposure)	gender, race	51.9%
Hou et al., 1995 (Sweden)	47 healthy non-smokers bus maintainance workers; 22 healthy non-smokers controls (Caucas.)	32P-postlabelling assay of PAH-DNA adducts in lymphocytes; mutant frequency in hprt gene	PCR	occupation (garage workers, mechanics, others)	GSTM1 polym., age (for mutant frequency only)	60.9%
Nielsen et al., 1996a (Denmark)	90 healthy non-smoking bus drivers, 60 healthy subjects from a rural area (Caucas.)	32P-postlabelling assay of PAH-DNA adducts in lymphocytes	PCR	smoking (smokers, non-smokers) for rural controls	race, GSTM1 polym., driving area (centre, suburban, dormitory) for bus drivers	51.1%
Oda et al., 1994 (Japan)	36 colorectal cancer histolog. confirmed (Asians)	K-ras mutations by PCR	RFLP		race	8.3%
Oyama et al., 1997 (Japan)	124 lung cancer histolog. confirmed (Asians)	p53 mutations by PCR	PCR		cancer histology, race, age (<65, >65 yrs)	11.0%
Romkes et al., 1996 (UK)	93 transitional cell bladder carcinoma histolog. confirmed (Caucas.?)	p53 and Rb mutations in tumour tissue by immunohistochemistry	dapsone 100 mg orally, blood collected after 8 hours; analysis performed by HPLC		tumour grade	
Scarpato et al., 1996 (Italy, Finland)	23 floriculturists occupationally exposed to pesticides; 22 bank clerks matched by gender, age and smoking (Caucas.)	SCE, CA and MN in lymphocytes	PCR	smoking, occupation	age, gender, race, GSTT1 and GSTM1 polym.	62.2%

Table 18 (Contd). Study design: NAT2 and outcomes other than cancer

Author	Subjects	Analysis	Phenotyping/ genotyping	Exposures	Covariates	NAT2 slow %
Sinues et al., 1992 (Spain)	70 textile workers exposed to arylamines, 83 non-expoxed subjects (Caucas.)	Ames assay in *Salmonella typhimurium* TA98 strain (number of revertant colonies per 100 ml urine)	isoniazid 10 mg/kg orally, urine collected after 8 hours; MR = 0.71; analysis performed by colorimetric method	occupation (high, moderate, no exposure to arylamines)	race	57.5%
Vineis et al., 1990 (Italy)	100 healthy male blood donors 45-64 yrs old (Caucas.)	4-aminobiphenyl-haemoglobin adduct level	70 mg caffeine orally, urine collected after 5 hours; analysis performed by HPLC; MR = 0.5 (AFMU/1MX)	smoking (type of tobacco, number of cig. smoked in the last 24 h)	age, race, place of birth, alcohol, medication use	65%
Vineis et al., 1994 (Italy)	100 healthy male blood donors 45-64 yrs old (Caucas.)	4-aminobiphenyl-haemoglobin adduct level; 32P-postlabelling assay of DNA adducts in exfoliated bladder cells	RFLP, 70 mg caffeine orally, urine collected after 5 hours; analysis performed by HPLC	smoking (smokers, non-smokers; cotinine and nicotine levels in urine)	gender, race	
Yu et al., 1994 (USA)	133 male healthy volunteers >35 yrs old (mixed)	3- and 4-aminobiphenyl-haemoglobin adduct level	MR = 0.6 (AFMU/1MX) 70 mg caffeine orally, urine collected after 12-15 hours; analysis performed by HPLC; MR = 0.34 (AAMU/AAMU+1MX+1 MU)	smoking (non-smokers, smokers 1-19, >9 cig./day)	gender, race	54% (Caucas.), 34% (Afric.-Americ.), 14% (Asians)

Table 19. Results: NAT2 and bladder cancer (case–case study shaded grey)

Author	OR - other cancer (slow vs. rapid acetylators)	OR - stratified by ethnicity	OR - stratified by smoking	OR - stratified by cancer histology	OR - interactions between polymorphisms	Other comments
Lower et al., 1979 (Sweden, Denmark)	1.35 (0.88-2.05), 1.74 (0.89-3.40) urban cases vs. urban controls, 1.13 (0.65-1.96) rural cases vs. rural controls					no significant difference in acetylator status in smokers vs. non-smokers cases
Cartwright et al., 1982 (UK)	1.51 (0.93-2.44), 1.52 (0.86-2.67) vs. hosp. controls, 1.50 (0.87-2.58) vs. healthy controls					no significant association with smoking status (p=0.40) or tumour stage (p=0.096) among cases; significant difference in acetylator status among chemical workers vs. other cases (p=0.0005)
Woodhouse et al., 1982 (UK)				1.60 (0.54-4.80) TCC		
Miller & Cosgriff, 1983 (USA)				0.38 (0.12-1.19) TCC		no significant difference in acetylator status in smokers vs. non-smokers cases and in occupationally exposed vs. non-exposed cases
Mommsen et al., 1985 (Denmark)	1.49 (0.92-2.40)					
Ladero et al., 1985 (Spain)				1.31 (0.82-2.12) TCC		no significant difference in acetylator status in smokers vs. non-smokers cases; significant differ. in acetyl. status in occupationally exposed cases vs. other cases (p=0.029)
Hanssen et al., 1985 (Germany)	2.17 (1.05-4.48), 2.81 (1.24-6.37) superficial, 1.59 (0.68-3.69) infiltrating, 4.67 (1.31-16.59) grade I, 2.22 (0.95-5.18) grade II, 1.56 (0.65-3.74) grade III					no significant difference in acetylator status in smokers vs. non smokers cases and in occupationally exposed vs. non exposed cases
Karakaya et al., 1996 (Turkey)				0.40 (0.16-1.01) TCC		
Kaisary et al., 1987 (USA, UK)			no significantly different NAT2slow frequency by smoking	1.57 (0.90-2.72) TCC, 1.89 (1.01-3.56) non-aggressive (stage I and II), 1.10 (0.51-2.40) aggressive (stage III)	no significant interaction between CYP2D6 and NAT2 polymorphisms	
Horai et al., 1989 (Japan)			no significantly different NAT2slow frequency by smoking	0.91 (0.16-3.50) TCC, no significantly different NAT2slow frequency by gender, age or tumour grade		

Table 19 (Contd). Results: NAT2 and bladder cancer (case–case study shaded grey)

Author	OR - other cancer (slow vs. rapid acetylators)	OR - stratified by ethnicity	OR - stratified by smoking	OR - stratified by cancer histology	OR - interactions between polymorphisms	Other comments
Hanke & Krajewska, 1990 (Poland)	2.82 (1.05-7.58)					significant difference in acetyl. status in occupationally exposed vs. non-exposed cases (p=0.02)
Hayes et al. 1993 (China)	0.29 (0.07-1.15) (phenotyping); 0.50 (0.15-1.62), 0.3 (0.0-2.2) low exp. to benzidine, 0.7 (0.1-4.5) medium exp., 0.6 (0.1-3.5) high exp. (genotyping)					no significant association with cancer risk after adjustment for smoking, age, weight, residence
Lee et al., 1994 (Korea)				0.98 (0.44-2.14) TCC, 1.07 (0.46-2.50) non-aggressive (stage I and II), 0.71 (0.19-2.72) aggressive (stage III)		no significant association with cancer risk after adjustment for gender, age and smoking status
Risch et al., 1995 (UK)	2.60 (1.43-4.72), 3.10 (1.46-6.58) likely exp. to bladder carcino., 2.39 (1.27-4.50) non-exp. to bladder carcino.		3.90 (1.69-9.06) smokers, 1.22 (0.31-4.74) non-smokers			no significant association with age and gender among cases
Brockmöller et al., 1996a (Germany)	1.21 (0.91-1.63), 1.16 (0.81-1.65) occupations not at risk for bladder cancer, 1.55 (0.89-2.72) occupations at risk for bladder cancer, 1.35 (0.94-1.93) male, 0.74 (0.44-1.24) female		0.82 (0.46-1.45) non-mokers, 1.43 (1.01-2.02) smokers, 1.27 (0.86-1.88) intermed. smokers, 2.23 (1.04-4.81) heavy smokers, 2.12 (1.13-3.97) smokers, 1.8 (0.8-3.7) intermediate smokers, 2.7 (1.0-7.4) heavy smokers (adjusted for age, gender, occupation and other polymorphisms)		significant interaction with GSTM1 polymorph. (p=0.007); no significant interaction with GSTT1, CYP2E1, CYP1A1 or CYP2D6 polym.	
Golka et al., 1996 (Germany)	no significant excess of NAT2slow in cases who worked in chemical production (p=0.123) or in chemical or rubber industry (p=0.141); almost significant excess in cases who worked in chemical or rubber industry in the Bayer Company (p=0.052)					no significant association with age, smoking status or tumour grade
Okkels et al. 1997 (Denmark)	1.22 (0.92-1.62) all, 1.23 (0.95-1.59) incid. cases, 1.08 (0.87-1.35) prev. cases (adjusted for gender, age and smoking)		1.04 (0.78-1.37) all, 1.34 (0.81-2.20) incident, 0.95 (0.70-1.30) prevalent (benign tumours); 1.35 (1.02-1.80) all, 1.50 (1.04-2.16) incident, 1.25 (0.87-1.80) prevalent (malignant tumours) (adjusted for age and gender)		1.51 (0.89-2.55) NAT2slow/GSTM1null vs. NAT2rapid/GSTM1+; 3.76 (1.07-13.31) NAT2slow/NAT1rapid vs. NAT2rapid/NAT1normal (adjusted for gender, age and smoking)	no significant association with cancer histology or tumour grade

Table 20. Results: NAT2 and colorectal cancer

Author	OR - colorectal cancer (rapid vs. slow acetylators)	OR - stratified by ethnicity	OR - stratified by smoking	OR - stratified by cancer histology	OR - interactions between polymorphisms	Other comments
Lang et al., 1986 (USA)	2.48 (1.02-6.03)					
Ilett et al., 1987 (Australia)	2.41 (1.18-4.95) vs. all controls, 3.80 (1.53-9.44) vs. older controls, 1.68 (0.74-3.80) vs. younger controls					
Kirlin et al., 1991 (USA)	0.31 (0.04-1.68)					
Ladero et al., 1991a (Spain)	1.14 (0.66-1.99)					no significant association with gender, surgery treatment or tumour site
Rodriguez et al., 1993 (USA)	0.96 (0.37-2.49)					
Shibuta et al., 1994 (Japan)	0.83 (0.48-1.57), 0.85 (0.41-1.78) <60 yrs, 1.09 (0.22-5.25) >60 yrs, 1.10 (0.52-2.33) colon, 0.66 (0.34-1.27) rectum			0.60 (0.29-1.23) well differentiated, 1.18 (0.52-2.65) moderately differ., 0.63 (0.07-5.39) poor differ.		
Oda et al., 1994 (Japan)	1.00 (0.19-5.32)					
Lang et al., 1994 (USA)	0.86 (0.39-1.90) colon cancer, 1.92 (0.92-4.03) colon polyps, 1.33 (0.76-2.34) combined cases				2.79 (1.69-4.47) NAT2rapid/CYP1A2rapid vs. NAT2 slow/CYP1A2slow (combined cases)	no significant association with age or smoking status
Spurr et al., 1995 (UK)	1.22 (0.65-2.29)					
Bell et al., 1995 (USA)	1.1 (0.71-1.80) AD, 0.48 (0.16-1.40) stage A, 0.96 (0.56-1.70) stage B, 1.47 (0.81-2.70) stage C (Duke's tumoral stage)				2.0 (1.1-3.8), 0.7 (0.2-2.3) stage A, 1.9 (1.1-3.4) stage B, 2.5 (1.3-4.7) stage C (NAT1rapid/NAT2rapid vs. NAT1slow/NAT2slow acetylators)	

Table 20 (Contd). Results: NAT2 and colorectal cancer

Author	OR - colorectal cancer (rapid vs. slow acetylators)	OR - stratified by ethnicity	OR - stratified by smoking	OR - stratified by cancer histology	OR - interactions between polymorphisms	Other comments
Roberts-Thompson et al., 1996 (Australia)	1.8 (1.0-13.3), 8.9 (2.6-30.4) <64 yrs, (colon cancer); 1.1 (0.6-2.1), 2.5 (0.7-9.4) <64 yrs (adenoma)					no significant association with gender, tumor site, cancer histology
Probst-Hensch et al., 1995 & 1996 (USA)	1.08 (0.83-1.4) incid. cases, 0.74 (0.41-1.33) incid. cases with negative sigmoidoscopy in last 5 yrs, 1.21 (0.90-1.63) small adenomas, 0.92 (0.62-1.39) large adenomas (adjusted for age, gender, date of sigmoidoscopy and clinic)	1.29 (0.9-1.84) Caucas., 0.44 (0.21-0.91) Afric.-Americ., 1.38 (0.72-2.67) Hispanics, 1.08 (0.40-2.39) Asians (adjusted for age, gender, date of sigmoidoscopy and clinic)			10.33 (1.94-55.04) NAT2rapid./GSTM1null vs. NAT2slow/GSTM1+ (Caucas. smokers) 1.11 (0.79-1.56) all cases 1.50 (0.73-3.10) incid. cases (NAT1rapid/NAT2rapid vs. NAT1slow/NAT2slow) (adjusted for age, gender, race, clinic and date of sigmoidoscopy)	

Table 21. Results: NAT2 and lung cancer

Author	OR - lung cancer (slow vs. rapid acetylators)	OR - stratified by ethnicity	OR - stratified by smoking	OR - stratified by cancer histology	OR - interactions between polymorphisms	Other comments
Burgess & Trafford, 1985 (UK)	1.10 (0.45-2.71)			1.18 (0.42-3.33) SQ, 0.48 (0.08-2.56) SC, 1.08 (0.11-14.68) AD		
Philip et al., 1988 (UK)	0.83 (0.55-1.27)		0.99 (0.56-1.74) smokers	0.98 (0.50-1.90) SQ, 0.85 (0.39-1.85) SC, 0.77 (0.34-1.75) AD		
Roots et al., 1988 (Germany) (part of Cascorbi et al., 1996)	0.89 (0.62-1.28)			0.96 (0.58-1.61) SQ, 0.77 (0.37-1.61) AD, 0.79 (0.42-1.51) SC, 1.09 (0.60-1.97) LC	2.13 (0.85-5.32) (NAT2slow/2D6 WW vs. NAT2rapid/2D6 MM)	
Martinez et al., 1995 (Spain)	1.31 (0.82-2.10)					no significant association between NAT2 genotypes and cancer histology, age, gender, or smoking status among cases; significantly higher risk for slow acetylators homozygous for variants 341C + 481T + 803G: OR=1.75 (0.99-3.12)
Cascorbi et al., 1996 (Germany)	0.90 (0.74-1.10), 0.95 (0.74-1.22) phenotyping, 0.91 (0.64-1.31) genotyping (slow vs. rapid); 2.37 (1.27-4.45) genotyp., 2.79 (1.16-6.82) genotyp. in males; (WWrapid vs. WMrapid + slow)		3.22 (1.27-7.92) smokers 20-50 PY (WWrapid vs. WMrapid + slow)	4.24 (0.84-1.72) LC male, 5.19 (1.00-22.0) mixed-cell tumours, male (WWrapid vs. WMrapid + slow)		
Oyama et al., 1997 (Japan)	1.33 (0.73-2.45)			0.71 (0.24-2.09) SQ, 1.82 (0.92-3.60) AD		no significant association between NAT2 genotypes and age, gender, smoking index or tumour stage

Table 22. Results: NAT2 and breast cancer

Author	OR - breast cancer (rapid vs. slow acetylators)	OR - stratified by ethnicity	OR - stratified by smoking	OR - stratified by cancer histology	OR - interactions between polymor-	Other comments
Bulovskaya et al., 1978 (USSR)	3.69 (1.46-9.37)					
Ladero et al., 1987 (Spain)	0.98 (0.52-1.86), 1.01 (0.38-2.63) pre-menop., 0.94 (0.44-2.24) post-menopausal					
Philip et al., 1987 (UK)	1.19 (0.83-1.69), 0.77 (0.41-1.43) stage I, 1.06 (0.66-1.71) stage II, 1.60 (0.61-4.15) stage III, 2.55 (0.75-8.65) stage IV (breast cancer); 1.44 (0.96-2.14) (benign disease)					significant trend for increasing propor-tion of NAT2 rapid in higher tumour stages (p<0.001); non-significant association with age or sex hormones receptor status among cancer cases
Webster et al., 1989 (UK)	1.09 (0.62-1.90)					
Ilett et al., 1990 (Australia)	1.46 (0.63-3.36)		4.00 (0.35-58.20) smokers, 1.12 (0.40-3.21) non-smokers			no significant association with tumour stage (p=0.26) or with sex hormones receptor status among cases (p=0.87)
Sardas et al., 1990 (Turkey)	2.83 (1.09-7.34)					
Agundez et al., 1995a (Spain)	0.91 (0.57-1.44)			0.82 (0.50-1.36) ductal carcinoma, 0.69 (0.06-6.22) in situ carcinoma, 0.69 (0.06-6.22) colloidal carcinoma; 0 slow acetylator among lobular carcinoma (p=0.014)		no significant association with menopausal status among cases (p=0.46)
Ambrosone et al., 1996 (USA)	0.99 (0.59-1.67) pre-menopausal, 0.86 (0.58-1.28) post-menopausal		0.83 (0.37-1.83) non-smokers, 0.90 (0.40-2.02) smokers (pre-menopausal); 1.24 (0.70-2.19) non-smokers, 2.06 (0.69-6.16) <15 cig/day, 0.51 (0.20-1.29) 16-20 cig/day, 0.11 (0.02-0.64) >20 cig/day (post-menopausal)			

Table 23. Results: NAT2 and other cancer

Author	OR - other cancer (slow vs. rapid acetylators)	OR - stratified by ethnicity	OR - stratified by smoking	OR - stratified by cancer histology	OR - interactions between polymorphisms	Other comments
Spigelman et al., 1994 (UK)	3.57 (1.09-11.74) FAP					
Hirvonen et al., 1995 (Finland)	mesothelioma: 2.08 (1.06-4.10) all, 1.19 (0.48-2.96) low/moderate exp. to asbstos, 3.69 (1.34-10.17) high exp. to asbestos				3.59 (1.35-9.58) all, 1.70 (0.46-6.31) low/moderate exp., 7.37 (1.60-33.98) high exp. to asbestos (GSTM1null/NAT2slow vs. GSTM1+/NAT2rapid)	no significant association with smoking status
Agundez et al., 1996 (Spain)	1.82 (1.12-2.96) HCC, 5.14 (1.13-23.41) HCC cases without HBV-HCV markers				2.65 (1.83-21.29), 5.70 (1.55-20.93) HCC cases without HBV-HCV markers (NAT2slow/CYP2D6WW vs. others combined); 6.24 (1.83-21.29) (NAT2slow/2D6 WW vs. NAT2rapid/2D6 MM+WM)	significantly increased risk for developing HCC with decreasing number of NAT2 functional alleles (test for trend: $p=0.015$)
Henning et al., 1996 (Germany)	1.30 (0.89-1.89) larynx cancer (rapid/slow); 1.95 (0.82-4.58) larynx cancer (WW/rapid vs. slow)					

Table 24. Results: NAT2 and outcomes other than cancer

Author	SCE	MN and CA (slow/rapid acetylator)	Mutagenicity (slow/rapid acetylator)	DNA adducts (slow/rapid acetylator)	Hb and proteins adducts (slow/rapid acetylator)	OR - Interactions between polymorphisms	Other comments
Badawi et al., 1995 (USA)				non-significant association between aromatic amines-DNA adduct level and NAT2 polym. (p=0.64)		non-significantly higher aromatic amines-DNA adduct level in NAT1rapid/NAT2 slow vs. NAT1slow/NAT2rapid (p=0.37)	no significant association with smoking
Degawa et al., 1994 (USA)				no appreciable NAT2 activity in larynx cytosol (<0.01 nmol/min/mg protein)			
Brockmöller et al., 1996b (Germany)			non-significantly different p53 mutations frequency (p=0.92); non-significant association of NAT2slow with transversions vs. transitions mutations (p=0.12)				
Hirvonen et al., 1994 (Finland)			no significantly different mean urinary mutagenicity on YG1024 strain in smokers (p=0.96), but almost significantly different in non-smokers (p=0.06)				
Hou et al., 1995 (Sweden)			no significantly different mutant frequency in hprt gene (p=0.8)	non-significantly different PAH-DNA adducts level (p=0.8); almost significantly higher PAH-DNA adducts level in garage workers (p=0.07)		significantly higher PAH-DNA adduct level in GSTM1null/NAT2slow vs. GSTM1+/NAT2rapid (p=0.03)	
Nielsen et al., 1996a (Denmark)				non-significantly higher PAH-DNA adduct level (p=0.24)		no significant interaction with GSTM1 polym. on PAH-DNA adduct level	
Gabbani et al., 1996 (Italy, Sweden)			significantly higher urinary mutagenicity among smokers (p<0.05)			significantly higher urinary mutagenicity in smokers GSTM1null/NAT2slow vs. GSTM1+/NAT2rapid (p<0.05)	
Oda et al., 1994 (Japan)			significantly higher K-ras mutations frequency in WWrapid vs. WMrapid-slow cases (p=0.033)				

Reference			
Oyama et al., 1997 (Japan)	non significantly different p53 mutations frequency (p=0.92)		no significant association with age or cancer histology
Romkes et al., 1996 (UK)	non-significant difference in SCE frequency (p=0.43)	non-significant differences in MN frequency (p=0.59) and CA frequency (p=0.23); non-significant association between NAT2 activity and p53 or Rb mutations	no significant association with tumour grade
Scarpato et al., 1996 (Italy, Finland)		non significant interactions between GSTM1, GSTT1 and NAT2 polymorph. in determining SCE, MN or CA frequency	no significant association with smoking status
Vineis et al., 1990 (Italy)		significantly higher Hb-adduct level either in all group (p=0.003, adjusted for type of tobacco and number of cig. smoked) or in smokers (p=0.046)	
Vineis et al., 1994 (Italy)	non-significantly different DNA adduct level	significantly higher NAT2 slow frequency in subjects with Hb-adducts above vs. below the median: 17.5 (2.0-153) if cotinine + nicotine=0 2.3 (0.8-7.0) if cotinine + nicotine>0	significant correlation between number of mutations and slow phenotype
Yu et al., 1994 (USA)		significantly higher level of 3-ABP Hb adducts (p<0.0005), but not of 4-ABP Hb adducts (p=0.19) (adjusted for smoking)	
Sinues et al., 1992 (Spain)	non-significant difference in mutagenicity in all group and in non-exposed workers; significant difference after incubation of urine with β-glucuronidase in subjects exposed to arylamines (p<0.01 in high, p<0.05 in moderate exposure groups)		

Table 25. Study design: CYP1A1 and AHH activity and inducibility and cancer (case–case studies shaded grey)

Author	# of cases	# of controls	Response	Genotype/ phenotype	Exposures	Covariates	Therapy	% variants in controls	Power (α=0.05, OR>2)
Abe et al., 1990 (Japan)	31 prev. lung cancer histolog. confirmed (Asians)	20 healthy volunteers and 5 hospital controls (Asians)		basal AHH activity in PAM; AHH inducibility in lymphocytes	smoking (non-smokers, current smokers, ex-smokers)	ethnicity, tumour location			
Alexandrie et al., 1994 (Sweden)	296 incid. lung cancer histolog. confirmed (Caucas.)	329 healthy controls from laboratory personnel, chimney sweeps and welders <65 yrs; 79 COPD patients (Caucas.)		PCR (MspI, Exon7)		ethnicity, age (<65, >65 yrs), gender, GSTM1 polym., cancer histology		15.8% WM, 0.3% MM (MspI); 7% WM (Exon7)	92.8% MspI, 51.0% Exon7 (WM+MM/WW)
Ambrosone et al., 1995 (USA)	176 incid. post-menopausal breast cancer histolog. Confirmed (Caucas.)	228 healthy controls frequency matched by age and county residence (Caucas.)		PCR (Exon7)	smoking (non-smokers, smokers <29, >29 PY)	ethnicity, GSTM1 polym., age (at diagnosis, menarche, first pregnancy and menopause), education, BMI, family history of breast cancer		15% (WM), 1% (MM)	75.0% (WM+MM/WW) 5.6% (MM/WW+WM)
Anttila et al., 1994 (Finland)	54 incid. lung cancer histolog. confirmed undergoing surgery, smokers (Caucas.)			CYP1A1 activity in normal lung tissue by immunohistochemistry		cancer histology, GSTM1 polym., tumour location			
Bouchardy et al., 1997 (France)	150 incid. lung cancer histolog. confirmed, smokers >5 cig./day x 5 yrs (Caucas.)	171 hospital controls, smokers >5 cig./day x 5 yrs (Caucas.)		PCR (MspI, Exon7)	smoking (smokers <20, 21-30, >30 g tobacco/day; ex-smokers), occupation (exp. to asbestos and to arsenic)	age, gender, ethnicity, cancer histology		19.3%, MspI (WM), 8.8% Exon7 (WM)	72.3% MspI, 45.3% Exon7 (WM+MM/WW)
Brockmöller et al., 1996a (Germany)	374 incid. + prev. bladder cancer histolog. confirmed (Caucas.)	373 hospital cancer-free controls (Caucas.)		PCR (MspI, Exon7)	smoking, occupation (>1 year in jobs at high risk for bladder cancer)	age, gender, ethnicity, cancer histology, tumour stage, tumour grade, GSTM1, GSTT1, NAT2, CYP2D6 and CYP2E1 polym.		16.2% (MspI), 5.6% (Exon7) (WM+MM)	96.2% MspI, Exon7 (WM+MM/WW); 64.7%
Drakoulis et al., 1994 (Germany)	142 incid. lung cancer histolog. confirmed (Caucas.)	171 healthy or hospital controls (Caucas.)		PCR (Msp I, Exon7)	smoking (for cases only)	gender, ethnicity, cancer histology		14.6% (WM) Msp I, 6.4% (WM) Exon7	62.2% Msp I, 34.0% Exon7 (WM+MM/WW)

Study	Cases	Controls	Response	Method	Factor	Factor	Treatment	Frequency	Frequency
Emery et al., 1978 (UK)	62 incid. SQ lung cancer histolog. confirmed, smokers >20 cig./day for at least 10 yrs (Caucas.)	62 hospital controls, smokers, matched by age, gender, social class and smoking history (Caucas.)		AHH Ratio (induced/basal) in lymphocytes; high AHH ratio: >4.0	smoking	ethnicity		34%	39.8%
Esteller et al., 1997 (Spain)	80 incid. endometrial cancer histolog. confirmed undergoing surgery (Caucas.)	60 healthy controls from the same area (Caucas.)		PCR (Mspl, Exon7)		ethnicity	no radiotherapy or treatment with hormones before genotyping	10% Mspl, 8.3% Exon7 (WM), 1.6% Exon7 (MM)	18.8% Mspl, 18.7% Exon7 (WM+MM+WW)
Gahmberg et al., 1979 (Finland)	90 incid. lung cancer (Caucas.)	404 healthy controls (Caucas.)		induced AHH activity in lymphoblasts; high AHH: relative value >1.5		ethnicity	no treatment before phenotyping	15%	64.3%
Goto et al. 1996 (Japan)	232 incid. lung cancer (non-SC) histolog. confirmed (Asians)			PCR (Mspl)	smoking (non-smokers, smokers)	age (<65, >65 yrs), gender, cancer histology, tumour stage and grade, GSTM1 polym., survival time, operability	no treatment before genotyping		
Guirgis et al., 1976 (USA)	11 prev. lung cancer histolog. confirmed, male smokers (Caucas.?)	11 healthy controls matched by age and gender (Caucas.?)		induced AHH activity in lymphocytes			no chemotherapy or radiotherapy before phenotyping		46.9%
Hamada et al., 1995 (Brazil)	99 incid. lung cancer histolog. confirmed (79 Caucas., 20 Afric.-Americ.)	108 hospital cancer-free patients matched by gender, age (3 yrs) and ethnicity (87 Caucas., 21 Afric.-Americ.)	80.5% cases, 99.1% controls	PCR (Exon7)	smoking (non-smokers, <40 PY, 40-59 PY, >59 PY) for cases only	age, gender, ethnicity, smoking		17% (WM+MM) White Brazilians 10% (WM+MM) Black Brazilians	38.4% White Brazilians 4.9% Black Brazilians (WM+MM+WW)
Hayashi et al., 1992 (Japan)	212 incid. lung cancer, 95 incid. stomach cancer, incid. 85 incid. colon cancer, 98 incid. breast cancer histolog. confirmed (Asians)	358 healthy controls from a cohort study (Asians)		PCR (Exon7)		ethnicity, cancer histology and GSTM1 polym. (for lung cancer)		30.2% (WM), 4.7% (MM)	97.2% lung, 81.8% stomach, 78.1% colon, 82.7% breast (WM+MM+WW); 45.4% lung, 27.7% stomach, 29.4% colon, 30.7% breast (MM/WM+WW)
Hirvonen et al., 1992a (Finland)	87 incid. lung cancer histolog. confirmed undergoing surgery (Caucas.)	121 healthy controls, 23 hospital controls with nonmalignant pulmonary diseases (Caucas.)		PCR (Mspl, Exon7)	smoking and occupation (for cases and hospital controls only)	ethnicity, cancer histology	no radio- or chemotherapy before genotyping	19.8% (WM), 1.7% (MM) Mspl; 7.4% (WM), 1.6% (MM) Exon7	53.9% Mspl (WM+MM+WW)
Hirvonen et al., 1993 (Finland)	74 incid. lung cancer histolog. confirmed undergoing surgery (Caucas.)	118 healthy controls (Caucas.)		PCR (Mspl)		ethnicity, cancer histology	no radio- or chemotherapy before genotyping	21.2% (WM), 1.7% (MM)	49.1% (WM+MM+WW)

Table 25 (Contd). Study design: CYP1A1 and AHH activity and inducibility and cancer (case–case studies shaded grey)

Author	# of cases	# of controls	Response	Genotype/phenotype	Exposures	Covariates	Therapy	% variants in controls	Power (α=0.05, OR>2)
Jacquet et al., 1996 (Belgium)	48 prev. lung cancer histolog. confirmed (Caucas.)	81 healthy blood donors (Caucas.)		PCR (MspI), AHH inducibility in lymphocytes		ethnicity, cancer histology		2.5% (MM), 18.5% (WM)	21.0% (WM+MM/WW)
Jahnke et al., 1996 (UK)	269 prev. laryngeal SQ histolog. confirmed undergoing surgery (Caucas.)	216 healthy controls (Caucas.)		PCR (MspI, Exon7)		ethnicity, cancer histology, tumour location (glottic, supra-glottic), grading and staging			
Kärki et al., 1987 (Finland)	30 prev. lung cancer histolog. confirmed (Caucas.)	80 hospital controls (Caucas.)		basal, induced & AHH Ratio (induced/basal) in lymphocytes; AHH activity corrected by 3H-TdR incorporation		ethnicity			
Katoh, et al., 1995 (Japan)	83 prev. TCC histolog. confirmed (65 of the bladder, 12 renal pelvis, 6 ureter) (Asians)	101 healthy controls (Asians)		PCR (Exon7)				38.6% (WM), 5.0% (MM)	58.2% (WM+MM/WW), 15.1% (MM/WM+WW)
Kawajiri et al., 1990 (Japan)	68 prev. lung cancer histolog. confirmed (Asians)	104 healthy controls (Asians)		PCR (MspI)		ethnicity, cancer histology		40.4% (WM), 10.8% (MM)	51.2% (WM+MM/WW), 28.2% (MM/WM+WW)
Kellermann et al., 1973 (USA)	50 incid. lung cancer histolog. confirmed, smokers (Caucas.)	85 healthy controls (Caucas.)		AHH ratio (induced/basal) in lymphocytes: low <2.5, intermed. 2.6-3.6, high >3.6		ethnicity		45.9% (intermediate), 10.9% (high)	19.8% (MM/WM+WW), 37.4% (WM+MM/WW)
Kelsey et al., 1994 (USA)	72 incid. lung cancer histolog. confirmed (African-Americans)	97 healthy controls matched by age (5 yrs) and gender (African-Americans)		PCR (AA)	smoking (non-smokers, smokers <25, 25-49, >49 PY)	ethnicity, cancer histology	no treatment before genotyping	21.6% (WM), 2.1% (MM)	47.2% (WM+MM/WW)
Kihara et al., 1995b (Japan)	118 incid. lung cancer histolog. confirmed, smokers (71 SQ, 47 SC) <70 yrs (Asians)	331 healthy controls <70 yrs, smokers (Asians)		PCR (MspI, Exon7)	smoking (non-smokers, ex-smokers, current smokers <800, >800, >1200 cig. per day x yrs), occupation (no exp. to lung carcinog.)	ethnicity, gender, GSTM1 polym., cancer histology		17.8% MspI, 6.0% Exon 7 (MM)	75.6% MspI, 40.6% Exon7 (MM/WM+WW)

Reference	Study population (cases/controls)	%	Method	Exposure	Adjustment factors	Results
Korsgaard et al., 1984 (Sweden)	21 incid. lung cancer, 34 prev. oral cancer, 41 prev. laryngeal cancer, 76 prev. urothelial TCC (30 renal pelvis and ureteral, 46 bladder) histolog. confirmed (Caucas.) / 92 healthy controls (hospital staff and workers exp. to asbestos) matched by age, gender and smoking (Caucas.)		AHH ratio (induced/basal) in lymphoblasts: low <2.5, intermed. 2.6-3.6, high >3.6		ethnicity	9.2% (high AHH ratio); 13.2% (oral), 18.6% (laryngeal), 16.9% (lung), 15.8% (renal), 19.6% (bladder)
Kouri et al., 1982 (USA)	21 incid. lung cancer histolog. confirmed (mixed) / 30 hospital patients with other pulmonary diseases, comparable to cases for age, ethnicity and smoking history (mixed)		induced AHH activity in lymphocytes; AHH activity (peak units of AHH per cytochrome c)	smoking	age, cancer histology, tumour location, family history of cancer	
Lear et al., 1996 (UK)	827 incid BCC histolog. confirmed (Caucas.)		PCR (MspI, Exon7)		gender, skin type, eye colour, number of BCC, BCC rate, GSTM1, GSTT1 and CYP2D6 polym.	no treatment before phenotyping
Lear et al., 1997 (UK)	74 prev. BCC histolog. confirmed with at least one truncal tumour (Caucas.) / 263 prev. BCC controls without truncal tumours (Caucas.)	100%	PCR (MspI, Exon7)		age, gender, ethnicity, cancer histology, BCC number, GSTT1, GSTM1, GSTM3 and CYP2D6 polym.	
Liu et al., 1988 (China)	53 prev. lung cancer histolog. confirmed (Asians) / 61 hospital patients with other pulmonary diseases (Asians)		basal AHH activity in lung tissue		age, gender, ethnicity, living conditions, medication history, smoking and occupation (exposure to PAH)	
London et al., 1995b (USA)	144 incid. lung cancer histolog. confirmed (African-Americans) / 230 healthy controls frequency matched by age, ethnicity and gender (African-Americans)A	86.2% cases, 89.1% controls	PCR (AA)	smoking (non-smokers, smokers 1-35, >35 PY), occupation (exposure to asbestos or motor vehicle exhaust)	ethnicity, cancer histology, intake of b-carotene, vitamin E and C	15.2% (WM+MM); 70.6% (WM+MMWW)
Lucas et al., 1996 (France)	62 prev. esophageal cancer, 96 prev. upper aerodigestive tract cancer (Caucas.) / 260 healthy controls (Caucas.)		PCR (Msp I)	alcohol	ethnicity	15.0% (WM), 1.2% (MM); 49.3% esophageal cancer, 62.8% upper aerodigestive cancer (WM+MM/WW)
McLemore et al., 1977 (USA)	47 incid. lung cancer histolog. confirmed (Caucas.?) / 56 hospital patients with other pulmonary diseases (Caucas.?)		basal AHH activity in PAM and AHH activity in lymphocytes; AHH Ratio (induced/basal) in lymphocytes	smoking (non-smokers, smokers)		

Table 25 (Contd). Study design: CYP1A1 and AHH activity and inducibility and cancer (case–case studies shaded grey)

Author	# of cases	# of controls	Response	Genotype/phenotype	Exposures	Covariates	Therapy	% variants in controls	Power ($\alpha=0.05$, OR>2)
McLemore et al., 1978 (USA)	14 lung cancer histolog. confirmed, smokers (Caucas.?)	15 hospital patients with other pulmonary diseases, smokers (Caucas.?)		basal and induced AHH activity in PAM and lymphocytes; AHH Ratio (induced/basal) in PAM and lymphocytes: high AHH ratio: >2	smoking		no chemotherapy or radiotherapy before phenotyping		
McLemore et al., 1979 (USA)	52 incid. lung cancer histolog. confirmed, smokers (Caucas.?)	52 hospital patients with other pulmonary diseases, smokers (Caucas.?)		basal AHH activity in PAM, high AHH >100mU; AHH ratio (induced/basal) in lymphocytes: high ratio >2 fold	smoking	age, family history of cancer	no treatment before phenotyping	28% (basal) 30.8% (ratio)	35.6% 37.3%
Morita et al, 1997 (Japan)	53 incid. oesophageal SQ histolog. confirmed undergoing surgery (Asians)	132 healthy controls (Asians)		PCR (Exon7)	smoking (non-smokers, smokers), alcohol (non-drinkers, drinkers)	ethnicity, gender, cancer histology, GSTM1 and CYP2E1 polym.	no treatment before phenotyping	2.3% (MM), 37.1% (WM)	7.5% (MM/WM+WW), 49.9% (WM-MM/WW)
Nakachi et al., 1991 (Japan)	151 incid. lung cancer histolog. confirmed (Asians)	375 healthy controls matched by age (1 year) and gender (Asians)		PCR (MspI)	smoking (< 41, 41-55 PY, >55 PY)	ethnicity, cancer histology		45.1% (WM) 10.6% (MM)	91.4% (WM+MM/WW), 68.6% (MM/WM+WW)
Nakachi et al., 1993 (Japan) (includes SQ cases from Nakachi et al., 1991)	85 incid. SQ lung cancer histolog. confirmed (Asians)	170 healthy controls from a cohort study, matched by age (1 year) and gender (Asians)		PCR (MspI, Exon7)	smoking (< 44 PY, >44 PY)	ethnicity, GSTM1 polym., cancer histology		42.9% WM, 8.8% MM (MspI); 31.8% WM 3.5% MM (Exon7)	15.9% Exon7 35.1% MspI (MM/WM+WW)
Okada et al., 1994 (Japan)	267 incid. lung cancer and 54 incid. pancreatic cancer histolog. confirmed undergoing surgery (Asians)	same as Nakachi et al, 1991		PCR (MspI)	smoking (non-smokers, <41 PY, >41 PY)	ethnicity, cancer histology, presence of metastasis		45.1% (WM) 10.6% (MM)	83.2% (MM/WM+WW)
Paigen et al., 1977 (USA)	12 incid. lung cancer histolog. confirmed (Caucas.?)	57 healthy controls (Caucas.?)		basal AHH activity in lymphocytes; AHH Ratio (induced/basal) in lymphocytes			no treatment before phenotyping		

Reference	Cases	Controls	Response	basal AHH activity in normal lung parenchyma	smoking	covariates	no treatment before phenotyping	genotype (het)	genotype frequency
Petruzzelli et al., 1988 (Italy)	49 incid. lung cancer histolog. confirmed (Caucas.)	16 hospital patients with other lung diseases (Caucas.)		PCR (Exon7)		ethnicity		0% (MM+WM)	N.D.
Rebbeck et al., 1994 (USA)	96 incid. breast cancer (Caucas.)	146 healthy controls (Caucas.)				ethnicity		30.4% (WM), 8.7% (MM) African-Americans; 20% (WM), 4.0% (MM) Caucas.	14.9% African-Americans, 12.9% Caucas. (WM+MM/WW)
Shields et al., 1993b (USA)	56 incid. lung cancer histolog. confirmed (mixed)	31 COPD and 15 controls with cancer at sites other than lung and bladder (mixed)	55.3%	Southern blot; PCR (MspI)	smoking (non-smokers, <40 PY, 40-59 PY, >59 PY)	ethnicity, age, gender, cancer histology, CYP2D6 polym.			
Sivaraman et al, 1994 (USA)	43 incid. colorectal AD in situ (mixed)	124 healthy controls matched by gender, age (5 yrs) and ethnicity (mixed)	73.4%	PCR (MspI, Exon7)		age, gender, ethnicity		47% (WM), 4% (MM) MspI, 30% (WM) Exon7	27.7% MspI 27.3% Exon7 (WM+MM/WW); 5.0% MspI (MM/WM+WW)
Sugimura et al., 1994 (Brazil)	110 incid. lung cancer histolog. confirmed (mixed)	112 hospital cancer-free outpatients controls matched by gender, age (3 yrs) and ethnicity (mixed)		PCR (MspI)	smoking (<40 PY, 40-60 PY >60 PY) for cases only	ethnicity, cancer histology		30% (WM), 8% (MM) White Brazilians; 27% (WM), 9% (MM) Black Brazilians	67.0% (WM+MM/WW), 28.3% (MM/WM+WW)
Taioli et al., 1995a (USA)	76 incid. lung cancer histolog. confirmed (African-Americans)	123 healthy controls (African-Americans)		PCR (AA)	smoking (non-smokers, eversmokers)	ethnicity, cancer histology		16.3%	43.4%
Taioli, et al., 1995b (USA)	51 breast cancer (mixed)	269 healthy controls matched by ethnicity (mixed)	96.1% cases, 94.8% controls	PCR (MspI, Exon7, AA)		ethnicity		36.5% (WM), 3.5% (MM) Afric.-Americ., 17.5% (WM), 2.7% (MM) Caucas. (MspI); 6.0% (WM) Afric.-Americ., 16.0% (WM), 1.1% (MM) Caucas. (Exon7); 16.2% (WM) Afric.-Americ. (AA)	21.5% African-Americans, 30.8% Caucas. (MspI); 27.7% Caucas. (Exon7); 17.6% African-Americans (AA); (WM+MM/WW)
Tefre et al., 1991 (Norway)	221 incid. lung cancer histolog. confirmed (Caucas.)	212 healthy controls (Caucas.)		PCR (MspI)		ethnicity, cancer histology		20.3% (WM), 0.9% (MM)	86.3% (WM+MM/WW), 6.3% (MM/WM+WW)

Table 25 (Contd). Study design: CYP1A1 and AHH activity and inducibility and cancer (case–case studies shaded grey)

Author	# of cases	# of controls	Response	Genotype/ phenotype	Exposures	Covariates	Therapy	% variants in controls	Power (α=0.05, OR>2)
Ward et al., 1978 (USA)	32 prev. lung cancer, 27 prev. laryngeal cancer histolog. confirmed (Caucas.?)	65 spouses of the cases, 17 healthy controls matched by age (Caucas.?)		basal AHH activity in lymphocytes; AHH ratio (induced/basal) in lymphocytes	smoking (>20, 20-40, >40 PY) for cases only	age (<57, >57 yrs), family history of cancer		12.3% (high), 35.1% (intermed.),	25.4% lung. 22.2% larynx (WM+MM/WW)
Xu et al., 1996 (USA)	207 incid. lung cancer histolog. confirmed (mixed)	93 healthy and 190 hospital controls (mixed)	77.8% cases, 97.2% controls	PCR (MspI)	smoking (non-smokers, smokers <35, >35 PY, ex-smokers, yrs since quitting), occupation (exp. to asbestos)	age, gender, education, ethnicity, cancer histology, family cancer history		0.7% (MM), 17.0% (WM)	87.1% (WM+MM/WW)
Yengi et al., 1996 (UK)	286 basal cell carcinoma (92 single BCC, 194 multiple BCC) histologic. confirmed (Caucas.)	300 cancer-free hospital controls (Caucas.)		PCR (MspI, Exon7)		age, gender, skin type, ethnicity, cancer histology, GSTM1, GSTM3, GSTT1 and CYP2D6 polym.		7.1% (WM), 1.2% (MM) Exon7; 13.4% (WM), 0.0% (MM) MspI	27.9% Exon7, 43.7% MspI (WM+MM/WW)
Yoshikawa et al., 1994 (Japan)	56 incid. lung cancer histolog. confirmed (Asians)	36 hospital controls deceased for causes other than pulmonary diseases (Asians)		basal AHH activity in normal lung tissue	smoking (non-smokers, smokers)	ethnicity, cancer histology			

Table 26. Study design: CYP1A1 and outcomes other than cancer

Author	Subjects	Analysis	Phenotyping/ genotyping	Exposures	Covariates	Variants (%)
Alexandrov et al., 1992 (Italy)	13 lung cancer (Caucas.)	BPDE-DNA adducts measured in normal parenchymal lung tissue by HPLC + fluorescence spectrometry	AHH activity in lung microsomes measured by fluorimetric assay		ethnicity	
Bartsch et al., 1992a (Italy, Finland)	60 lung cancer, 20 other thoracic diseases (Caucas.)	32P-postlabelling assay of DNA adducts in bronchial and parenchymal lung tissue	AHH activity in bronchial and parenchymal lung microsomes measured by fluorimetric assay	smoking (smokers, non-smokers)	ethnicity	
Bartsch et al., 1995 (Finland)	230 patients undergoing surgery for lung cancer or other thoracic diseases (Caucas.)	32P-postlabelling assay of PAH-DNA adducts and BPDE-DNA adducts in parenchymal lung tissue	AHH activity in lung microsomes	smoking (smokers, non-smokers, ex-smokers)	ethnicity	
Brockmöller et al., 1996b (Germany)	69 bladder cancer histolog. confirmed (Caucas.)	p53 mutations by PCR	PCR (Exon7, MspI)		ethnicity	
Cheng et al., 1995a (USA)	78 healthy controls (95% Caucas.)	SCE in lymphocytes	PCR (Msp I, Exon 7)	smoking (current, former, never smokers), alcohol	age, gender, diet (vit. A, C, E, folate)	10% MspI, 20% Exon7 (WM+MM)
Degawa et al., 1994 (USA)	25 laryngeal cancer patients (Caucas.?)	32P-postlabelling assay of total DNA adducts in normal laryngeal mucosa	AHH activity in laryngeal microsomes measured by immunoblotting	smoking (smokers, non-smokers)		
Gallagher et al., 1994 (USA)	10 US pregnant women, 8 Taiwanese non-smoking pregnant women	32P-postlabelling assay of total DNA adducts in placental tissue	AHH activity in placental microsomes	smoking (smokers, non-smokers) for US women, exp. to PCB and PCDF for Taiwanese women	ethnicity	
Hemminki et al., 1997 (Finland, USA)	100 foundry workers (Caucas.)	32P-postlabelling assay of PAH-DNA adducts in lymphocytes	PCR (Exon 7, Msp I)		ethnicity, smoking, occupation (exp. to PAH), diet (charcoal broiled food)	5.2%WM+MM (Exon7); 11.5% WM+MM (MspI)
Ichiba et al., 1994 (Sweden)	69 male chimney sweeps, 35 male healthy controls lacking a definite PAH exposure (Caucas.)	32P-postlabelling assay of PAH-DNA adducts in total WBC; micronuclei in B- and T-lymphocytes	PCR (Msp I, Exon 7)	smoking, occupation (exp. to PAH)	ethnicity, gender	25.6% (WM)
Kato et al., 1995a (USA)	90 cancer-free autopsy donors (mixed)	32P-postlabelling assay of PAH-dGMP) in parenchymal lung tissue	PCR (Exon 7)	smoking (serum cotinine levels)		15.5% (WM+MM)
Kawajiri et al., 1996 (Japan)	187 non-SC lung cancers: 75 SQ, 112 AD (Asians)	p53 mutations by PCR	PCR (Msp I, Exon 7)	smoking (current or ex-smokers, non-smokers)	ethnicity, GSTM1 polym.	8.1% (MM), 32.4% (WM) Exon7, 14.9% (MM), 46.6% (WM) MspI

Table 26 (Contd). Study design: CYP1A1 and outcomes other than cancer

Author	Subjects	Analysis	Phenotyping/ genotyping	Exposures	Covariates	Variants (%)
Manchester et al., 1992 (USA)	16 healthy women at delivery (mixed)	BPDE-DNA adducts measured in placental tissue by immunoaffinity chromatography + fluorescence spectrometry	AHH activity in placental microsomes	smoking (cig./day, cord blood cotinine levels)		
Mooney et al., 1997 (USA)	159 heavy smokers enrolled in a smoking cessation program (mixed, 90% Caucas.)	PAH-DNA adducts in WBC by ELISA	PCR (Exon7, MspI)	smoking (>20 cig./day for >1 year)	GSTM1 polym., serum levels of retinol, β-carotene and α-tocopherol	6.3% WM (Exon7); 1.2% MM, 16.4% WM (MspI)
Ohshima et al., 1997 (Japan)	35 prev. SQ lung cancer histolog. confirmed (Asians)	p53 mutations by PCR	PCR (Exon7)		ethnicity, family history of cancer	5.7% MM, 45.7% WM (Exon7)
Rebbeck et al., 1996 (USA)	28 prev. ductal breast cancer histolog. confirmed	LOH in tumour tissue	PCR (Exon7)			
Rothman et al., 1995 (USA)	47 non-smoking fire-fighters (mixed)	PAH-DNA adducts in WBC by ELISA	PCR (Exon7)	smoking (non-smokers)	ethnicity, age, gender, season of blood collection, alcohol (drinks per week), GSTM1 polym.	19.1% Exon7 (WM+MM)
Shields et al., 1993a (USA)	38 cancer-free autopsy donors (12 Afric.-Americ., 26 Caucas.)	32P-postlabelling assay of PAH-DNA adducts in parenchymal lung tissue	PCR (Exon7)	smoking (serum cotinine levels) for 30 cases	age, gender, ethnicity	5.3% (WM) 10.5% (MM)
Wang et al., 1997 (Japan)	192 healthy male workers employed in a food products factory (Asians)	32P-postlabelling assay of PAH-DNA adducts in lymphocytes	PCR (Exon7)	smoking (smokers, non-smokers)	ethnicity, gender, serum levels of β-carotene and α-tocopherol	

Table 27. Results: CYP1A1 and AHH activity and inducibility – lung cancer (case-case studies shaded grey)

Author	OR - Lung cancer	OR - stratified by ethnicity	OR - stratified by smoking	OR - stratified by cancer histology	OR - interactions between polymorphisms	Other comments
Guirgis et al., 1976 (USA)	significantly higher AAH activity in cases than controls (p<0.025)			3.70 (1.25-10.96) SQ, 2.42 (0.68-8.64) SC, 1.99 (0.57-6.98) AD (MM/WM+WW); 2.20 (0.84-5.79) SQ, 1.20 (0.44-3.29) SC, 1.56 (0.60-4.09) AD (WM+MM/WW)		
Kawajiri et al., 1990 (Japan)	Msp I: 2.60 (1.12-6.02) (MM/WM+WW); 1.76 (0.94-3.31) (WM+MM/WW)					
Kellermann et al., 1973 (USA)	19.40 (4.48-172.21) (WM+MM/WW), 4.13 (1.46-12.21) (MM/WM+WW)					
McLemore et al., 1977 (USA)	significantly higher PAM AAH activity in cases than controls (p>0.05)		AHH lymphocyte activity significantly higher in cases than controls for non-smokers (p<0.001), but not for smokers (p>0.1); significantly lower AHH induction in cases than controls for non-smokers (p<0.001), but not for smokers (p>0.1)			
Paigen et al., 1977 (USA)	significantly lower induced AHH activity in cases than controls (p<0.001)					
Emery et al., 1978 (UK)			significantly greater proportion of high AHH inducers in cases than controls (p<0.001)			
McLemore et al., 1978 (USA)			no significantly different basal or induced AHH activity (in both PAM and lymphocytes) in cases compared to controls			
Ward et al., 1978 (USA)	AHH activity: 0.76 (0.32-1.83) (WM+MM/WW); 1.65 (0.50-5.41) (MM/WM+WW)					no significantly different AHH activity between younger vs. older cases and between cases with positive vs. negative family history of cancer

Table 27 (Contd). Results: CYP1A1 and AHH activity and inducibility – lung cancer (case–case studies shaded grey)

Author	OR - Lung cancer	OR - stratified by ethnicity	OR - stratified by smoking	OR - stratified by cancer histology	OR - interactions between polymorphisms	Other comments
Gahmberg et al., 1979 (Finland)	significantly higher AHH activity after induction in cases than controls (p<0.0001)					significantly lower age among cases with high AHH activity (p<0.01)
McLemore et al., 1979 (USA)			significantly greater proportion of cases compared to controls with high AHH induction ratio in lymphocytes (p<0.05), but not in PAMs (p>0.2)			significantly higher AHH induction ratio in lymphocytes between cases with positive vs. negative family history of cancer (p=0.02)
Kouri et al., 1982 (USA)	significantly higher AHH/cytochrome c activity in cases than controls (p<0.001)					no significant association of AHH activity with age (p=0.45), cancer family history (p=0.38), cancer histology (p=0.13), tumour location (p=0.80) or smoking history (p=0.80) among cases
Korsgaard et al., 1984 (Sweden)	11.07 (3.74-32.75) (high vs. low + intermediate AHH ratio)					
Kärki et al., 1987 (Finland)	no significantly different AHH activity ratio between cases and controls (p=0.47)					
Liu et al., 1988 (China)	significantly higher AHH activity (p<0.05) in cases compared to controls (adjusted for age, gender, living conditions, occupational exposure, smoking and medication history)					
Petruzzelli et al., 1988 (Italy)	no significantly different AHH activity between cases and controls (p=0.47)		significantly higher AHH activity among smoking cases compared to smoking controls (p<0.01)			
Abe et al., 1990 (Japan)	no significantly different AHH activity (p=0.51) or AHH inducibility (p=1.00) between cases and controls		no significantly different AHH activity (p=0.88) or AHH inducibility (p=0.21) between smoking cases and smoking controls			no significant association of AHH activity with age (p=0.21); significantly higher AHH activity in cases with central compared to peripherical cancers (p<0.001)

Reference	Genotype OR (95% CI)	By smoking (PY)	By histology	Gene–gene interaction	Comments
Nakachi et al., 1991 (Japan)	MspI: 2.25 (1.35-3.75) (MM/WM+WW)	2.85 (1.18-6.88) smokers, 7.31 (1.85-28.86) <41 PY, 2.00 (0.42-9.55) 41-55 PY, 1.13 (0.20-6.39) >55 PY (MM/WM+WW)	2.99 (1.52-5.87) SQ, 3.45 (1.35-8.82) SC, 2.09 (0.43-10.20) LC, 3.00 (1.70-5.30) Kreyberg I, 1.29 (0.57-2.91) AD (MM+WM+WW)		no significant association of MspI polymorphism with age (p=0.52), gender (p=0.60), cancer histology (p=0.56), family history of cancer (p=0.57) or smoking history (p=0.58) among cases (WM+MM/WW)
Tefre et al, 1991 (Norway)	Msp I: 0.96 (0.13-6.87) (MM/WM+WW), 1.06 (0.67-1.67) (WM+MM/WW) Exon7: no significant association between Exon7 polymorph. and lung cancer		1.32 (0.73-2.40) SQ, 0.82 (0.39-1.76) SC, 0.78 (0.34-1.79) AD (WM+MM/WW)		
Hayashi et al., 1992 (Japan)	Exon 7: 2.80 (1.48-5.30) (MM/WM+WW)		3.52 (1.53-8.07) SQ, 3.21 (1.57-6.58) Kreyberg I, 2.33 (1.03-5.28) AD (MM/WM+WW)	5.83 (2.38-14.28), 9.07 (2.95-27.93) SQ, 3.45 (1.04-11.49) AD, 7.94 (2.99-21.08) Kreyberg I (GSTM1null/Exon7 MM vs. GSTM1+/Exon7 WW)	no significant association of MspI or Exon7 polymorphisms with occupational exposure to asbestos
Hirvonen et al., 1992a (Finland)	MspI: 1.24 (0.65-2.37) (WM+MM/WW); Exon7: no significant association between Exon7 polymorph. and lung cancer	1.39 (0.34-5.73) smokers, 0.40 (0.02-8.07) <25 PY, 1.45 (0.25-8.27) >25 PY, 0.83 (0.04-17.00) non-smokers, 1.57 (0.07-37.94) ex-smokers (MspI, WM+MM/WW)	1.71 (0.79-3.68) SQ, 1.46 (0.31-7.97) SC, 0.84 (0.31-2.26) AD (MspI, WM+MM/WW)		
Hirvonen et al., 1993 (Finland)	Msp I: 0.70 (0.34-1.46) vs. all controls, 0.65 (0.31-1.38) vs. healthy controls (WM+MM/WW)		0.82 (0.33-2.03) SQ, 0.79 (0.28-2.24) AD, 0 MM or WM among SC cases (p=0.54) (vs. all controls); 0.76 (0.30-1.92) SQ, 0.73 (0.25-2.11) AD, 0 MM or WM among SC cases (p=0.56) (vs. healthy controls)		
Nakachi et al., 1993 (Japan)	MspI: 2.97 (1.43-6.21) SQ, Exon7: 3.24 (1.11-9.42) SQ (MM/WM+WW)	MspI: 7.62 (2.96-19.58) < 44 PY, 1.22 (0.32-4.63) >44 PY; Exon7: 7.38 (1.94-28.08) < 44 PY, 1.21 (0.19-7.56) >44 PY (MM/WM+WW)		20.67 (3.60-118.50) < 44 PY, 1.83 (0.15-21.64 >44 PY, (GSTM1null/Exon7 MM vs. GSTM1+/Exon7 WW+WM); 23.20 (5.13-104.85) < 44 PY, 1.82 (0.30-11.02) >44 PY, (GSTM1null/MspI MM vs. GSTM1+/MspI WW+WM)	

Table 27 (Contd). Results: CYP1A1 and AHH activity and inducibility – lung cancer (case-case studies shaded grey)

Author	OR - Lung cancer	OR - stratified by ethnicity	OR - stratified by smoking	OR - stratified by cancer histology	OR - interactions between polymorphisms	Other comments
Shields et al., 1993b (USA)	Mspl: 0.67 (0.28-1.59), 0.76 (0.3-2.2) adjusted for age, ethnicity, smoking habit, gender and CYP2D6 polymorphism (WM+MM/WW); 0.56 (0.09-3.47) (MM/WM+WW)	0.9 (0.3-2.7) African-Americans, 0.4 (0.1-1.6) Caucas. (WM+MM/WW)	0.7 (0.2-3.3) <40 PY, 1.5 (0.2-9.9) 40-59 PY, 0.4 (0.1-2.0) >59 PY (WM+MM/WW)	0.6 (0.2-2.2) AD, 1.0 (0.4-2.7) SQ (WM+MM/WW)		100% concordance between PCR and Southern blot
Alexandrie et al., 1994 (Sweden)	Mspl: 0.99 (0.66-1.48), Exon7: 0.78 (0.41-1.46) (WM+MM/WW) vs. all controls			Mspl: 1.20 (0.68-2.11) SQ, 0.83 (0.37-1.86) SC, 0.95 (0.49-1.85) AD; Exon7: 1.22 (0.55-2.73) SQ, 0.23 (0.03-1.76) SC, 0.84 (0.31-2.28) AD (WM+MM/WW)	1.23 (0.69-2.19), 1.14 (0.54-2.41) SQ, 2.30 (0.76-5.40) SQ <65 yrs, 0.70 (0.25-1.96) SQ >65 yrs, 1.55 (0.56-4.25) SC, 1.20 (0.48-3.04) AD (GSTM1null/Mspl WM+MM vs. GSTM1+/Mspl WW)	no significant association of Mspl or Exon7 polymorph. with gender
Antilla et al., 1994 (Finland)	significant association of CYP1A1 inducible phenotype with peripheral tumour location (p=0.001), but non-significant with cancer histology (WM+MM/WW)				no significant association between GSTM1 polymorph. and cancer histology among CYP1A1 inducible polymorph. (p=0.064); significant association between GSTM1 polymorph. and tumour location among CYP1A1 inducible polymorph. (p=0.037)	
Drakoulis et al., 1994 (Germany)	1.13 (0.61-2.09) Mspl, 1.98 (0.89-4.37) Exon7 (WM+MM/WW)			Mspl: 1.65 (0.73-3.57) SQ, 1.21 (0.29-3.75) LC, 0.78 (0.14-2.69) SC, 0.79 (0.19-2.41) AD; Exon7: 2.51 (0.85-7.05) SQ, 2.10 (0.36-8.36) LC, 1.84 (0.32-7.29) SC, 2.39 (0.63-7.75) AD (WM+MM/WW)	1.18 (0.46-2.99) WM+MM vs. WW (Mspl+Exon7)	significantly lower frequency of Exon7 allele M in smokers compared to non-smokers (p=0.044); no significant association of Mspl or Exon7 polymorphisms with gender
Kelsey et al., 1994 (USA)	AA polymorphism: 0.64 (0.30-1.40) Afric.-Americ. (WM+MM/WW)		2.00 (0.34-11.76) <24 PY, 0.63 (0.09-4.22) 25-49 PY, 0.27 (0.03-2.19) >49 PY			no significant association of AA variants with any histological subtype of lung cancer

Reference					Comments
Okada et al., 1994 (Japan)	Msp I: 1.70 (1.07-2.69) (MM/WM+WW)	1.70 (0.90-3.20) smokers, 2.97 (1.27-6.95) <41 PY, 0.85 (0.33-3.23) >41 PY, 1.85 (0.66-5.17) AD <41 PY, 0.67 (0.21-2.16) AD>41 PY, 4.60 (1.69-12.55) SQ <41 PY, 0.75 (0.22-2.57) SQ >41 PY	1.24 (0.69-2.23) AD, 2.22 (1.20-4.10) SQ, 3.35 (1.23-9.12) LC, 0.49 (0.03-8.60) SC, 2.21 (1.27-3.85) Kreyberg I		significantly lower Mspl MM frequency among smokers cases (p=0.026) and SQ cases (p<0.05) with metastasis compared to corresponding cases without metastasis
Sugimura et al., 1994 (Brazil)	Msp I: 0.99 (0.57-1.71) (WM+MM/WW)	0.90 (0.49-1.65) White Brazilians, 1.46 (0.44-4.88) Black Brazilians (WM+MM/WW)	0.94 (0.52-1.68) Kreyberg I 1.19 (0.49-2.42) AD (WM+MM/WW)		no significantly different Mspl genotype frequency between cases with a smoking history <50 PY and >50PY (p=0.20)
Yoshikawa et al., 1994 (Japan)	significantly higher AHH activity in cases compared to controls (p<0.01)	significantly higher AHH activity in smoking cases compared to non-smoking controls (p<0.01) and in non-smoking cases compared to non-smoking controls (p<0.05)	no significant difference in AHH activity between SQ or AD cases and controls (stratified by smoking)		
Hamada et al., 1995 (Brazil)	Exon 7: 2.22 (1.13-4.36), 2.26 (1.14-4.49) adjusted for gender, age and ethnicity (WM+MM/WW)	2.35 (1.14-4.88) non-Blacks, 1.68 (0.25-11.27) Blacks; 2.40 (1.15-4.98) non-Blacks, 1.60 (0.23-11.1) Blacks (adjusted for age and gender) (WM+MM/WW)			no significant association between Exon7 genotype and smoking history among cases (p=0.75)
Kihara et al., 1995b (Japan)		Mspl: 0.91 (0.47-1.75), 0.84 (0.28-2.52) <800 SI, 1.02 (0.43-2.38) >800 Si; Exon7: 0.86 (0.29-2.56) (MM/WM+WW) (male smokers)	Mspl: 0.90 (0.42-1.96) SQ, 0.92 (0.35-2.39) SC; Exon7: 0.55 (0.12-2.53) SQ, 1.41 (0.37-5.34) SC; (MM/WM+WW) (male smokers)	1.95 (0.82-4.61) (GSTM1null/Mspl MM vs. GSTM1+/Mspl WM+WW)	
London et al., 1995b (USA)	AA polymorphism: 1.1 (0.63-1.96); 1.3 (0.7-2.4), 2.7 (0.6-11.8) possible exp. to motor vehicle exhausts. 2.2 (0.8-6.1) possible exp. to asbestos (adjusted for age, gender and smoking history) (WM+MM/WW)	1.5 (0.8-3.1) all smokers, 1.3 (0.6-3.2) 1-35 PY, 2.2 (0.6-7.8) >35 PY, (adjusted for age, gender) (WM+MM/WW)	1.3 (0.5-3.2) AD, 2.1 (0.8-5.9) SQ, 1.0 (0.2-5.4) SC, (adjusted for age, gender and smoking history) (WM+MM/WW)		no significant association of AA variants with intake of b-carotene, vitamin C or E
Taioli et al., 1995a (USA)	AA polymorphism: 1.1 (0.5-2.3) African-Americans (WM+MM/WW)	12.0 (0.7-197.4) AD, non-smokers, 2.28 (0.63-8.23) AD, smokers (WM+MM/WW)	2.6 (1.1-6.3) AD, 0.4 (0.1-2.0) SQ, 0.39 (0.02-7.60) SC (WM+MM/WW)		

Table 27 (Contd). Results: CYP1A1 and AHH activity and inducibility – lung cancer (case–case studies shaded grey)

Author	OR - Lung cancer	OR - stratified by ethnicity	OR - stratified by smoking	OR - stratified by cancer histology	OR - interactions between polymorphisms	Other comments
Goto et al., 1996 (Japan)	significant association of Mspl polymorph. with cancer histology (p=0.033), performance status (p=0.03), T-factor (p<0.001) and operability (p=0.037); almost significant with tumour stage (p=0.084), N-factor (p=0.057) and survival time (p=0.005) (WM+MM/WW)		significant association between Mspl polymorph. and survival time in smokers (p=0.024), but not in non-smokers (p=0.10)		significantly shorter survival time in GSTM1null/Mspl WM+MM vs. GSTM1+/Mspl WW (p=0.017)	significantly shorter survival time of non-resectable advanced-stage cases Mspl WM+MM vs. WW (p=0.005), adjusted for age, sex, smoking, cancer histology, performance status, clinical stages, GSTM1 polymorph.
Jacquet et al., 1996 (Belgium)	Msp I: 0.71 (0.27-1.87) (WM+MM/WW)			0.68 (0.14-3.35) SQ, 0.94 (0.24-3.72) AD, 3.76 (0.49-28.58) mixed (WM+MM/WW)		significant association between AHH hyperinducibility (90th percentile inducibility) and lung cancer: 3.41 (1.19-9.75) all, 5.29 (1.27-22.00) AD, 3.52 (0.77-16.03) SQ, 1.51 (0.16-14.05) SC
Xu et al., 1996 (USA)	Msp I: 1.01 (0.64-1.62) crude; 2.08 (1.15-3.73) adjusted for age, gender, ethnicity, education, family cancer history, smoking, asbestos exposure (WM+MM/WW)	1.94 (1.06-3.54) Caucas. (adjusted for age, gender, education, family cancer history, smoking, asbestos exposure) (WM+MM/WW)	1.81 (0.87-3.77) <35 PY, 1.54 (0.54-4.39) 35+ PY (crude); 2.16 (0.90-4.99) <35 PY, 2.03 (0.61-6.78) 35+ PY (adjusted for age, gender, ethnicity, education, family cancer history, asbestos exposure) (WM+MM/WW)	0.82 (0.39-1.71) SQ, 1.10 (0.63-1.94) AD (crude); 2.05 (0.72-5.82) SQ, 1.75 (0.90-3.42) AD (adjusted for age, gender, ethnicity, smoking, education, family cancer history, asbestos exposure) (WM+MM/WW)		
Bouchardy et al., 1997 (France)			Mspl: 1.0 (0.4-2.1) current smokers, 0.9 (0.3-2.6) ex-smokers, Exon7: 0.6 (0.2-1.8) current smokers, 1.7 (0.3-11.8) ex-smokers (adjusted for age, gender, age at start smoking, inhalation and occupational exposure) (WM+MM/WW)	Mspl: 1.2 (0.6-2.3) SQ, 0.7 (0.2-1.8) SC, Exon7: 0.8 (0.3-1.9) SQ, 1.1 (0.4-3.1) SC (smokers) (adjusted for age, gender, age at start smoking, inhalation and occupational exposure) (WM+MM/WW)		

Table 28. Results: CYP1A1 and AHH activity and inducibility – other cancers (case-case study shaded grey)

Author	OR - other cancers	OR - stratified by ethnicity	OR - stratified by smoking	OR - interactions between polymorphisms	Other comments
Ward et al., 1978 (USA)	AHH activity: 0.65 (0.26-1.67) larynx cancer (WM+MM/WW); 0.57 (0.11-2.96) larynx cancer (MM/WM+WW)				no significantly different AHH activity between younger vs. older cases and between cases with positive vs. negative family history of cancer
Korsgaard et al., 1984 (Sweden)	5.32 (2.09-13.57) larynx, 5.03 (1.88-13.45) oral cavity, 1.42 (0.40-4.99) renal pelvis and ureter, 1.38 (0.46-4.15) bladder (high vs. low+intermediate AHH ratio)				
Hayashi et al., 1992 (Japan)	Exon 7: 0.88 (0.29-2.68) stomach; 1.25 (0.45-3.50) colon; 0.85 (0.28-2.60) breast (MM/WM+WW)				
Okada et al., 1994 (Japan)	MspI: 0.65 (0.23-1.95) pancreas (MM/WM+WW)				
Rebbeck et al., 1994 (USA)	breast cancer no significant difference in Exon 7 mutant allele frequency between cases and controls (p=0.186)				
Sivaraman et al., 1994 (USA)	colon cancer in situ MspI: 6.82 (1.40-33.21) Exon7: 5.72 (0.27-122.65) (MM/WM+WW), MspI: 0.83 (0.36-1.91), Exon7: 0.81 (0.32-2.05) (WM+MM/WW)	MspI: 7.9 (1.4-44.4), Exon7: 5.7 (0.5-66.3) (MM/WM+WW)(Asians); 0 MspI MM among controls (p<0.001) (Hawaiians)			significant correlation between MspI and Exon7 polymorphisms (r=0.69, p<0.001); no changes in risk estimate after adjustment for age and gender
Ambrosone et al., 1995 (USA)	breast cancer 1.52 (0.90-2.56); 1.61 (0.94-2.75) adjusted for age (at diagnosis, menarche, first pregnancy and menopause), education, BMI, family history of breast cancer (WM+MM/WW); 2.85 (0.59-16.56) (MM/WM+WW)		1.30 (0.62-2.70) non-smokers, 5.22 (1.16-23.56) smokers <29 PY, 0.86 (0.24-3.09) smokers >29 PY, adjusted for age (at diagnosis, menarche, first pregnancy and menopause), education, BMI, family history of breast cancer (WM+MM/WW)	1.69 (0.82-3.48) (GSTM1null/Exon7WM+MM vs. GSTM1+/Exon7WW)	no significant association of Exon7 polymorph. with age: 1.57 (0.77-3.20) <64 yrs, 1.36 (0.63-2.95) >64 yrs (WM+MM/WW)

Table 28 (Contd). Results: CYP1A1 and AHH activity and inducibility – other cancers (case-case study shaded grey)

Author	OR - other cancers	OR - stratified by ethnicity	OR - stratified by smoking	OR - interactions between polymorphisms	Other comments
Taioli et al., 1995b (USA)		breast cancer Mspl: 3.00 (1.10-8.20) 1.43 (0.59-3.48) Caucas. (WM+MM/WW), 6.43 (1.32-31.40) (MM/WM+WW); AA: 1.21 (0.35-4.14) African-Americans (WM/WW); Exon7: 1.01 (0.36-2.85) Caucas. WM+MM/WW)		no significant interaction between CYP1A1 polymorphisms (AA, Mspl, Exon7)	
Katoh et al., 1995 (Japan)	colon cancer in situ Exon7: 0.86 (0.47-1.54) (WM+MM/WW); 0.72 (0.17-3.11) (MM/WM+WW)				
Lucas et al., 1996 (France)	no significant association of Mspl poly-morph. with esophageal cancer (p=0.09) or with upper aerodigestive cancer (p=0.20)				
Brockmöller et al, 1996a (Germany)	bladder cancer Mspl: 0.92 (0.61-1.41), Exon7: 0.67 (0.33-1.39) (WM+MM/WW) adjusted for age, gender, smoking and occupation			no significant interaction between polymorphisms on bladder cancer risk	no significant association of CYP1A1 genotype frequency (Mspl and Exon7) with cancer histology, tumour stage and grade
Yengi et al., 1996 (UK)	Exon7: 2.32 (1.01-5.37) total BCC, 2.17 (0.84-5.62) single BCC, 2.41 (1.01-5.74) multiple BCC Mspl: 1.41 (0.69-2.86) total BCC, 1.27 (0.55-2.96) single BCC, 1.48 (0.70-3.12) multiple BCC (WM+MM/WW)			significant interaction between GSTM3 and CYP1A1Mspl polymorph. on the number of tumours (p<0.001) (adjusted for age and gender)	significant association of CYP1A1 WW genotype with the number of tumours (p<0.001) (adjusted for age and gender)
Jahnke et al., 1996 (UK)	no significant association of Mspl or Exon7 polymorphisms with larynx cancer				

Lear *et al.*, 1996 (UK)	significant association of MspI WW with number of BCC (p=0.004) or with green-blue eye colour and number of BCC (p=0.002)(adjusted by age); almost significant association of Exon7 WW with BCC rate (p=0.079)	no significant higher risk of increased number of BCC in MspI MM/CYP2D6 WW vs. MspI WM+WW/CYP2D6 WW+MM (p=0.095); no significant interactions between polymorphisms in determining BCC rate
Esteller *et al.*, 1997 (Spain)	MspI: 3.67 (1.21-13.26), Exon7: 3.67 (1.21-13.26) endometrial cancer (WM+MM/WW)	
Lear *et al.*, 1997 (UK)	Exon7: 1.51 (1.29-1.77) truncal BCC, adjusted for age, gender and BCC number (WW/WM+MM); MspI: no significant association between MspI polymorph. and presence of truncal BCC	3.56 (1.52-8.34) (Exon7 WW/GSTT1null vs. Exon7 WM+MM/GSTT1+) adjusted for age, gender and BCC number
Morita *et al.*, 1997 (Japan)	oesophageal cancer Exon 7: 0.83 (0.02-10.58) SQ (MM/WM+WW), 1.01 (0.53-1.94) SQ (WM+MM/WW)	no significant interaction between CYP1A1 Exon7, CYP2E1 and GSTM1 polymorphisms on cancer risk

Table 29. Results: CYP1A1 and outcomes other than cancer

Author	SCE	MN and CA	Mutagenicity	DNA adducts	Interactions between polymorphisms	Other comments
Alexandrov et al., 1992 (Italy)				positive linear correlation between BPDE-DNA adducts level and AHH activity (r=0.91, p<0.001)		
Bartsch et al., 1992a (Italy, Finland)				positive linear correlation in smokers between total DNA-adduct level and AHH activity (r=0.69, p<0.001)		
Manchester et al., 1992 (USA)				significantly higher AHH activity in placentas with detectable compared to non-detectable BPDE-DNA adducts (p=0.03)		significant association between AHH activity and blood cotinine level (p<0.05)
Shields et al., 1993a (USA)				no significant association of PAH-DNA adduct level with Exon7 polymorph. (p=0.77), adjusted for age, gender, ethnicity, serum cotinine levels and GSTM1 polymorph.		
Degawa et al., 1994 (USA)				positive linear correlation in smokers between total DNA adduct level and AHH activity (r=0.67, p<0.05)		
Gallagher et al., 1994 (USA)				no significant correlation between AHH activity and total DNA adducts (p=0.51 among US smoking women, p=0.16 among Taiwanese non-smoking women exposed to PCB/PCDF)		
Ichiba et al., 1994 (Sweden)		no significant association of MN frequency with MspI or Exon7 polymorphisms		significantly higher DNA adduct level among sweeps with MspI WW compared to WM genotype (p=0.01); no significant association with Exon7 polymorph.		significant correlation between DNA adducts and MN levels in T-lymphocytes (r=0.30, p=0.04)
Bartsch et al., 1995 (Finland)				significant correlation in smokers of AHH activity with aromatic DNA adducts (r=0.64, p<0.001) and BPDE-DNA adducts (r=0.91, p<0.001)		
Cheng et al., 1995a (USA)	no significant association between SCE frequency and CYP1A1 MspI or Exon7 polymorphisms					
Kato et al., 1995a (USA)				no significant association of Exon7 polymorph. with PAH-DNA adduct level (p=0.92)		

Study			
Rothman et al., 1995 (USA)	no significant association of PAH-DNA adduct level with Exon7 polymorphism (p=0.12)		almost significantly higher PAH-DNA adduct level in GSTM1+/Exon7 WW vs. GSTM1 null/ Exon7 WM+MM (p=0.06)
Brockmöller et al., 1996b (Germany)	no significant association between p53 mutation frequency and MspI (p=0.64) or Exon7 (p=1.00) polymorphisms		
Kawajiri et al., 1996 (Japan)	significant association in smokers of p53 mutation frequency and MspI or Exon7 polymorph.: 3.50 (1.36-9.00) all, 2.06 (0.65-6.57) SQ, 7.08 (1.26-39.78) AD (MspI MM/WM+WW); 5.68 (1.47-21.99) all, 4.11 (0.66-43.85) SQ, 7.80 (0.57-417.10) AD (Exon 7 MM/WM+WW)	9.24 (2.38-35.93) (MspI MM/GSTM1- vs. MspI WW/GSTM1+); 8.17 (1.74-38.47) (Exon7 MM/GSTM1- vs. Exon7 WW/GSTM1+) (p53 mutations)	
Rebbeck et al., 1996 (USA)	non significant association between LOH and CYP1A1 Exon7 polymorph. (p=0.85)		
Hemminki et al., 1997 (Finland, USA)	no significant association of PAH-DNA adduct level with Exon7 (p=0.45) or MspI (p=0.86) polymorphisms;	almost significantly higher PAH-DNA adduct level for Exon7 WM+MM vs. WW among subjects with MspI WM or MM genotype (p=0.08)	no significant association of PAH-DNA adduct level with Exon7 or MspI polymorphisms after adjustment for smoking, occupational exp. and diet
Mooney et al., 1997 (USA)	significantly higher PAH-DNA adduct level for Exon7 WM vs. WW genotype (p<0.01); no significant association with Msp I polymorphism (p=0.25) (smokers)	no significant interaction of GSTM1 with CYP1A1 Exon7 or MspI polymorph. on PAH-DNA adduct level	significantly higher PAH-DNA adduct levels for Exon7 WM vs. WW among subjects GSTM1+ (p=0.004)
Ohshima et al., 1997 (Japan)	no significant association between p53 mutation frequency and Exon7 WM+WM compared to subjects with WW genotype (p=0.63)		no significant association of Exon7 polymorph. with family history of cancer (p=0.90)
Wang et al., 1997 (Japan)	no significant association of Exon7 polymorph. with PAH-DNA adducts		

Table 30. Study design: CYP1A2 and cancer

Author	# of cases	# of controls	Response	Genotyping/phenotyping	Exposures	Covariates	Therapy	Rapid variants among controls	Power (α=0.05, OR>2)
Lang et al., 1994 (USA)	41 incid. colorectal polyp and 34 colorectal cancer histolog. confirmed (mixed)	205 healthy controls randomly digit dialling selected (mixed)		caffeine 100 mg orally, urine coll. after 5 hours; analysis performed by HPLC; MR 17X+17U/137X = 4, 10		age (<35, >35 yrs, <60, >60 yrs), NAT2 polym., ethnicity, smoking		41%	67.8% all; 39.0% colon cancer; 45.5% colon polyps
Spigelman et al., 1994 (UK)	29 prev. familial adenomatous polyposis (Caucas.)	54 healthy volunteers matched by age and sex (Caucas.)		caffeine 300 mg orally, urine coll. after 2-6 hours; analysis performed by HPLC; MR = AAMU+1MX+1MU / 1,7 dimethylurate			no significant difference in CYP1A2 activity before and after colectomy		
Lee et al., 1994 (Korea)	100 prev. bladder cancer histolog. confirmed (Asians)	84 outpatients from the same department matched by age and sex (Asians)		theophylline 150 mg orally, urine coll. after 8 hours; analysis performed by HPLC	smoking, occupation (no exp. to bladder carcinogens)	age, sex, tumour grade (I, II, III)	no drugs known to influence the CYP1A2 metabolism		

Table 31. Study design: CYP1A2 and outcomes other than cancer

Author	Subjects	Analysis	Genotyping	Exposures	Covariates	CYP1A2 variants
Landi et al., 1996 (Italy)	100 healthy male blood donors 45-64 yrs old (Caucas.)	4-aminobiphenyl-haemoglobin adduct levels	70 mg caffeine orally, urine collected after 5 hours; analysis performed by capillary GC; MR = 4.6;	smoking (smokers, non-smokers, cotinine and nicotine in urine)	NAT2 polym., GSTM1 polym. (only 45 subjects)	65.2% (WM+MM)

Table 32. Results: CYP1A2 and cancer

Author	OR - digestive cancer (CYP1A2rapid/slow)	OR - other cancers (CYP1A2rapid/slow)	OR - interaction between polymorphisms	Other comments
Lang et al., 1994 (USA)	1.91 (1.20-2.87) all; 1.44 (0.70-2.98) colorectal cancers, 2.50 (1.25-5.00) colorectal polyps		2.79 (1.69-4.47) (CYP1A2rapid/NAT2rapid vs. CYP1A2slow/NAT2slow)	
Spigelman et al., 1994 (UK)	CYP1A2 activity significantly higher in FAP patients than controls (p=0.007)			
Lee et al., 1994 (Korea)		CYP1A2 activity significantly higher in bladder cancer cases than controls (p=0.006)		

Table 33. Results: CYP1A2 and outcomes other than cancers other than cancer

Author	Hb and albumin adducts (OR = WM+MM/WW)	OR - interactions between polymorphisms (OR = WM+MM/WW)
Landi et al., 1996 (Italy)	non-significant association between Hb-adducts and CYP1A2 polym. in non-smokers (p=0.70), but significant association in smokers (<1.5 mmol NICO: p=0.043; >1.5 mmol NICO: p=0.046)	no significant increase of ABP-Hb adduct level in CYP1A2rapid/NAT2slow vs. CYP1A2slow/NAT2rapid, nor in CYP1A2rapid/GSTM1null vs. CYP1A2slow/GSTM1+

Table 34. Study design: CYP2D6 and cancer (case–case studies shaded grey)

Author	# of cases	# of controls	Response	Phenotyping/genotyping	Exposures	Covariates	Therapy	MM in controls	Power (α=0.05, OR>2)
Agundez et al., 1994 (Spain)	89 incid. lung cancer histolog. confirmed (Caucas.)	98 healthy volunteers (Caucas.)		PCR		ethnicity, cancer history		7.0%	9.9% (WW+WM/MM)
Agundez et al., 1996 (Spain)	100 incid. HCC histolog. confirmed	258 healthy volunteers, 40 cirrhotic patients (Caucas.)	100% cases, 98% controls	PCR		ethnicity, cancer history, NAT2 polym., HBV-HCV markers		3.1%	56.5% (WW/WM+MM); <5% (WW+WM/MM)
Anwar et al., 1996 (Egypt)	22 prev. bladder cancer histolog. confirmed (Caucas.)	21 healthy controls matched by age and smoking (Caucas.)		PCR		ethnicity, CYP2E1 and GSTM1 polym.		52.4%	12.1% (WW+WM/MM)
Ayesh et al., 1984 (UK)	245 prev. lung cancer histolog. confirmed, smokers (Caucas.)	234 COPD smokers matched for gender, age, smoking history (Caucas.)		DBQ 10 mg administration and 8 hours urine collection; analysis performed by electron capture GC; MR = 1.0, 12.6 (DBQ/4-OH-DBQ)	smoking (>20 PY), occupation (exp. to asbestos and PAH)	ethnicity, gender, age, cancer histology	no surgery, radio- or chemotherapy before phenotyping	9%	39.0% (WW+WM/MM)
Caporaso et al., 1989 (UK, USA)									
Benhamou et al., 1996 (France)	140 incid. laryngeal SQ histolog. confirmed, male smokers >5 cig./day x 5 yrs (Caucas.)	154 hospital controls, male smokers >5 cig./day x 5 yrs (Caucas.)		dextromethorphan 25 mg administration and 8-12 hours urine collection; analysis performed by HPLC/fluorescence; MR=0.16, 0.08	smoking (smoking status, duration of smoking and age at start, inhalation, daily consumpt.), alcohol (drinking status, duration and daily consumption)	ethnicity, gender, age, tumor location (glottic, supraglottic), medication use	no drugs known to influence the phenotyping	32.5%	68.3% (WW+WM/MM)
Benitez et al., 1990 (Spain)	125 prev. transitional cell bladder cancer histolog. confirmed (Caucas.)	556 healthy controls having no use of drugs (Caucas.)		DBQ 10 mg administration and 8 hours urine collection; analysis performed by flame ionization GC; MR = 12.6 (DBQ/4-OH-DBQ)	smoking (<10, 10-19, 20-24, >24 cig./day), alcohol (<40, >40 g/day), occupation (exp. to bladder carcinog.) for cases	gender, ethnicity, cancer histology		6.1%	14.4% (WW+WM/MM)

Table 34 (Contd). Study design: CYP2D6 and cancer (case–case studies shaded grey)

Author	# of cases	# of controls	Response	Phenotyping/ genotyping	Exposures	Covariates	Therapy	MM in controls	Power (α=0.05, OR>2)
Benitez et al., 1991 (Spain)	84 prev. lung cancer histolog. confirmed, all ex- or current smokers, except two (Caucas.)	143 healthy male smokers, similar to cases for gender and smoking history (Caucas.)		DBQ 10 mg administration and 8 hours urine collection; analysis performed by flame ionization GC; MR = 12.6 (DBQ/4-OH-DBQ)	smoking (former-current)	ethnicity, cancer histology		7.0%	9.6% (WW+WM/MM)
Bouchardy et al., 1996 (France)	128 incid. lung cancer histolog. confirmed, smokers >5 cig./day x 5 yrs (Caucas.)	157 hospit. controls, smokers >5 cig/day x 5 yrs (Caucas.)		dextromethorphan 25 mg administration and 8-12 hours urine collection; analysis performed by HPLC/fluorescence; MR = 0.3	smoking (smoking status, duration of smoking, g./day of tobacco), occupation (exp. to asbestos or arsenic)	age, ethnicity, cancer histology, medication use		7.6%	35.9% (WW+WM/MM)
Brockmöller et al, 1996a (Germany)	374 incid. bladder cancer histolog. confirmed (Caucas.)	373 hospital cancer-free controls (Caucas.)		PCR; dextromethorphan 30 mg or DBQ 5 mg administration and 0-5 hours urine collection; analysis performed by HPLC/fluorescence; MR=12.6 (DBQ), 0.3 (dextromethorphan)	smoking, occupation (>1 year in jobs at high risk for bladder cancer)	age, gender, ethnicity, cancer histology, tumour stage and grade, NAT2, GSTT1, GSTM1, CYP2E1 and CYP1A1 polym.		5.9%	40.3% (WW+WM/MM) 99.5% (WW/WM+MM)
Buchert et al., 1993 (USA)	167 incid. + prev. breast cancer (Caucas.)	114 healthy controls (Caucas.)		PCR, RFLP		age (<40, 40-49, 50-59, >60 yrs), ethnicity, menopausal status (pre-, post-)		6.1%	24.9% (MM/WW+WM)
Caporaso et al., 1990 (USA)	96 incid. lung cancer histolog. confirmed (mixed)	55 COPD and 37 controls with cancers other than lung and bladder (mixed)	26%	DBQ 10 mg administration and 8 hours urine collection; analysis performed by electron capture GC; MR = 4.8, 11.7 (Caucas.), 4.2, 26.4 Afric.-Americ. (DBQ/4-OH-DBQ)	smoking (< or > median), alcohol, occupation (exp. to lung carcinog.)	age (<64, >64 yrs), gender, ethnicity, cancer histology, educational level, hospital	no radio- or chemotherapy before phenotyping	20% (Caucas.), 5% (African-Americ.)	38.0% (WW/WM+MM) 19.6% (WW+WM/MM)
Sugimura et al., 1990 (USA)									

Reference	Cases	Controls	%	Method	Smoking / exposure	Medication / treatment	Matching / adjustment variables	PM	Frequency (genotype/phenotype)
Cartwright et al., 1984 (UK)	122 prev. bladder cancer (Caucas.?)	94 hospital controls (Caucas.?)		DBQ 10 mg administration and 8 hours urine collection; analysis performed by alkali-flame ionization gas-liquid chromatography; MR = 12.6 (DBQ/4-OH-DBQ)	occupation (exp. to benzidine)		tumour grade and stage, cancer histology	2%	8.8% (WW+WM/MM)
Chingwundoh & Kalsary, 1996 (UK)	126 TCC of the bladder (Caucas.?)			PCR	smoking				
Dolzan et al., 1995 (Slovenia)	200 prev. lung cancer histolog. confirmed <75 yrs (Caucas.)	107 blood donors controls (Caucas.)		PCR			ethnicity, cancer histology	6.5%	18.5% (WW+WM/MM)
Duche et al., 1991 (France)	153 prev. lung cancer histolog. confirmed, smokers >20 PY (Caucas.)	135 COPD, smokers >20 PY, similar to cases for age and smoking history; 119 healthy controls (Caucas.)		DBQ 10 mg administration and 8 hours urine collection; analysis performed by flame ionization GC; MR = 13.18 (DBQ/4-OH-DBQ)	smoking (smokers) for cases and COPD controls		ethnicity	6.7%	19.5% (WW+WM/MM)
Elexpuru-Camiruaga et al., 1995 (UK)	109 incid. astrocytoma, 49 incid. meningioma histolog. confirmed (Caucas.)	577 hospital cancer-free controls (Caucas.)	100% cases	PCR			gender, age, ethnicity, cancer histology, CYP2D6 and GSTT1 polym	4.4%	32.9% (astrocytoma), 19.6% (meningioma) (MM/WW+WM)
Heagerty et al., 1996 (UK)	599 incid. BCC (396 single, 203 multiple) histolog. confirmed (Caucas.)	310 hospital controls (Caucas.)		PCR	smoking (never, former, current)		gender, ethnicity, skin type, hair and eye colour, GSTM1 and GSTT1 polym.	5.5%	45.3% (WW+WM/MM)
Hirvonen et al., 1993b (Finland)	106 incid. lung cancer histolog. confirmed (Caucas.)	122 blood donors controls (Caucas.)		DBQ 10 mg administration and 6 hours urine collection; analysis performed by GC; MR = 12.6 (DBQ/4-OH-DBQ); PCR, RFLP	smoking (non-smokers, ex-smokers, smokers <25, 26-50, >50 PY) for cases	no radio- or, chemotherapy or surgery before genotyping	ethnicity, cancer histology	5.7%	9.7% (WW+WM/MM)
Horai et al., 1989 (Japan)	51 prev. transitional cell bladder cancer histolog. confirmed (Asians)	203 healthy controls (Asians)		metoprolol 100 mg administration; 8 hours urine collection; analysis performed by HPLC	smoking (none, <20, >20 cig/day) and occupation for cases only (no exp. to b-naphthylamine, benzidine, 4-ABP)	no drugs known to influence the phenotyping	ethnicity, gender, age, tumour grade, cancer histology	0.5%	<5% (WW+WM/MM)

Table 34 (Contd). Study design: CYP2D6 and cancer (case–case studies shaded grey)

Author	# of cases	# of controls	Response	Phenotyping/ genotyping	Exposures	Covariates	Therapy	MM in controls	Power (α=0.05, OR>2)
Horsmans et al., 1991 (Belgium)	91 prev. lung cancer histolog. confirmed <80 yrs (Caucas.)	167 healthy controls (Caucas.)		DBQ 10 mg administration and 8 hours urine collection; analysis performed by flame-ionization GC; MR = 12.6 (DBQ/4-OH-DBQ)	smoking (never, light, moderate, heavy); alcohol (never, light, moderate, heavy)	ethnicity, cancer histology	14 cases had radiotherapy and 6 had chemotherapy more than 4 weeks before	7.2%	11.1% (WW+WM/MM)
Jahnke et al., 1996 (UK)	269 prev. laryngeal SQ histolog. confirmed undergoing surgery (Caucas.)	216 healthy controls (Caucas.)		PCR		ethnicity, cancer histology, tumour location (glottic, supraglottic), grading and staging			
Jennings et al., 1996 (UK)	105 incid. breast cancer histolog. confirmed (mixed)	223 women with benign breast disease (mixed)		DBQ 10 mg administration and 8 hours urine collection; analysis performed by GLC; MR=12.6 (DBQ/4-OH-DBQ); PCR	occupation (no exp. to known bladder carcinogens)		no radio- or chemotherapy before phenotyping	12.0%	53.9% (MM/WW+WM)
Kaisary et al., 1987 (USA)	98 prev. transitional cell bladder cancer histolog. confirmed (Caucas.)	110 urolog. patients (Caucas.)		DBQ 10 mg administration and 8 hours urine collection; analysis performed by electron capture GC; RR = 0.12 (4-OH-DBQ/4-OH-DBQ + DBQ)	gender, age, ethnicity, smoking, alcohol, cancer histology, tumour stage, NAT2 polym.		no drugs known to influence the dapsone metabolism before phenotyping	5.2%	35.9% (MM/WM+WW)
Ladero, et al., 1991b (Spain)	98 incid. breast cancer histolog. confirmed, mastectomized (Caucas.)	446 healthy controls (Caucas.)		DBQ 10 mg administration and 8 hours urine collection; analysis performed by flame ionization GC; MR = 12.6 (DBQ/4-OH-DBQ)		ethnicity	no radio- or chemotherapy before phenotyping		
Ladona et al., 1996 (Spain)	187 incid. + prev. breast cancer histolog. confirmed (Caucas.)	151 healthy controls from the same geographical area matched by gender and ethnicity (Caucas.)		PCR		ethnicity, cancer histology, menopausal status (pre-, post-) for cases only		2.7%	13.7% (MM/WW+WM)

Reference	Cases	Controls	Method	Exposure (smoking)	Adjustment factors	Treatment	%	%
Law et al., 1989 (UK)	104 incid. lung cancer histolog. confirmed, smokers >10 PY (Caucas.)	82 healthy and 22 hospital controls, smokers >10 PY, matched by gender, age, smoking history (Caucas.)	DBQ 10 mg administration and 8 hours urine collection; analysis performed by electron capture GC; MR = 12.6 (DBQ/4-OH-DBQ)	smoking (smokers)	ethnicity		8.7%	14.9% (WW+WM/MM)
Lear et al., 1996 (UK)	827 incid BCC histolog. confirmed (Caucas.)		PCR		sex, skin type, eye colour, cancer histology, number of BCC; BCC rate, GSTM1, GSTT1 and CYP1A1 polym.			
Lear et al., 1997 (UK)	74 prev. BCC histolog. confirmed with at least one truncal tumour (Caucas.)	263 prev. BCC controls without truncal tumours (Caucas.)	100%	PCR		age, gender, ethnicity, cancer histology, BCC number, CYP1A1, GSTM1, GSTM3 and CYP1A1 polym.		
Lee et al., 1994 (Korea)	100 prev. transitional cell bladder cancer histolog. confirmed (Asians)	84 outpatients from the same department, matched by age and gender (Asians)	metoprolol 100 mg orally, urine coll. after 8 hours; analysis performed by HPLC; MR=12.6 (metoprolol/ a-hydroxymetoprolol)	occupation (no exp. to bladder carcinogens)	age, gender, ethnicity, tumour stage (I, II, III), cancer histology, smoking	no drugs known to influence the CYP2D6 metabolism	1.2%	<5% (WW+WM/MM)
London et al., 1997 (UK)	341 incid. lung cancer histolog. confirmed (mixed)	710 healthy controls frequency matched by age, gender and ethnicity (mixed)	69.8% cases, 75.1% controls	PCR	smoking (nonsmokers, smokers <35, >35 PY), occupation (exp. to PAH and asbestos)	age, gender, ethnicity, cancer histology		4.9% all, 5.8% Caucas., 3.3% Afric.-Americ.	37.0% all, 22.0% Caucas., 8.3% Afric.-Americ. (WW+WM/MM); 99.6% all, 94.7% Caucas., 73.1% Afric.-Americ. (WW/WM+MM)
Roots et al., 1988 (Germany)	270 prev. lung cancer histolog. confirmed <80 yrs (Caucas.)	270 hospital controls <80 yrs (Caucas.)	DBQ 5, 7.5 or 10 mg administration in relation to age and body weight; 5 hours urine collection; analysis performed by GC; MR = 12 (DBQ/4-OH-DBQ)		ethnicity, age (<50, >50 yrs) for cases, cancer histology, NAT2 polym.	no therapy before phenotyping	11.1%	52.5% (WW+WM/MM)
Samanis et al., 1996 (UK)	83 incid. epithelial ovarian cancer histolog. confirmed (Caucas.)	280 hospital controls (Caucas.)	PCR		ethnicity	no treatment before genotyping	5.0%	63.7% (WW+WM/MM), 5.9% (WW/WM+MM)
Shaw et al., 1995 (USA, Canada)	335 incid. Lung cancer histolog. confirmed (Caucas.)	135 outpatients and 238 inpatients, matched for 5-yrs age group and gender (Caucas.)	80.5% cases, 59% outpat, 98% inpatients	DBQ 10 mg administration and 8 hours urine collection; analysis performed by HPLC; MR = 7.39 (DBQ/4-OH-DBQ)	smoking (non-smokers, 1-30, 31-49, >50 PY), occupation (exp. to asbestos)	age, gender, ethnicity, education, cancer histology, tumour stage, hospital, medication use	7.0%	43.7% (WW+WM/MM)

Table 34 (Contd). Study design: CYP2D6 and cancer (case-case studies shaded grey)

Author	# of cases	# of controls	Response	Phenotyping/genotyping	Exposures	Covariates	Therapy	MM in controls	Power (α=0.05, OR>2)
Speirs et al., 1990 (UK)	82 prev. lung cancer histolog. confirmed (Caucas.)			DBQ 1 mg administration and 8 hours urine collection; analysis performed by GC-mass spectroscopy. MR = 12.6 (DBQ/4-OH-DBQ)		cancer histology	most cases treated with drugs, surgery, radio- or chemotherapy		
Spurr et al., 1995 (UK)	126 prev. bladder cancer (Caucas.)	132 outpatient controls (Caucas.)		PCR		ethnicity, tumour grade		6.1%	12.7% (WW+WM/MM)
Stucker et al., 1995 (France) Legrand et al., 1996 (France)	249 incid. lung cancer histolog. confirmed, male <75 yrs (Caucas.)	271 hospital controls matched by age, gender, hospital and residence (Caucas.)		PCR	smoking (smoking status, duration of smoking, g/day and kind of tobacco)	age, ethnicity, gender, residence, hospital, cancer histology, lung cancer family history	no radio- or chemotherapy before phenotyping	5.5%	48.5% (WW+WM/MM)
Tefre et al., 1994 (Norway)	204 incid.non operable lung cancer histolog. confirmed (Caucas.)	117 healthy controls (Caucas.)		PCR	smoking (non-smokers, <20, 20-40, >40 PY) for 165 cases	age, gender, ethnicity, cancer histology		5.1%	15.2% (WW+WM/MM)
Warwick et al., 1994a (UK)	175 prev. uterus CIN, 77 prev. uterus SQ (Caucas.)	180 cancer-free controls affected by menorrhagia (Caucas.)		PCR	smoking (non-smokers, smokers: >10 cig./day for at least 5 yrs)	GSTM1 polym., ethnicity, cancer histology		7.2%	62.0% SQ, 84.6% CIN (WW/WM+MM); 8.7% SQ, 21.0% CIN (WW+WM/MM)
Wolf et al., 1992 (UK)	361 prev. lung cancer, 184 prev. bladder cancer, 313 prev. breast cancer (Caucas.)	720 healthy and 151 COPD controls (Caucas.)		PCR		ethnicity, cancer histology (for lung cancer cases only)	no radio- or chemotherapy or surgery before genotyping	4.3%	33.8% (lung), 14.6% (bladder), 68.6% (breast) (WW+WM/MM)
Wundrack et al., 1994 (Germany)	31 prev. meningioma (Caucas.)	720 healthy controls from Wolf et al., 1992 (Caucas.)		PCR		ethnicity		4.3%	24.5% (WW/WM+MM), <5% (WW+WM/MM)
Yengi et al., 1996 (UK)	286 prev. basal cell carcinoma (92 single BCC, 194 multiple BCC) histolog. confirmed (Caucas.)	300 cancer-free hospital controls (Caucas.)		PCR		age, gender, ethnicity, skin type, cancer histology, CYP1A1, GSTM1, GSTM3 and GSTT1 polym.		2.5%	88.5% (all BCC), 60.9% (single BCC), 79.4% (multiple BCC) (WW/WM+MM)

Table 35. Study design: CYP2D6 and outcomes other than cancer

Author	Subjects	Analysis	Phenotyping/ genotyping	Exposures	Covariates	MM in controls (%)
Brockmöller et al., 1996b (Germany)	69 bladder cancer histologic. confirmed (Caucas.)	p53 mutations by PCR	PCR		ethnicity	
Cheng et al., 1995 (USA)	78 healthy controls (95% Caucas.)	SCE in lymphocytes	PCR	smoking (current, former, never smokers), alcohol	age, gender, ethnicity, diet (vit. A, C, E, folate)	40% (MM+WM)
Kato et al., 1995a (USA)	90 cancer-free autopsy donors (mixed)	32P-postlabelling assay of PAH-DNA adducts (PAH-dGMP) in parenchymal lung tissue	PCR	smoking (serum cotinine levels)		10.6%
Perrett et al., 1995 (UK)	136 pituitary tumours histologically confirmed (Caucas.)	p53 mutations by immunohistochemical analysis	PCR		ethnicity	5%
Romkes et al., 1996 (UK)	93 transitional cell bladder carcinoma histolog. confirmed (Caucas.?)	p53 abd Rb mutations in tumour tissue by immunohistochemistry	DBQ 10 mg orally and 8 hours urine collection; analysis performed by capillary GC			
Sarhanis et al., 1996 (UK)	64 epithelial ovarian cancer histolog. confirmed, 20 hospital controls (Caucas.)	p53 mutations by immunohistochemical analysis (monoclonal antibody DO-7)	PCR		ethnicity, gender, cancer histology, stage and grade, GSTT1 and GSTM1 polymorph.	5%
Weston et al., 1991 (USA)	53 lung cancer, 33 COPD controls, 23 non-pulmonary cancer controls (mixed)	4-aminobiphenyl-haemoglobin adducts	DBQ 10 mg orally and 8 hours urine collection; analysis performed by electron capture GC; MR = 4.8, 11.7 (Caucas.), 4.2, 26.4 (Afric.-Amer.)	smoking (number of cig. smoked in the last 24 h, urine and plasma cotinine levels)	age (<64, >64 yrs), gender, ethnicity, cancer histology, education, hospital	5.8%

Table 36. Results: CYP2D6 and lung cancer (case–case study shaded grey)

Author	OR - lung cancer	OR - stratified by ethnicity	OR - stratified by smoking	OR - stratified by cancer histology	OR - interactions between polymorphisms	Other comments
Ayesh et al., 1984 (UK)			5.94 (1.95-24.10) smokers (WW+WM/MM)			
Roots et al., 1988 (Germany)	1.65 (0.91-3.01) (WW+WM/MM)			1.42 (0.63-3.22) SQ; 1.23 (0.45-3.31) SC; 4.50 (0.70-188.62) AD	2.13 (0.85-5.32) (2D6 WW/NAT2slow vs. 2D6 MM/NAT2rapid)	no significantly different CYP2D6 frequency between <50 years vs. >50 years cases (p=0.20)
Caporaso et al., 1989 (UK, USA)	6.6 (3.9-11.3), 4.0 (1.9-8.3) males, 10.5 (4.7-23.5) females, 14.8 (6.44-34.08) exp. to PAH, 12.78 (4.33-37.69) exp. to asbestos (WW/WM+MM); 2.86 (0.76-10.82) non occup. exposed (WW+WM/MM)			7.8 (4.0-15.4) SQ; 8.4 (3.5-20.4) SC; 2.5 (0.9-7.2) AD (WW/WM+MM)		
Law et al. 1989 (UK)	4.83 (0.96-46.77) (WW+WM/MM)					
Caporaso et al., 1990 (USA)	5.93 (2.15-16.36); 6.1 (2.2-17.1) adjusted for age, ethnicity, smoking, asbestos exposure (WW/WM+MM); 13.20 (1.68-103.81) (WW+WM/MM)	4.81 (1.12-28.58) African-Americans; 7.58 (1.53-72.28) Caucas. (WW/WM+MM)		7.94 (1.8-71.86) SQ, 0 MM among SC, p=0.37, 4.76 (1.05-43.97) AD (WW/WM+MM); 14.75 (0.85-254.87) SQ, 2.95 (0.16-53.92) SC, 4.20 (0.52-33.79) AD (WW+WM/MM)		
Speirs et al., 1990 (UK)	no significant association of CYP2D6 polymorphism with cancer histology (p=0.37)					
Sugimura et al., 1990 (USA) (part of Caporaso et al., 1990)	0 MM among cases, p=0.04 (vs. healthy controls), p=0.004 (vs. hosp. controls) (WW+WM/MM)					
Benitez et al., 1991 (Spain)			1.5 (0.42-6.78) smokers (WW+WM/MM)	3.31 (0.45-146.78) SQ; 4.48 (0.26-78.74) SC; 0.30 (0.05-3.32) AD		
Duche et al., 1991 (France)	1.22 (0.56-2.69); 1.03 (0.39-2.70) vs. healthy controls (WW+WM/MM)		1.40 (0.58-3.34) vs. COPD controls (smokers) (WW+WM/MM)			no changes in phenotype in 14 cancer patients after surgery

Study	OR (WW+WM/MM)	Histology-specific OR	Smoking-stratified OR	Comments
Horsmans et al., 1991 (France)	1.33 (0.42-4.98) (WW+WM/MM)	0 MM among SQ, p=0.13; 0.54 (0.15-2.48) SC; 0.70 (0.08-33.05) AD		
Wolf et al., 1992 (UK)	1.15 (0.60-2.20) vs. all controls; 1.2 (0.62-2.33) vs. healthy controls; 0.92 (0.32-2.62) vs. COPD controls (WW+WM/MM)	1.25 (0.46-3.30) SQ; 1.06 (0.32-3.57) AD (vs. healthy controls)		
Hirvonen et al., 1993b (Finland)	6.39 (0.79-290.74) (WW+WM/MM)	0 MM among SQ, p=0.098; 0 MM among SC, p=1.00; 2.19 (0.27-101.46) AD		no significantly different CYP2D6 frequency in smokers vs. non-smokers cases
Agundez et al., 1994 (Spain)	2.55 (0.58-15.33); 0 MM among cases, p=0.015, considering CYPD26(C) as an active allele (WW+WM/MM)	0 MM among SQ, p=0.09; 0 MM among SC, p=0.59; 0 MM among AD, p=0.6 (considering CYPD26(C) as an active allele)		
Tefre et al., 1994 (Norway)	0.50 (0.19-1.28) (WW+WM/MM)	0.59 (0.18-1.92) SQ; 0.45 (0.14-1.39) SC; 0.42 (0.11-1.58) AD		no significantly different CYP2D6 frequency by age (p=0.24), gender (p=0.99) and smoking status (p=1.00) among cases
Dolzan et al., 1995 (Slovenia)	2.73 (0.72-11.13) (WW+WM/MM)	2.87 (0.52-28.91) SQ, 3.43 (0.42-157.69) SC, 2.24 (0.27-104.06) AD, 2.85 (0.70-13.58) Kreyberg		
Shaw et al., 1995 (USA, Canada)	0.82 (0.48-1.42); 0.64 (0.34-1.19); 0.77 (0.36-1.72) stage I or II, 0.86 (0.41-1.86) stage III or IV (adjusted for age, gender, smoking, education and clinic) (WW+WM/MM)	–	0.42 (0.08-1.54) smokers; 0.37 (0.37-0.10-1.39) 1-30 PY; 1.74 (0.39-8.75) 31-49 PY; 0.73 (0.23-2.04) 50+ PY; 0.41 (0.07-4.55) non-smokers; 0.81 (0.36-1.81) ex-smokers	
Stucker et al., 1995 (France)	0.80 (0.37-1.73) (WW+WM/MM)	0.43 (0.15-1.22) AD, 1.31 (0.49-3.64) SQ+SC	0.95 (0.37-2.45) all smokers, 1.44 (0.41-6.39) <30 PY, 0.44 (0.12-2.03) AD <30 PY, 6.71 (0.39-116.16) SQ+SC <30 PY; 0.55 (0.13-1.90) >30 PY, 0.38 (0.06-2.81) AD >30 PY, 0.80 (0.16-3.51) SQ+SC >30 PY (WW+WM/MM)	no significantly different CYP2D6 frequency after adjustment for age, hospital and residence
Bouchardy et al., 1996 (Spain)		no significantly different CYP2D6 frequency by cancer histology	0.98 (0.41-2.34) all smokers, 0.42 (0.10-1.71) <20 g/day tobacco, 3.15 (0.60-16.50) >20 g/day tobacco (WW+WM/MM)	no significantly different CYP2D6 frequency after adjustment for age, smoking and occupational exposure

Table 36 (Contd). Results: CYP2D6 and lung cancer (case–case study shaded grey)

Author	OR - lung cancer	OR - stratified by ethnicity	OR - stratified by smoking	OR - stratified by cancer histology	OR - interactions between polymorphisms	Other comments
Legrand et al., 1996 (France) (same cases and controls as Stucker et al., 1995)	1.2 (0.5-2.9) (presence/absence C mutation) adjusted for age, hospital and smoking history		1.3 (0.4-3.8) <30 PY, 1.7 (0.5-5.9) >30 PY (presence/absence C mutation) adjusted for age, hospital and smoking history	1.74 (0.6-4.8) SQ, 0.9 (0.2-3.9) AD, 0.98 (0.2-4.9) SC (presence/absence C mutation) adjusted for age, hospital and smoking history		
London et al., 1997 (UK)	1.13 (0.61-2.11) (WW+WM/MM); 1.33 (1.00-1.78) (WW/WM+MM)	0.98 (0.47-2.01) Caucas., 1.29 (0.38-4.37) African-Americans, 0.80 (0.36-1.78) Caucas. smokers, 1.34 (0.37-4.86) African-American smokers (WW+WM/MM); 1.05 (0.73-1.52) Caucas., 1.70 (1.01-2.88) African-Americans, 1.01 (0.68-1.50) Caucas. smokers, 1.89 (1.07-3.36) African-American smokers (WW/WM+MM)	0.98 (0.58-1.93) smokers, 2.01 (0.54-11.19) <35 PY, 0.69 (0.24-1.89) >35 PY (WW+WM/MM); 1.10 (0.87-1.38) smokers, 1.78 (1.08-2.93) <35 PY, 0.98 (0.63-1.55) >35 PY (WW/WM+MM)	0.99 (0.41-2.42) AD, 1.05 (0.43-3.13) SQ+SC, (WW+WM/MM); 1.62 (1.02-2.58) AD, 1.09 (0.72-1.66) SQ+SC (WW/WM+MM);		no significantly different CYP2D6 genotype by age, gender or occupational exposure

Table 37. Results: CYP2D6 and bladder cancer [*] (case-case study shaded grey)

Author	OR - bladder cancer	OR - interactions between polymorphisms	Other comments
Cartwright et al., 1984 (UK)	1.30 (0.09-18.28); 0 WM or MM, p=0.04 among cases with past benzidine exposure (WW+WM/MM)		
Kaisary et al., 1987 (USA)	significantly higher frequency of WW in aggressive cases (p=0.006), but not in non-aggressive cases (adjusted for age, gender, smoking status, alcohol intake)	no significant interaction between CYP2D6 and NAT2 polymorphisms	no significant association among smokers
Horai et al., 1989 (Japan)	TCC: non-significant association of WW status and cancer (P=1.0); no significantly different CYP2D6 frequency by gender, age or tumour grade (WW+WM/MM)		no significant difference in CYP2D6 status by smoking (p=0.75)
Benitez et al., 1990 (Spain)	TCC:2.65 (0.81-13.68) (WW+WM/MM)		no significant difference in CYP2D6 status in smoking and alcohol subgroups; significant difference in occupationally exposed vs. non exposed cases (p=0.03)
Wolf et al., 1992 (UK)	0.99 (0.45-2.19) (WW+WM/MM); 0.60 (0.43-0.83) (WW/WM+MM)		
Lee et al., 1994 (Korea)	TCC:0.59 (0.05-6.50), 0.40 (0.006-7.83) non-aggressive (stage I and II), 0 MM among aggressive cancer (stage III) (p=0.56) (WW+WM/MM)		CYP2D6 activity significantly higher in cases than controls (p=0.027); no significant association with cancer risk after adjustment for gender, age and smoking status
Spurr et al., 1995 (UK)	0.61 (0.22-1.68) (WW+WM/MM)		no significantly different CYP2D6 genotype frequency by tumour grade (p=0.16)
Brockmöller et al., 1996a (Germany)	1.05 (0.57-1.95) (WW+WM/MM); 0.98 (0.74-1.31) (WW/WM+MM)	no significant interaction with NAT2, GSTT1, GSTM1, CYP2E1 or CYP1A1 polymorphisms in determining bladder cancer risk	no significantly different CYP2D6 genotype frequency by age, gender, tumour stage and grade, smoking status and occupational exposure

Table 37 (Contd). Results: CYP2D6 and bladder cancer (case-case study shaded grey)

Author	OR - bladder cancer	OR - interactions between polymorphisms	Other comments
Anwar et al., 1996 (Egypt)	2.36 (0.68-9.90) (WW+WM/MM)	non-significant interaction between CYP2D6 and CYP2E1 polymorphisms; 8.4 (1.26-56.03) (2D6WW+WM/GSTM1null vs. 2D6MM/GSTM1+)	
Chinegwundoh & Kaisary, 1996 (UK)			no significantly different CYP2D6 frequency in smokers compared to non-smokers (p=0.92); no significantly different CYP2D6 frequency by tumour grade among smokers (p=0.35)

Table 38. Results: CYP2D6 and breast cancer

Author	OR - breast cancer	OR - interactions between polymorphisms	Other comments
Ladero et al., 1991b (Spain)	2.09 (0.96-4.55) (MM/WM+WW)		
Wolf et al., 1992 (UK)	0.92 (0.45-1.87) (MM/WM+WW)		no significantly different CYP2D6 frequency by age groups
Buchert et al., 1993 (USA)	1.18 (0.45-3.10), 1.54 (0.42-5.64) pre-menop., 0.61 (0.14-2.65) post-menop. (MM/WM+WW)		
Ladona et al., 1996 (Spain)	1.43 (0.41-4.98), 0.97 (0.24-3.94) ductal infiltrating, 3.94 (0.84-18.56) other histologies (MM/WM+WW)		significant association between CYP2D6 B allele frequency and breast cancer: p=0.018 all cases, p=0.0086 post-menopausal, p=0.003 non-ductal infiltrating; no significantly different PM frequency in pre-menopausal vs. post-menopausal cases (p=0.35)
Jennings et al., 1996 (UK)	0.94 (0.45-1.93) (MM/WM+WW)		no significantly different frequency of CYP2D6 B allele

Table 39. CYP2D6 and other cancers (case-case study shaded grey)

Author	OR - other cancers	OR - interactions between polymorphisms	Other comments
Warwick et al., 1994a (UK)	0.76 (0.29-2.01) SQ, 1.01 (0.44-2.32) CIN (WW+WM/MM); 1.28 (0.74-2.22) SQ, 2.54 (1.64-3.93) CIN, 2.68 (1.40-5.13) high-grade CIN in smokers (WW/WM+MM)	1.60 (0.43-6.78) low-gr. CIN, 0.44 (0.07-2.87) high-gr. CIN, 0.34 (0.10-1.13) SQ (non-smokers); 2.22 (0.69-7.94) low-gr. CIN, 1.92 (0.71-5.37) high-gr. CIN, 2.17 (0.61-8.97) SQ (smokers) (2D6 WW/GSTM1null vs. 2D6 WM+MM/GSTM1+)	
Wundrack et al., 1994 (Germany)	meningioma 0.65 (0.15-2.86) (WW+WM/MM); 0.71 (0.34-1.47) (WW/WM+MM)		no significantly different CYP2D6 frequency by age and gender
Elexpuru-Camiruaga et al., 1995 (UK)	2.96 (1.40-6.26) astrocytoma, 3.13 (1.18-8.31) meningioma (MM/WW+WM); 0.34 (0.16-0.71) astrocytoma, 0.32 (0.12-0.85) meningioma (WW+WM/MM)	no significant interactions between CYP2D6 and GSTT1 or GSTM1 polymorphisms	
Agundez et al., 1996 (Spain)	4.12 (1.90-8.92) HCC 1.03 (0.27-3.98) (WW+WM/MM) WW/WM+MM (considering C and L alleles as active)	2.65 (1.83-21.29), 5.70 (1.55-20.93) HCC cases without HBV-HCV markers (NAT2slow/CYP2D6 WW vs. others combined); 6.24 (1.83-21.29) (NAT2slow/CYP2D6 WW vs. NAT2rapid/CYP2D6 WM+MM)	
Benhamou et al., 1996 (France)	laryngeal SQ: 1.05 (0.64-1.70) smokers, 0.71 (0.33-1.54) <20 cig/day, 2.19 (0.75-6.33) 21-30 cig./day, 1.03 (0.45-2.36) >30 cig/day (WW+WM/MM)		increased risk with increased level of smoking among WW (trend test, p<0.06), but not among WM or MM; no significantly different CYP2D6 frequency after adjustment for age, smoking, alcohol and medication use
Heagerty et al., 1996 (UK)	0.75 (0.42-1.34) all BCC, 0.66 (0.36-1.21) single BCC, 1.01 (0.46-2.21) multiple BCC (WW+WM/MM)	no significant interactions with GSTT1 and GSTM1 polymorphisms	no significantly different CYP2D6 frequency by skin type; no significant association between CYP2D6 and BCC in smokers
Jahnke et al., 1996 (UK)	laryngeal SQ: no significantly different CYP2D6 genotype frequency between cases and controls		
Lear et al., 1996 (UK)	significant association of CYP2D6 WW with number of BCC (p<0.001) and BCC rate (p<0.001), with green-blue eye colour and number of BCC (p=0.046) and with male gender and number of BCC (p=0.049) (adjusted by age)	almost significant higher risk of increased number of BCC in MspI MM/2D6 WW vs. MspI WM+WW/2D6 WM+MM (p=0.095); no significant interactions with GSTM1, GSTT1 or CYP1A1 polymorphisms in determining BCC rate	

Table 39 (Contd). CYP2D6 and other cancers (case-case study shaded grey)

Author	OR - other cancers	OR - interactions between polymorphisms	Other comments
Sarhanis et al., 1996 (UK)	epithelial ovarian cancer 0.82 (0.14-4.80) (WW+WM/MM) 0.84 (0.36-1.94) (WW/WM+MM)		
Yengi et al., 1996 (UK)	0.60 (0.20-1.78) all BCC, 0.54 (0.14-2.04) single BCC, 0.64 (0.19-2.13) multiple BCC (WW+WM/MM); 1.01 (0.68-1.49) all BCC, 0.85 (0.50-1.41) single BCC, 1.12 (0.72-1.73) multiple BCC; 1.61 (1.25-2.07) multiple BCC (adjusted for age, gender and skin type) (WW/WM+MM)	no significant interactions with CYP1A1, GSTM1, GSTM3 or GSTT1 polymorphisms	
Lear et al., 1997 (UK)	no significant association between CYP2D6 polymorph. and presence of truncal BCC	no significant interactions with CYP1A1, GSTM3, GSTT1 and GSTM1 polymorphisms	

Table 40. Results: CYP2D6 and outcomes other than cancer

Author	SCE	MN and CA	Mutagenicity	DNA adducts	Hb adducts
Weston et al., 1991 (USA)					no significantly different Hb-adduct level in WW/WM+MM
Cheng et al., 1995 (USA)	no association between SCE frequency and CYP2D6 polymorphism				
Kato et al., 1995a (USA)				7-methyl-dGMP adducts significantly higher in WW+WM vs. MM carriers for all subjects (p=0.01) and for subjects with cotinine levels below the median (p=0.004)	
Perrett et al., 1995 (UK)			almost significantly lower frequency of MM vs. WW+WM in p53 negative tumours (p=0.055)		
Brockmöller et al., 1996b (Germany)			non-significantly different p53 mutations frequency in WW vs. WM+MM (p=0.45)		
Romkes et al., 1996 (UK)			significant association between Rb mutations and CYP2D6 activity (p=0.025); no significant association between p53 mutations and CYP2D6 activity		
Sarhanis et al., 1996 (UK)			non-significant association between p53 positivity and CYP2D6 polymorph.		no significant association with tumour grade (p=0.99)

Table 41. Study design: CYP2E1 and cancer

Author	# of cases	# of controls	Response	Phenotyping/ genotyping	Exposures	Covariates	Therapy	CYP2E1 variants in controls	Power (α=0.05, OR>2)
Anwar et al., 1996 (Egypt)	22 prev. bladder cancer histol. confirmed (Caucas.)	21 healthy controls matched by age and smoking (Caucas.)		PCR (Pst I)		ethnicity, GSTM1 and CYP2D6 polym.		4.7% (WM)	8.1% (WM/WW)
Brockmöller et al., 1996a (Germany)	374 incid. + prev. bladder cancer histolog. confirmed (Caucas.)	373 hospital cancer-free controls (Caucas.)		PCR (Rsa I, Dra I, Taq I)	smoking, occupation (>1 year in jobs at high risk for bladder cancer)	age, gender, ethnicity, cancer histology, tumour stage, tumor grade, GSTM1, GSTT1, CYP2D6, NAT2 and CYP1A1 polym.		6.3% (Rsa I), 27.0% (Taq I), 12.7% (Dra I) (WM+MM)	69.1% (Rsa I), 98.8% (Taq I), 88.6% (Dra I) (WM+MM/WW)
El-Zein et al., 1997 (USA)	52 incid. lung cancer histolog. confirmed undergoing surgery, smokers (Caucas.?)	48 healthy controls matched by smoking habit, age (5 yrs) and gender (Caucas.?)		PCR (Pst I)	smoking	cancer histology	no radiotherapy or chemotherapy before genotyping	4.1% (WM+MM)	5.4% (MM+WM/WW)
Hamada et al., 1995 (Brazil)	113 incid. lung cancer histolog. confirmed (88 Caucas., 22 African-Americans)	108 hospital cancer-free controls matched by gender, age and ethnicity (90 Caucas., 22 African-Americans)	80.5% cases, 99.1% controls	PCR (Rsa I)	smoking	age, gender, ethnicity, smoking		10.2% (WM)	34.5% (WM/WW)
Hildesheim et al., 1995 (Taiwan, USA)	50 incid. nasopharyngeal carcinoma histolog. confirmed <75 yrs (Asians)	50 healthy controls matched by age, gender, residence (Asians)		PCR (Rsa I, Dra I)		ethnicity	no treatment before genotyping	32.0% (Rsa I WM), 2.0% (Rsa I MM), 34.0% (Dra I WM), 4.0% (Dra I MM)	31.7% (Dra I), 31.1% (Rsa I) (MM+WM/WW)
Hirvonen et al., 1993d (Finland)	101 incid. lung cancer histolog. confirmed (Caucas.)	94 healthy controls, 40 controls with pulmonary diseases other than lung cancer (Caucas.)		PCR (Dra I)	smoking (never, ex-, current smokers <26, 26-50, >50 PY) for cases and hospital controls	ethnicity, cancer histology	no radio- or chemotherapy before genotyping	19.8% (WM), 0.8% (MM) (Dra I)	56.4% (Dra I) (WM+MM/WW)
Jahnke et al., 1996 (UK)	269 prev. laryngeal SQ carcinoma histolog. confirmed undergoing surgery (Caucas.)	216 healthy controls (Caucas.)		PCR	smoking (never, light, moderate, heavy); alcohol (never, light, moderate, heavy)	ethnicity, cancer histology, tumour grading, staging and location (glottic, supraglottic)			
Kato et al., 1992 (USA)	67 incid. lung cancer histolog. confirmed (mixed)	41 COPD patients, 20 patients with cancer other than lung and bladder (mixed)		PCR (Pst I and Rsa I)	smoking (smokers <53, >53 PY), occupation (exp. to asbestos)	age, gender, ethnicity, cancer histology		6.6% (Pst I polymorphism) (WM)	12.0% (Pst I polymorphism) (WM/WW)

Table 41 (Contd). Study design: CYP2E1 and cancer

Author	# of cases	# of controls	Response	Phenotyping/ genotyping	Exposures	Covariates	Therapy	CYP2E1 variants in controls	Power (α=0.05, OR>2)
Kato et al., 1994 (USA)	58 incid. lung cancer histolog. confirmed (mixed)	38 COPD patients, 18 patients with cancers other than lung and bladder (mixed)		PCR (Dra I)	smoking (smokers <53, >53 PY), occupation (exp. to asbestos)	age, gender, ethnicity, cancer histology		14.0% (WM)	21.8% (WM/WW)
Kato et al., 1995b (Japan)	150 incid. gastric cancer, 16 incid. HCC, 48 incid. liver cirrhosis histolog. confirmed (Asians)	203 controls with benign gastric disease (Asians)		PCR (Rsa I)		gender, ethnicity, cancer histology (for liver cancer)		34.0% (WM), 7.0% (MM)	87.2% (gastric cancer, 18.8% (HCC), 51.2% (liver cirrhosis) (MM+WM/WW)
Kato et al., 1996 (Japan)	82 incid. gastric cancer histolog. confirmed who did not undergo gastrectomy (Asians)	151 controls affected by benign gastric diseases matched by age (3 yrs) and gender (Asians)		PCR (Rsa I)		gender, age, ethnicity, cancer histology, pepsinogen I levels, pepsinogen I/II ratios, H. pylori IgG, L-myc and GSTM1 genotypes		41.0% (MM+WM)	66.0% (MM+WM/WW)
Lucas et al., 1996 (France)	62 prev. oesophageal cancer, 96 prev. upper aerodigestive tract cancer (Caucas.)	260 healthy controls (Caucas.)		PCR (Rsa I, Dra I)	alcohol	ethnicity		4.2% WM, 0.4% MM (Rsa I); 14.3% WM, 0.8% MM (Dra I)	21.1% Rsa I, 61.1% Dra I (WM+MM/WW)
Morita et al., 1997 (Japan)	53 incid. oesophageal SQ histolog. confirmed undergoing surgery (Asians)	132 healthy controls (Asians)		PCR (5'-flanking region)	smoking (non-smokers, smokers), alcohol (non-drinkers, drinkers)	ethnicity, cancer histology, GSTM1 and CYP1A1 polymorphisms		3.8% (MM), 31.8% (WM)	12.1% (MM/WM+WW), 49.8% (WM+MM/WW)
Oyama et al., 1997 (Japan)	126 incid. lung cancer histolog. confirmed undergoing surgery (Asians)	612 healthy factory workers (Asians)	82.9% cases	PCR (Rsa I)	smoking for cases only	ethnicity, age, gender, cancer histology, tumour stage		32.0% (WM), 4.1% (MM)	92.9% (MM+WM/WW), 37.9% (MM/WM+WW)
Persson et al., 1993 (Sweden)	195 prev. lung cancer histolog. confirmed (Caucas.)	152 healthy controls, 55 COPD controls (Caucas.)		PCR (Dra I, Taq I, 5'-flanking region)		ethnicity		18.0% (Dra I WM), 1.2% (Dra I MM), 18.3% (Taq I WM), 0.5% (Taq I MM), 9.4% (5'-fr WM), 0.5% (5'-fr MM)	82.2% Dra I, 81.7% Taq I, 60.0% 5'-fr (WM+MM/WW); 62.3% Dra I, 61.4% Taq I, 35.3% 5'-fr (WW/WM+MM)

Author	Cases	Controls	Phenotyping/genotyping	Exposures	Covariates	CYP2E1 variants	Results
Shields et al., 1996 (USA)	272 incid. breast cancer histolog. confirmed (Caucas.)	334 healthy controls randomly selected, frequency matched by age and residence (Caucas.)	PCR (Dra I)	smoking	menopausal status (pre-, post-), age (at diagnosis, menarche, first pregnancy, menopause), ethnicity, BMI, education, family history of breast cancer	14.7% WM+MM (Dra I)	90.0% all, 48.3% pre-menopausal, 70.6% post-menopausal (WM+MM/WW)
Uematsu et al., 1994 (Japan)	91 prev. lung cancer, 45 prev. digestive cancer (14 gastric, 10 colorectal, 10 oesophageal) histolog. confirmed (Asians)	76 healthy controls (Asians)	PCR (Dra I)	smoking (smokers <20, >20 PY) for lung cancer cases	ethnicity, cancer histology	28.9% (WM), 14.5% (MM)	53.7% (lung cancer), 37.0% (digestive cancer) (MM+WM/WW)
Watanabe et al., 1995 (Japan)	316 prev. lung cancer histolog. confirmed (Asians)	503 healthy controls (Asians)	PCR (Rsa I)	smoking, alcohol for cases only	ethnicity, cancer histology	31.8% (WM), 3.2% (MM)	99.7% (MM+WM/WW), 46.7% (MM/WM+WW)
Wu et al., 1997 (USA)	137 incid. lung cancer (mixed)	206 healthy controls frequency matched by age (5 yrs), gender, ethnicity and residence (mixed)	PCR (Pst I and Rsa I)	smoking (current, former, never smokers)	ethnicity, gender, mutagen sensitivity	29.3% Mexican-Americans, 13.2% African-Americans (WM+MM)	53.6% all, 24.7% (Mexican-Americans), 21.6% (African-Americans)
Yu et al., 1995 (Taiwan, USA)	30 incid. HCC histolog. confirmed, males, HBV carriers (Asians)	150 healthy controls, male, from a cohort study, matched by age, HBV carriers (Asians)	PCR (Pst I and Rsa I, Dra I)	smoking (non-smokers, smokers 1-17.4 PY, 17.5-29.2 PY, >29.2 PY)	ethnicity, gender, GSTM1 genotype, HBV status	32.7% (Rsa I WM), 4.0% (Rsa I MM), 31.5% (Dra I WM), 6.9% (Dra I MM)	22.8% Rsa I, 24.0% Dra I (WW/WM+MM); 33.7% Rsa I, 33.6% Dra I (WM+MM/WW)

Table 42. Study design: CYP2E1 and outcomes other than cancer

Author	Subjects	Analysis	Phenotyping/genotyping	Exposures	Covariates	CYP2E1 variants
Brockmöller et al., 1996b (Germany)	69 bladder cancer histologic. confirmed (Caucas.)	p53 mutations by PCR	PCR (Rsa I, Dra I)		ethnicity	
Degawa et al., 1994 (USA)	25 laryngeal cancer patients (Caucas.)	32P-postlabelling assay of total DNA adducts in normal laryngeal mucosa	immunoblot analysis with anti-P4502E1 antibodies			
Kato et al., 1995a (USA)	90 cancer-free autopsy donors (mixed)	32P-postlabelling assay of 7-methyl-dGMP adducts in parenchymal lung tissue	PCR (Dra I)	smoking (serum cotinine levels)		21% (WM)
Oyama et al., 1997 (Japan)	126 lung cancer patients (Asians)	p53 mutations by PCR	PCR (Rsa I)		ethnicity, cancer histology	32.0% (WM), 4.1% (MM)

Table 43. Results: CYP2E1 and lung cancer

Author	OR - lung cancer (5'-flanking region polymorphism: Rsa I, Pst I)	OR - stratified by ethnicity	OR - stratified by smoking	OR - stratified by cancer histology	OR - interactions between polymorphisms	Other comments
Kato et al., 1992 (USA, Japan)	0.9 (0.2-2.8) Rsa I, 0.7 (0.2-5.4) Pst I (WM/WW)	0.2 (0.02-2.43) African-Americans, 4.28 (0.35-50.6) Caucas. (Rsa I); 0.19 (0.03-1.38) African-Americans, 4.13 (0.34-48.8) Caucas. (Pst I) (WM/WW)				no significantly different CYP2E1 genotype frequency by cancer histology or smoking status
Persson et al., 1993 (Sweden)	0.41 (0.18-0.96) vs. all controls, 0.40 (0.17-0.98) vs. healthy controls (WM+MM/WW); 2.42 (1.04-5.63) vs. all controls, 2.48 (1.02-6.02) vs. healthy controls (WW/WM+MM)					
Hamada et al., 1995 (Brazil)	0.86 (0.36-2.05), 0.85 (0.36-2.02) adjusted for age, gender and ethnicity (WM/WW)					no significant difference in risk after adjusting for ethnicity and smoking history
Watanabe et al., 1995 (Japan)	1.31 (0.62-2.75) (MM/WM+WW), 0.98 (0.73-1.31) (MM+WM/WW)			0.83 (0.52-1.30) SQ, 0.77 (0.41-1.45) SC, 1.06 (0.72-1.56) AD (MM+WM/WW)		non-significant difference in cigarette and alcohol consumption over lifetime between cases with different Rsa I genotype
El-Zein et al., 1997 (USA)			3.58 (0.70-18.2) smokers (MM+WM/WW)	8.47 (1.61-44.56) AD, 0.41 (0.02-8.97) SQ (MM+WM/WW)		significantly lower proportion of CYP2E1 WM+MM among SQ compared to AD cases (p=0.036)
Oyama et al., 1997 (Japan)	1.38 (0.58-3.27), (MM/WM+WW); 0.79 (0.53-1.20), (MM+WM/WW)			0.66 (0.15-2.85) AD, 2.45 (0.90-6.68) SQ, (MM/WM+WW); 0.98 (0.59-1.62) AD, 0.58 (0.30-1.10) SQ (MM+WM/WW)		no significant association among cases of CYP2E1 genotype frequency with age, gender, smoking index, tumour stage

Author	OR - lung cancer (5'-flanking region polymorphism: Rsa I, Pst I)	OR - stratified by ethnicity	OR - stratified by smoking	OR - stratified by cancer histology	OR - interactions between polymorphisms	Other comments
Wu et al., 1997 (USA)	1.94 (1.04-3.61) (WW/WM+MM); 0.52 (0.28-0.96) (WM+MM/WW)	2.7 (1.0-7.1) crude, 14.0 (1.9-101.5) adjusted for age, gender, smoking and mutagen sensitivity (Mexican-Americans); 1.2 (0.5-2.9) crude, 1.5 (0.4-5.5) adjusted for age, gender, smoking and mutagen sensitivity (African-Americans) (WW/WM+MM); 0.80 (0.34-1.89) African-Americans, 0.37 (0.14-0.98) Mexican-Americans (WM+MM/WW)	1.5 (0.4-5.6) smokers, 2.3 (0.1-47.4) never smokers, 15.4 (1.8-134.9) ex-smokers (Mexican-Americans); 2.1 (0.5-8.2) smokers, 0.3 (0.0-3.9) never smokers, 1.0 (0.3-3.8) ex-smokers (African-Americans) (WW/WM+MM); 0.67 (0.18-2.50) smokers, 0.43 (0.02-8.64) never smokers, 0.07 (0.01-0.57) ex-smokers (Mexican-Americans); 0.49 (0.12-1.95) smokers, 3.08 (0.26-37.09) never smokers, 0.97 (0.26-3.55) ex-smokers (African-Americans) (WM+MM/WW)			

Author	OR - lung cancer (Dra I polymorphism)	OR - stratified by ethnicity	OR - stratified by smoking	OR - stratified by cancer histology	OR - interactions between polymorphisms	Other comments
Hirvonen et al., 1993d (Finland)	0.72 (0.36-1.44) vs. healthy controls, 0.89 (0.33-2.35) vs. hospital controls (MM+WM/WW)		4.13 (0.51-33.72) smokers, 4.55 (0.19-106.59) <25 PY, 2.20 (0.25-19.02) >25 PY, 0.75 (0.06-9.27) ex-smokers, 0.10 (0.005-2.19) never smokers (MM+WM/WW)	0.67 (0.28-1.59) SQ, 0.36 (0.10-1.27) AD, 3.84 (0.90-16.44) SC (MM+WM/WW)		
Persson et al., 1993 (Sweden)	0.86 (0.51-1.42) vs. all controls, 0.87 (0.50-1.52) vs. healthy controls (MM+WM/WW); 1.17 (0.70-1.94) vs. all controls, 1.14 (0.66-1.98) vs. healthy controls (WW/WM+MM)					
Kato et al., 1994	1.57 (0.59-4.18), 1.93 (0.66-5.65) adjusted for age, ethnicity, smoking and gender (WW/WW)	1.24 (0.25-6.14) African-Americans, 1.94 (0.54-6.92) Caucas. (WM/WW)	1.41 (0.35-7.51) smokers >53 PY (WW/WW)	1.15 (0.34-3.91) SQ, 1.60 (0.42-6.07) AD, 0 WM among SC cases (p=1.00) (WW/WW)		no significant difference in risk after adjusting for age, ethnicity, gender and smoking status
Uematsu et al., 1994	0.13 (0.03-0.62) (MM/WW+WM); 1.22 (0.66-2.25) (MM+WM/WW)			0.93 (0.37-2.36) SQ, 1.18 (0.45-3.12) SC, 1.46 (0.66-3.23) AD (MM+WM/WW)		significantly different MM+WM frequency between cases who smoked <20 PY and >20 PY (p<0.05)

Table 43 (Contd). Results: CYP2E1 and lung cancer

Author	OR - lung cancer Taq I polymorphism	OR - stratified by ethnicity	OR - stratified by smoking	OR - stratified by cancer histology	OR - interactions between polymorphisms	Other comments
Persson et al., 1993 (Sweden)	0.99 (0.59-1.67) vs. all controls, 0.92 (0.53-1.60) vs. healthy controls, (MM+WM/WW); 1.01 (0.60-1.69) vs. all controls, 1.09 (0.63-1.89) vs. healthy controls (WW/WM+MM)					

Table 44. Results: CYP2E1 and other cancers

Author	OR - digestive cancer (Dra I polymorphism)	OR - digestive cancer (5'-flanking region polymorphism)	OR - digestive cancer (Taq I polymorphism)	OR - interactions between polymorphisms	Other comments
Uematsu et al., 1994 (Japan)	0.74 (0.24-2.28) (MM/WM+WW), 1.95 (0.92-4.13) (MM+WM/WW) (all digestive cancer)				no significant association with liver cirrhosis (p=0.91); no significantly different CYP2D6 genotype frequency by gender between gastric cancers and controls
Kato et al., 1995b (Japan)		0.96 (0.63-1.48) (MM+WM/WW), 0.57 (0.22-1.50) (MM/WM+WW) (gastric cancer); 0.96 (0.12-7.88) (MM/WM+WW), 0.72 (0.24-2.19) (MM+WM/WW) (HCC)			
Yu et al., 1995b (Taiwan, USA)	1.63 (0.68-3.94) (WW/WM+WM), 0.61 (0.25-1.48) (MM+WM/WW) (HCC)	2.89 (1.05-8.00), 1.1 (0.3-3.3) non-smokers, 24.25 (1.37-428.22) smokers, (WW/WM+MM); 0.35 (0.13-0.95) (WM+MM/WW) (HCC)		1.86 (0.38-9.10) (GSTM1null/2E1 WW vs. GSTM1+/2E1 WM+MM)	significant correlation between Dra I and Rsa I polymorphisms: r=0.68 (p<0.01) among controls and r=0.61 (p<0.01) among cases; 100% concordance between Pst I and Rsa I genotypes; significant dose-response relationship between PY of smoking and HCC risk (p=0.02, trend test) in WW, but not in WM or MM Rsa I genotype
Kato et al., 1996 (Japan)		0.78 (0.45-1.36), 0.66 (0.28-1.56) adjusted for age, gender, pepsinogen I levels, pepsinogen I/II ratios, IgG anti-H. pylori, L-myc and GSTM1 polym. (MM+WM/WW) (gastric cancer)			

Author	OR - bladder cancer (Dra I polymorphism)	OR - bladder cancer (5'-flanking region polymorphism)	OR - bladder cancer (Taq I polymorphism)	OR - interactions between polymorphisms	Other comments
Lucas et al., 1996 (France)	no significant association between oesophageal or upper aerodigestive tract cancer and Dra I polymorph.				
Morita et al., 1997 (Japan)		no significant association between esophageal or upper aerodigestive tract cancer and Rsa I polymorph. — 0.49 (0.06-4.28) SQ (MM/WM+WW); 1.01 (0.52-1.97) SQ, 1.5 (0.6-3.7) male smokers SQ, 0.7 (0.3-1.5) male drinkers SQ (WM+MM/WW) (oesophageal cancer)			no significant interactions between CYP1A1 Exon7, CYP2E1 and GSTM1 polym.
Anwar et al., 1996 (Egypt)		0 MM or WM genotype among cases (p=0.48)		no significant interaction between CYP2E1 and GSTM1 or CYP2D6 polym.	
Brockmöller et al., 1996a (Germany)	1.16 (0.73-1.82) (WM+MM/WW)	0.54 (0.27-1.08) (WM+MM/WW)	0.76 (0.54-1.08) (WM+MM/WW)	no significant interaction between CYP2E1 and GSTM1, GSTT1, NAT2, CYP1A1 or CYP2D6 polym.	no significantly different CYPE1 genotype frequency between cases and controls, by age, gender, smoking and occupation

Author	OR - other cancers (Dra I polymorphism)	OR - other cancers (5'-flanking region polymorphism)	OR - other cancers (Taq I polymorphism)	OR - interactions between polymorphisms	Other comments
Hildesheim et al., 1995 (Taiwan)	4.96 (0.86-50.89) (MM/WW), 4.80 (0.96-23.90) (MM/WM+WW), 1.50 (0.67-3.35) (MM+WM/WW) (nasopharyngeal cancer)	7.70 (0.88-357.31) (MM/WW), 8.37 (0.99-70.82) (MM/WM+WW), 1.16 (0.51-2.66) (MM+WM/WW) (nasopharyngeal cancer)			significant correlation between Dra I and Rsa I plymorphisms: $r=0.91$ ($p<0.001$) among controls, $r=-0.86$ ($p<0.001$) among cases
Jahnke et al., 1996 (UK)		non significantly different CYP2E1 genotype frequency between cases and controls (larynx cancer)			

Table 44 (Contd). Results: CYP2E1 and other cancers

Author	OR - other cancers (Dra I polymorphism)	OR - bladder cancer (5'-flanking region polymorphism)	OR - bladder cancer (Taq I polymorphism)	OR - interactions between polymorphisms	Other comments
Shields et al., 1996 (USA)	1.08 (0.53-2.21) all, 3.00 (0.91-9.88) smokers, 2.13 (0.60-7.59) smokers, adjusted for age, education, age at menarche and first pregnancy, BMI, family history of breast cancer (pre-menopausal); 0.94 (0.52-1.69) all, 1.01 (0.47-2.16) smokers (post-menopausal) (WM+MM/WW) (breast cancer)				

Table 45. Results: CYP2E1 and outcomes other than cancer

Author	SCE	MN and CA	Mutagenicity	DNA adducts	Hb and albumin adducts
Degawa et al., 1994 (USA)				no significant correlation between total DNA adduct level and P4502E1 activity	
Kato et al., 1995a (USA)				significantly higher levels of 7-methyl-dGMP adducts in carriers of Dra I WM compared to WW, at low cotinine levels (p=0.05)	
Brockmöller et al., 1996b (Germany)			no significant association between p53 mutations and Rsa I (p=1.00) or Dra I polymorph. (p=0.33)		
Oyama et al., 1997 (Japan)			significantly higher p53 mutations frequency among Rsa I MM vs. WM+WW (p<0.01)		

Metabolic Polymorphisms and Susceptibility to Cancer
W. Ryder
IARC Scientific Publications No. 148
International Agency for Research on Cancer, Lyon, 1999

Index

Achevé d'imprimer sur rotative par l'imprimerie Darantiere
à Dijon/Quetigny en juin 1999.

Dépôt légal : 2ᵉ trimestre 1999.
N° d'impression : 99-0175.